T0200642

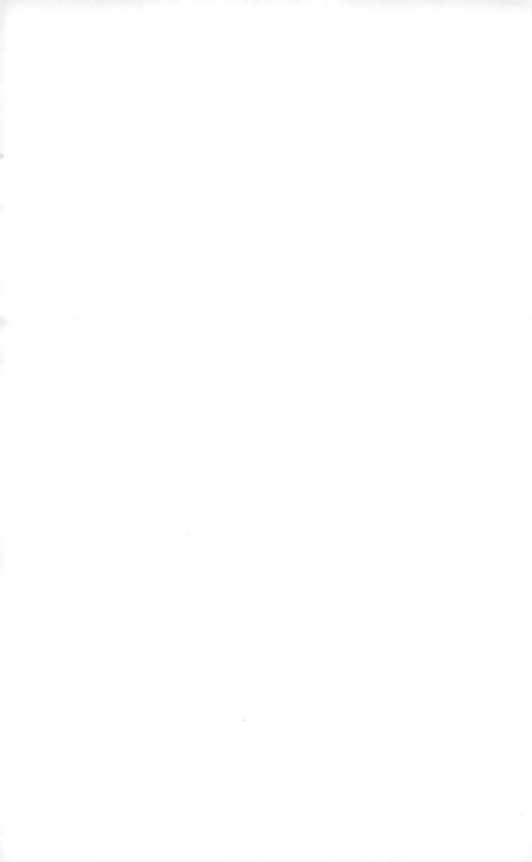

DISSECTION IN CLASSICAL ANTIQUITY

Dissection is a practice with a long history stretching back to antiquity and has played a crucial role in the development of anatomical knowledge. This absorbing book takes the story back to Classical antiquity, employing a wide range of textual and material evidence. Claire Bubb reveals how dissection was practiced from the Hippocratic authors of the fifth century BC, through Aristotle and the Hellenistic doctors Herophilus and Erasistratus, to Galen in the second century AD. She focuses on its material concerns and social contexts, from the anatomical subjects (animal or human) and how they were acquired, to the motivations and audiences of dissection, to its place in the web of social contexts that informed its reception, including butchery, sacrifice, and spectacle. The book concludes with a thorough examination of the relationship of dissection to the development of anatomical literature into Late Antiquity.

CLAIRE BUBB is an assistant professor of Classical Literature and Science at the Institute for the Study of the Ancient World, New York University.

DISSECTION IN CLASSICAL ANTIQUITY

A Social and Medical History

CLAIRE BUBB

New York University

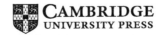
CAMBRIDGE
UNIVERSITY PRESS

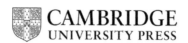

CAMBRIDGE
UNIVERSITY PRESS

Shaftesbury Road, Cambridge CB2 8EA, United Kingdom

One Liberty Plaza, 20th Floor, New York, NY 10006, USA

477 Williamstown Road, Port Melbourne, VIC 3207, Australia

314–321, 3rd Floor, Plot 3, Splendor Forum, Jasola District Centre, New Delhi – 110025, India

103 Penang Road, #05–06/07, Visioncrest Commercial, Singapore 238467

Cambridge University Press is part of Cambridge University Press & Assessment, a department of the University of Cambridge.

We share the University's mission to contribute to society through the pursuit of education, learning, and research at the highest international levels of excellence.

www.cambridge.org
Information on this title: www.cambridge.org/9781009159470

DOI: 10.1017/9781009159494

© Claire Bubb 2022

First published 2022

Printed in the United Kingdom by TJ Books Limited, Padstow Cornwall

A catalogue record for this publication is available from the British Library.

Library of Congress Cataloging-in-Publication Data
NAMES: Bubb, Claire, author.
TITLE: Dissection in classical antiquity : a social and medical history /
Claire Bubb, New York University.
DESCRIPTION: Cambridge, United Kingdom ; New York, NY :
Cambridge University Press, 2022. | Includes bibliographical references and index.
IDENTIFIERS: LCCN 2022022845 | ISBN 9781009159470 (hardback) |
ISBN 9781009159494 (ebook)
SUBJECTS: LCSH: Dissection – Greece – History – To 400. | Dissection – Rome –
History – To 400. | Human anatomy – Greece – History – To 400. | Human anatomy –
Rome – History – To 400. | Medicine, Greek and Roman.
CLASSIFICATION: LCC QM33.4 .B83 2022 | DDC 611.00938–dc23/eng/20220713
LC record available at https://lccn.loc.gov/2022022845

ISBN 978-1-009-15947-0 Hardback

Contents

Figures

Acknowledgments

This book has its origins in my doctoral dissertation; it has since grown considerably and changed shape several times, but I am deeply grateful to my primary advisor, Mark Schiefsky, and my committee members, Kathleen Coleman and Emma Dench, for seeing the project along the first leg of its journey and for their continued advice, feedback, and support as it (and I) branched out. I would also like to thank David Konstan, who first suggested that I work on Galen as an undergraduate – little did either of us know where that would lead! – Gisela Striker, who introduced me to the pleasures of reading Aristotle, and Yvona Trnka-Amrhein, colleague and friend, who helped kindle my interest in the intellectual culture of the second century. This book would not be what it is had I written it outside of the stimulating and supportive environment at the Institute for the Study of the Ancient World, and I am grateful to my colleagues and students both there and at the New York University Department of Classics for their enriching company. At an individual level, I would like to thank Sebastian Heath, Amber Jacob, Alexander Jones, Candida Moss, Michael Peachin, Caroline Petit, Luis Salas, and Colin Webster for their comments, help, and advice along the course of this project. Particular thanks to Vivian Nutton for allowing me an advanced look at his work on Galen's *De voce*, as well as providing thoughtful comments and suggestions on the manuscript. I am also very grateful for the guidance of Michael Sharp and his team at Cambridge and for the anonymous feedback that I received through the review process. Finally, my eternal gratitude goes to my entire family, especially my mother, an abiding academic inspiration and cheerleader, my husband, a loving support and fount of good advice, and my children, who were (mostly unwittingly) my near constant companions during the completion of this book and who always bring me joy.

A Note on Citations, Abbreviations, and Dates

Abbreviations for Galenic titles follow those in the appendix to Singer and van der Eijk (2018), which also includes a list of modern editions and translations; to the degree to which anything about the Galenic corpus is standardized, these abbreviations are the standard ones – they are just about identical, for example, to those in the appendix to Hankinson (2008*a*). Similarly, for the sake of both simplicity and flexibility for the reader, all citations to Galen refer to the pervasively available pagination from Kühn (1821–33). I supply chapter or page numbers from other editions only in cases where the text or specific passage is not included in the Kühn numeration. I have, however, consulted modern critical editions wherever available; in cases where textual differences become pertinent, I cite the relevant edition(s) in the footnotes. The only exceptions to this practice are references to *On the Usefulness of the Parts* (*UP*) and *On the Doctrines of Hippocrates and Plato* (*PHP*). For *UP*, I include the pagination in Helmreich (1907–9) (H) after the Kühn numbers to facilitate reference to May (1968); for *PHP*, I include the chapter numbers from De Lacy (1978–84) after the Kühn numbers to facilitate reference to the *Thesaurus Linguae Graecae*.

For passages from the latter books of Galen's *Anatomical Procedures* (*AA*), which survive only in Arabic, I use the pagination from Simon (1906) (S) and the translation from Duckworth, Lyons, and Towers (1962). For other texts that survive only in Arabic, the cited edition is also the source of any quoted translations. Unless otherwise indicated, all other translations are my own.

Hippocratic abbreviations follow those in Craik (2015); all other abbreviations are according to *The Oxford Classical Dictionary* (4th ed.) (2012), as available. The abbreviation *CMG* refers to the *Corpus Medicorum Graecorum* series, *TLG* refers to the *Thesaurus Linguae Graecae*, and *DK* refers to the numeration in Diels and Kranz (1951–2).

For the convenience of the reader, I have included dates for all major figures when they are first handled; these are according to *The Oxford Classical Dictionary* (4th ed.) (2012), *The Oxford Dictionary of Late Antiquity* (2018), or *The Oxford Dictionary of Byzantium* (1991), as appropriate, unless otherwise noted.

CHAPTER I

Introduction

"But then", he says, "for what reason save an evil one did you cut up
the fish which the slave Themison brought you?" As if I had not just
said that I write about the little bits of all the animals – about their
situation, size, and purpose – and studiously investigate and add to
the books of anatomy by Aristotle. And, in fact, I am most astonished
that you know about a single little fish inspected by me when I have
likewise inspected many, in whichever place they can be obtained,
and all the more so because I do none of this secretly, but all of it in
the open, so that whoever desires, even strangers, may attend.... This
little fish, which you called a sea hare, I showed to many who were
present.

Apuleius, *Apology*[1]

Apuleius of Madaurus (b. *c.* AD 125) may not seem a likely person to open
a book on dissection. A novelist and orator from Northern Africa, he is
known best for his sharp wit and rhetorical panache. Yet, in the passage
above, he presents himself as a dissector. Not just a dissector, but a public one. With the assistance of Themison, his medically trained slave, he
pursues his passion for anatomy "in the open," welcoming any passers-by
to observe the bone formations and other notable features of rare aquatic
species. So passionate is his interest in this topic that he has an open call
to friends and local fishermen to bring him any unusual specimens so that
he can put them under the knife.[2] Further, he reads anatomical texts with

---

[1] Apuleius, *Apol.* 40 ("at enim" inquit "piscem cui rei nisi malae proscidisti, quem tibi Themis[c]on
seruus attulit?" quasi uero non paulo prius dixerim me de particulis omnium animalium, de situ
earum de[ni]que numero de[ni]que causa conscribere ac libros ἀνατομῶν Aristoteli et explorare
studio et augere. atque adeo summe miror quod unum a me pisciculum inspectum sciatis, cum iam
plurimos, ubicumque locorum oblati sunt, aeque inspexerim, praesertim quod nihil ego clanculo,
sed omnia in propatulo ago, ut quiuis uel extrarius arbiter adsistat ... hunc adeo pisciculum, quem
uos leporem marinum nominatis, plurimis qui aderant ostendi).

[2] Apuleius, *Apol.* 33.

I

assiduous attention and even produces both Greek and Latin anatomical writing of his own.[3] Certainly, Apuleius has an agenda in describing these activities: He is defending himself on charges of magic, which included, among other things, an allegedly sinister interest in fish. Yet, the rhetorical felicity of his defense need not detract from its credibility. In fact, this speech dates to the period when interest in anatomy was at its peak in the ancient Mediterranean, when intellectuals were reading anatomical books for pleasure and the public dissection of animals for scientific ends was indeed a comparatively common occurrence.

Just a year before Apuleius' defense, and a bit further along the African coast, a young Galen (AD 129-c. 216) left Alexandria, where he had been studying, and returned to his hometown of Pergamon.[4] There, he leveraged his anatomical prowess and performative acumen to attain a coveted medical position from under the noses of more established doctors; soon he moved on to Rome, where his skill as a dissector earned him access to the social elite and eventually helped bring him to the notice of the emperor himself. Like Apuleius, he put his name around appropriate circles as someone on the look-out for choice anatomical specimens – and his appetite for them was insatiable. Across the Mediterranean, Galen's colleagues and rivals were similarly employed. The second century AD saw a burgeoning of dissection, both private and performative, and a surge in the production and circulation of anatomical texts. Apuleius is a powerful witness to this trend. Even outside the context of the medical world and in North African Oea, a comparative backwater of the Roman Empire, he attests to the fascination that dissection held across the social spectrum and to the diversity of interest in anatomical writing; further, his legal predicament reminds us that dissection was embedded in a nexus of other associations, some of them uncomfortable.

This book follows the development of the practice of dissection, including its social contexts, and traces the concomitant evolution of anatomical texts from fifth century BC Greece to Galen and Apuleius' day in the Roman period. No such comprehensive history of dissection in antiquity has yet been attempted. Scholarly work in this area has typically approached ancient dissection through the overlapping, but by no means

---

[3] Apuleius, *Apol.* 36–8.
[4] Apuleius' trial, if it was indeed a historical event, occurred in the winter of AD 158/9; see Hunink (1997), vol. I, p. 12. For a timeline of Galen's life, see Boudon-Millot (2012), 345–9.

identical, topic of ancient anatomy.[5] Anatomy consists of the arrangement and characteristics of the parts of the body, both external and internal. The science or study of anatomy therefore cultivates a knowledge of these topics, and anatomical texts, by my definition, include any text that engages with them, either exclusively or in a sustained way. Writing the history of anatomy involves mapping the evolution of anatomical thought over time: that is, chronicling the ways in which people conceive of the structures of the parts of the body and their interconnections. C. R. S. Harris' study of the vascular system from Alcmaeon to Galen is an excellent example of an in-depth history of anatomy: He articulates the details of different attempts throughout Classical antiquity to describe the structure, position, and relationship of the heart and the veins and arteries, including also a discussion of their function or physiology.[6] This book is not a history of anatomy; it will not address the details and development of anatomical data. Rather, it is a study of how these anatomical data were obtained and how this impacted the ways in which they were shared.

While the modern study of anatomy is predicated more or less exclusively on dissection, this is not an inevitable predication, and it has not always held true. There are, in short, other ways of conceiving of anatomy. Shigehisa Kuriyama's comparative study of Greek and Chinese medicine beautifully highlights the fact that dissection was not a foreordained anatomical methodology.[7] Even just within the Classical world, it did not hold continuous or universal sway. Brooke Holmes has demonstrated a marked shift around the fifth century BC, when the Greeks began approaching the interior of the body as a more knowable space, using exterior symptoms and observations to conceptualize its depths.[8] Colin Webster has now shown how ancient conceptions of the body depended on preexisting understandings of the physics of the natural world: Thus, technological developments shifted the ways in which the ancients conceived of the

---

[5] Several histories of early anatomy and dissection of varying length and focus have been written over the last century, including Singer (1925) and (1957), Edelstein (1932) and (1935), Kudlien (1968*a*) and (1969), May (1968), 13–38, Lloyd (1975*a*) and (1979), 156–69, Potter (1976), Vegetti (1979), 13–53, von Staden (1989), 138–53 and (1992*a*), Annoni and Barras (1993), Malomo, Idowu, and Osuagwu (2006), Byl (2011), 117–28, Rocca (2016), and Dean-Jones (2018). In addition, the Greco-Roman period often occupies the first section of books dealing with the history of anatomy in other periods, though often in an uncritical way; see Cole (1944), 24–47, Kevorkian (1959), 1–30, Persaud (1984), 29–69 and Persaud, Loukas, and Tubbs (2014), 3–45, Le Breton (1993), 25–35, Wootton (2006), 46–8, and Quigley (2012), 13.
[6] Harris (1973); Solmsen (1961) does the same for the nerves.
[7] Kuriyama (1999), 116–29.
[8] Holmes (2010); cf. Holmes (2018).

component parts of bodies and their functions.[9] More linguistically, Mary Beard has queried the ways in which anatomical vocabulary itself both reflected and molded ancient perceptions of bodily composition.[10] Ancient thinkers approached anatomy through analogy, through theoretical models, and through sheer conjecture.[11] Indeed, throughout the history of the development of dissection as a practice, alternative methods of anatomical insight continued to contest its primacy, its necessity, and even its reliability.

Nevertheless, Greek doctors and natural philosophers began experimenting with dissection at an early date, and it steadily gained importance as the most potent heuristic in the study of anatomy. Dissection, by my definition, consists in the cutting open of bodies and the observation of their component parts for the express purpose of adding to, confirming, or contesting anatomical knowledge; vivisection is a special type of dissection practiced on living bodies in order to ascertain both structure and, more particularly, function. Motivation critically underlies this definition of dissection: There are other ways of cutting into and observing bodies that are not dissective. Divinatory examination of animal entrails, for example, despite the keen and expert observations it requires, is not dissection because its practitioners are looking for divine, not anatomical data. Indeed, although the modern ubiquity of basic anatomical knowledge has homogenized our conception of bodily interiors, cutting open a body is a messy and multivalent activity. When first approaching an opened abdomen, it is very difficult to know what you are seeing until you have been told what you are looking at. Dissection, in short, requires a special type of looking.[12] Greek thinkers began to cultivate this way of viewing the

---

[9] Webster (forthcoming).

[10] Beard (2002).

[11] The Hippocratic idea of the womb as a cupping vessel or jar (e.g., *VM* 22 [I.626 Littré], *Mul.I* 33 [VIII.78 Littré]) and the popular conception of the heart and vessels as an irrigation system (e.g., Plato, *Ti.* 77c6–d8, Aristotle, *PA* 668a11–32) are good examples of anatomy by analogy; for more discussion of analogical approaches to the body, see Holmes (2010), 108–16. Theoretical models, for example of symmetry and the primacy of the center, similarly drove many of the early conceptions of the body (e.g., Diogenes' system of paired vessels at DK 64B 6[7] and Aristotle's three-chambered heart at *PA* 666b21–667a6). Plausible conjecture was a constant feature of ancient anatomy, underlying everything from the Methodists' pervasive system of pores or channels (Tecusan [2004], 11–12) to Erasistratus' *triplokia* (see Chapter 2, "Herophilus and Erasistratus" at p. 39) and Galen's assertion of a permeable interventricular septum in the heart (*Nat.Fac.* II.207–8).

[12] I am here following Kuriyama (1999), 111–29, who distinguishes dissection in these terms; he also broaches the assumptions and goals behind the move to dissection, a question which represents a distinct, philosophical dimension of the history of anatomy that I have not had space to engage with in a sustained way here.

interior at some point in the early fifth century in the context of a burgeoning desire to organize and understand the natural world; by the fourth century it had become a fully operative methodology.

Ancient dissection occurred almost exclusively on animal bodies, and throughout this book all unqualified references to dissection presume animal subjects. Some – notably Aristotle and those, like Apuleius, working in his tradition – were interested in animal anatomy on its own terms; most, however, used animals as a proxy for understanding human anatomy. This comparative anatomy is already visible among the authors of the Hippocratic Corpus, and they are fully aware of the limitations intrinsic to it: A goat's innards, when all is said and done, are not the same as a human's. Galen, our most extensive source, is also alert to comparative anatomy's potential to be misleading, but his confidence in the close homology between monkeys and humans forestalls any serious misgivings. This was for the best because the dissection of human bodies was not a routine occurrence in Greco-Roman antiquity; the only names securely associated with the practice are the early Hellenistic doctors Herophilus and Erasistratus. Nevertheless, historians have been perennially keen to focus on the availability of human subjects, perhaps in reaction to the fact that it was Vesalius' transition from the animal to the human body that ushered the science of anatomy into the modern era.

This book seeks to offer a complete picture of the practice of dissection in Classical antiquity. In doing so, it redresses imbalances in the attention paid to dissection in some previous work on the history of anatomy, namely a tendency to downplay the importance of the dissection of animals compared with that of humans and, relatedly, to overemphasize the Hellenistic period at the expense of the Roman one. Influentially, Ludwig Edelstein framed the Hellenistic switch from animal to human subjects as "the crucial question in the history of anatomy," but this focus on the human strikes me as ahistorical.[13] From the modern perspective animal dissection naturally seems a paltry substitute for human dissection, but the ancients did not feel this way. Certainly, they acknowledged that human

---

[13] Edelstein (1932), 97 ("diese Frage ist die entscheidende in der Geschichte der Anatomie"). In addition to a perennial fascination with the question in more general histories of anatomy, human dissection in antiquity has also been the subject of numerous dedicated articles, most recently Kudlien (1969), von Staden (1992*a*), Annoni and Barras (1993), and Dean-Jones (2018). I certainly do not dispute that human dissection is an interesting and worthwhile topic – nor that it was implicated in the leap forward in anatomical sophistication in the Hellenistic period – but simply assert that animal dissection is equally worthy of interest and plays a far more significant role overall in the history of ancient anatomical study.

subjects would provide the most accurate window into human anatomy, and later authors respected the privileged findings of Herophilus and Erasistratus accordingly. However, they were confident in their extensive use of animal dissection as a reliable proxy, and with good reason.[14] By the Roman period, despite never having dissected a human body, Galen exhibits a nuanced and expert understanding of anatomy in its minutest details.[15] Though he is respectful of the anatomical legacy of Herophilus and Erasistratus, it is manifest across his anatomical writings that his nearer contemporaries' work on animals, like his own, has advanced anatomical knowledge past their observations. Charles Singer's assertion that after the work of Herophilus and Erasistratus in the Hellenistic period "anatomy did not revive till the rise of the mediaeval universities" epitomizes the distorting effect of a disproportionate focus on human dissection.[16] When animal dissection receives its due share of the attention, a widespread, vibrant, and sophisticated surge in anatomical activity in the first two centuries of the Common Era comes into clearer focus: one that surpasses its Hellenistic antecedent in both its scale and its influence on the history of anatomical study. Indeed, I would argue that its reliance on animal subjects, which were both abundantly available and uncontroversial to kill, spurred rather than curbed its success and productivity.

I have taken a twofold approach to the history of dissection, reflected in the two-part structure of this book. In Part I, I consider what one might call the social history of the practice of dissection: who was doing it, how, and in what contexts. Although the answers to these questions lie mostly in texts, I have taken material culture and archaeological finds into account

[14] Indeed, anyone with access to their writing would have been perfectly aware that Herophilus and Erasistratus themselves contextualized their human dissections within a broader program of animal dissection.

[15] Galen, of course, knows full well that his simian-based anatomy is not exactly the same as human anatomy; indeed, he describes the monkey body as a "caricature" of the human body at *UP* III.80 (I.59H) (μίμημα γελοῖόν) and he is fully aware that the proportions as well as some of the details are different. Nevertheless, by cross-referencing his intimate knowledge of simian and other animal anatomy with his medical experience of human bodies, he arrives at what he is satisfied is a globally accurate picture of human anatomy. In general, when I speak of the anatomical knowledge derived from dissection in this book, I am referring to this amalgamation of animal data, as cast onto the human frame.

[16] Singer (1957), 38; cf. his claim on p. 46 that "it would seem that neither Lycus nor any of the other second century anatomists were able to use the human subject, and it is clear that Anatomy was in headlong decay. For all his greatness the only result of Galen's work was to codify the researches of antiquity for after ages." Authors since Singer have generally been more favorably disposed toward the anatomical work of Galen and his peers, but I hope that my intensive handling of the Roman period will offer a still more robust and multifaceted picture of the anatomical richness of the late first and second centuries AD than has yet been achieved.

wherever possible. Chapter 2 offers evidence for the practice of Dissection in the Classical and Hellenistic periods, terms which I use as rough but convenient markers for the fifth century BC and the fourth to first centuries BC, respectively; in light of the highly performative character that dissection would later come to adopt, I also include discussion of the range of public contexts within which the practice would have fallen in each of these periods. Chapter 3 turns to the Roman period (a moniker of convenience for the first and second centuries AD) and catalogues the motivations for and public-facing dimensions of dissective activity in Rome and across the Mediterranean. Chapter 4 gets into the practical details that underlay dissection in the ancient world: what subjects anatomists used and how they obtained them – including an in-depth discussion of the question of human dissection – and what further equipment and support was required and how easy it was to procure. Finally, Chapter 5 considers dissection in its broader social contexts. As Apuleius demonstrates, dissection operated within a wider world of bodily manipulations, and it would have been perceived with different valences by different people in different places. Though by no means exhaustive, this chapter seeks to contextualize dissection beyond the medical and philosophical circles where it was at home.

Part II of the book gauges the impact that dissection had on the field of anatomy by tracing the development of anatomical literature, including the diversity of its authorship, the evolution of its subgenres, and its variable relationship to the practice of dissection. Chapter 6 begins with anatomical writing in the Classical and Hellenistic periods. These texts mirror the development of dissection in these centuries: Few of the early texts are exclusively anatomical and, even in the Hellenistic period when more dedicated texts become popular, multiple approaches to anatomy remain vibrant. Chapter 7 surveys anatomical authors of the Roman period other than Galen. Though the bulk of the writing about anatomy from this time is lost, textual references and the papyrological record combine to reveal a wide and diverse field of anatomical literature, paralleling the popularity of dissection in this period as described in Chapter 3. Chapter 8 discusses Galen's minor anatomical writings, both those that survive and those that do not; it highlights the role that Galen apportions to dissection in these texts, as well as how he deploys it across his wider oeuvre. Chapter 9 focuses on Galen's *Anatomical Procedures*, a detailed set of instructions for the dissection of animals and the only text surviving from antiquity that seamlessly fuses dissection and anatomical writing. I consider Galen's purposes in writing this text and the audience he envisions using it and how, ending the chapter with broad conclusions on the history of dissection in antiquity as a whole. Finally, a brief epilogue in Chapter 10 provides a coda of sorts, following the history of dissection and anatomical writing into Late Antiquity and offering a bridge from the Classical anatomical world to the medieval one.

PART I

Practice

CHAPTER 2

Dissection in the Classical and Hellenistic Periods

> Alcmaeon of Croton, a man versed in natural philosophy, who first
> dared to attempt dissection, and Callisthenes, student of Aristotle,
> and Herophilus brought many remarkable things to light.
>
> Calcidius, *Commentary on Plato's* Timaeus[1]

Anatomy had a long history in the ancient world. Even before dissection
emerged as an investigative methodology, the Greeks had an operative
understanding of the interiors of bodies, including a functional vocabulary for the bones and internal viscera.[2] The anatomical descriptions in
the Homeric poems are detailed enough to have led scholars of the early
twentieth century to suggest that the Greeks of the Archaic period engaged
in dissection, but there is insufficient evidence to make this claim compelling.[3] The anatomical knowledge in Homer more likely results from animal sacrifice, butchery, and the familiarity with open wounds and corpses
that warfare entails. Indeed, the bulk of the anatomical terms occur in
passages describing violent wounds, suggesting that this was indeed a productive source of knowledge.[4] The collection of corpses for burial, from

---

[1] Calcidius, *In Tim.* 279 (Alcmaeo Crotoniensis in physicis exercitatus quique primus exectionem
aggredi est ausus, et Callisthenes, Aristotelis auditor, et Herophilus multa et praeclara in lucem
protulerunt).

[2] For catalogues of anatomical terminology in the Homeric poems, see Körner (1929), 13–31, and Lind
(1978), 39–44; for an attempt to map these onto modern anatomical understanding, see Saunders
(1999). Holmes (2010), 58–69 offers a more theoretical discussion of Homeric conceptualizations of
the body, which augments this picture of anatomical knowledge.

[3] Körner (1922) and (1929), 6–13 argues that Homeric doctors practiced not just dissection, but human
dissection, while Fuld (1922) goes so far as to suggest that pre-Homeric human sacrifice contributed
to anatomical knowledge. As I will explore later in this chapter in "Herophilus and Erasistratus" and
in Chapter 4, "Anatomical Subjects: Humans" at pp. 110–18, human dissection is an unusual exception to the rule in antiquity.

[4] Indeed, the Empiricist school of medicine would much later argue that the study of wounds ought to
be sufficient for medical understanding of human anatomy; see this chapter, "The Later Hellenistic
Period" at pp. 42–4 and Chapter 7, "Anatomy in the Roman Intellectual Scene" at pp. 267–9.

the battlefield and other catastrophic events, such as shipwrecks, would also have offered enough insight into skeletal and gross anatomy to make the basic homologies between human and animal bodies apparent. It is not until the fifth century BC that the earliest evidence for the intentional collection of data from bodies emerges. Herodotus (mid-fifth century BC) confirms that the activities just noted could offer direct insight into human anatomy in its own right, describing how later Plataeans observed anatomical anomalies in the bones unearthed from the Battle of Plataea.[5] Herodotus also reveals that the idea to cut open animals in order to learn about their interiors was considered unremarkable in his day, explaining quite matter of factly how it is possible to conclude the bile-producing effect of Scythian grass "from the opened up bodies of herd animals."[6] Indeed, at around this time, certain groups begin to evince great curiosity about the interior of the body, and we can find intimations of dissection among both philosophers and doctors of the Classical period.

The "Pre-Socratics"

The philosopher Alcmaeon (fifth century BC) is the earliest name to have garnered a reputation for anatomical investigation with his dissection of the eye, as reported in the Calcidius passage that forms the epigraph to this chapter. Lloyd, however, has convincingly cast doubt on the significance to be attached to this claim, suggesting that this "dissection" was quite limited in scope, confined, perhaps, to the simple excision of the eyeball from the head of an animal.[7] Anaxagoras of Clazomenae (500–428 BC), who apparently used the evidence of a goat brain to advocate for rational over divine explanation for natural occurrences, is another name mentioned in the early history of anatomy.[8] Diogenes of Apollonia (later fifth century BC), too, often finds a place on modern lists of early anatomists, but his description of the human vascular system – mostly a series of symmetrical pairs of vessels

---

Aristotle (*HA* 511b21–3) also describes how some of his predecessors contented themselves with examining the surface anatomy of extremely skinny patients, which would have yielded a reasonable amount of skeletal and vascular observations.

[5] Herodotus, IX.83.

[6] Herodotus, IV.58 (ἀνοιγομένοισι δὲ τοῖσι κτήνεσι). Vegetti (1979), 28–9 argues, in contrast, that there was something transgressive, bordering on impious, about the act of opening animals only for the sake of seeing what was inside (cf. Lloyd [1975a], 118); he does not discuss this passage. One could certainly argue that the anatomical observations here were incidental to the slaughter of the animals for food, but it nevertheless points to a habit of critical anatomical observation.

[7] Lloyd (1975a), 113–28. Longrigg (1993), 59–60 prefers the suggestion that Alcmaeon excised a human eye during the course of a "daring" medical treatment and thus made his anatomical observations incidentally.

[8] Plutarch, *Per.* 6.2 (DK 59A 16).

running from head to toe – smacks far more of abstract theory than of observation.[9] Democritus of Abdera (b. 460–457 BC) had already achieved a reputation as an expert anatomist in the Hellenistic period. One of the pseudepigraphic letters of Hippocrates describes him sitting surrounded by dismembered animals whose entrails he was examining in order to trace the locations of bile and discover the psychosomatic key to madness.[10] While it is unlikely that this Hellenistic testimony reflects any actual knowledge of Democritus' practices, it is certainly the case that his interests included anatomical and physiological topics.[11] Aelian records Democritus' opinions on uterine shapes in pigs, dogs, and mules and their impact on the animals' fecundity, and on the skulls and veins of deer, oxen, and bulls and how they contribute to the growth of horns.[12] Empedocles (*c.* 492–432 BC), too, focuses a great deal on the body, particularly its physiology, as the extensive passages that discuss breathing and vision indicate.[13] In both of those, though, his theories derive from comparison with the physics of inanimate objects – a clepsydra and a lantern – rather than more biological or anatomical observations.[14] In general, the fragmentary nature of the evidence for these early philosophers renders any detailed claims about their investigative methodology difficult to defend, but, while we do not have compelling evidence that dissection was a common productive tool in philosophical circles of this period, it is certainly the case that there was a widespread interest both in the structure and in the function of bodies.

Hippocratic Doctors[15]

On the medical side, the evidence for anatomical study is more robust thanks to the breadth of the Hippocratic Corpus, but it nevertheless

---

[9] Diogenes' description of the vascular system is quoted in full by Aristotle at *HA* 511b31–512b11 (DK 64B 6[7]); see Lloyd (2006).

[10] Ps.-Hippocratic *Ep.* 17.2–3 (IX.352, 356 Littré) (cf. DK 68C 3).

[11] On the Democritus letters, including their dating and historical reliability, see Smith (1990), 20–34, especially 24–6. For Democritus as a zoologist, see Perilli (2006). It is worth noting that Aristotle (*PA* 665a32–4) passes along, albeit critically, Democritus' belief that bloodless creatures have viscera that are simply too small to see, suggesting that Democritus had gone and looked for them.

[12] Aelian, *HN* XII.16, 18–20 (DK 68A 151, 153–5). Perilli (2006), 172–5 suggests that the most anatomically detailed of these topics, namely the discussion of the growth of horns, is reliant for its anatomical facts on Hippocratic sources.

[13] Breathing at Aristotle *Resp.* 473b9–4a6 (DK 31B 100); vision at Aristotle *Sens.* 437b25–8a2 (DK 31B 84).

[14] See Webster (forthcoming) for an analysis of how Empedocles' vision of the body was shaped by the technologies of his world.

[15] I use the terms "Hippocratic doctors" and "Hippocratic authors" simply as a concise way to refer to the people responsible for contributing to the texts that comprise the modern Hippocratic Corpus,

remains largely tantalizing.[16] The authors in the corpus display a general understanding of and vocabulary for the skeleton and the internal organs of the body.[17] The precision and confidence with which these terms are deployed, however, varies from text to text. Diverse theories for the structure and function of the vascular system are also evident in the corpus; at a minimum, there is a pervasive concept of special "wide" or "hollow" vessels that are important, typically including one in each arm that are linked to the spleen and the liver, respectively.[18] While in most cases this anatomical information occurs in passing or is presented without any explanation, there are a few instances where the authors engage with their methods for acquiring knowledge about the body.

Some authors resign themselves to a largely theoretical anatomy. After a brief and quite idiosyncratic résumé of human internal organs, the author of the Hippocratic *Art* adds,

> Certainly, it is not possible for any of these things here described to be seen by anyone looking with their *eyes*, which is why I have called them obscure … but it is possible [to understand them] insofar as the natures of the ill lie open for investigation and the natures of the investigators bend towards inquiry. Indeed, they are understood with greater work and no less time

particularly those that date to the fifth and early fourth centuries BC. I do not mean to imply that they constituted a single unified and self-identifying group in their own time.

[16] Evidence for the interests of contemporary medical authors not included in the Hippocratic Corpus is more tantalizing still; see van der Eijk (2016), especially 27–34. One can, however, infer at least some level of anatomical interest there as well from the fact that Rufus cites Philistion of Locri (*c.* 427–347 BC), the Sicilian doctor often cited as an influence on Plato, for a vascular term (*Nom.Part.* 201), and Plutarch and Aulus Gellius discuss his opinion on the anatomy of the throat (Plutarch, *Quaest.Conv.* 699C; Gellius, *NA* 17.11).

[17] On Hippocratic anatomical vocabulary, see Chantraine (1975), Irigoin (1980), and Irmer (1980). Certainly, many authors in the corpus demonstrate more interest in the humors or fluids within the body than the structures of the body itself, but, as Gundert (1992) shows, this did not preclude engagement with the parts. For a broader perspective on Hippocratic approaches to the body, see Holmes (2010) and (2018).

[18] For the vascular system in the Hippocratic corpus, see Harris (1973), 29–96 and Duminil (1983). References to "wide" (παχείη) vessels occur at *Epid.II* 6.19 (V.136 Littré), *Coac.* 430, 499 (V.680, 698 Littré), *Nat.Hom.* 11 (VI.58–60 Littré), *Morb.I* 21 (VI.182 Littré), *Morb.II* 8 (VII.16 Littré), *Prorrh.II* 12 (IX.34 Littré), *Oss.* 5, 7–9, 12–15, 18 (IX.170–6, 182–8, 192 Littré); to "hollow" (κοίλη) vessels at *Loc.Hom.* 3 (VI.282 Littré), *Int.* 18 (VII.210 Littré), *Carn.* 5 (VIII.590 Littré); to the splenetic and/or hepatic vessels at *Epid.II* 2.22 (V.94 Littré), *Nat.Hom.* 11 (VI.60 Littré), *Morb.I* 26 (VI.194 Littré), *Loc.Hom.* 3 (VI.282 Littré), *Morb.Sac.* 6 (VI.366 Littré), *Int.* 19, 28 (VII.214, 242 Littré), *Oss.* 10 (IX.178 Littré) (cf. *Epid.II* 4.1 [V.120–2 Littré]). There are also a handful of mentions of named vessels, including the jugulars (αἱ σφάγιαι καλεόμεναι) at *Morb.IV* 7, 9 (VII.554, 560) (cf. *Acut. B* 9 [II.410 Littré]) and the acromial (ἡ ἐπωμιδίη ὀνομαζομένη) at *Oss.* 12 (IX.182 Littré).

than if they were seen by the eyes themselves. For, whatever things escape the vision of the eyes, are conquered by the mind's eye.[19]

This author clearly leaves the door open to inferences based on internal structures seen in the course of medical practice; it is less straightforward to understand what he means by "inquiry" on the part of the doctors. It is most natural to take the two halves of the clause together and assume that the possibility of looking into a patient's body is only as fruitful as the determination of the practitioner to do it. There is no indication that he has considered the dissection of animals as a productive avenue of "inquiry," and, interestingly, unlike some later authors, he does not express any wish to view the insides of the body, priding himself instead on the powers of inductive reasoning. His near contemporary, the author of *Ancient Medicine*, takes a similar view, saying that one must base theories about the obscure internal organs on analogies to "external things that are visible," such as lips, cupping vessels, and sponges.[20]

In contrast, the author of *On Joints* is more up front about his opinion on the potential of dissection, proffering two different imaginary scenarios for cutting open humans. In the first, he is recounting his frustration with a public situation in which he found himself: He was arguing against other physicians that a certain case was not a forward dislocation of the shoulder joint – and indeed that such a dislocation is an impossibility – and he was scarcely able to gain any credibility at all. In order to convince his readers of the same fact, he jumps straight into a hypothetical dissection, explaining what the joint would look like "if one were to strip bare the shoulder from the flesh of the arm."[21] Later, contemplating the equally improbable scenario of an inwardly fractured spine, he entertains an intentionally fantastic solution, saying that such an injury would obviously not be possible to reduce, "unless someone, cutting open the man, then kneading his way through the bowels, should push from the inside to the outside with his hand; and this might be possible to do in a dead man, but definitely not

---

[19] *Art.* 11 (VI.18 Littré) (οὐ γὰρ δὴ ὀφθαλμοῖσί γε ἰδόντι τούτων τῶν εἰρημένων οὐδενὶ οὐδέν ἐστιν εἰδέναι· διὸ καὶ ἄδηλα ἐμοί τε ὠνόμασται ... δυνατὸν δέ, ὅσον αἵ τε τῶν νοσεόντων φύσιες ἐς τὸ σκεφθῆναι παρέχουσιν, αἵ τε τῶν ἐρευνησόντων ἐς τὴν ἔρευναν πεφύκασιν. μετὰ πλείονος μὲν γὰρ πόνου καὶ οὐ μετ᾽ ἐλάσσονος χρόνου, ἢ εἰ τοῖσιν ὀφθαλμοῖσιν ἑώρατο, γινώσκεται· ὅσα γὰρ τὴν τῶν ὀμμάτων ὄψιν ἐκφεύγει, ταῦτα τῇ τῆς γνώμης ὄψει κεκράτηται); the emphasis is in the Greek (γε).

[20] *VM* 22 (I.626 Littré) (ἔξωθεν ἐκ τῶν φανερῶν); on this author's conception of the body, see Schiefsky (2005), 321–7 and Webster (forthcoming). All dating for the Hippocratic Corpus is according to Craik (2015) unless otherwise noted.

[21] *Artic.* 1 (IV.80 Littré) (εἴ τις τοῦ βραχίονος ψιλώσειε μὲν τῶν σαρκέων τὴν ἐπωμίδα). Interestingly, it is in just this type of conflictual public situation that Galen would have had recourse to an actual dissection (see Chapter 3, "Performance to Discredit Rivals").

in a living one."[22] The evident sarcasm of the final clause, which highlights the futility of such a suggestion given that the entire point of the operation is to cure a living patient, underscores the fact that this is merely a hypothetical procedure.[23] Nevertheless, it is striking that he is thinking about the body in such "dissective" terms. Indeed, the fact that he mentions, only a dozen lines later, that man has the narrowest body cavity of all the animals suggests that the intentional observation of animal anatomy for comparative purposes has colored his attitude toward the human body.[24]

The multiple references to animal anatomy throughout the Hippocratic Corpus confirm that comparative anatomy was an operative method for conceptualizing the insides of the human body for these authors. Some of the animal anatomy could certainly have been acquired through the course of routine observations. Familiarity with the viscera of the more common herd animals would have been a natural by-product of animal sacrifice and the eating of meat; indeed, the author of *Fleshes* suggests that one might conveniently observe how blood congeals "whenever one slaughters a sacrificial animal."[25] Similarly, familiarity with these animals' bones requires no special explanation. The size of a sheep's vertebra, for example, is such general knowledge that the author of *Internal Affections* uses it as a unit of measure.[26] The Hippocratic doctor could also become familiar with the organs of animals unlikely to have been sacrificed through the course of his practice; *Diseases of Women II* and *III* contain recipes that require the doctor to "burn separately the head of a hare and three mice and remove the bowels of two mice, but not their liver and kidneys" and to "cut open as young a puppy as possible ... taking out [its] innards."[27] It could certainly be from activity like this that the author of *Epidemics VI* is able to assert that "[man] has bowels like a dog's, but bigger."[28]

---

[22] *Artic.* 46 (IV.198 Littré) (εἰ μή τις διαταμὼν τὸν ἄνθρωπον, ἔπειτα ἐσμασάμενος ἐς τὴν κοιλίην, ἐκ τοῦ εἴσωθεν τῇ χειρὶ ἐς τὸ ἔξω ἀντωθέοι· καὶ ταῦτα νεκρῷ μὲν οἷόν τε ποιέειν, ζῶντι δὲ οὐ πάνυ).

[23] Di Benedetto (1986), 240–1, however, reads it as an endorsement of human dissection, arguing that the author himself practiced it.

[24] *Artic.* 46 (IV.198 Littré); alternatively, Annoni and Barras (1993), 195–6 point out that the handling of the human body that the author hypothesizes has interesting parallels to the way in which a *mageiros* opens and disembowels a sacrificial animal.

[25] *Carn.* 8 (VIII.595 Littré) (ὁκόταν σφάξῃ τις ἱερεῖον).

[26] *Int.* 20 (VII.216 Littré).

[27] *Mul.II* 76 (VIII.366 Littré) (κεφαλὴν λαγωοῦ καὶ μύας τρεῖς κατακαῦσαι χωρὶς, καὶ τῶν δύο μυῶν ἐξελεῖν κοιλίην, ἧπαρ δὲ καὶ νεφροὺς μή); *Mul.III* 18.3 (VIII.440 Littré) (σκυλάκιον ὅτι νεώτατον ἀνασχίσας ... τὰ ἐντοσθίδια ἐξελών). Puppies also come up throughout the corpus as a dish for sick patients, as at *Epid.VII* 62 (V.428 Littré), *Morb.II* 56 (VII.88 Littré), *Int.* 27 (VII.240 Littré), *Mul. III* 5 (VIII.420 Littré), *Superf.* 29 (VIII.496 Littré).

[28] *Epid.VI* 4.6 (V.308 Littré) (τὰ κῶλα ἔχει οἷα κυνός, μείζω δέ).

The continuation of the passage in *Epidemics VI*, however, suggests a more intentional program than the mere accumulation of chance anatomical observations. The author goes on to say that "[man's] bowels are hung from the mesocolon, and that [is hung] by sinews from the backbone under the stomach."[29] Whether this statement was drawn from critical attention during medical practice or, more likely, from extrapolation from the purposeful dissection of animals, it indicates that the author is a motivated student of anatomy, interested in the arrangement and details of the body *in situ*, not just in the general shape of the organs. Many of his peers in the Hippocratic Corpus exhibit similar interest. Some authors describe manipulating parts of the body, often leaving ambiguous the circumstances and the species. The author of *Wounds in the Head* describes moist, fleshy pockets in the skull that produce blood "if someone rubs them with his fingers," while the author of *Glands* describes cutting and touching glands, and adds what happens "if you knead one with your fingers, exerting a good deal of strength."[30] In *Fleshes*, we find the even more aggressive suggestion to burn a spinal cord in order to evaluate what type of material it is made of.[31] Perhaps the most famous such moment is that in *On the Sacred Disease*, when the author suggests dissection as a means of proving that seizures have physical rather than divine causation: "If you cut open the head [of an affected goat], you will discover that the brain is moist and full of dropsy and smells bad, and from this you will know clearly that it is not a god that harms the body, but a disease."[32] This particular dissection, however, does not appear to have proceeded much farther than the opening of the skull and examination of the surface of the brain, leaving the connections described between it and the rest of the body at a theoretical level.[33]

Several of the various authors in the compilation known as *On the Nature of Bones* also exhibit marked interest in anatomical research. One

---

[29] *Epid. VI* 4.6 (V.308 Littré) (ἤρτηται ἐκ τῶν μεσοκώλων· ταῦτα δὲ ἐκ νεύρων ἀπὸ τῆς ῥάχιος ὑπὸ τὴν γαστέρα.).

[30] *VC* 1 (III.188 Littré) (εἴ τις αὐτὰ διατρίβοι τοῖσι δακτύλοισιν); *Gland.* 1 (VIII.566 Littré) (κἢν ὀργάσῃς τοῖς δακτύλοις ἐπιπουλὺ βιησάμενος).

[31] *Carn.* 4 (VIII.598 Littré).

[32] *Morb. Sac.* 11 (VI.382 Littré) (ἢν διακόψῃς τὴν κεφαλήν, εὑρήσεις τὸν ἐγκέφαλον ὑγρὸν ἐόντα καὶ ὕδρωπος περίπλεων καὶ κακὸν ὄζοντα, καὶ ἐν τούτῳ δηλονότι γνώσῃ ὅτι οὐχ ὁ θεὸς τὸ σῶμα λυμαίνεται, ἀλλ' ἡ νοῦσος). Note the parallel to Anaxagoras' goat dissection (see above, "The 'Pre-Socratics'" at p. 12).

[33] Compare the brief and similarly superficial statement on the same topic at *Morb. Sac.* 3 (VI.366 Littré), where the author says "the brain of man is two-fold just like also for all other animals; a fine

opens his enumeration of the vertebrae by saying "these are the things that *we ourselves* observed from the bones of man," using the personal pronoun and the emphatic demonstrative, both grammatically superfluous, in order to underscore his own verification of these facts.[34] Another qualifies his description of the vessels of the kidneys, adding that these are the only ones "as far as *I* know," again using a personal pronoun to add emphasis.[35] Most compellingly, the author of the most extensive description of the vascular system in *On the Nature of Bones* – and the entire corpus – is clearly practicing dissection:

> The diaphragm grows upon the liver, and they are not easy to separate. Pairs [of vessels run] from the collarbones, some on the inside, others on the inside but under the chest and into the abdomen; where they go from there, I do not yet know.... Somewhere around this place, the hepatic vessel, having run back again from the heart, terminates.... There are many branches [of the hepatic vessel] through the diaphragm ... and these ones are rather more visible.[36]

This author has almost certainly had his hands inside an animal, pulling things apart, following the paths of veins, and doing his best to descry features of variable visibility. More strikingly, he views this as a work in progress: He is not *yet* aware of the exact paths or locations of some of the vessels he describes, but he exudes confidence that his methodology will eventually lead him to this knowledge.

There is, then, good reason to believe that animal dissection was the basis for some of the anatomical knowledge in the Hippocratic Corpus.[37] Indeed, several authors are thoughtful about the trade-offs of using this knowledge gained from animals as a proxy for knowledge about their

membrane separates the middle of it" (ὁ ἐγκέφαλος τοῦ ἀνθρώπου ἐστὶ διπλόος ὥσπερ καὶ τοῖσιν ἄλλοισι ζώοισιν ἅπασιν· τὸ δὲ μέσον αὐτοῦ διείργει μῆνιγξ λεπτή); see Lloyd (1975a), 130–1.

[34] *Oss.* 1 (IX.168 Littré) (ἃ δ' ἡμεῖς αὐτοὶ ἐξ ἀνθρώπου ὀστέων κατεμάθομεν); the emphasis is implicit in the Greek. There is nothing here, however, that could not have been observed on a skinny patient.

[35] *Oss.* 4 (IX.170 Littré) (ὅσον ἐγὼ οἶδα); again, the emphasis is implicit in the Greek construction.

[36] *Oss.* 10 (IX.180 Littré) (φρένες δὲ προσπεφύκασι τῷ ἥπατι, ἃς οὐ ῥάδιον χωρίσαι. δισσαὶ δ' ἀπὸ κληΐδων, αἱ μὲν ἔνθεν, αἱ δὲ ἔνθεν ὑπὸ στῆθος ἐς ἦτρον· ὅποι δὲ ἐντεῦθεν, οὔπω οἶδα ... ταύτῃ πη παλινδρομήσασα ἀπὸ καρδίης ἡ ἡπατῖτις ἔληγεν ... πολυσχιδεῖς δὲ διὰ τῶν φρενῶν εἰσιν ... αὗται δὲ μᾶλλόν τι ἐμφανέες); compare the parallel passage at *Epid.II* 4.1 (V.122 Littré).

[37] Suggestively, the author of *Anatomy*, an extremely truncated work, frequently reaches for animal comparisons; cf. *Anat.* 1, 3–5, 10 (VIII.538–40 Littré) (following the chapter divisions in Craik [2006]). There are also moments of surprisingly accurate human anatomy there as well: The lobes of the lungs and of the liver are unambiguously human (*Anat.* 2, 4 [VIII.538 Littré]); cf. Craik (2006), 133, 140. The description of the heart (*Anat.* 3), in contrast, bears no resemblance to human cardiac structure, despite being pointedly compared to the hearts of other animals. On the dating of this text, see Chapter 6, n. 12.

human patients. The author of *Nature of the Child* uses bird eggs to understand human fetal development, saying that they offer "as clear a way of discerning as is possible for human understanding for all those who want to know about this."[38] He proposes that the reader set twenty eggs under a hen and crack one open each day in order to track the progression of the external development of the chick, which will allow him to understand human fetal development, at least "as far as one ought to compare the nature of a bird with the nature of man."[39] He certainly recognizes both the value and the pitfalls of this comparative methodology. Similarly, the author of *On Joints* hesitates aloud as to whether a veterinary comparandum is appropriate for a work on human joints, but comes down in the affirmative.[40] The author of *Internal Affections* is also careful about justifying his use of animal dissection to discuss human disease, saying:

> The proof for me that dropsy also arises from tubercules is from cattle and dogs and pigs; for, of the quadrupeds, tubercules in the lung containing fluid come about most of all in these, and, cutting through them, you would know this straightaway, for fluid will flow out. And it seems that this sort of thing would also happen in humans, to a greater degree than in animals since we use an unhealthier diet.[41]

This author is operating on an understanding of an essential homology between animals and humans, while conceding that differences must still be accounted for.

In addition to the dissection of animals as a comparative proxy and to the mostly passive observation of patients' injuries and of unburied corpses, a Hippocratic doctor with an interest in empirical anatomy may also have taken advantage of his comparatively easy access to human fetuses and stillborn infants.[42] The author of *Fleshes* describes his own personal experience on this front, explaining:

---

[38] *Nat.Pue.* 18 (29L) (VII.530 Littré) (τὴν διάγνωσιν ... ὡς ἀνυστὸν ἀνθρωπίνῃ γνώμῃ ἐμφανέα ἐοῦσαν παντὶ τῷ θέλοντι εἰδέναι τούτου πέρι).

[39] *Nat.Pue.* 18 (29L) (VII.530 Littré) (ὡς χρὴ ὄρνιθος φύσιν ξυμβάλλειν ἀνθρώπου φύσει).

[40] *Artic.* 8 (IV.96 Littré); see also the comparison of human and animal bones at *Artic.* 13 (IV.116 Littré) and *Mochl.* 1 (IV.344 Littré). However, this author is clearly reliant on animal anatomy, as his description of the lower jaw at *Artic.* 34 (IV.154 Littré) confirms; cf. *Loc.Hom.* 6 (VI.284–6 Littré).

[41] *Int.* 23 (VII.224 Littré) (ὡς δὲ γίνεται καὶ ἀπὸ φυμάτων ὕδερος, τόδε μοι μαρτύριον καὶ ἐν βοΐ καὶ ἐν κυνὶ καὶ ἐν ὑΐ· μάλιστα γὰρ τῶν τετραπόδων ἐν τούτοισι γίνεται φύματα ἐν τῷ πλεύμονι ἅπερ ἔχει ὕδωρ, διαταμὼν δ' ἂν γνοίης τάχιστα, ῥεύσεται γὰρ ὕδωρ· δοκέει δὲ καὶ ἐν ἀνθρώπῳ ἐγγίνεσθαι τοιαῦτα πολλῷ μᾶλλον ἢ ἐν προβάτοισιν, ὁκόσῳ καὶ τῇ διαίτῃ ἐπινούσῳ χρεόμεθα μᾶλλον).

[42] It is impossible to completely rule out surreptitious dissection of the adult human corpse among these doctors, a periodically recurring claim in Hippocratic scholarship since Littré; see, for example, Menetrier (1930) and Craik (2006), 159. However, there is also no clear evidence to support it and, given human dissection's controversial status in antiquity, it seems to me to bear the burden

[W]hen once the seed comes into the uterus, in seven days it has all the parts of the body that there are. But someone might wonder how I know this: I have seen many, in the following way. The common prostitutes, the ones who have frequent experience with such things, whenever they lie with a man, know when they have conceived, and then they destroy [the pregnancy]. And once destroyed, it falls out like flesh. Putting this flesh into water, and looking at it in the water, you discover that it has all the limbs and places for the eyes and the ears and the hands. And the fingers on the hands and the legs and feet and toes and private parts and all the rest of the body are evident.[43]

The author of this text is in general seized with a desire to offer proof for his assertions, but this particular proof clearly takes pride of place.[44] Fetal development, like internal anatomy, is an area of obscurity that receives a significant amount of attention in the Hippocratic Corpus. While this author has found an active means of lifting the veil and seeing into the process, it falls short of invasive. He is interested only in observing surface anatomy and makes no move to dissect – an undertaking that would anyway have been futilely minute. The author of *Nature of the Child* finds himself in a similar situation. He, too, describes in detail his personal witnessing of the putative abortion of a prostitute and his chance to observe what he believes to be the six-day-old fetus, though he does not describe manipulating the fetus in any way, and all that he claims to be able to discern is the umbilicus.[45]

In addition to these two extraordinary first-person narratives, there are other indications that Hippocratic doctors were indeed able to handle aborted or miscarried fetuses. Later in *Nature of the Child*, the author describes the periods within which fetal limbs and genitals become articulated, using the evidence of abortions of both genders and different gestational ages as proof.[46] The author of *Epidemics II* also records the

---

of proof. The most suggestive piece of data on this front has been provided by Dean-Jones (2018), 230, n. 4, who argues that the knowledge of the human lungs in *Anat.*, which are described in a way befitting a diseased specimen, resulted from the dissection of a slave from silver mines; however, a more passive observation of such a patient, if violently wounded, could also yield the same results.

[43] *Carn.* 19 (VIII.610 Littré) (ἐπὴν ἐς τὰς μήτρας ἔλθη ὁ γόνος, ἐν ἑπτὰ ἡμέρῃσιν ἔχει ὁκόσα περ ἐστὶν ἔχειν τοῦ σώματος· τοῦτο δέ τις ἂν θαυμάσειεν ὅκως ἐγὼ οἶδα· πολλὰ δὲ εἶδον τρόπῳ τοιῷδε· αἱ ἑταῖραι αἱ δημόσιαι, αἵτινες αὐτέων πεπείρηνται πολλάκις, ὁκόταν παρὰ ἄνδρα ἔλθῃ, γινώσκουσιν ὁκόταν λάβωσιν ἐν γαστρί· κἄπειτ' ἐνδιαφθείρουσιν· ἐπειδὰν δὲ ἤδη διαφθαρῇ, ἐκπίπτει ὥσπερ σάρξ. ταύτην τὴν σάρκα ἐς ὕδωρ ἐμβαλών, σκεπτόμενος ἐν τῷ ὕδατι, εὑρήσεις ἔχειν πάντα μέλεα καὶ τῶν ὀφθαλμῶν τὰς χώρας καὶ τὰ οὔατα καὶ τὰ γυῖα· καὶ τῶν χειρῶν οἱ δάκτυλοι καὶ τὰ σκέλεα καὶ οἱ πόδες καὶ οἱ δάκτυλοι τῶν ποδῶν, καὶ τὸ αἰδοῖον καὶ τὸ ἄλλο πᾶν σῶμα δῆλον).

[44] The author also discusses or provides proof at *Carn.* 4, 6, 8, 9, 15, and 18 (VIII.590–6, 604–8 Littré).

[45] *Nat.Pue.* 2 (13L) (VII.490–2 Littré).

[46] *Nat.Pue.* 7 (18L) (VII.504 Littré).

development and gender of miscarried fetuses.[47] Though interesting for embryological theory, none of this activity would have had much bearing on internal anatomy. It does, however, suggest a willingness to allow physicians to handle and manipulate human fetal material. In addition, three different Hippocratic gynecological texts discuss embryotomy, the practice of dismembering and/or selectively crushing a stillborn child that could not otherwise be removed from the laboring mother. *Diseases of Women I* instructs the doctor faced with a dead fetus whose arm or leg is protruding from the vagina to

> cut it up in the following way: having severed the head with a knife, crush it with a press in such a way that it is not ruptured, and draw out the bones with a bone forceps … when you have pulled these parts out and it is at the point of its shoulders, cut off both the arms at the shoulder joints…. If it [still] does not obey, split the entire chest up to the jugulars, but be careful that you do not cut below the stomach or strip off any part of the embryo, for then the stomach and the bowels and the feces come out.[48]

Superfetation has a similar passage, which also instructs to the doctor to remove the arms, but this time has him "extract the innards, having carefully cut open [its belly]."[49] The author of *Excision of the Fetus* suggests that the doctor should first "cover up the head [of the mother] with a cloth, so that she not be frightened, seeing whatever you do," and then "taking up the arm [protruding from the vagina], attempt to pull it out as far as possible, and then skin the arm, also laying bare the bone … and, making an incision all around the shoulder, pull it away at the joint."[50]

These doctors are without doubt – and with a socially legitimized medical purpose – cutting up dead human bodies. The freedom with which they handled early stage aborted fetuses suggests that their manipulation of dismembered bodies of these full-term fetuses need not have been entirely cursory. While the mother was understandably shielded from the distressing sight, it is difficult to imagine that a physician with the intellectual

---

[47] *Epid.II* 2.4, 2.13 (V.84–6, 90 Littré).

[48] *Mul.I* 70 (VIII.148 Littré) (τάμνειν τῷδε τῷ τρόπῳ· σχίσαντα τὴν κεφαλὴν μαχαιρίῳ ξυμφλάσαι, ἵνα μὴ θράσσῃ, τῷ πιέστρῳ, καὶ τὰ ὀστέα ἕλκειν ὀστεολόγῳ … ὅταν δὲ ταῦτα μὲν ἔξω εἰρύσῃς, ἐν δὲ τοῖσιν ὤμοισιν ἔῃ, τάμνειν τὰς χεῖρας ἄμφω ἐν τοῖσιν ἄρθροισι μετὰ τῶν ὤμων … ἢν δὲ μὴ ἐνακούσῃ, τὸ στῆθος πᾶν μέχρι τῶν σφαγέων σχίζειν, φυλάσσεσθαι δὲ ὡς μὴ κατὰ τὴν γαστέρα τάμῃς, καὶ ψιλώσῃς τι τοῦ ἐμβρύου, ἔξεισι γὰρ ἡ γαστὴρ καὶ τὰ ἔντερα καὶ κόπρος).

[49] *Superf.* 7 (VIII.480 Littré) (ἀνασχίσαντα ἡσυχῇ ἐξελεῖν τὰ ἐντοσθίδια).

[50] *Foet.Exsect.* 1 (VIII.512 Littré) (τὴν κεφαλὴν κατακαλύψαι χρὴ τῇ σινδόνι, ὅκως μὴ ὁρῶσα φοβῆται ὅ τι ἂν ποιήσῃς … τῆς χειρὸς ἐπιλαβόμενος προάγειν ἔξω ἐπιχείρει ὡς μάλιστα, παραδεῖραι δὲ τὸν βραχίονα, καὶ ἀποψιλώσας τὸ ὀστέον … τὸν ὦμον περισάρκισον καὶ ἄφελε κατὰ τὸ ἄρθρον).

curiosity of those encountered here would have passed up an opportunity like this to peek at the obscurities of human anatomy, should a stillbirth come his way. This is, therefore, another potential source of human information; certainly, it would, at the very least, have confirmed the general homology of humans to animals.[51]

There is thus sufficient – though by no means abundant or unambiguous – evidence to assert that dissection was a legitimate anatomical tool in use in the Classical period. Hippocratic references to animal anatomy certainly incorporate observations from quotidian encounters with animal bodies, but also go beyond them, into intentional animal dissection. The authors that employ it present a reasonably sophisticated awareness of the methodological limits and pitfalls of using animal anatomy as a comparative proxy for that of humans, and they likely also took observant advantage of professional moments that allowed them access to the viscera of humans themselves. Nevertheless, anatomy was neither a strongly developed field nor a topic of pervasive interest across the Hippocratic Corpus. Of those who do take an interest, only a fraction show evidence of engagement with dissection, while the rest are content to rely on more theoretical models.

Medical Performance in the Classical Period

Despite this evidence for dissection in the Classical period, we have little detail about how it was practiced. There is nothing to suggest whether it was purely private research or whether it might in some way have been a forerunner of the unabashedly performative dissections of the Roman period. A survey of the performative aspects of medical practice during this period must therefore offer the context and parameters within which dissection would have fallen. It is certainly the case that the medical profession had a public and performative element, dating back to the beginnings of attested Greek medicine. The very act of consulting and treating a patient was a semipublic event: Between competing doctors and interested friends and family members, the practicing physician was afforded little privacy. The opening of the Hippocratic *On Affections* outright encourages this behavior, exhorting the intelligent layman to "understand the

---

[51] The medical rather than investigative motivations preclude embryotomy from counting as dissection by my definition (see Chapter 1), though it is certainly an example of a case where motivations might begin to multiply and boundaries to blur, not least because the subjects themselves were dead at the time of incision.

things said by the physician and the things applied to his body and to understand each of these things to the degree suitable to a layman … and to be able to contribute [an opinion] about the things said and done with a degree of judgement."[52] Patients were evidently liable to fall short of this ideal, however, and to be attracted by impressive cures more than by sound ones, leading the author of *Precepts* to counsel his fellow doctors to try to tactfully dissuade such misguided people for their own good.[53] Many less scrupulous physicians embraced this tendency and cultivated skills and treatments designed to be eye-catching and memorable, to the chagrin of some of their peers. There was apparently a proliferation of fancy ways to wrap bandages, denounced by more than one author as useless, even potentially harmful, pageantry.[54] On a larger scale, the various machines used to reduce fractures were known for drawing a crowd. The author of *On Joints* repeatedly expresses distaste for their use. In one case, he derides the use of succussion to straighten hunchbacks, a process that involves tying the patient to a ladder and then dropping him down the side of a high building:

> First of all, succussions on a ladder have never straightened out anyone, that I am aware of; and, further, those doctors use it most of all who desire to make a big crowd gape and stare – for to those kinds of people it is amazing to see someone suspended or thrown down or whatever seems fitting in these sorts of cases, and they always applaud these things and it has never

---

[52] *Aff.* 1 (VI.208 Littré) (ἐπίστασθαι δὲ τὰ ὑπὸ τῶν ἰητρῶν καὶ λεγόμενα καὶ προσφερόμενα πρὸς τὸ σῶμα τὸ ἑωυτοῦ καὶ διαγινώσκειν· ἐπίστασθαι δὲ τούτων ἕκαστα, ἐς ὅσον εἰκὸς ἰδιώτην … περὶ δὲ τούτων καὶ τῶν λεγομένων καὶ τῶν ποιευμένων οἷόν τε εἶναι τὸν ἰδιώτην γνώμῃ τινὶ ξυμβάλλεσθαι).

[53] *Praec.* 5 (IX.256–8 Littré).

[54] *Off.* 7 (III.290–2 Littré) recommends that bandaging be neat and tidy and describes several different styles, including "simple, oblique, uphill, eye, rhomboid, and lozenge" (ἁπλοῦν, σκέπαρνον, σιμόν, ὀφθαλμὸς, ῥόμβος, καὶ ἡμίτομον); cf. 4 (III.288 Littré) where he counsels doctors to incise "gracefully" (εὐρύθμως). The author of *Morb.I* 10 (VI.158 Littré) seems to have this type of advice directly in mind when he says that, while dexterity is necessary for good medical practice, "holding [a scalpel?] with the fingers elegantly, well or not well, extended or shortened, or bandaging well and with all sorts of bandagings, these are not considered to be part of the art under the heading of dexterity, but are something else" (τὸ δὲ τοῖσι δακτύλοισιν εὐσχημόνως λαμβάνειν, ἢ καλῶς ἢ μὴ καλῶς, ἢ μακροῖσιν ἢ βραχέσιν, ἢ καλῶς ἐπιδεῖν, καὶ ἐπιδέσιας παντοίας, οὐ πρὸς τῇ τέχνῃ κρίνεται εὐχειρίης πέρι, ἀλλὰ χωρίς). The authors of *Medic.* and *Artic.* are more openly scornful. *Medic.* 4 (IX.210 Littré) calls this kind of bandaging "graceful and theatrical" and rejects it as "vulgar and entirely for charlatans," claiming that it is not helpful and often quite harmful (εὐρύθμους … καὶ θεητρικὰς; φορτικὸν … καὶ παντελῶς ἀλαζονικὸν); *Artic.* 35 (IV.158 Littré) describes the joy of unscrupulous doctors who "uncritically rejoice in beautiful bandaging" when they get the chance to apply a tricky but useless nose bandage, "gladly practicing their mindless skill" and "strut[ting]" about their useless accomplishments (οἱ χαίροντες τῇσι καλῇσιν ἐπιδέσεσιν ἄνευ νόου.τὴν ἀνόητον εὐχειρίην ἐπιτηδεύοντες ἄσμενοι … ἀγάλλεται μὲν ὁ ἰητρός).

yet been a matter of concern to them what sort of outcome results from this treatment, whether good or bad … These sorts of methods are mostly the remit of charlatans.[55]

This particular physician is certainly bearing witness to a school of thought holding that using machines when not strictly necessary is a "shameful" spectacle and "in rather bad taste," but, of course, this very position implies that others were not so reluctant to embrace spectacle in their medical cures.[56]

Beyond these opportunities for display arising in the course of normal medical duties, there were also more explicitly performative moments. To be engaged in the post of public physician, for example, candidates had to make a case for themselves before the city council. At a minimum, this would have required presenting the names of their teachers and information on previous successful cures. Plato's *Gorgias* riffs on this requirement in order to provide a cautionary tale: "if a rhetorical man and a doctor, entering any city you wish, had to argue, in the assembly or in some other gathering, which of them ought to be chosen as the doctor, the doctor would not even make a showing, but the one clever at speaking would be chosen, if he wished it."[57] Though this is, fittingly, a rhetorical exaggeration, it does suggest that more oratorical self-promotion would not have gone amiss.[58] Even those doctors not putting their names forward for a specific post could maintain a public image. Indeed, those arriving in a new city were well advised to do so, both to establish a professional presence and to stake out their ground vis-à-vis local rivals. Several of the texts in the Hippocratic Corpus bear signs of having been produced for a wider, nonmedical audience, and may even have been performed before large crowds.[59] Others furnish the reader with the wherewithal to engage in

---

[55] *Artic.* 42 (IV.182–4 Littré) (τοῦτο μὲν γὰρ, αἱ ἐν τῇ κλίμακι κατασείσιες οὐδένα πω ἐξίθυναν, ὧν γε ἐγὼ οἶδα· χρέονται δὲ οἱ ἰητροὶ μάλιστα αὐτῇ οὗτοι οἱ ἐπιθυμέοντες ἐκχαυνοῦν τὸν πολὺν ὄχλον· τοῖσι γὰρ τοιούτοισι ταῦτα θαυμάσιά ἐστιν, ἢν ἢ κρεμάμενον ἴδωσιν, ἢ ῥιπτεόμενον, ἢ ὅσα τοῖσι τοιούτοισιν ἔοικε, καὶ ταῦτα κληΐζουσιν αἰεὶ, καὶ οὐκέτι αὐτοῖσι μέλει, ὁκοῖόν τι ἀπέβη ἀπὸ τοῦ χειρίσματος, εἴτε κακὸν, εἴτε ἀγαθόν … πρὸς ἀπατεώνων μᾶλλον οἱ τοιοῦτοι τρόποι); cf. 70 (IV.288–90 Littré) where he says that seeing people hanging upside down "is rather impressive, at least for those who take pleasure in these sorts of clever contrivances" (τι καὶ ἀγωνιστικὸν ἔχουσα, ὅστις γε τοῖσι τοιούτοισιν ἥδεται κομψευόμενος).

[56] *Artic.* 44 (IV.188 Littré) (αἰσχρὸν); *Fract.* 15 (III.472 Littré) (σολοικότερον); cf. *Artic.* 78 (IV.312 Littré).

[57] Plato, *Grg.* 456b–c ([φημὶ δὲ καὶ] εἰς πόλιν ὅπῃ βούλει ἐλθόντα ῥητορικὸν ἄνδρα καὶ ἰατρόν, εἰ δέοι λόγῳ διαγωνίζεσθαι ἐν ἐκκλησίᾳ ἢ ἐν ἄλλῳ τινὶ συλλόγῳ ὁπότερον δεῖ αἱρεθῆναι ἰατρόν, οὐδαμοῦ ἂν φανῆναι τὸν ἰατρόν, ἀλλ' αἱρεθῆναι ἂν τὸν εἰπεῖν δυνατόν, εἰ βούλοιτο).

[58] On the hiring of public physicians, see also Jouanna (2017), 113–16, and Massar (2001), 179–84.

[59] Jouanna (2017), 117 and 653, n. 19; see also Lloyd (1987), 83–102 for a broader discussion of the performative and competitive nature of medical practice in this period. For further argument for

a debate with a medical colleague, most explicitly *Diseases I*, which opens, "whoever wishes to both interrogate properly and, on being interrogated, to reply and dispute properly concerning the method of healing ought to take to heart the following."[60] The author of *On Joints* gives a window into such a situation, describing, as we saw earlier, his difficulty convincing both a group of other doctors and "the public" that his diagnosis was to be preferred to his interlocutor's.[61] Interestingly, however, the explicit mentions in the Hippocratic Corpus of medical lectures and large attracted crowds occur in the texts that are generally dated to the Hellenistic or even Roman periods.[62]

In short, a doctor from this period would have been called on to display his skill and knowledge when he chose, or was obliged, to treat patients in a public or semipublic venue and when he chose to debate with colleagues or, perhaps, deliver rhetorical lectures. None of these circumstances suggest that dissections would have been anything but private inquiries. Indeed, the efforts that some Hippocratic doctors took to distance themselves from religion and magic may have rendered them hesitant to publicly perform these new dissective activities, which would no doubt have been most immediately evocative of animal sacrifice and divination.[63]

Aristotle and the Fourth Century

It is in the fourth century BC that the practice of animal dissection really began to flourish. Somewhere in the middle of that century the physician Diocles wrote what Galen describes as the first anatomical handbook.[64] Though only a handful of fragments from his anatomical writing survives, it is sound to assume that he dissected for the sake of compiling the knowledge he conveys within: A fragment preserved in ps.-Plutarch purports to be a verbatim quote of Diocles saying, "in dissections I have often seen

---

the oral dimension of these texts, see Kollesch (1992) and Cross (2018); Dean-Jones (2003), however, suggests that such texts were not performed, but rather were circulated to attract students.

[60] *Morb.I* 1 (VI.140 Littré) (ὃς ἂν περὶ ἰήσιος ἐθέλῃ ἐρωτᾶν τε ὀρθῶς, καὶ ἐρωτῶντι ἀποκρίνεσθαι, καὶ ἀντιλέγειν ὀρθῶς, ἐνθυμέεσθαι χρὴ τάδε).

[61] *Artic.* 1 (IV.78–80 Littré) (τῶν δημοτέων).

[62] See *Praec.* 12–13 (IX.266–8 Littré) and *Decent.* 2 (IX.228 Littré).

[63] *Morb.Sac.* is particularly vocal in this regard. On the parallels between dissection and sacrifice, see Chapter 5, "Religious Practices" at pp. 152–3.

[64] Werner Jaeger argued in the 1930s and 1940s for a significantly later date for Diocles, *c.* 340–260 BC, but his reasoning has since been seriously doubted; see von Staden (1989), 44–46, and (1992*b*) and van der Eijk (2000–1), vol. II, xxxi–viii. On Galen's attribution of the handbook to Diocles, see *AA* II.281–2 and Chapter 6, "Diocles of Carystus" at p. 182.

that the uterus of mules is [small, bent, and narrow]."[65] In addition to Diocles, Galen also names several other doctors from this period who were noteworthy in the field of anatomy, though remains of their work and evidence for their precise dates are scanty.[66]

The towering figure in anatomy of this century was, of course, Aristotle (384–322 BC); it is from him that we have the first surviving evidence of an explicit and defined program of dissection. While he does say that his predecessors engaged in dissection, he also takes some pains to justify and proselytize the practice, suggesting that it was by no means a mainstream endeavor.[67] Indeed, he explicitly tells us that only some of his predecessors approached vascular anatomy through dissection, while others were content to extrapolate based on surface observations in emaciated people.[68] Regardless of its contemporary popularity, he sees dissection as an important tool in the accumulation of knowledge about the natural world. Aristotle believes that any study of the natural world must be predicated on the collection of observations, which can then in turn give rise to theories of causal explanation. He indicates in *Prior Analytics* that this is the correct approach "for any sort of art or science whatever," and he follows through with this methodology in his biological writings.[69] In *Generation of Animals*, for example, he outlines a theory for the generation of bees, but cautions that he is working from insufficient facts and that if ever more reliable data should come to light, "perception must be trusted over theories."[70]

Aristotle's two main zoological texts nicely illustrate this approach to the natural world: *History of Animals* collects and organizes data, while

[65] Ps.-Plutarch, *Plac.* V.14 (van der Eijk [2000–1], fr. 24b) (ἐν ταῖς ἀνατομαῖς πολλάκις ἑωράκαμεν τοιαύτην μήτραν τῶν ἡμιόνων); for the anatomical fragments as a group, see van der Eijk (2000–1), 22–39.

[66] Galen's longest list of doctors who anatomize "both more and less exactly" occurs at *HNH* XV.135–36 (οὔτε τῶν ἧττον οὔτε τῶν μᾶλλον ἀκριβῶς ἀνατεμνόντων); the dating of these figures is notoriously difficult, but names from roughly the mid-fourth century include Diocles (van der Eijk [2000–1]), Dieuches (Bertier [1972]), and Mnesitheus (Bertier [1972]), and from roughly the late-fourth/early third century include Praxagoras (Steckerl [1958] and Lewis [2017]), Pleistonikus (Steckerl [1958], 3, 124–6), Phylotimus (Steckerl [1958], 2–4, 108–23), Chrysippus (von Staden [1989], 46–7), Aristogenes, and Medius. For more on these minor figures, see Chapter 6, "Diocles of Carystus" at p. 183 and "Praxagoras" at pp. 194–5.

[67] He is explicit about his predecessors dissecting at *HA* 511b13–21 and implies it at 496b4–7; his famous defense of the study of the body and lower order creatures is at *PA* 644b22–645a30.

[68] *HA* 511b21–2.

[69] *An.pr.* 46a21–2 (περὶ ... ὁποιανοῦν ... τέχνην τε καὶ ἐπιστήμην); for Aristotle's biology within his larger philosophy of science, see, for example, Balme (1987), Kullmann (1990), Lennox (2001*b*) and (2001*c*), and many of the essays in Connell (2021).

[70] *GA* 760b31–2 (τῇ αἰσθήσει μᾶλλον τῶν λόγων πιστευτέον).

Parts of Animals builds on this data in order to uncover the logical organization of living things. Thus, *History of Animals* is conceptually prior to *Parts of Animals*; one cannot understand how to classify the world without first knowing all the particulars of the things that occur in it. Because of his interest in categorization and organization, a key driver of Aristotle's information-gathering process is the uncovering of similarities and differences. Thus, he says, "one must first consider the parts out of which animals are composed – for it is through these, most of all and primarily, that the entireties of the animals also differ."[71] While the external parts are easily perceptible, an accurate enumeration of the internal parts requires systematic dissection, and the goal of observing the parts of all living creatures demands a research program of enormous scale.

History of Animals offers ample evidence of this ambitious program, testifying to Aristotle and his colleagues' active research in these areas.[72] The descriptions of the internal organs display a detailed familiarity with the anatomy of a large variety of animals, indicating careful and extensive dissection. In comparing the spleens and gallbladders of different blooded animals, for example, he refers in passing to the anatomical vagaries of forty different species.[73] He often compares the organs of more obscure

---

[71] *HA* 491a14–16 (ληπτέον δὲ πρῶτον τὰ μέρη τῶν ζῴων ἐξ ὧν συνέστηκεν. κατὰ γὰρ ταῦτα μάλιστα καὶ πρῶτα διαφέρει καὶ τὰ ὅλα).

[72] The collection of data for *HA* was very likely a group effort. On the level of composition, since the mid-nineteenth century scholars have seen reason to doubt the authenticity of various passages in the text, some suggesting a gradual accretion of Peripatetic additions; for a survey, see Peck (1965), lv–lx. This proposed diversity of authorship is difficult to prove one way or the other. Even for the clearly anomalous Book X, which is generally recognized to not be part of the original text, an Aristotelian authorship has continued to be defended by some; see Dean-Jones (2012), 180–2 for the state of the question. What is more secure than the question of composition, however, is the diversity of the sources of research. Pliny (*NH* VIII.44) offers the story that Alexander the Great ordered "some thousands of men in all of Asia and Greece" engaged in animal-related pursuits to report zoological findings to Aristotle "so that no creature born anywhere would be unknown to him," and that *HA* was the result of Aristotle's deployment of this massive team (aliquot milia hominum in totius Asiae Graeciaeque … ne quid usquam genitum ignoraretur ab eo). Certainly, Aristotle is in some cases quite transparent about gathering information from others; for instance, he directly references the observations or opinions of "fishermen" twenty times; see Lehoux (2017) and Leunissen (2021) for his relationship to these sources. Kollesch (1997), 371–2 has also suggested that he made liberal use of existing medical literature, perhaps even that of Diocles in particular, in his descriptions of human anatomy. Beyond this catholic collection of reported information, one wonders how much of a collaborative effort the dissections themselves also were. Surely Aristotle did not, for example, personally bisect every known variety of insect (*HA* 531b31)? While Lones (1912), 102–6 and Ross (1995), 118 attribute all of the work to Aristotle himself, most scholars, including Lloyd (1975a), 129, 138, Stückelberger (1993), 141, French (1994), 14–15, 40, 44, 51, and Kollesch (1997), 367, assume a fairly large collaborative team of researchers.

[73] *HA* 506a13–b24.

animals to those of more familiar ones, especially dogs and pigs, suggesting that these were frequently or familiarly dissected creatures that could serve as benchmarks.[74] There are several instances, too, where he refers tellingly to the difficulty of observing various aspects of internal anatomy. He complains that in smaller animals some organs are so minute as to be very hard to see.[75] He evinces particular frustration in the case of the serpent, because "on account of its narrowness and length, all the viscera are narrow and long, so that they can even escape detection because of the similarity of their shapes."[76] While some observations may have been made incidentally in the course of butchery or sacrifice, this particular gripe about this particular animal speaks strongly to dissection as a deliberate and methodical undertaking.[77]

Indeed, over and above all this suggestive but more circumstantial evidence, Aristotle offers explicit references to dissection and vivisection. His descriptions of the blood vessels are clearly based on personal inspection. He says that his anatomy of the vascular system is superior to those that came before because he dissects animals that have been purposefully starved and then strangled, rather than just looking into any chance animal whose blood loss at death has caused the vessels to collapse.[78] That he has based his findings on numerous dissections, spanning numerous species, is evident from his comment that the arrangement of the vessels "is not similarly clear in all animals, but most of all in those that are largest and most full of blood; for in small ones and those that have scant blood, either because of their nature or because of the fattiness of their parts, it is not similarly possible to examine closely."[79]

In addition to this type of large-scale survey work for the purpose of sketching out the parts that are generally similar in all animals, he also

---

[74] See especially *HA* 507b22–7, but also 495b24–7, 496b20–1, 502b23–4, 507b37–8a2, 508a6–8, 28–9; the passages in Aristophanes of Byzantium's *Epitome* that may derive from Aristotle's *Anatomies* (see Chapter 6, "Aristotle" at p. 186) display a similar comparative tendency, also dominated by the dog and the pig (*Ep.* II.138, 210, 245, 248, 309, 390, 410, 437). Other animals he compares to repeatedly include the ox (*HA* 496b23–4, 507b38; Aristophanes, *Ep.* II.328) and the horse (500b6–7, 502a14–15; Aristophanes, *Ep.* II.425).

[75] For example, the diaphragm at *HA* 506a7–8, the spleen at 506a13–17, and the membranes surrounding bones and viscera at 519b1–2.

[76] *HA* 508a15–17 (ἅπαντα διὰ τὴν στενότητα καὶ τὸ μῆκος στενὰ καὶ μακρὰ τὰ σπλάγχνα, ὥστε καὶ λανθάνειν διὰ τὴν ὁμοιότητα τῶν σχημάτων).

[77] Observations that seem to clearly stem from sacrifice or butchery include *HA* 496b19–21 and 559b20, where anomalous findings are couched in the language of monstrosities; cf. *PA* 667a34–b2.

[78] *HA* 511b10–23.

[79] *HA* 515a19–23 (οὐ μὴν οὐδ' ὁμοίως ἐν ἅπασίν ἐστι φανερόν, ἀλλὰ μάλιστα ἐν τοῖς μάλιστα πολυαίμοις καὶ μεγίστοις. ἐν γὰρ τοῖς μικροῖς καὶ μὴ πολυαίμοις ἢ διὰ φύσιν ἢ διὰ πιότητα τοῦ σώματος οὐχ ὁμοίως ἔστι καταμαθεῖν).

engages in dissection to address specific questions. For example, he settles the seeming exception to his observation that all viviparous creatures have eyes, by explaining that, though no eyes are visible in the mole externally, "when the skin has been removed, it has a place for the eyes and the blacks of the eyes are in their [expected] position."[80] Further, he describes touching, smelling, and even perhaps blowing into various internal organs, and in a few instances specifically details what the inside of an animal looks like "when it has been cut open."[81]

Aristotle's anatomical activities included a significant focus on aspects of the body related to generation, a subject of considerable interest to him and one in which little can be gleaned without dissection of some kind. He reports dissecting testicles, pregnant uteri, eggs, and embryos.[82] Most strikingly, like the Hippocratic authors of *Nature of the Child* and *Fleshes*, he, or someone reporting to him, had the opportunity to examine aborted human fetuses. He reports that when a male embryo is aborted after forty days of gestation,

> If someone puts it into something else, it is dissolved and disappears, but if into cold water, it sets as if in a membrane; when this is picked apart, the embryo appears, in size similar to a large ant, and the parts are distinct, both all the other ones and the genitals, and the eyes are the largest part, just like in other animals.[83]

Aristotle would have had less professional access to human fetuses than his medical counterparts, but this passage is certainly suggestive that he may have been able to handle them. Further, it is possible that he went farther than his predecessors and actually dissected them. In *Parts of Animals*, he adds that the heart is visible "in aborted embryos," a turn of phrase that

---

[80] *HA* 491b30–32 (ἀφαιρεθέντος δὲ τοῦ δέρματος ἔχει τήν τε χώραν τῶν ὀμμάτων καὶ τῶν ὀφθαλμῶν τὰ μέλανα κατὰ τὸν τόπον).

[81] Touching at *HA* 494b34 and 495b34 (though both of these instances ostensibly describe the human brain, it is safe to infer that these descriptions are by animal proxy, as he indicates just before at 494b22–4); smell at 594b27–8; blowing at 495b14–16 and 510b32. He uses a few different verbs to indicate dissection, including ἀνατέμνειν (*HA* 503b23, 565b9, *PA* 667b9), ἀνοίγειν (*HA* 497b17, 531a16, 594b27), and διαιρεῖν (*HA* 496a11, 496b6, 502b25–6, 510a23, 511b20, 520b17, 531b30–2, 559b18, 565b15, *Incess.* 707a25–9, *Juv.* 468a27, *Long.Vit.* 467a19, *Resp.* 474b18, 479a3).

[82] Testicles at *HA* 510a23; pregnant uteri at *GA* 764a33–6 and 771b32; eggs and embryos at *HA* 565b9–17 (cf. 565a3–12).

[83] *HA* 583b14–20 (ἐὰν μὲν εἰς ἄλλο τι ἀφῇ τις, διαχεῖταί τε καὶ ἀφανίζεται, ἐὰν δ' εἰς ψυχρὸν ὕδωρ, συνίσταται οἷον ἐν ὑμένι· τούτου δὲ διακινσθέντος φαίνεται τὸ ἔμβρυον τὸ μέγεθος ἡλίκον μύρμηξ τῶν μεγάλων, τά τε μέλη δῆλα, τά τε ἄλλα πάντα καὶ τὸ αἰδοῖον, καὶ οἱ ὀφθαλμοὶ καθάπερ ἐπὶ τῶν ἄλλων ζῴων μέγιστοι). This entire section appears heavily influenced by the Hippocratic gynecological writings, which report similar times for the articulation of female and male fetuses.

suggests human rather than animal subjects.[84] However, this claim could also result from simple surface observation: A fetus of the size described here would still be sufficiently translucent to allow a dark spot to be visible in the thoracic cavity through the skin, and suspending the embryo in water would further enhance this effect, as well as somewhat magnifying the fetus as a whole.[85] Elsewhere, he asserts that the human kidney is lobulated, as in an ox, which is not generally true in adults, but is true for a period in fetal development.[86] The proposal that his erroneous description of the heart's cavities is based on the dissection of human infants is elegant, but to my mind not convincing.[87] The heart of a newborn infant is very small – on average about 50 mm (less than 2 inches) – making it unlikely that this was a more productive source of information than the hearts of larger, adult animals, which are, in fact, what he says that his anatomy of the cardiovascular system is based on.[88] In general, the small size of human fetuses and neonates – and all the more so those aborted or miscarried early in gestation, like the ant-sized one he actually describes – suggests that any fetal dissection that Aristotle might have engaged in would have remained mostly at the level of gross anatomy, allowing him simply to confirm or modify in a general way the parallels that he had drawn from animal subjects. Indeed, Aristotle himself does not consider human fetal

---

[84] *PA* 665b1–2 (ἐν τοῖς ἐκβολίμοις τῶν ἐμβρύων); as Ogle (1882), 149 has already pointed out, Aristotle felt no need to wait for animals to abort their fetuses in order to dissect them.

[85] See Seneca, *QNat.* I.6.5 for ancient awareness of water's optic effects; cf. Salas (2020), 106–7.

[86] *PA* 671b6; Menetrier (1930), 260, and Peck and Forster (1937), *ad loc.* make this observation, and Shaw (1972), 361–70 incorporates it into an extended argument that Aristotle dissected human fetuses. Normally developing fetal kidney lobes become visible at ten weeks gestation and fuse during the late second trimester, so this observation, if fetal, would have to derive from an abortion or miscarriage, not a stillbirth or exposed infant; see Patriquin et al. (1990), 193. Peck adds a second observation, that at *PA* 676b30 Aristotle describes the gallbladder as present in some humans but missing in others; he notes "its absence is rare; and Aristotle's statement may well be derived from his observation of aborted embryos, in which the gall-bladder develops somewhat late" (p. 307, n. *a*). This example is less convincing, however, as the fetal gallbladder is discernible as early as fifteen weeks gestation and throughout the second and third trimesters; see Chan et al. (1995), 421, 425.

[87] This solution was current as early as the late nineteenth century (see Ogle [1882], 149) and has remained a part of the debate: see Shaw (1972), 361–70, who argues that he inspected the surface, but not the internal, anatomy of the fetal heart, and Dean-Jones (2017), 132–40.

[88] Dimensions of the fetal heart from Burnard and James (1961), 732, using the average transverse diameter of the control groups; indeed, Aristotle explicitly says that the heart of an aborted fetus is "very small" (πάμμικρα) and comparable to that in a bird embryo, which is "the size of a period" (στιγμῆς ἔχοντα μέγεθος) at *PA* 665a35–b1. For Aristotle on the use of dissected animals for research into the vascular system, see *HA* 511b10–23. The same structural arguments about the anatomical identity of the cavities Aristotle describes could be made by claiming that he dissected fetal *animal* hearts; the objection remains, however, that adult animal hearts are much larger and easier to examine.

dissection to merit discussion as a viable avenue of research: He is explicit that the internal parts of humans rest in obscurity, and that to gain any sense of them, "it is necessary to refer to the parts of the other animals, looking at those that are most similar in nature."[89]

In addition to this work on dead bodies, Aristotle exhibits a hands-on inquisitiveness that stretches to deliberate interference with living creatures; he describes the difficulties one faces when attempting to pull apart two copulating flies, the altered gait of a millipede whose feet have been selectively mutilated, the ubiquity of blood no matter where you cut an animal, and the fact that, though it is possible to drown tortoises, frogs, and similar creatures by holding them down under water, it is impossible to drown a fish, "no matter how one tries it."[90] This willingness to mutilate and kill in the name of scientific discovery leads to the first description of vivisection. A remarkable passage describes the anatomy of the chameleon, beginning with the easily observable external anatomy, but then moving to the internal organs, including a description of the anatomy of the eyes "when the outer skin has been stripped off," and concluding with the observation that "after having been completely cut open for a long time, it even operates with its breath, with an exceedingly small movement still continuing in it around the heart, and, while it contracts the parts around lungs especially, it certainly contracts the other parts of the body as well."[91]

---

[89] *HA* 494b21–4 (δεῖ πρὸς τὰ τῶν ἄλλων μόρια ζῴων ἀνάγοντας σκοπεῖν, οἷς ἔχει παραπλησίαν τὴν φύσιν). It is certainly possible that he is ambivalent about the social reception of fetal dissection rather than about its potential as a methodology, though his willingness to talk about fetal manipulation at *HA* 583b14–20 suggests that practicalities rather than social boundaries are what is holding him back. Note that Galen says that those of his nearer contemporaries who allegedly dissected exposed infants did so only to confirm human-animal homology (*AA* II.386 and Chapter 4, "Anatomical Subjects: Humans" at pp. 115–17): Whether because of their small size or dissectors' moral reticence, they do not seem to have materially forwarded anatomical knowledge.

[90] Copulating flies at *HA* 542a6–7; mutilating millipedes at *Prog.An.* 708b4–11; ubiquity of blood at *HA* 520b15–17 (cf. *PA* 668a31); drowning fish at *Resp.* 471b3–5 (πειρωμένοις πάντα τρόπον).

[91] The chameleon passage occurs at 503a15–b28; the flaying of the eye is described at 503b19 (περιαιρεθέντος δὲ τοῦ ἔξωθεν δέρματος); the quoted passage is 503b23–7 (ἐνεργεῖ δὲ καὶ τῷ πνεύματι ἀνατετμημένος ὅλος ἐπὶ πολὺν χρόνον, βραχείας ἰσχυρῶς ἔτι κινήσεως ἐν αὐτῷ περὶ τὴν καρδίαν οὔσης, καὶ συνάγει διαφερόντως μὲν τὰ περὶ τὰ πλευρά, οὐ μὴν ἀλλὰ καὶ τὰ λοιπὰ μέρη τοῦ σώματος); earlier in the passage, at 503b9–11, he also observes the color change that occurs as the creature dies. Regenbogen (1956) has argued for discrepancies in language and content that signal that this passage is a later Peripatetic interpolation. Though the sentence at 503a18–19 comparing the face (πρόσωπον – a word he explicitly denies to nonhuman animals at 491b9–11) of the chameleon to that of the baboon (χοιροπίθηκος – an animal not mentioned elsewhere) is clearly suspect (cf. Thompson [1910], *ad loc.* for an alternative reading), there seem to me insufficient grounds for dismissing the passage as a whole; cf. Balme (1987), 17. Certainly, Regenbogen's suggestion that it was drawn from Theophrastus' work on animals that change color does not seem plausible, given that Aristotle's vivisectory interests are far better attested than those of Theophrastus, whose work on animals seems to have centered largely on behavior rather than anatomy (see this chapter, n. 150).

Although this is the most explicit description of vivisection in Aristotle's works, there is evidence of it elsewhere as well.[92] As with dissection, he is particularly keen to use this tool in the area of embryology. He reports that, though infant animals spend an inordinate amount of time asleep, he has witnessed in dissections that they do have periods of wakefulness, even in the womb.[93] Any such observation, of course, necessitates the vivisection of the pregnant mother. He also greatly expands on the vivisectory chicken egg observations described in the Hippocratic *Nature of the Child*. While the Hippocratic author mentions only the membranes of the chicks, Aristotle charts a detailed embryological development, including the gradual elaboration of the vascular system from the initial, pulsating blood spot that is the heart.[94] He describes the characteristic disproportionately large eyes of the early fetal chick and adds: "[W]hen the skin has been peeled off [them] there is a moisture inside, white and cold and very glittering in the light, but nothing solid."[95] His vivisections continue to the twenty-day fetal chick, which, "moving, peeps if you touch it" and whose stomach he dissects, and onto a chick ten days after hatching, which, "if someone cuts [it] open," still has residues of yolk in its stomach.[96] In addition to those at the beginning of their lives, he took a more medical interest in those at the end, reporting the state of the internal organs of animals that he dissected while they were dying from evident diseases.[97]

Even with all of this evidence, however, we have but a diminished picture of Aristotle's engagement with dissection since his main text dealing with the topic, to which he frequently alludes, has been lost. This text, which he typically refers to as *Anatomies* (ἀνατομαί), was a multivolume work that illustrated and, perhaps, described the results of his anatomical activities.[98] From his own cross-references to it and from citations that

---

[92] Compare the less elaborated statement that tortoises continue to move after their heart has been removed (*Juv.* 468b15).

[93] *GA* 779a7–10; he similarly reports that dissections refute the commonly held belief that fetuses suck on the flesh of the uterus in order to practice for nursing, since he has never come across an animal fetus doing this (*GA* 746a20–2).

[94] *HA* 561a4–562a21; pulsating heart at *HA* 561a11–15.

[95] *HA* 561a30–2 (ἀφαιρουμένου δὲ τοῦ δέρματος ὑγρὸν ἔνεστι λευκὸν καὶ ψυχρόν, σφόδρα στίλβον πρὸς τὴν αὐγήν, στερεὸν δ' οὐδέν).

[96] *HA* 561b27–8 (φθέγγεταί τε κινούμενος ἔσωθεν, ἐάν τις θίγῃ διελών) (following Peck [1970], *ad loc.*), 562a11 (ἄν τις ἀνασχίσῃ).

[97] *PA* 667b8–10, 677a7–11; it is ambiguous from the text whether these animals were dissected or vivisected, but it is noteworthy that in the earlier instance the deliberate dissection of sick animals is contrasted with the routine observation of the organs of dead sacrificial animals.

[98] For more detailed discussion of this text, see Chapter 6, "Aristotle" at pp. 185–7. The suggestion in Longrigg (1993), 161–2 that Aristotle's references to this work actually refer to Diocles' anatomical handbook has been rightly refuted by Kollesch (1997), 370–1.

may derive from it, we learn that Aristotle and his colleagues performed carefully documented dissections of a wide variety of mammals, fish, and other sea creatures.[99] The text appears to have encouraged comparison of structures across species and included detailed drawings of specific structures in specific animals. We learn, for example, that it contained illustrations of the uteri of a number of different creatures, the multiple stomachs of ruminants, the various possible arrangements of gills, and the internal structure of each kind of hard- and soft-shelled sea creature.[100] The reputed length for *Anatomies* of six or seven books is credible, given the enormous anatomical detail preserved in the extant works, and is indicative of the extent of Peripatetic activity in the field of dissection.[101]

Praxagoras and the Hippocratic *On the Heart*

It is not surprising, then, that authors from the turn of the fourth century BC to the third show considerably more anatomical sophistication than their predecessors. It would seem that by this time dissection had become a routine avenue of scientific research. Praxagoras of Cos, whose prime can be plausibly conjectured to be around 300 BC, was the first to clearly map out distinct venous and arterial systems.[102] There has been some hesitancy, however, to attribute this pathbreaking differentiation to accurate anatomical observation, on two main counts. First, Galen tells us that Praxagoras believes that the arteries taper off into the nerves, allowing the heart to be at the center of the nervous system, in keeping with Aristotelian cardiocentrism, but contrary to the actually observable situation in the

[99] For the collected references, see Gigon (1987), fr. 295–324, as well as the two additional fragments discussed in Hellmann (2004), 67. Animals mentioned include cuttlefish (*HA* 525a7–9), limpets (*HA* 529b18–19), hermit crabs (*HA* 530a30–31), hard-shelled sea creatures (*PA* 679b37–80a3), soft-shelled sea creatures (*PA* 684b1–5), selachians (*HA* 566a13–15, *GA* 719a8–10), ruminants (*PA* 674b15–17), and multiple unspecified varieties of fish (*Resp.* 478a34–b1, *HA* 509b21–4, 511a11–14, 565a12–13, *PA* 696b14–16) and of mammals (*Resp.* 478a26, *HA* 497a31–3, *PA* 650a31–2, 689a17–20, *GA* 746a14–15). Potential citations of the work in Aristophanes of Byzantium's *Epitome* of *HA* (see this chapter, "The Later Hellenistic Period" at p. 47 and Chapter 6, "Minor Hellenistic Authors" at pp. 209–12) include lions (II.138), dogs (II.168), wolves (II.210), leopards (II.248), hyenas (II.309), bears (II.328), field mice (II.373), weasels (II.378), foxes (II.390), hares (II.410, 418), hedgehogs (II.425), bats (II.437), and camels (II.451).

[100] For a tabulation of all the topics and types of animals covered in the text, see Hellmann (2004), 71–3.

[101] Ancient testimony suggest that it was somewhere from six to possibly even eight books; for the various citations of the work in later lists and a discussion of the differing book numbers attributed to it, see Hellmann (2004), 66, n. 5.

[102] For discussion of his dates, see Lewis (2017), 1–3; for his distinction between veins and arteries, see Harris (1973), 108–9, and Lewis (2017), 215–19.

body.[103] Second, his famous distinction between the two sets of vessels – that the veins contained blood, while the arteries contained no humors, but only *pneuma* – is not consistent with careful observation, as Galen later takes great pains to point out.[104] Orly Lewis, the most recent scholar on Praxagoras, has carefully addressed these criticisms, however, and has defended the consistency of his theories with an acutely observed practice of dissection, for which there is also ancient testimony.[105]

Most strikingly, Praxagoras was the author of a text called *Anatomy*, of which at least one fragment, related to the arrangement of the trachea, esophagus, epiglottis, and uvula, remains.[106] Further, Praxagoras' differentiation of the two types of vessels is based on some of their anatomical characteristics: He accurately describes the sinewy character of the arteries, their hollow structure, and the coherent, branching unity of the system.[107] Though Galen, who is our source for these observations, criticizes Praxagoras' results and conclusions, he does not entertain any doubt that Praxagoras based them on real dissections. Galen tells us that Praxagoras and Aristotle had "observed many other things accurately in dissections," and he says that, in making his claims for the nerves sprouting from the arteries, Praxagoras "surely does not plead dim-sightedness, but professes to see sharply."[108] Indeed, Galen implies that Praxagoras also attempted vivisectory experiments. He says that Praxagoras offers as proof that the arteries pulsate independently of the heart the observation that "if someone, having cut away the flesh of an animal, should put it down, quivering, on the ground, the movement of the arteries would be obvious to see,"

---

[103] Galen, *PHP* V.187–200 (I.6.11–7.55 De Lacy) (Steckerl 11; Lewis 3); though Praxagoras' theories are recognizably influenced by those of Aristotle, there is no evidence that directly connects him to the Peripatetic school.

[104] See Galen, *Dig.Puls.* VIII.941, 950 (Steckerl 9, 84; Lewis 12, 14) and *Plen.* VII.573–4 (Steckerl 85; Lewis 13). Scholars have pointed out that the collapsed state of the arteries in a dead animal might be the observational grounds of such a claim (see Harris [1973], 92–3), suggesting either that he did not cross check with vivisections (or, indeed, with patients in his medical practice) or that, like Erasistratus, he had a theoretical reason to discount the evidence of the wounded body; cf. Lewis (2017), 249–50.

[105] On the first objection, see Lewis (2017), 234–9, 278–84; on the second, Lewis (2017), 229–31, 246–50; on his practice of dissection generally, Lewis (2017), 105, 236–9.

[106] For discussion of the text and the fragment, see Chapter 6, "Praxagoras" at pp. 193–4.

[107] Galen, *PHP* V.188 (I.6.18 De Lacy) (Steckerl 11; Lewis 3.19–24).

[108] Galen *PHP* V.187 (I.6.14 De Lacy) (Steckerl 11; Lewis 3.9–10) (ὅτι μὲν γὰρ ἄλλα πολλὰ τῶν κατὰ τὰς ἀνατομὰς ἀκριβῶς ἑωράκασιν) and 192 (I.7.17 De Lacy) (Steckerl 11; Lewis 3.64–6) (οὐκ ἀμβλυωπίαν ὑποτιμᾶται δήπουθεν, ἀλλ' ὀξὺ βλέπειν ἐπαγγέλλεται). Note that the passage at *UP* III.671 (I.487H) where Galen complains about "ignorance of the very things made evident in dissections" of the brain is directed at the later school of Praxagoreans, not at Praxagoras himself (αὐτῶν τῶν ἐν ταῖς διαιρέσεσι φαινομένων τῆς ἀγνοίας).

suggesting that Praxagoras himself employed this sort of vivisection to support his theories.[109] Thus, Praxagoras appears to have been a dissector of a caliber in keeping with the other anatomical work we know to have been going on at this time.

The Hippocratic treatise *On the Heart*, whose date has been vigorously contested but most convincingly hovers in the first half of the third century, near to that of Praxagoras, presents an extremely detailed description of the heart, which is clearly the result of dedicated and observant dissection.[110] It offers three particularly striking examples of heuristic investigations.[111] In the first, the author suggests an experiment to prove his Platonic assertion that some liquid enters the trachea during drinking.[112] The experiment is couched as a hypothetical:

> If one were to give water, having mixed it with blue or red, to a very thirsty animal to drink, especially to a pig, since it is neither a fastidious nor an elegant beast, and if you then were to cut its neck while it was still drinking, you would find [the trachea] stained by the drink. But surgery is not for everyone.[113]

The final rider adds to the ambiguity of whether the author has actually attempted – and is actually actively recommending – this vivisection or is merely speculating. The details of the second instance, however, though also framed hypothetically, more clearly indicate that the author himself has performed the dissection repeatedly and observed the details of various methods of proceeding first hand: "The mouths into [the ventricles] are not patent unless one cuts off the tip of the auricles and the head of the heart; if one clips them, double mouths will even be apparent for the

---

[109] Galen, *PHP* V.560–2 (VI.7.3–4 De Lacy) (Steckerl 28b; Lewis 10) (εἰ σάρκα τις ἐκτεμὼν ζῴου καταθείη παλλομένην ἐπὶ τῆς γῆς, ἐναργῶς ὁρᾶσθαι τὴν κίνησιν τῶν ἀρτηριῶν); see the discussion in Lewis (2017), 242–6.

[110] For the history of the scholarship dating *Cord.*, see Duminil (2003), 175–81. Of the most recent opinions, Lonie (1973), 152 suggests that "a date in the first half of the third century BC ... would seem to create the fewest problems"; Duminil (2003), 181 declines to propose a date herself, but says "il faut encore insister sur les liens de l'auteur de *Coeur* avec l'école d'Alexandrie, liens dont il est impossible d'expliquer la nature et les modalités"; in keeping, Craik (2015), 56 feels that "a date of around 300 BC is possible but somewhat later, between 300 and 250, is perhaps more likely."

[111] There is also a fourth instance of dissection at *Cord.* 11, which describes the left ventricle as empty of blood in the heart of an animal that has already become stiff after death.

[112] Plato puts forth a version of this surprisingly long-lived view at *Ti.* 91a; there had already been a lively repudiation of it in Aristotle *PA* 664b3–19 and in the Hippocratic *Morb.IV* 56. On the Roman reception of this passage, see Chapter 6, "Minor Hellenistic Authors" at pp. 205–6.

[113] *Cord.* 2 (ἢν γάρ τις κυάνῳ ἢ μίλτῳ φορύξας ὕδωρδοίη δεδιψηκότι πάνυ πιεῖν, μάλιστα δὲ συΐ, τὸ γὰρ κτῆνος οὐκ ἔστιν ἐπιμελὲς οὐδὲ φιλόκαλον, ἔπειτα δὲ εἰ ἔτι πίνοντος ἀνατέμνοις τὸν λαιμὸν, εὕροις ἂν τοῦτον κεχρωσμένον τῷ ποτῷ· ἀλλ' οὐ παντὸς ἀνδρὸς ἡ χειρουργία.).

two ventricles—the thick vein running up from one of them deceives the vision if it is cut."[114] The last instance confirms not just dissection but also experimental manipulation: "And if someone thoroughly acquainted with the old order, having removed the heart of a dead [animal], should bend away one [of the valves] and flatten down the other, neither water nor forced air would enter the heart."[115] This unattributed text offers here one of the first descriptions of the cardiac valves, including a basic understanding of their function – a healthy reminder that today's surviving evidence is tied to a mere handful of famous individuals and that only lucky accidents, such as the Hippocratic attribution of this text, can offer glimpses into the breadth of anatomical activity beyond these names.[116]

---

[114] *Cord.* 7 (στόματα δ' αὐτέῃσιν οὐκ ἀνεώγασιν, εἰ μή τις ἀποκείρει τῶν οὐάτων τὴν κορυφὴν καὶ τῆς καρδίης τὴν κεφαλήν· ἢν δ' ἀποκείρῃ, φανήσεται καὶ δισσὰ στόματα ἐπὶ δυσὶ γαστέροιν· ἡ γὰρ παχείη φλὲψ ἐκ μιῆς ἀναθέουσα, πλανᾷ τὴν ὄψιν, ἢν ἀνατμηθῇ); text according to Potter (2010), 62; for alternative readings, see Duminil (2003), 192.

[115] *Cord.* 10 (καὶ τὴν καρδίην ἀποθανόντος ἢν τις ἐξεπιστάμενος τὸν ἀρχαῖον κόσμον ἀφελὼν, τῶνδε τὸν μὲν ἀποστήσῃ, τὸν δὲ ἐπανακλίνῃ, οὔτε ὕδωρ ἂν διέλθοι εἰς τὴν καρδίην οὔτε φῦσα ἐμβαλλομένη). Several scholars have taken this passage as evidence that this treatise describes human dissection, owing to the obscure phrase that I have translated as neutrally as possible as "the old order" (τὸν ἀρχαῖον κόσμον). Lonie (1978), 350 translates it "the original arrangement," as in the way the heart lay *in situ*; Duminil (2003), 194 and Potter (2010), 67, however, have it as "l'ancienne pratique" and "the ancient rite" respectively, and Duminil speculates (p. 253, n. 46) that this could refer to either the traditional Greek practice of examining the entrails of sacrificial animals or to the still more ancient Egyptian practice of mummification; see also Harris (1973), 89 for similar arguments. This latter option potentially opens up the door for the deceased possessor of the heart, described only with a masculine (or neuter) participle, to have been human; Harris (1973), 83 and 89 ("the heart of a dead man") upholds this opinion and offers some scholarly history (cf. Duminil [2003], 167 and Potter [2010], 54 and 67 ["the heart of a man who had died"]). This interpretation would raise many questions: Did the author himself engage openly in human dissection? If so, is this the first documented instance or is this grounds to date the treatise to a later period when we already know human dissection to have been openly occurring? Alternatively, does the mention of the "ancient rite" imply that human dissection had hither-to unsuspected ancient roots, but has now become clandestine? My own opinion is that Lonie's uncontroversial translation, though still quite awkward, is closest to the truth, and that this passage describes the dissection of an animal heart. Apart from this passage and what can best be described as hunches (Wellmann [1901], 94; Potter [2010], 67), the only explicit grounds for taking this as human dissection that have been put forward are that the description of the position of the heart in the thorax, leaning to the left, is recognizably human (Bidez and Leboucq [1944], 26–7), a level of observation about human organs that does not go much past that evinced by some of the earlier Hippocratic treatises and is indeed already alluded to in Aristotle (*HA* 495b13–18). The evidence that Duminil (2003), 166–7 gives to insist that the author is discussing hands-on dissection seems to me indicative simply of hands-on dissection on the part of the author, not of human dissection per se.

[116] Galen implies that Erasistratus was the discoverer of the valves of the heart (especially at *PHP* V.548–50 [VI.6.4–11 De Lacy]), but his precise meaning is debatable; Lonie (1973), 13–14, 136–40, 152 evaluates the evidence for and against *Cord.* preceding Erasistratus and comes down cautiously in favor of dating it before, "though it cannot be by much" (p. 152).

Herophilus and Erasistratus

The pinnacle of pre-Roman anatomy was undoubtedly reached in Alexandria in the early to mid-third century. Herophilus (*c.* 330–260 BC) and Erasistratus (*c.* 330–255/50 BC) represent a watershed in the history of dissection.[117] They were the first, and seemingly also the last, anatomists of antiquity to openly dissect – and likely even vivisect – the human body.[118] Galen describes Herophilus as having obtained his superior anatomical knowledge "not from irrational animals, like most people, but from humans themselves," and other sources support this claim.[119] Celsus (*fl.* AD 14–37) describes how Herophilus and Erasistratus "cut into criminal men, accepted from the kings (*sc.* Ptolemy I Soter and Ptolemy II Philadelphus) out of prison, while they were alive … while breath still remained"; though it has sometimes been dismissed as sensationalism, there are no solid grounds on which to discredit this assertion.[120] In addition to these innovative and memorably daring feats, Herophilus and Erasistratus each, as we shall see, also continued the dissection of animal subjects.

Herophilus, hailed as the "founder of anatomy as a scientific discipline," did indeed bring the field forward in decisive ways.[121] His work on the anatomy and function of the brain and nerves was particularly groundbreaking, and was considered so in the Roman period: He appears to have been the first to describe the ventricles of the brain and the first to differentiate

---

[117] On Herophilus, including a discussion of his dates and a collection of the fragments, see von Staden (1989). On Erasistratus, see Garofalo (1988) for the fragments and, for his life and date, Wellmann (1907), 333–36, Fraser (1969), Longrigg (1981), 177–8, Garofalo (1988), 17–22, and von Staden (1989), 47, who proposes the dates provided here; Fraser (1969) also defends the controversial claim that he was based in the Seleucid court rather than in Alexandria, a view that has since been rebutted by Harris (1973), 177–8 and, pointedly, Lloyd (1975*b*).

[118] See Edelstein (1932), 78–106, Kudlien (1969), French (1978), 153–5, Longrigg (1981), 162–4 and (1993), 184–90, 218–19, von Staden (1992*a*), 231–7, Annoni and Barras (1993), 204–15, Flemming (2003), 451–7, and Byl (2011), 117–28 for discussion of the reasons for the brief exception in Alexandria and for its almost immediate reversal; Dean-Jones (2018) has now offered rebuttal to this position (see my response in Chapter 4, "Anatomical Subjects: Humans" at pp. 110–18).

[119] Galen, *Ut.Diss.* II.895 (οὐκ ἐπὶ ἀλόγων ζῴων καθάπερ οἱ πολλοί, ἀλλ' ἐπ' αὐτῶν τῶν ἀνθρώπων). See von Staden (1989), 139–53 for a thorough discussion of all the passages relevant to Herophilus. For Erasistratus, see Galen *UP* III.673 (I.488H) and *PHP* V.602 (VII.3.6 De Lacy) for descriptions of the human brain in contrast to those "of other animals" (τῶν ἄλλων ζῴων; τῶν λοιπῶν ζῴων) and the discussions at Harris (1973), 177–8, 195, Lloyd (1975*b*), and Longrigg (1981), 158–60, all of whom firmly reject the doubts raised by Fraser (1969) on Erasistratus' experience with human bodies.

[120] Celsus, *DM* proem.23–4 (Herophilum et Erasistratum, qui nocentes homines a regibus ex carcere acceptos vivos inciderint … etiamnum spiritu remanente); for a survey of the skeptical scholarship and a defense of Celsus' reliability, see von Staden (1989), 144–53; for the possible identity of the kings, ibid., 37 and 142.

[121] Sarton (1927), 159.

and describe the nerves.[122] He also made major strides in the anatomy and physiology of the eye, of the vascular system, and of the male and female genitalia, including more medically focused work on gynecology. In addition, he proposed theories of physiology and pathology in keeping with these findings, including the most detailed explanation to date of the brain and nervous system and a hugely influential theory of the pulse. All of this progress was predicated on a program of meticulous dissection.

Three fragments remain from Herophilus' book on anatomy, of which the longer two incorporate both human and animal elements. The first provides a brief but precise account of the veins by the collarbones.[123] In the second, he gives what is probably the first description of the ovaries and fallopian tubes, offering a great deal of detail; the implication is that he is describing human female anatomy, which he supplements and confirms by pointing out that "in mares they are also very much present, being of a good size."[124] The final passage, which Galen presents as a direct quote, handles the liver and makes it clear that humans were but one of the many species that Herophilus carefully dissected:

> The human liver is of a good size, even larger than that in some other creatures of a size comparable to man. The part where it abuts the diaphragm bulges and is smooth; the part where it abuts the digestive tract is concave and uneven. It is comparable in this part to the sort of fissure though which the umbilical vein in embryos also grows into it. The liver is not similar in all creatures, but varies from one to another in its width, length, thickness, height, number of lobes, unevenness at the front, where it is thickest, and in the rounded tops, as to their thinness. For in some it does not have lobes, but is completely round and unarticulated, in others it has two lobes, in others even more, and in many it even has four.[125]

---

[122] Galen indicates his opinion of Herophilus as a groundbreaker at *HNH* XV.136 (von Staden T69).

[123] Galen, *Hipp.Epid.II* 4.1 (*CMG Suppl.Or.* V.2, p. 645; von Staden T62).

[124] Galen, *Sem.* IV.596–8K (von Staden T61) (ταῖς δὲ ἵπποις καὶ πάνυ εἰσὶν εὐμεγέθεις); see the commentary at von Staden (1989), 232–3.

[125] Galen, *AA* II.570–1 (von Staden T60.4–15) (ἔστι δ' εὐμέγεθες τὸ τοῦ ἀνθρώπου ἧπαρ, καὶ μεῖζον τοῦ ἔν τισιν ἑτέροις ζώοις ἰσοπαλέσιν ἀνθρώπῳ. καὶ καθ' ὃ μὲν ταῖς φρεσὶ προσψαύει, κεκύρτωται καὶ λεῖόν ἐστι· καθ' ὃ δὲ τῇ κοιλίᾳ [καὶ τῷ κυρτῷ τῆς κοιλίας] προσψαύει, ἔνσιμον καὶ ἀνώμαλον. ἀφωμοίωται δὲ κατὰ τοῦτο διασφαγῇ τινι, καθ' ὃ καὶ τοῖς ἐμβρύοις ἡ ἐκ τοῦ ὀμφαλοῦ φλὲψ εἰς αὐτὸ ἐμπέφυκεν. οὐχ ὅμοιον δ' ἐστὶν ἐν ἅπασιν, ἀλλὰ καὶ πλάτει καὶ μήκει καὶ πάχει καὶ ὕψει καὶ λοβῶν πλήθει καὶ ἀνωμαλίᾳ τῇ ἐκ τοῦ ἔμπροσθεν, καθ' ὃ παχύτατόν ἐστι, καὶ τοῖς ἄκροις τοῖς κύκλῳ κατὰ τὴν λεπτότητα, ἄλλοις ἀλλοῖον. λοβοὺς γάρ τισι μὲν οὐδ' ἔχει, ἀλλ' ἔστιν ὅλον στρογγύλον καὶ ἄναρθρον, τοῖς δὲ δύο, τοῖς δὲ καὶ πλείους, καὶ πολλοῖς καὶ τέσσαρας ἔχει); following the text in Garofalo (1986–2000). Galen adds a few lines later (von Staden T60.17–20) that he mentions that the liver can extend over to the left side of the body "in a few humans, but more than a few animals," though he specifically singles out only the hare (ὀλίγων μὲν ἐπ' ἀνθρώπων, οὐκ ὀλίγων δ' ἐπ' ἄλλων ζώων).

Thus, Herophilus, while clearly breaking new ground and advancing ana-tomical knowledge to an unprecedented level, is working firmly within the zoocentric anatomical tradition that had already developed in the fourth century.[126]

Erasistratus, sometimes described as a younger contemporary of Herophilus, attempted to create a physiological system for the body based entirely on mechanical principles.[127] As a result, unlike Herophilus, he is par-ticularly known for his physiology and theoretical anatomy rather than his anatomical observations. Most notable among his doctrines are his theory of the heart as a double pump, his development of Praxagoras' bloodless, pneuma-filled arterial system, his use of *horror vacui* to explain various pro-cesses, including digestion and nutrition, and his contention that every nerve, vein, and artery was composed of miniscule nervlets, veinlets, and arterioles wound together into a constructive fiber, known as the "triplokia."[128] In addi-tion to this more theoretical turn, he was an able and active dissector.

Like Herophilus, Erasistratus grounded his work on humans in a pro-gram of animal dissection and vivisection. In keeping with his interest in function, we know of several vivisectory experiments he performed on animals: In one, he observes the effects on an ox of damage to specific parts of the brain; in another, he performs a tricky operation in which a reed is inserted into an artery in order to observe the source of arterial pulsation.[129] His vivisectory work on humans no doubt also sought physiological infor-mation, and even his human dissections may have focused on process as well as structure, since he seems to have used them to understand inter-nal causes of death.[130] Galen, who provides the richest testimonia to his

---

[126] In addition to the two passages quoted here, animal dissection is implied by the nonhuman anat-omy underlying the description of the *rete mirabile* attributed to his school at *Us.Puls.* V.155 (von Staden T121) and by the statements at *Sem.* IV.597 (von Staden T61) and Rufus, *Nom.Part.* 186 (von Staden T105).

[127] Erasistratus as a younger contemporary at Wellmann (1907), 333, l. 34, Harris (1973), 179, and Longrigg (1981), 177 and (1993), 205, 211; for details on the relative dating of the two figures, which is more complex than this label would suggest, see Garofalo (1988), 21–2, and von Staden (1989), 46–8.

[128] For overviews of Erasistratus' theories, see Harris (1973), 195–233, Longrigg (1981), 177–186, and Garofalo (1988), 22–58, as well as Lonie (1964), specifically on his theories of the heart and blood-flow.

[129] The ox experiment is at *PHP* V.610 (VII.3.32 De Lacy) and the other (which Galen, at least, per-formed on a goat) is at *AA* II.648–9. The Anonymous London Papyrus describes another experi-ment, albeit not vivisectory, on a bird (XXXIII.44–51); see also Garofalo (1988), 27–9, and von Staden (1989), 140, n. 3. The evidence that Fraser (1969), 532, n. 37 uses to support his claim that Erasistratus never vivisected animals (*PHP* V.604 [VII.3.13 De Lacy]), refers to his failure to have done one specific vivisectory experiment that Galen came up with, not a general abstention from the activity. On Erasistratus' experimentation, see Salas (2020), 257–64.

[130] Ps.-Dioscorides, *Ther.* 15.5 (cf. Paul of Aegina, V.18) cites Erasistratus on the effects of the venom of a certain snake, claiming that he dissected people killed by it and found their livers and bladders destroyed.

anatomical work, credits him with the first accurate description of the valves of the heart and with careful dissection of the human brain, albeit allegedly done late in life, after having earlier propounded false views.[131] Galen's report of the cardiac work indicates that it was done for the purpose of elucidating physiological function, with a focus as much on the valves' role in dictating the direction and timing of the flow of substances into and out of the heart as on their appearance.[132] His description of Erasistratus' work on the human brain includes an extended direct quotation that reveals both his comparative approach to anatomy and his careful observations:

> And we also observed the nature of the brain, and the brain was bipartite, just like in other animals, and there were cavities situated there, elongated in form. And these opened into one [cavity] at the conjunction of the parts and, from that point, [the single cavity] led into the so-called cerebellum and there was another small cavity there. And each of the parts had been divided off by membranes: the cerebellum had been divided off all by itself and the brain, being very similar to the jejunum, was full of convolutions. But the cerebellum was provided to an even greater degree with numerous intricate windings. So, the observer learns from these things that, just as it stands for the other animals—the deer and the hare and any other animal that greatly excels other animals in running [does so] by means of being well provided with the things useful for running, that is muscles and nerves—it is just so for humans as well: since they far surpass the other animals in thinking, this [their brain] is exceedingly full of convolutions. And all the branches of the nerves stem from the brain; to speak generally, the brain seems to be the source of the nerves in the body. For the perception arising from the nostrils opens into it and also those from the ears. And offshoots from the brain lead also into the tongue and the eyes.[133]

---

[131] For the debate around the pioneering status of his work on the valves, see this chapter, n. 116; for his work on the brain, see Galen, *PHP* V.602 (VII.3.7 De Lacy).

[132] Galen, *PHP* V.548–50 (VI.6.4–11 De Lacy).

[133] Galen, *PHP* V.602–4 (VII.3.8–13 De Lacy) (ἐθεωροῦμεν δὲ καὶ τὴν φύσιν τοῦ ἐγκεφάλου καὶ ἦν ὁ μὲν ἐγκέφαλος διμερής, καθάπερ καὶ τῶν λοιπῶν ζῴων, καὶ κοιλίαι παραμήκεις τῷ εἴδει κείμεναι· συντέτρηντο δ' αὗται εἰς μίαν κατὰ τὴν συναφὴν τῶν μερῶν· ἐκ δὲ ταύτης ἔφερεν εἰς τὴν ἐπεγκρανίδα καλουμένην καὶ ἐκεῖ ἑτέρα ἦν μικρὰ κοιλία. διαπέφρακτο δὲ ταῖς μήνιγξιν ἕκαστον τῶν μερῶν· ἥ τε γὰρ ἐπεγκρανὶς διετέφρακτο αὐτὴ καθ' ἑαυτὴν καὶ ὁ ἐγκέφαλος παραπλήσιος ὢν νήστει καὶ πολύπλοκος, πολὺ δ' ἔτι μᾶλλον τούτου ἡ ἐπεγκρανὶς πολλοῖς ἑλιγμοῖς καὶ ποικίλοις κατεσκεύαστο. ὥστε μαθεῖν <ἐκ> τούτων τὸν θεωροῦντα ὅτι ὥσπερ ἐπὶ τῶν λοιπῶν ζῴων, ἐλάφου τε καὶ λαγωοῦ καὶ εἴ τι ἄλλο κατὰ τὸ τρέχειν πολύ τι τῶν λοιπῶν ζῴων ὑπεραίρει τοῖς πρὸς ταῦτα χρησίμοις εὖ κατεσκευασμένον μυσί τε καὶ νεύροις, οὕτω καὶ ἀνθρώπῳ, ἐπειδὴ τῶν λοιπῶν ζῴων πολὺ τῷ διανοεῖσθαι περίεστι, πολὺ τοῦτ' ἔστι <καὶ> πολύπλοκον. ἦσαν δὲ καὶ ἀποφύσεις τῶν νεύρων αἱ πᾶσαι ἀπὸ τοῦ ἐγκεφάλου, καὶ καθ' ὅλον εἰπεῖν ἀρχὴ φαίνεται εἶναι τῶν κατὰ τὸ σῶμα ὁ ἐγκέφαλος. ἥ τε γὰρ ἀπὸ τῶν ῥινῶν γιγνομένη αἴσθησις συντέτρητο ἐπὶ τοῦτον καὶ αἱ ἀπὸ τῶν ὤτων. ἐφέροντο δὲ καὶ ἐπὶ τὴν γλῶσσαν καὶ ἐπὶ τοὺς ὀφθαλμοὺς ἀποφύσεις ἀπὸ τοῦ ἐγκεφάλου).

Once again, questions of physiology motivate this description to some degree, and it is clear why even Galen, who does not always look charitably on Erasistratus, considers him to be an anatomical authority on a par with Herophilus.[134]

The Later Hellenistic Period

After these two giants in the field, however, the Hellenistic period appears to have run dry: There is little evidence for anatomical practice on animal let alone human subjects in the two centuries that followed their deaths. The only name of note to succeed them in this period is that of a certain Eudemus, a rough contemporary of Herophilus and Erasistratus, who appears several times in Galen as an accomplished dissector and is credited, along with Herophilus, with initiating the study of glands and carefully investigating the nerves, including the optic nerves.[135] He is clearly closely linked with Herophilus, and the suggestion that he is his student, though conjectural, is not without temptation.[136] Indeed, the dramatic decrease of individual figures of note in this period is consistent with the rising dominance of schools or sects in Hellenistic medicine after the mid-third century.[137] This rise of the sects, however, seems to have ushered in a concomitant and steep decline in the practice of dissection. Herophilus and Erasistratus both had major schools of followers, but neither emulated their leader's emphasis on anatomy. The Erasistrateans, a long-lived and faithful sect, focused in large part on developing his therapeutics and on pharmacology; on the topic of physiology, they seem to have confined themselves to textual exegesis of the work Erasistratus had already done, and there is little evidence for interest in anatomy, at least during the Hellenistic period.[138] The Herophileans, too, largely abandoned the

---

[134] On Galen's opinion of Erasistratus as an anatomist, see Chapter 6, "Erasistratus" at pp. 200–3.

[135] For a differentiation of the various figures named Eudemus, see von Staden (1989), 62–3. Galen calls this Eudemus, along with Herophilus and Phylotimus, a contemporary of Erasistratus at *Hipp.Aph.* XVIIIa.7. For the glands, see *Sem.* IV.646; for the nerves, see *Loc.Aff.* VIII.212 and *Lib.Prop.* XIX.30 (optic nerve); he is also mentioned in connection with osteological questions (Galen, *UP* III.203 [I.148–9H] and Rufus, *Nom.Part.* 73) and with embryonic vasculature (Soranus, *Gyn.* 1.57).

[136] Fraser (1972), II.1112–13.

[137] Smith (1979), 177–246 discusses the rise of the medical sects in this period; indeed, he suggests that Herophilus and Erasistratus may have intentionally set out to create schools of their own, after the manner of the philosophers (pp. 194, 196); see also Gourevitch (1998).

[138] For the limitation of physiology to exegetical work, see Garofalo (1988), 4. The only hint we have for Erasistratean work in this area is the mention in ps.-Galen, *Int.* XIV.699–700 that, after Aristotle, doctors became concerned with the precision of nomenclature for the exterior of the body and

practice of anatomy that was so central to their master's discoveries.[139] Of the eighteen Herophileans of whom we have any trace, only one, Hegetor, appears to have had an interest in anatomy, and the evidence for his interest occurs in the context of his arguing just for its basic utility.[140] He does not even suggest that his opponents practice dissection, but simply urges them to avail themselves of the anatomical knowledge that has already been discovered. After its moment of spectacular success, dissection very soon found itself embattled.

The sect that proved to be the most outspoken and influential opponent of dissection was that of the Empiricists, who rapidly rose to prominence at some point in the middle of the third century BC.[141] According to the anonymous second century AD text *Doctor: Introduction*, the sect was founded by Philinus of Cos (*fl. c.* 240 BC), a renegade student of Herophilus.[142] Celsus relates in the preface to his work on medicine that the sect values experience and the cumulative observation of successful cures over reasoning based on unseen causes.[143] Further, he reports at some length their views on dissection. Though they are willing to countenance chance views of the viscera during medical treatment, they maintain that

that the most active of these were "those in the school of Erasistratus, like Apollonius of Memphis and Xenophon before him" (οἱ περὶ Ἐρασίστρατον ... ὡς Ἀπολλώνιος ὁ Μεμφίτης καὶ Ξενοφῶν ὁ πρὸ αὐτοῦ) (cf. ps.-Galen, *Def.Med.* XIX.347 and the notes in Petit [2009], 23, 132–3); however, this activity seems to fall more in the realm of scholarly work than of anatomical research. There is also a small papyrus fragment on osteology (P.Iand. 5.82) dating to the second or first century BC whose editor has suggested might be the work of an Erasistratean, perhaps this same Apollonius (see Chapter 7, n. 194); however, his rationale – that it refers to a Herophilean term as one used by others – is hardly sufficient to prove an Erasistratean origin. In the second century AD, Galen reports that one of his Erasistratean contemporaries, Martianus or Martialios, wrote an anatomy in two books, a development in keeping with the general revival of interest (Galen, *Lib.Prop.* XIX.13, *Praen.* XIV.615); see Chapter 7, "Anatomy in the Roman Intellectual Scene" at p. 265. On the faithfulness of the Erasistrateans, see Galen, *Nat.Fac.* II.67, 90 (albeit with a heavily polemical slant), and Lonie (1964), 440.

[139] On the Herophileans, including their general abandonment of anatomy, which he calls "perhaps the single most striking development" (p. 445) in the Herophilean sect after the death of Herophilus, see von Staden (1989), 445–62.

[140] On Hegetor, see von Staden (1989), 512–14; his defense of anatomy against the Empiricists is quoted, with hostile intent, at Apollonius of Citium, *InHipp.Artic.* 23.

[141] On the Empiricists, see Deichgräber (1965) (with collected fragments), Frede (1987), 243–60, and Hankinson (1995).

[142] Ps.-Galen, *Int.* XIV.683; while some other sources confirm the information there, the historical record is mixed. Celsus (*DM* proem.10), for example, ascribes the founding of the sect to Serapion of Alexandria, whom the passage in *Int.* names as Philinus' successor. That there is still a lack of agreement on the dating and leadership of the beginning of the Empiricist sect can be seen by comparing the conflicting statements on the subject in Frede (1987), 245, Hankinson (1995), 64, and Nutton (2013a), 149–50; for the relevant sources, see Deichgräber (1965), fr. 5–8.

[143] Celsus, *DM* proem.27–44.

[T]he color, smoothness, softness, hardness, and everything similar are not such in a cut-open body as they are in a whole one, for, even when bodies are unhurt, they may yet often be changed by fear, pain, fasting, indigestion, weariness, and a thousand other ordinary affections; by how much more is it likely that the internal parts, to which there is a greater susceptibility and to which the light itself is strange, are changed by exceptionally serious wounds and downright butchery. Nor is anything more stupid than to believe that whatever is the case for a living man will be just the same for a dying one, let alone one already dead.[144]

This Schrödinger's cat scenario obviously negates any value attributed to dissection: If the very act of looking inside changes what is inside, how can one ever be certain of what lies within the living body? The Empiricists were thus vocal critics of dissection, and their rise must have both diminished the overall popularity of anatomical research within a now more starkly diversified medical community and also pushed the Rationalists or Dogmatists, as the non-Empiricist came to be known by contrast, toward forms of argumentation less susceptible to this attack.

The Empiricists were also invested in the establishment of the Hippocratic Corpus as a textual canon for medicine.[145] Beginning at around the time of Herophilus and in keeping with the general literary and philological interests of the Hellenistic period, there was an increasing engagement with Hippocratic texts, in the form of lexica, commentaries, and other secondary literature.[146] This trend to "textualize" medical education and literature, which rapidly came to dominate from this period onwards, effectively canonized the medical knowledge of the past and likely served to pull the field further from experimental work; the Empiricists' aggressive activity in this area cannot have done dissection any favors either. The only exemplum of this kind of scholarship that we are fortunate enough

---

[144] Celsus, *DM* proem.41–2 (… colorem, leuorem, mollitiem, duritiem, similiaque omnia non esse talia inciso corpore, qualia integro fuerint, quia, cum corpor<a> inuiolata sint, haec tamen metu, dolore, inedia, cruditate, lassitudine, mille aliis mediocribus adfectibus saepe mutentur; multo magis ueri simile esse interiora, quibus maior mollities, lux ipsa noua sit, sub grauissimis uulneribus et ipsa trucidatione mutari. Neque quicquam esse stultius, quam quale quidque uiuo homine est, tale existimare esse moriente, immo iam mortuo); for the acceptability of anatomical data learned in passing, see *DM* proem.43 and ps.-Galen, *Def.Med.* XIX.357. Compare Galen, *Sect.Int.* I.77, where he says that "the Empiricists concede neither that dissection discovers anything nor, even if it were to discover something, that it would be necessary for the art [of medicine]" (τῶν δ' ἐμπειρικῶν μήθ' εὑρίσκειν τι τὴν ἀνατομὴν συγχωρούντων μήτ', εἰ καὶ εὑρίσκοιτ', ἀναγκαῖον εἰς τὴν τέχνην εἶναι τοῦτο); cf. Cicero, *Acad.* II.122.

[145] Indeed, Smith (1979), 204–15 argues that they were the pioneers of this endeavor.

[146] On Herophilus' exegetical activities, as well as those of his follower Bacchius, who wrote what appears to have been the first Hippocratic lexicon, see von Staden (1989), 427–42, 484–500. For other early figures, see also Wellmann (1931) and Smith (1979), 199–215.

to have is Apollonius of Citium's (*c.* 90–15? BC) work on the Hippocratic *On Joints*.[147] Despite the obvious opening that the topic of this text provides for a discussion of more recent anatomical findings – an opening that Galen takes full advantage of in his own commentary on the text two centuries later – the only reference that Apollonius makes to dissection is decidedly disparaging, in keeping with his clear Empiricist sympathies.[148]

The dampening effect of sectarian politics on the activity of dissection was not just limited to medical circles. Natural philosophy, too, heretofore an active contributor to anatomical progress, saw a major decline in interest over the course of the Hellenistic period. While a few philosophical questions, notably the location of the soul and the identity of the ruling part of the body, continued to bear relevance to anatomy, the philosophers were for the most part ready to debate on theoretical grounds rather than engage with the results of anatomical investigations.[149] The Peripatetics did maintain Aristotle's strong interest in biology in the generation or two immediately after his death, but do not appear to have made any major contributions to anatomical questions. Theophrastus (372/1 or 371/70–288/7 or 287/6 BC), Aristotle's immediate successor as head of the Lyceum, continued to cultivate Aristotle's interest in natural history. Though he is best known for his lengthy surviving works on plants, his

---

[147] Though Apollonius' text is traditionally referred to as a commentary, this is generally understood to be a misnomer (see Deichgräber [1965], 321, Smith [1979], 212, and Potter [1993], 117); it is, rather, a distillation of the practical information in the Hippocratic text, with a generally panegyric attitude.

[148] Apollonius of Citium, *InHipp.Artic.* 23, where he refers to dissection derisively as "much-spoken-of" or, even, "notorious" (πολυθρύλητον), in the context of his attack on Hegetor the Herophilean; Dean-Jones (2018), 233 has proposed that this be read as evidence that Apollonius' contemporaries were engaged in the "notorious" pursuit of human dissection, but I find the context to be more suggestive of a derogatory remark on what he views to be a pointless hobby-horse of the Herophilean sect (cf. Galen's similar use of the word at *MMG* XI.6 to refer to a Methodist practice that he despised). Though Deichgräber (1965), 321–2 suggests it to be likely that Apollonius was himself an Empiricist, Smith (1979), 214–15 argues against this reading, proposing that he would have thought of himself rather as a "Hippocratean." For anatomy in Galen's commentary, see, for example, *Hipp. Art.* XVIIIa.524–5 (which includes a pointed attack on Empiricist interpretations of Hippocrates), 528–9, 627, and 639. Empiricist rhetoric notwithstanding, the utility of anatomical knowledge generally for surgical operations was by no means lost on Hellenistic doctors, as evidenced by the major advances in Hellenistic surgical techniques, discussed in Michler (1968) (for the influence of anatomy, see especially pp. 7–11). Michler emphasizes, however, the effects of anatomical advances in the early Hellenistic period; there is no evidence for any notable interest in further active study of the subject among surgeons after the period of Herophilus and Erasistratus.

[149] For example, Galen sets up the Stoic Chrysippus' (*c.* 280–207 BC) theory of the commanding location of the soul in contrast to Erasistratus', but he also quotes him as candidly admitting that he is "inexperienced in anatomy" at *PHP* V.185, 187 (ὁμολογεῖ γὰρ ἀπείρως ἔχειν τῶν ἀνατομῶν), 281 (I.6.3, 13, II.8.38 De Lacy) (cf. *Foet.Form.* IV.674, where he discusses Stoic and Peripatetic theories of cardiocentrism more broadly); see Cambiano (1999), 599–602.

interests also stretched to animals and to physiology.[150] Indeed, there has been debate as to whether the eighth and ninth books of *History of Animals* were in fact the work of Theophrastus rather than Aristotle.[151] Similarly, the Aristotelian *Problemata*, which likely began under Aristotle and continued to be produced and added to under Theophrastus' leadership and in the generations that followed, show a marked interest in the body.[152] It provides many fascinating insights into medical and physiological theories of the period, and the tenth book in particular betrays a definite interest in animals and topics relevant to Aristotle's zoological interests.[153] There is little, however, that suggests anatomical research.[154]

From among Aristotle's other surviving associates and students more indications of potentially anatomical interests can be teased out. Clearchus of Soli, a student, has left behind fragments from treatises on a variety of relevant topics, including botany and aquatic life, as well as some physiological remarks in his work *On Ways of Life*, for example the statement that cowardice results from the physical condition of the liver.[155] Most strikingly, we have multiple references to his work *On Skeletons*, which survived long enough to be criticized by Rufus in the first century AD; this is our one solid example of a Peripatetic anatomical text from the generation after Aristotle, though the suggestion that it was based on the study of mummies is untenable.[156] Meno, another pupil, is reputed to have written

[150] For Theophrastus' interest in animals and physiology, see Fortenbaugh, Huby, Sharples, and Gutas (1992), fr. 350–83 and 328–48, respectively, with the commentary in Sharples (1995). None of the fragments suggests a specific interest in anatomy, with the possible exception of fr. 370A (Pliny, *NH* VIII.128), which asserts that a hibernating bear has no food to be found in its stomach nor blood to be found in its body – a claim whose framing gestures toward dissection as a basis for knowledge, but whose substance indicates that no dissection was actually performed.

[151] For a summary of the debate, see Sharples (1995), 33–4; for a defense of Aristotelian authorship, see Balme (1991), 1–13.

[152] For a résumé of the issues surrounding the dating and authorship of the *Problemata*, see Mayhew (2011), xvi–xxi; he gives his own theory on the date at xviii.

[153] Indeed, Apuleius, at *Apol.* 36.5, appends the *Problemata* to a list of Aristotle's zoological works, describing it as "the countless problems by the same man and then by others from the same sect, in which various topics of this sort are handled" (problemata innumera eiusdem, tum ex eadem secta ceterorum, in quibus id genus varia tractantur).

[154] Though I found no evidence for new anatomical research or dedicated interest in anatomy, mentions of anatomical topics occur at II.14, 17, III.14, 31, IV.26, V.19, 26, 40, IX.13, X.3, 14, 18, 20, 44, XI.34, 44, XIII.2, XXXI.5, 7, 21–2, XXXII.6, 12–13, XXXIII.1, 10, 12, XXXIV.4, 9, XXXVI.2.

[155] Botany: Wehrli (1944–59), v. 3, fr. 100; fish: Wehrli (1944–59), v. 3, fr. 101–104; on the liver in cowardice: Wehrli (1944–59), v. 3, fr. 40; on his biological interests generally, see Hellmann (2006), 330.

[156] See Wehrli (1944–59), v. 3, fr. 106–110, including the comment at Rufus, *Nom.Part.* 192 (Wehrli v. 3, fr. 106b) that he incorrectly described the names of the muscles along the spine; on the fragments, see Chapter 6, "Aristotle" at pp. 192–3. The title uses the unusual word "skeleton" (σκελετῶν), which means "dried up" or "withered," and can, according to the *LSJ*, apply as a substantive to either

a large medical doxography, his *Iatrika*, from which large sections of the Anonymous London Papyrus seem to derive; however, Galen describes this as a scholarly endeavor, without giving any indication that Meno himself conducted any biological research.[157] Eudemus of Rhodes, another candidate for taking over the Lyceum after Aristotle's death, appears have written a zoological treatise of some kind.[158] Strato of Lampsacus, who succeeded Theophrastus as head of the Lyceum from 287 to 269 BC, known most for his work on physics and cosmology, also produced various works with a psychological, physiological, or zoological focus, including treatises on puzzling animals, on mythological animals, on diseases, and on *pneuma*, of which there remain little trace outside their titles, and a treatise on the generation of animals, which remained accessible in some form in the Roman

skeletons, in the modern sense, or to desiccated corpses, including mummies. Kudlien (1968a), 42 and (1969), 88–9, and Potter (1976), 58 latched on to this last possibility and suggested that Clearchus took a major step forward in anatomical methodology by using human mummies, pointing out that later references to the text cite its description of muscles, rather than just bones. However, a closer look at the evidence discredits this interpretation. First, this is not the normal term by which Greeks referred to Egyptian mummies: It does not appear in the famous accounts of mummification in Herodotus (II.85–90) and Diodorus Siculus (I.91), for example, which rely on derivatives of the verb for embalming (ταριχεύειν). Teles (XXXI.9–10), though using a verbal cognate of σκελετός, does not use it as a recognizable term for mummy, but rather as a generic descriptor of the process: "we [the Greeks] shrink from both looking at and touching them, but they [the Egyptians], drying them out, keep corpses inside like a good thing and use them as financial sureties" (ἡμεῖς μὲν καὶ ἰδεῖν καὶ ἄψασθαι ὀκνοῦμεν· οἱ δὲ σκελετεύσαντες ἔνδον ἔχουσιν ὡς καλόν τι καὶ ἐνέχυρα τοὺς νεκροὺς λαμβάνουσιν). More significantly, according to the *TLG* database, the word σκελετός occurs only thirty-four times in the textual tradition between the fifth century BC and the third century AD (excluding duplicate entries). Of these instances, only a single one seems like it might plausibly refer to a mummy and it is explicitly described as an "Egyptian *skeletos*" (Plutarch, *Sept.Sap.Conv.* 148A [ὁ δ' Αἰγύπτιος σκελετός]). The remainder refer to the word's fundamental meaning of dry or withered (e.g., Nicander, *Ther.* 696 and Herodian 122), to emaciated *living* people (e.g., Plato [comic.], Fr. 184 [Kock], Posidippus, *Epig.* 95, and *Anthologia Graeca* XI.392), or to skeletons in the modern, bony sense (e.g., Democritus, fr. 1a [DK] and Phlegon, *Mirab.* 17–19). Further, Galen explicitly defines σκελετός as "the complete collection of all the bones in the human body connected to each other" (*Oss.* II.734; cf. II.777) – using it in this way numerous times throughout his corpus – and tells us that it is a common title for osteological texts (*AA* II.220, *Oss.* II.734). I therefore see no persuasive grounds on which to link Clearchus' *On Skeletons* to mummies nor to claim that it was anything other than a work on bones, albeit one with some extra-osteological comments.

[157] *HNH* XV.26; for the relationship between this work and the Anonymous London Papyrus, where it is attributed rather to Aristotle, see Manetti (1999), 98–9, who takes issue with Galen's (and Diels') assumption that it should actually by ascribed to Meno.

[158] Apuleius cites him, together with Lyco, as being in the company of Aristotle and Theophrastus as authors of books on the generation, life, parts, and differences of animals at *Apol.* 36 (Wehrli [1944–59], v. 8, fr. 125). Numerous references to Eudemus in Aelian's work on animals confirm a zoological interest on his part: *NA* III.20, 21, IV.8, 45, 53, 56, V.7 (Wehrli [1944–59], v. 8, fr. 126–32); however, all of the citations pertain to animal behavior, especially anthropomorphic behavior and interactions with humans, rather than to anatomy (which, it should be noted, is not the case for Aelian's work in general). For a more detailed discussion of Eudemus' interests in natural philosophy, see White (2002).

period.[159] Of the anatomical interests of Callisthenes (d. 327 BC) mentioned in the Calcidian epigraph to this chapter, there is no other trace.[160] Similarly, Apuleius' claim that Lyco (*c.* 300/298–*c.* 226/4 BC), the successor to Strato, performed zoological work in the style of Aristotle is usually considered erroneous; even if accurate, the complete lack of evidence for this interest elsewhere inclines one to suspect that Cicero's damning evaluation of Lyco as "rich in style, but rather barren in content" might apply here too.[161] All told, the little evidence we have from these early Peripatetic figures suggests that, with the exception of Clearchus, they were more interested in collecting the habits and characteristics of animals than in producing new research on the comparative arrangement of their organs.

About half a century later in Alexandria, in the same academic spirit as Apollonius' subsequent work on Hippocrates there, Aristophanes of Byzantium (*c.* 257–180 BC) compiled his *Epitome* of Aristotle's zoological works, which collects information from the Aristotelian corpus (and, possibly, elsewhere) and rearranges it into species-by-species order, rather than the anatomical order that Aristotle followed.[162] This editorial decision exposes Aristophanes' interests: He was driven by organizational rather than anatomical motivations, striving, essentially, to turn an insightful work of comparative zoology into an easily navigable animal reference book.[163]

---

[159] For the relevant fragments, see Sharples (2011), fr. 55–81. There is a list of his complete works at Diogenes Laertius, *VP* V.59 (Sharples [2011], fr. 1); his text *On the Generation of Animals* (Περὶ ζωογονίας) is likely what is cited by Galen at *Sem.* II.5 (Wehrli [1944–59], v. 5, fr. 95; Sharples [2011], fr. 71); see also Hellmann (2006), 330–1.

[160] Calcidius, *In Tim.* 279 (24A.10 D-K); see Lloyd (1975a), 117, n. 19.

[161] Cicero, *Fin.* 5.5.13 (oratione locuples, rebus ipsis ieiunior). As we just saw in n. 158 of this chaper, Apuleius mentions a zoological treatise by Lyco at *Apol.* 36 (Wehrli [1944–59], v. 6, fr. 30, where it is listed under "zweifelhaftes"). Owing to a lack of any other indication that Lyco had biological interests, scholars have suggested that Apuleius was actually thinking of Strato's treatise on generation (Capelle [1927], 2306, l. 45–54) or that he meant instead the ethnographer and historian Lycus of Rhegium (*fl. c.* 300 BC), whom we know to have incorporated some information on animals into his works on Sicily and Libya (White [2002], 209, n. 6); see also Sharples (2006), 308–9, and Hellmann (2006), 331–2.

[162] The *Epitome* survives in excerpts in a Byzantine compilation, as well as in a single, small papyrus fragment (*P.Lit.Lond.* 164); see Chapter 6, "Minor Hellenistic Authors" at p. 209.

[163] He basically says as much at II.1, where he explains that he wrote the text "so that you might not march through the work by Aristotle on animals, which is divided into many parts, but that you might have all the information about each single animal gathered together at the same place" (ἵνα μὴ διηρημένην ἐν πολλοῖς τὴν ὑπὸ Ἀριστοτέλους περὶ ζῴων πραγματείαν ἐπιπορεύῃ, συνηγμένην δὲ ὁμοῦ πᾶσαν τὴν ἐφ' ἑνὶ ἑκάστῳ ζῴῳ ἱστορίαν ἔχῃς.). Hellmann (2006), 346 adds that "one may certainly agree that Aristophanes did not do any biological research himself, and that he had no scientific ambitions in this field" and comes to conclude that he likely created the *Epitome* to be a reference book or lexicon for those, such as *poetae docti*, seeking details about a specific animal (354); see also Hatzimichali (2021), 235–9 for Aristophanes' slightly different goals in the first book of the *Epitome*.

In the broader context, this is not surprising. By and large, by the time of the deaths of Herophilus and Erasistratus in the middle of the third century BC, the Peripatetic school was waning and those who remained appear to have simply lost interest, not just in anatomy, but in biology altogether.[164]

In sum, the study and practice of dissection developed enormously both in the acceptance and frequency of its use and in its technical and theoretical sophistication from the faint and unsystematic hints of it that we can descry at the turning of the fifth century to the renowned, highly accurate, and detailed work of the mid-third century. Yet the surviving evidence supports Galen's claim that it then experienced a prolonged and widespread lull from those heady times in the early Hellenistic period until its revival under the aegis of the Roman Empire in the late first century AD, where we will pick up its trail again in due course.[165]

Medical Performance in the Hellenistic Period

In tandem with this surge in anatomical activity, the performative aspects of medical practice became increasingly formalized with the transition from the Classical to the Hellenistic period.[166] We must therefore consider anew the professional contexts of these dissections and query the existence of a performative strand of anatomy in anticipation of its large role in the later Roman revival. Several inscriptions mentioning public displays by doctors survive. In a clear case of a candidate applying for the role of public physician, an inscription from Istros records that a certain Diocles of Cyzicus, was "summoned by the popular assembly and, having given many lectures (ἀκροάσεις) and [interpretations] on all topics … was thought worthy on account of these things to receive a salary from the state."[167] Similarly, at Elatea the doctor Asklepiodorus "performed

---

[164] The Lyceum famously went into decline in the second century BC. On the decrease in interest in natural history specifically, which he describes as "one of the striking features in the history of the Peripatetic school," see Sharples (2006); cf. Lennox (1994), Hellmann (2006), 329–32, and Hatzimichali (2021).

[165] On Galen's claim about this lull, see Chapter 3, n. 2, and Chapter 7, "Rufus of Ephesus" at pp. 226–8 and "Marinus" at p. 231.

[166] For the epigraphic evidence on doctors in this period, see Cohn-Haft (1956), 76–85, Massar (2001), and Samama (2003); for performance specifically, see Nutton (1979), 187–8.

[167] SEG 19.467 (Samama 098) (… Διοκλῆς Ἀρτεμιδώρου Κυζ(ζ)ικηνὸς ἰατρὸς μεταπεμφθεὶς ὑπὸ τοῦ [δή]μου καὶ ποιησάμενος ἀκροάσεις [καὶ συνκρί]σεις πλείονας ἐμ πάσαις [εὐδοκίμησεν, ἀ]ξιωθεὶς τε διὰ ταῦτ[α ὑπὸ τῶν πολιτ]ῶν ἐδημοσίευσε [δωρεὰν ἐν ἄλλαις νόσοις(?) –]προ). For more details and an image, see Popescu (1956), 346–8; for discussion of the restoration of the lacunae, see Robert and Robert (1958), no. 336 (pp. 280–2). Compare IG 12 Suppl. 249 (Samama 163), ln. 18, in conversation with which the pair ἀκροάσεις [καὶ συνκρί]σεις is restored.

lectures over several days concerning things related to his profession" and did "many useful things for the citizens," resulting in his being accorded "privileges fitting to his profession," including tax exemption, immunity, and other privileges appropriate for public benefactors.[168] In both of these cases the vocabulary suggests that the public performances were restricted to purely oral lectures.

In a different vein, a double inscription by the citizens of Perge and the citizens of Seleucia praises the doctor Asklepiades. The section from Perge describes how Asklepiades "has made great demonstrations (ἀ[πο]δείξεις) of his own skill and, through his lectures (ἀκροάσεων) in the gymnasium, has provided great service here towards the health of the citizens, and has provided care of the suffering worthy of himself and of his ancestors."[169] The section from Seleucia also mentions that he

> made great demonstrations (ἀ[ποδ]είξεις) of his treatment, presenting surpassing experience in the art, and he saved many citizens and dwellers in the city who were in danger, applying suitable remedies with the utmost zeal, and in the matters related to surgery, having exhibited (ἀναδεξάμενος) many incredible treatments, he made his proficiency clear, and having described in his lectures (ἀκρο]άσεσιν) many things contributing towards health, he also acquired praise from these things.[170]

It is noteworthy that Asklepiades appears to have done all of these activities in Seleucia after "having previously been furnished with one thousand drachmas for several years," indicating that his performances were part of his normal practice, not a preliminary audition.[171]

---

[168] SEG 3.416 (IG IX, 1.104; Samama 051) (Ἀσκ[λαπιόδωρος … ἀκροάσεις ἐποιή|σατο ἐπὶ] ἁμέρας πλείονας περὶ τῶν κατὰ τὸ ἐπιτάδευμ[α καὶ πολλὰ χρήσιμα τοῖς πολίταις διαθέμε|νος ἀξί]ω παρὰ τᾶς πόλιος τὰ τῷ ἐπιταδεύματι καθήκοντα [ἀπολαβεῖν φιλάνθρωπα … κα]ὶ δεδόσθαι αὐτῶι καὶ ἐκγόνοις αὐτοῦ προξενίαν, π[ολιτείαν, ἀσφάλειαν, ἀσυλί]αν, ἐπιν]ομίαν, προεδρίαν, ἀτέλειαν καὶ κατὰ γᾶν [κα]ὶ κατὰ θάλ[ασσαν καὶ τἆλλα πάντα, ὅσα] καὶ τ]οῖς ἄλλοις προξένοις καὶ εὐεργέταις τᾶς πόλιος τῶ[ν Ἐλατέων). See also Wilhelm (1974), II.174–6.

[169] IK Perge 12.5–12 (Samama 341.5–12) (ἀ[πο]δείξεις μεγάλας πεποίηται τῆς ἑαυτοῦ ἐνπειρίας, διά τε τῶν ἐν τῶι γυμνασίωι ἀκροάσεων πολλὰ χρή[σι]μα διατέθειται ἐν αὐταῖς πρὸς ὑγείαν τοῖς πολίται[ς] ἀνήκοντα, τήν τε τῶν καμνόντων ἐπιμέλειαν πεποίηται ἀξίαν ἑαυτοῦ καὶ τῶν προγόνων). On this inscription, see Wilhelm (1974), I.227–31, 334–5, Sahin (1999), 14–16, and Samama (2003), 439–42.

[170] IK Perge 12.26–36 (Samama 341.26–36) (μεγάλας ἀ[ποδ]είξεις ἐποιήσατο τῆς ἑαυτοῦ ἐπιμελείας, διαφέρουσαν παρασ[χ]όμενος τὴν διὰ τῆς τέχνης ἐνπειρίαν, πλείονάς τε τῶν πολιτῶν καὶ τῶν κατοικούντων ἐν τῆι πόλει διατεθέντας ἐπισφαλῶς διέσω[σε] τὰς ἁρμοζούσας θεραπείας προσαγαγὼν με[τὰ πά]σης προθυμίας, ἔν τε τοῖς κατὰ τὴν χειρουργ[ίαν πολλὰ] καὶ παράδοξα ἀναδεξάμενος θεραπεύ[ματα διάδη]λον κατέστησεν τὴν αὐτοῦ προκοπ[ήν, ἔν τε ταῖς ἀκρο]άσεσιν πολλὰ τῶν πρὸς ὑγείαν συντε[λούντων διατιθέ]μενος καὶ τὸν ἐκ τούτων ἔπαινον πε[ριεποιήσατο).

[171] IK Perge 12.25–26 (Samama 341.25–26) (πρότερον μὲν ὀψωνι[ασ]θεὶς δραχμὰς χιλίας ἐφ᾽ ἔτη πλέονα). On the salary, see Wilhelm (1974), I.230–34, 334–5.

The repeated contrast between the language of lecturing and the language of demonstrating in the Perge-Seleucia inscription has led to the claim that hands-on demonstrations of skills, of the sort that Galen describes in the second century, were already occurring in the Hellenistic period.[172] While it is certainly possible that this is the case, it seems to me more likely that these particular demonstrations of medical skill were noticed over the course of Asklepiades' regular practice. Variations on the phrase "make great demonstrations of his own skill" appear as something of a stock element in several other inscriptions that lack any suggestions of performative contexts.[173] Further, in the Perge section, the mention of demonstration is preceded by the identifying nominative phrase "a well-reputed citizen of our city and practicing the medical art," which has more of a circumstantial force than the simple attributive "doctor" in the second line of the inscription and implies that his demonstrations of skill were linked to his ongoing practice.[174]

The emphasis on demonstration, however, does merit further probing. Asklepiades' medical credentials were continually under scrutiny by the public. Indeed, he seems to have encouraged and played toward the inevitability of this fact of Hellenistic medical practice. Even if his public demonstrations were of practical medical utility rather than sheerly performative, he was nevertheless deliberately showcasing his professional abilities. The inscription takes care to mention his demonstrations of skill as distinct from other cures that he performed, suggesting a triad of activities: his unmarked, daily care of patients, his advertised (and perhaps publicly executed) cures and surgeries, and his lectures for public benefit in the gymnasium.

Unlike the citizens of Perge and Seleucia, who were delighted with their lectures, however, Polybius (c. 200–c. 118 BC) takes issue with a system that was open to abuse:

---

[172] Nutton (1979), 187 and n. 5.

[173] SEG 41:680 (Samama 137) (πλείονα ἀπόδειξιν ἐποιήσατο πολλῶι μᾶλλον τᾶς τε κατὰ τὰν τέχναν ἐμπειρίας καὶ τᾶς κατὰ τὸν βίον εὐταξίας), SEG 33:673 (Samama 133) ([πολλὰς καὶ μεγάλας πεπ]οιημένον ἀποδείξεις ἐ[μπειρίας τῆς κατὰ τὴν τέχνην]); see also IG XII.5 824 (Samama 166) (π[ολλ]ὰ[ς ἀποδείξεις ποιησάμενος] καὶ κατὰ τὴν τέχνην καὶ κατὰ τὴν λ[οιπ]ὴν [ε]ὔνοιαν) and SEG 30:1051 (πολλὰς ἀ[ποδείξεις ἐποιήσατο τᾶς αὐτοῦ ἐπιμελείας]), which have been restored on the strength of the foregoing examples.

[174] IK Perge 12.4–5 (Samama 341.4–5) (πολίτης ἡμῶν εὔδοξ[ος] καὶ μεταχειριζόμενος τὴν ἰατρικὴν τέχνην). For other examples of μεταχειρίζω being used in inscriptions to denote medical practice, see IG V,1 1145.23 (Samama 035.23) and BCH 52 (1928) 174[2].9 (Samama 060.9); in both cases the phrase emphasizes ongoing practice rather than simple identification as a doctor.

[The theoretical part of medicine], through display and advertisement, attracts such ostentation that none of the other [types of] doctors seem to prevail in the business. But whenever you entrust a sick person to [doctors who specialize in theoretical display], bringing them to face with reality, they are discovered to hold back their hand in just the way that those who have never read a single medical treatise would. Indeed, some ill people, turning themselves over to such men on account of the power of their speech, despite having nothing serious the matter with them, ran risks often and at every turn. For [these doctors] are truly like pilots who steer from a book. But, nevertheless, such men, traversing the cities with ostentation, whenever they have gathered a crowd *** †to their name†, drive those [doctors] who have offered a true test of themselves in the affairs themselves to the utmost difficulty and contempt at the hands of the audience, so often does the persuasiveness of speech prevail against the scrutiny of deeds themselves.[175]

Here, as earlier in Plato's *Gorgias*, opening the door to rhetoric and performance in medicine produces anxiety about how to evaluate members of the medical profession. Polybius agrees with the citizens responsible for these honorific plaques that the cumulative demonstration of successful practice is key to judging medical competency. The trend toward increased rhetorical showmanship, such as that practiced by Asklepiades, may have "gathered a crowd," but it veered from the practical and the testable in way that made Polybius understandably uneasy.

Nor was Polybius alone. His same distrust of doctors who put emphasis on show over skill continues as a trope into the Roman period. Lucian (b. *c.* AD 120) juxtaposes the flashy, chryselephantine tools of the quack with the patinated but effective tool of the learned practitioner.[176] Dio Chrysostom (*c.* AD 40/50–110/120) has a very similar passage to the one in Polybius, in the context of deriding the impressive, but unsound, volubility of the extemporaneous sophist:

This sort of recitation, being a sort of spectacle and pomp, bears a certain resemblance to the displays of the so-called doctors, who, sitting in

---

[175] Polybius, 12.25d2–6 (κατὰ δὲ τὴν ἐπίφασιν καὶ τὴν ἐπαγγελίαν τοιαύτην ἐφέλκεται φαντασίαν ὥστε δοκεῖν μηδένα τῶν ἄλλων κρατεῖν τοῦ πράγματος· οὓς ὅταν ἐπὶ τὴν ἀλήθειαν ἀπαγαγὼν ἄρρωστον ἐγχειρίσῃς, τοσοῦτον ἀπέχοντες εὑρίσκονται τῆς χρείας ὅσον [καὶ] οἱ μηδὲν ἀνεγνωκότες ἁπλῶς ἰατρικὸν ὑπόμνημα· οἷς ἤδη τινὲς τῶν ἀρρώστων ἐπιτρέψαντες αὐτοὺς διὰ τὴν ἐν λόγῳ δύναμιν οὐδὲν ἔχοντες δεινὸν τοῖς ὅλοις πολλάκις ἐκινδύνευσαν. εἰσὶ γὰρ ἀληθῶς ὅμοιοι τοῖς ἐκ βυβλίου κυβερνῶσιν· ἀλλ' ὅμως οὗτοι μετὰ φαντασίας ἐπιπορευόμενοι τὰς πόλεις, ἐπειδὰν ἀθροίσωσι τοὺς ὄχλους *** †ἐπ' ὀνόματος†, τοὺς ἐπ' αὐτῶν τῶν ἔργων ἀληθινὴν πεῖραν δεδωκότας αὐτῶν εἰς τὴν ἐσχάτην ἄγουσιν ἀπορίαν καὶ καταφρόνησιν παρὰ τοῖς ἀκούουσι, τῆς τοῦ λόγου πιθανότητος καταγωνιζομένης πολλάκις τὴν ἐπ' αὐτῶν τῶν ἔργων δοκιμασίαν).

[176] Lucian, *Ind.* 29.

state in the middle [of a crowd] go through in detail the attachments of the joints and the junction and juxtaposition of the bones and other such things: pores and breaths and filterings. And the crowds are agape and are bewitched more than children. But the true doctor is not of this sort and does not thus lecture to those actually in need. Why should he? Rather he prescribes what it is necessary to do, and he hinders the [patient] desiring to eat or to drink, and, taking hold, he cuts off some problematic part of the body.[177]

Interestingly, though he maintains the same general contrast between rhetoric and action, Dio provides more details about the content of the speech of the specious doctor. These details accord nicely with the type of contemporary medical conversations we know to have been going on: Questions of an anatomical and physiological nature had become increasingly popular testing grounds for doctors in the Roman period, as Galen describes it. Ultimately, however, the concerns raised here center on rhetoric and shallow but flashy gimmicks. The trend of performative dissection that emerges in the early empire does not fall easily into either of those categories and would surely not fit the scorn that Dio or Polybius unleashes. The feats described by Galen, as we shall soon see, could never be dismissed as unskilled, unpracticed, or irrelevant.

Nothing here offers a definitive answer to the question of the visibility of the practice of dissection during the Hellenistic period. There is no indication that it was staged publicly in the way that it came to be under the Roman Empire or that it occurred outside the comparatively private spheres of research and teaching, where it was popular, at least in some circles, in the fourth and early third centuries. Even there, given the sharp decline in interest in the practice from the middle of the third century BC until the middle of the first century AD, it is unclear how ingrained it ever became in the tradition of medical education.[178] However, though there

---

[177] Dio Chrysostom, *Or.* 33.6 (ἡ μὲν οὖν τοιάδε ἀκρόασις θεωρία τις οὖσα καὶ πομπὴ παραπλήσιον ἔχει τι ταῖς ἐπιδείξεσι τῶν καλουμένων ἰατρῶν, οἳ προκαθίζοντες ἐν τῷ μέσῳ ξυμβολὰς ἄρθρων καὶ ὀστέων συνθέσεις καὶ παραθέσεις καὶ τοιαῦθ᾽ ἕτερα ἐπεξίασι, πόρους καὶ πνεύματα καὶ διηθήσεις. οἱ δὲ πολλοὶ κεχήνασι καὶ κεκήληνται τῶν παιδίων μᾶλλον. ὁ δ᾽ ἀληθὴς ἰατρὸς οὐκ ἔστι τοιοῦτος οὐδὲ οὕτως διαλέγεται τοῖς ὄντως δεομένοις· πόθεν; ἀλλὰ προσέταξε τί δεῖ ποιεῖν, καὶ φαγεῖν βουλόμενον ἢ πιεῖν ἐκώλυσε, καὶ λαβὼν ἔτεμεν ἀφεστηκός τι τοῦ σώματος).

[178] See, for example, the papyrus fragment (BKT 3.22–26 [MP³ 2354]) from the latter half of the first century AD on the topic of surgical education, which describes the foundational knowledge required for surgery as knowing things like "the varieties of lint wads [and] the uses of sponges" (Col II, ll. 15–16). While a lack of anatomy in this list is not terribly surprising given the markedly Empirical character of the text, the polemic, at least in this surviving part of the text, is squarely directed against excessive book-learning, not against any elementary study of dissection; cf. Marganne (1998), 13–34. Rufus of Ephesus, however, may offer some indication that there was sustained interest in the use of

is no concrete evidence for staged practical displays of medical skill in the Greek world, public lectures on medical topics were a routine event and the practice of medicine included public evaluation, based not just on professional success rate, but also, perhaps to a variable degree, on more formal public practice of the art, setting the stage for the performative dissections to come. Indeed, despite the largely negative conclusions here, the open nature of medical practice generally and the professional exigencies of the Hellenistic physician suggest that dissection may have been accessible, for those with an interest, when it did occur.

dissection for medical education, though he leaves it ambiguous whether the practice he describes was in continuous use from the third century BC or was a modified revival of the practice in the first or second century AD; see Chapter 7, "Rufus of Ephesus" at pp. 219–20.

CHAPTER 3

Dissection in the Roman Period

The crowds are agape and are bewitched more than children.

Dio Chrysostom, *Oration* 33

The spectators are still more amazed.

Galen, *Anatomical Procedures*[1]

Under the Roman Empire, near the beginning of the second century AD, dissection took a major turn. Galen tells us that it was then that Marinus "reviv[ed] anatomical study after the ancients, as it had been neglected in the intervening time."[2] Marinus likely does not deserve exclusive credit. While certainly the most famous and influential name, he seems to have been part of a larger groundswell of interest in anatomy that developed at the end of the first century AD and spread to intellectual centers across the Roman Empire. Dissections became an increasingly visible aspect of medical education and intellectual life; by the mid-second century, when Galen's writings allow us an unprecedentedly intimate look, dissection was a prominent pastime in certain medical circles and had been for nearly fifty years.[3] Most notably, an unambiguously public and performative variety of dissection emerged alongside the research- and education-oriented types that predominated in the Classical and Hellenistic periods. Galen casually reveals the existence of these different registers of dissective activity in his world, distinguishing among private dissections, semiprivate educational displays, and their more public and spectacular counterparts:

> And it is possible for you, in your demonstrations, to do just as you have
> seen me also do whenever the thorax was suggested for dissection: 1) you

---

[1] Dio Chrysostom, *Or.* XXXIII.6 (οἱ δὲ πολλοὶ κεχήνασι καὶ κεκήληνται τῶν παιδίων μᾶλλον); Galen, *AA* II.669 (μᾶλλον οἱ θεαταὶ θαυμάζουσι).
[2] *PHP* V.650 (VIII.1.6 De Lacy) (ὁ μετὰ τοὺς παλαιοῦς ἐν τῷ μεταξῦ χρόνῳ τὴν ἀνατομικὴν θεωρίαν ἠμελημένην ἀνακτησάμενος). On Marinus more broadly, see Chapter 7, "Marinus" at pp. 231–7.
[3] For a deeper discussion of the claims here and in the previous sentence, which depend on analyses of anatomical texts, see Chapter 7.

yourself giving the speech about the things that are going to be demonstrated, *having ordered others to expose the nerves* in the meantime and to make a demonstration of each to those present. 2) If, however, I am *demonstrating a dissection single-handed to a few lovers of knowledge*, I think it is quite clear, even I were not to say it, that it is necessary, first, to select a house full of light and, next, to have a very sharp lancet, as sharp as possible... 3) And I think it is particularly important that, in your initial tries, *when you are practicing by yourself*, you cut in the way that has been described, but that, later, you cut in the opposite way, as I will shortly explain.[4]

This single set of instructions for a thoracic dissection runs the gamut of dissection possibilities: 1) Galen dissects in front of a crowd, on a scale that requires theatrical speech making and a retinue of assistants to make sure that everything runs smoothly and at a pace suited to impressing an audience more motivated by a desire to be entertained than a thirst for anatomical knowledge; 2) he dissects in an intimate setting with only a few onlookers, who themselves are eager to learn all the details; and 3) he dissects alone, practicing.[5] In this chapter, I will address all three of these possible circumstances, grouping my analysis according to the motivations of the dissector, which could range from moments of practice and research to spectacular displays, advertisement, formal evaluation, and the discrediting of rivals. Although Galen's own experiences, largely centered on Rome, provide the bulk of the evidence, I have done my best to uncover the scope of the practice beyond him and to highlight as many voices from as many places as the sources allow.

Private Practice and Research

The most essential, and least glamorous, type of dissection is the last mentioned in Galen's passage here: practice. No doubt a large number of the animal dissections performed in the Roman period were done to hone skills, whether those required for surgery or those required for

---

[4] *AA* II.672–3 (καί σοι δυνατὸν ἐν ταῖς ἐπιδείξεσιν, ὥσπερ ἐθεάσασθε κἀμέ, προβληθέντος ποτὲ τοῦ θώρακος εἰς ἀνατομήν, αὐτὸν μὲν αὐτίκα *λέγοντα τοὺς λόγους* τῶν δειχθησομένων, *ἑτέροις δὲ ἐν τῷ τέως ἐκλαβεῖν τὰ νεῦρα προστάξαντα* τὴν ἐπίδειξιν ἰδιοποιῆσαι τοῖς παροῦσιν. εἰ μέντοι *κατὰ μόνας ὀλίγοις τῶν φιλομαθῶν ἐπιδείκνυμεν τὴν ἀνατομήν*, εὔδηλον οἶμαι, κἂν ἐγὼ μὴ λέγω, πρῶτον μὲν ἐπιλέξασθαι χρῆναι μεστὸν αὐγῆς οἶκον, εἶτα τὴν σμίλην ἔχειν ὀξυτάτην, ὡς ἔνι μάλιστα ... καὶ μάλιστά σε τέμνειν ἀξιῶ, τὰ μὲν πρῶτα *γυμναζόμενον ἐπὶ σαυτοῦ*, καθ' ὃν εἴρηται τρόπον, ὕστερον δ' ἐναντίως, ὡς ἐφεξῆς ἐρῶ...); my numeration and emphasis. See also *AA* II.669.
[5] Anderson (1989), 89–92 suggests a similar three-tiered structure for the audiences of sophists, though his categories (public, semiprivate tutorial of students, private displays before patrons) will end up being slightly different than mine. For the private/public dichotomy in audiences of medical performance specifically, see Debru (1995), 73, von Staden (1995), 52–3 and (1997), 44–7, and Mattern (2008), 16.

high-pressure, high-stakes public displays. Galen stresses that success in dissection is achieved only by repetition; he urges would-be dissectors "to practice often on many subjects."[6] In addition, anyone wishing to practice vivisection is particularly well advised to master the dissection of the relevant areas in dead specimens first, as the high-speed and bloody nature of vivisection makes it overwhelming for anyone not intimately acquainted with the structures already.[7]

Though preparation for surgery and performance was clearly a dominant aspect, dissection in private was not just a matter of developing competency. A truly dedicated doctor or natural philosopher would require multiple dissections on multiple subjects in order to be sure that he had truly understood a structure in all its possible variations: "it is best and most preferable to repeat frequently the dissection of every single organic part, in order that if in one animal or in two something remains obscure, and we do not see it clearly, we may observe it in the third, fourth, or following animal which we subsequently dissect."[8]

Similarly, even with the rich inheritance of anatomical information from the Hellenistic period, some dissections were for purely heuristic purposes. Galen describes using animal dissection to confirm theories of human physiology as well as his philosopho-religious views on teleology:

> Ants, mosquitos, fleas, and other small animals, I have never at all attempted to dissect. But the creeping animals, like weasels and mice, and the crawling ones, like snakes, and all the types of birds and fish and other sea creatures, I have often dissected, in order to be firmly convinced that it was a single mind that made these things and that in all of them the body is suited to the character of the animal.[9]

Further, he avails himself of the homologies underlying the heterogeny of animal forms to test and evaluate his anatomical research. For example, he describes using the elongated necks of cranes and ostriches as a natural extreme case to test whether he truly understood the arrangement of

---

[6] AA II.289 (πολλάκις ἐπὶ πολλῶν γεγυμνάσθαι); cf. AA II. 384–5, 674, S146.

[7] AA S159–60, 661–2, 694, S16, 106, 109, 128.

[8] AA S159–60; compare II.621.

[9] AA II.537 (μύρμηκας μὲν οὖν καὶ κώνωπας καὶ ψύλλας, ὅσα τ' ἄλλα τῶν ζώων μικρά, τὴν ἀρχὴν οὐδ' ἐπεχείρησά ποτ' ἀνατέμνειν· ὅσα δ' ἕρπει ζῷα, καθάπερ αἱ γαλαῖ τε καὶ οἱ μύες, ὅσα τ' εἰλυσπᾶται, καθάπερ οἱ ὄφεις, ὀρνίθων τε γένη πολλὰ καὶ ἰχθύων, ὅσα τἄλλα θαλάττια, πολλάκις ἀνέτεμον, ἕνεκα τοῦ πεισθῆναι βεβαίως, ἕνα τὸν νοῦν εἶναι τὸν διαπλάττοντα αὐτά, καὶ ὡς τῷ ἤθει τοῦ ζῴου τὸ σῶμά ἐστιν οἰκεῖον ἐν πᾶσιν); following the text in Garofalo (1986–2000). At PHP V.540 (VI.5.9 De Lacy) he further adds that the only thing holding him back from dissecting insects is the fear that they are too small to offer reliably discernible evidence. For using dissection to confirm theories of physiology, see Nat.Fac. II.147.

one of his discoveries – the recurrent laryngeal nerves, which loop back through the neck.[10]

Vivisection was also a powerful tool for discovery. Galen describes multiple experiments performed on living animals in order to answer both anatomical and physiological questions.[11] In one case, he ligates an animal's carotid arteries, investigates the immediate effects, and then patches up its wound, with the ligature still in place, and lets it wander around for the rest of the day, observing its health and behavior in order to deduce the details of the functional interdependence of the heart and the brain.[12] In another, he reproduces a delicate experiment that he attributes to Erasistratus for discovering the source of arterial pulsation; he inserts a reed or bronze tube into an animal's artery and ligates the substance of the vessel against it, while still allowing the contents to pass through, thus isolating the effect of the arterial coat on the pulse.[13] Some of these experiments were dead ends: He exerted considerable creative effort in an attempt to find a way to demonstrate that the liver is the seat of the appetitive soul, but none of his ligations, insections, or other interventions proved productive.[14] Unlike the examples I will discuss in the next section, most of this activity would not have been particularly exciting to watch. It represents the purely research oriented manifestation of Roman dissection, which, in Galen's case at least, must have constituted a solid amount of his anatomical energies.

Yet even these repetitive and heuristic forms of dissection and vivisection would not always have been solitary. Though he does not usually comment on the fact, a wealthy doctor such as Galen would rarely have been working alone. He likely had students eager to watch him in action, whether on patients, live animals, or carcasses, and he certainly had servants and slaves at hand to help with any and every aspect of his work, from holding open dismembered bodies to transcribing his dictated observations.[15] Nevertheless, these dissections were not overtly performative, unlike the remaining categories to be considered.

---

[10] *AA* S108.
[11] Debru (1994) offers a full catalogue of Galen's experiments, mostly vivisectory.
[12] *Ut.Resp.* IV.502–3 (cf. *Us.Puls.* V.154–5, *PHP* V.263–5 [II.6.1–12 De Lacy]); see the notes in Furley and Wilkie (1984), 48–50.
[13] *Art.Sang.* IV.733–4 (cf. *AA* II.646–8); see the notes in Furley and Wilkie (1984), 51–3 and the discussion in Salas (2020), 196–226.
[14] *PHP* V.519–21 (VI.3.2–6 De Lacy).
[15] For more on the role of assistants and the frequent tacit presence of slaves, see Chapter 4, "Other Requirements: Assistants" at pp. 136–9.

Performance for Public Display

The line between the other two, performative, types of dissection itemized in Galen's passage quoted earlier – dissecting for a small, scientifically oriented audience and dissecting for a larger, entertainment-seeking crowd – is not as bright as it might appear; indeed, it is often quite difficult to gauge which scenario any given dissection that Galen describes belonged to.[16] One natural assumption would be that the intimate, nonspectacular dissections constituted student–teacher interactions. In many instances this was likely so. Galen recalls witnessing his own teachers in Asia Minor dissecting before him. He mentions that his teachers "demonstrated and showed to [him] that breath is moved by the thorax," training that informed his own spectacular demonstrations on the voice.[17] In a larger and still more memorable display, his teacher Satyrus demonstrated muscular anatomy to his students in a hands-on lesson that took advantage of an epidemic of a necrotizing skin disease to use living patients as their subjects.[18] Though he indicates in that passage that not all doctors teaching students in Pergamon at the time were forward-thinking enough to include dissection and anatomy in their tuition, the story nevertheless suggests that a fair number of anatomical displays would have fallen into the category of professional education.

Though students are obvious candidates as audience members for the more intimate type of dissection, they were by no means the only ones. It is in this period that dissection as a performative event appears to have unfurled and truly blossomed. In *Anatomical Procedures*, Galen describes how to dissect the arm and, particularly, how to do the skinning that necessarily precedes dissection:

> This task requires a lot of time. Therefore, whenever you show the parts of the arm to some other intellectual, pre-strip off the membranes of the skin beforehand, as has been explained, before your audience member arrives. But if you wish to share the dissection with one of your companions who will himself at some point wish to demonstrate it to another, do the skinning while he is present. For it is a task requiring much exactitude, suitable to an intellectual and hard-working man.[19]

---

[16] Salas (2020), 36–44, which became available after my own manuscript was completely drafted, tackles this question from a different angle; our conclusions complement each other well.

[17] *AA* II.660 (ὅτι μὲν ὑπὸ τοῦ θώρακος ὁ πνεύμων κινεῖται … ἀποδειξάντων τε καὶ δειξάντων ἡμῖν).

[18] *AA* II.224–5. For more detailed discussion of this passage, see Chapter 4, "Anatomical Subjects: Humans" at pp. 119–20.

[19] *AA* II.351 (δεῖται δὲ τὸ ἔργον τοῦτο χρόνου πλείονος. ὅθεν, ὅταν ἑτέρῳ τινὶ τῶν φιλομαθῶν ἐπιδεικνύῃς τὰ κατὰ τὴν χεῖρα, φθάνων προαπόξυε τὸν ὑμένα τοῦ δέρματος, ὡς εἴρεται, πρὶν ἀφικέσθαι τὸν θεώμενον. εἰ δέ τινι τῶν ἑταίρων ἐθέλοις κοινωνῆσαι τῆς ἀνατομῆς, ὃς καὶ αὐτὸς ἄλλῳ ποτὲ δεῖξαι βουλήσεται, παρόντος αὐτοῦ ποιοῦ τὴν ἐγχείρησιν. ἔστι γὰρ τὸ ἔργον ἀκριβείας πολλῆς δεόμενον, ἀνδρὶ φιλοπόνῳ τε καὶ φιλομαθεῖ πρέπον.).

In the second scenario, the fellowship between the performer and the witness is emphasized. The latter is a "companion" and shares the same goals as the dissector – he, too, wants to learn this anatomy so that he can show it to other people. Not just an observer, he "shares" even the boring parts of the dissection, as the students discussed earlier no doubt did with their teachers.[20] In the first scenario, however, the dissector is performing for someone of an equally high intellectual status, but who is interested only in observing rather than doing; he comes across as a sort of client. Described by the word typically used for an audience member (τὸν θεώμενον), he will arrive at a given location and expect an interesting demonstration to be prepared for him and ready to begin, an expectation emphasized by the three different ways of expressing "before" in the instructions for preparation (φθάνων προαπόξυε … πρὶν).[21] In both cases, it is striking that Galen expects anatomists to be giving demonstrations as a matter of course: Either one is dissecting before others or one is training to do so. Over and above its practical utility to the training surgeon, this is a performative skill.

Among the small-scale dissections, then, some, as in the latter case in the passage quoted earlier, were aimed at a student or specialist audience, while others, like the former, were for laymen. Indeed, the main difference between smaller scale dissections and their larger counterparts seems to have been their size and exclusivity rather than their content or audience composition. Whether large-scale or intimate, open-door or closed, demonstrations aimed primarily at other doctors or anatomists allowed the dissector to debate findings and advocate for his own techniques and theories, while those aimed at the general public were more geared toward revealing marvelous or spectacular things about the body. Yet, given the public nature of medical care in antiquity, it is unlikely that the two types of audience members described here – the "professional" and the lay – were ever so neatly divided.[22]

Sometimes a dissection that started as a professional debate could end up providing entertainment for a broader audience. Galen describes one occasion on which he got into a heated argument about the kidney's role in urine production with some doctors from the Asclepiadean sect. Though several

---

[20] Indeed, ἑταῖρος is an ambiguous word, which Galen uses to refer to both students and friends; see Garofalo (2006), 64–5 and Mattern (2008), 16–21.

[21] Compare *AA* II.564 where the reader is instructed how to proceed if he wants only to see something for himself or demonstrate it to one other person (αὐτόν τε γνῶναι καὶ δεικνύειν ἑτέρῳ).

[22] See, for example, *AA* S233, where Galen says that he has repeatedly exposed some of Marinus' anatomical errors "in the city of Rome in distinguished company in the presence of all the notable surgeons," suggesting that his audience contained both preeminent surgeons and preeminent Romans.

hardened partisans refused to even engage with him on the question, some "submitted to the ureters, growing from the kidneys into the bladder, being demonstrated in their presence."[23] Even after witnessing – or putting up with – this demonstration, they persisted in interpreting the anatomy to suit their own theory, leading Galen to further anatomical demonstrations and eventually causing him, in increasing frustration, to escalate to vivisection, demonstrating "in the still living animal" that urine flowed through the ureters.[24] He describes this vivisection in detail, urging his readers to try it in order to confirm his view; it is a rigorous and multistep process, very well suited to impressing the wavering doubter. The showstopping moment comes when the dissector pierces a ureter that had previously been ligated off from the bladder, causing it to become distended with urine. At this, "the urine spurts out of it, like blood in venesection."[25] One can imagine the delight of dissector and spectator alike if he were able to build enough pressure for a truly impressive gush of urine. Though the context Galen describes here is that of a professional debate, this demonstration was likely too good to have been wasted on doctors alone – indeed, he describes the humiliation of his rivals here as occurring before "everyone who happened to be present," indicating a scene perhaps open to the curious passerby.[26]

Indeed, we know that there were nonprofessional audiences eager to witness such demonstrations. The single layman audience member about whom we know the most is Flavius Boethus. Boethus, as we learn from Galen, was a Syrian who served as consul and was later governor of Syria Palaestina.[27] In addition to these political demands on his time, he was also an avid fan of Aristotelian philosophy and, probably not coincidentally, he had a keen interest in anatomy. In fact, he appears to have been actively seeking out anatomical performances prior to Galen's arrival in Rome. When a mutual acquaintance, Eudemus, praises Galen's skill as a doctor, it transpires that Boethus had already been in contact with him:

> Boethus, having heard that I was trained to the highest degree in anatomical theory,[28] happened to have already invited me to demonstrate something on

[23] *Nat.Fac.* II.35 (δειχθῆναι παρόντων αὐτῶν τοὺς ἀπὸ τῶν νεφρῶν εἰς τὴν κύστιν ἐμφυομένους οὐρητῆρας ὑπομείναντες).

[24] *Nat.Fac.* II.36 (ἐπὶ ζῶντος ἔτι τοῦ ζῴου).

[25] *Nat.Fac.* II.37 (ἐξακοντίζεται τὸ οὖρον ἐξ αὐτοῦ, καθάπερ ἐν ταῖς φλεβοτομίαις τὸ αἷμα).

[26] *Nat.Fac.* II.34 (ἁπάντων … τῶν παρατυγχανόντων).

[27] On Boethus, all references to whom appear in Galen, see Halfmann (1979), no. 95, Nutton (1979), 164, and Mattern (2013), 141.

[28] The Greek for "anatomical theory" (τὴν ἀνατομικὴν θεωρίαν) could also be translated "anatomical spectacle"; given the context, it probably conveys a bit of both meanings here.

the voice and breathing, how they come about and through which organs. So, when he realized my name [in connection with the doctor Eudemus was praising], he told this to Paulus, too, and said that after the trial he would invite me to show something to him too. For Paulus said that he absolutely stood in need of seeing the things made visible by dissection. Similarly, also Barbarus, the uncle of the Emperor Lucius, who was prefect of the area called Mesopotamia, requested edification also for himself, just like Paulus. And later Severus did too, being both a consul and eagerly interested in Aristotle's philosophy.[29]

This passage is revealing in several ways.

First, the anecdote recounted here occurred within the first year of Galen's arrival in Rome in AD 162.[30] Even before firmly establishing his reputation as a physician, he appears to have made a public impression as a new and exciting performer of dissections. Further, Boethus requests a demonstration on the voice. Galen talks about this demonstration more than any other and in the most openly audience-focused way, and we know him to have been working on it already as a student in Smyrna.[31] All of this rather suggests that this was his debut public demonstration in the city as a new doctor and that someone in the crowd relayed an account of it to Boethus, knowing he would be interested. Second, the anecdote implies that Boethus was already interested in dissection prior to hearing of Galen. He is someone to whom people report anatomical goings-on. His passion for Aristotelian philosophy was no doubt the cause of this interest and also provided a circle of like-minded people through whom to receive such reports.[32] Yet, Boethus is not so eager that he is not choosy. He invites Galen to perform for him privately, an

---

[29] *Praen.* XIV.612–13 (ὁ δ' οὖν Βοηθός, ἀκηκοὼς εἰς ἄκρον ἠσκῆσθαί με τὴν ἀνατομικὴν θεωρίαν, ἔτυχεν ἤδη παρακαλῶν ἐπιδεῖξαί τι περὶ φωνῆς τε καὶ ἀναπνοῆς, ὅπως τε γίνοιτο καὶ διὰ τίνων ὀργάνων. ὡς οὖν ἐγνώρισέ μου τὸ ὄνομα καὶ τοῦτ' αὐτὸ τῷ τε Παύλῳ διηγήσατο καὶ μετὰ τὴν πεῖραν ἔφη παρακαλεῖν με δεῖξαί τι καὶ αὐτῷ· πάνυ γὰρ ἔφη δεῖσθαι τῆς θέας τῶν κατὰ τὰς ἀνατομὰς φαινομένων ὁ Παῦλος. ὁμοίως δὲ καὶ Βάρβαρος ὁ θεῖος τοῦ βασιλεύοντος Λευκίου, κατὰ τὴν Μεσοποταμίαν ὀνομαζομένην ὄντος ἐπάρχου, ἐδεῖτο τοῦ μαθήματος καὶ αὐτός, ὥσπερ ὁ Παῦλος. ὕστερον δὲ καὶ Σεβῆρος ὕπατος μὲν ὤν, ἐσπουδακὼς δὲ περὶ τὴν Ἀριστοτέλους φιλοσοφίαν); following the text in Nutton (1979).

[30] On the timing of the demonstration for Boethus within Galen's career, see Nutton (1979), 49 and 187, and Hankinson (2008*b*), 11–12.

[31] We know Galen to have been working on this topic as a student because he gave a copy of the accompanying speech to a student friend so that he, too, could use it as an advertising tool upon going home to set up practice. Indeed, variations on the same theme seem to have been popular display procedures among anatomists of Galen's time and the generation before; see this chapter, "Performance for Advertisement" at pp. 78–9 and Chapter 7, "Quintus and His Students: Numisianus, Heracleianus, Pelops, and Aelianus" at p. 246.

[32] For the surge in anatomical interest among Aristotle's readers, see Chapter 7, "Anatomy in the Roman Intellectual Scene" at pp. 272–3.

event that he calls a "trial." Only if he performs up to satisfaction, we can infer, will Boethus engage to offer a platform for him to dissect in front of other noteworthy Romans. This implies both that Boethus had some experience with witnessing, and therefore judging, dissection and that he had ambitions to become a sort of gatekeeper and patron in the field.[33] His Aristotelian-leaning friends agree that witnessing the kinds of things that Aristotle describes in his anatomical works is a desideratum. Assuming that Paulus' enthusiasm is not exaggerated to curry favor with his more genuinely interested friend, this passage also indicates that there were social dynamics at play in the composition of audiences in various venues: Galen and his ilk had been performing dissections of this sort in Rome for several decades, but Paulus, despite his professed interest, has never witnessed one before.[34] A hangout for physicians was not necessarily a milieu in which a man who was about to become prefect of the city of Rome would have deigned to appear.[35]

Perhaps in reaction to this last point, Galen is very keen to telegraph in this anecdote (and others like it) that his audience was elite, comprising the cream of Roman society. The four figures mentioned in this passage, Boethus, Paulus, Barbarus, and Severus, all held exalted political positions in the empire and had connections directly to the Emperor himself; they appear by name elsewhere in Galen's works as well.[36] In addition to the political elite, he also mentions the intellectual elite taking an interest in his work, including well-known sophists, such as Adrian of Tyre and Demetrius of Alexandria.[37] Sometimes, he sets the stage more

---

[33] Boethus' status as employer of Alexander of Damascus and patron of Adrian of Tyre, two famous intellectuals of the day, (see this chapter, n. 54) make it clear that he was a leading figure in Roman social and philosophical circles; cf. the suggestion in Jones (1986), 113–14 that Lucian alludes to him as a patron so famous that his name need not even be mentioned. His assiduous collection of anatomical texts indicates that he had ambitions of becoming a leader on this topic specifically. The texts that stemmed directly from the performances he facilitated would serve as a permanent record of his impact on the field, while the specialized collection as a whole, in a world where books were not always easy to find or readily accessible (see Chapter 4, "Other Requirements: Books" at pp. 127–36), would have made him a central figure in the intellectual circle; on this role of the private library generally, see Marshall (1976), 257.

[34] Quintus, who practiced in Rome and died in c. 145 AD, was a public dissector and may have been the among the first to develop thoracic vivisection as a spectacle; see Chapter 7, "Quintus and his Students" at pp. 237–9, 246, as well as the discussion of Quintus later in this section.

[35] On Paulus, see *Praen.* XIV.312 (cf. *AA* II.218) and Nutton (1979), 163.

[36] Boethus, with whom Galen had the closest relationship, comes up most frequently, appearing on numerous occasions in *Praen.*, *AA*, and *Lib.Prop.*; Paulus appears at *Praen.* XIV.612–13, 629, *AA* II.218; Barbarus at *Praen.* XIV.612–13, 629 (cf. Nutton [1979], 165); Severus at *Praen.* XIV.612–13, 629, 647, 653–6 and possibly at *Lib.Prop.* XIX.38 (cf. Nutton [1979], 166–7).

[37] For Adrian of Tyre and Demetrius of Alexandria, see this chapter, n. 54; he also alludes to a conversation with one of the most preeminent sophists of the time, Herodes Atticus, at *Opt.Med.*

generally, alluding to an audience of "office-holding men" or "distinguished company."[38]

Galen's popularity, however, was not limited to this elite clientele. He describes dissections before crowds, making it clear that entertainment, not just philosophical interest, was often their main selling point. He tells us that he performs before "large audiences" and he specifies that he performed one of his multiday anatomical exhibitions in "one of the large auditoria."[39] We can only speculate on the order of magnitude of these crowds. One potential gauge is the audience size of contemporary sophists, which is slightly less opaque to estimate. The suggested upper bound for these audiences ranges from five hundred to over a thousand, but an anecdote from Aelius Aristides more firmly pegs the lower bounds: He makes it clear that an audience of seventeen was pathetically small.[40] Like the sophists, doctors could have taken advantage of a variety of spaces for their public displays.[41] Philostratus and Aristides between them describe sophists declaiming in stoas, temples, theaters, council chambers, and odea.[42] In keeping, Plutarch describes doctors performing public surgeries in the theater, and Galen indicates that the Temple of Peace in Rome was a frequent location for medical disputations.[43] There were also dedicated lecture halls (*auditoria*/ἀκροατήρια), presumably identical to Galen's "*auditoria*" (ἀκουστήρια), which latter is an unusual, though perfectly intelligible,

---

[38] *AA* II.218 (ἀνδρῶν ἐν τέλει) and S233.

[39] *AA* S233 and *Lib.Prop.* XIX.21 (τι τῶν μεγάλων ἀκουστηρίων). He also mentions at *Sem.* IV.595 that he has demonstrated one anatomical point "to thousands" (μυρίοις), though there he is underscoring not just the size of his audiences but also the frequency with which he demonstrates.

[40] For discussions of the audience size and venues of sophists, see Russell (1983), 75–7, Anderson (1989), 91–2, Schmitz (1997), 160–1, and Whitmarsh (2005), 19–20; on the audience of seventeen (in contrast to his own packed event), see Aristides, *Ier.Log.* V.34 (354 Jebb). Galen indicates that philosophers' daily lectures could routinely expect audiences of "twenty or thirty or sometimes even more" (ὁ μὲν εἴκοσιν, ὁ δὲ τριάκοντα καί ποτε καὶ πλείονας) (*Pecc.Dig.* V.92).

[41] For brief discussion of various places that doctors might have performed, see Nutton (1979), 188, von Staden (1995), 61, Boudon-Millot (2012), 137.

[42] Stoa: Aristides, *Ier.Log.* IV.15–18 (324 Jebb); temples: Philostratus, *VS* 493, 618–19, Aristides, *Ier. Log.* II.31, IV.15–18 (298, 324 Jebb); theaters: Philostratus, *VS* 482, 571, 579, Aristides, *Ier.Log.* II.30 (297 Jebb); council chambers: Philostratus, *VS* 580, Aristides, *Ier.Log.* IV.95, V.16, 31–34 (343, 349, 353–4 Jebb); odea: Aristides, *Ier.Log.* V.30, 34 (353–4 Jebb). The tendency to adapt various locations intended for other purposes into venues for performance is parodied by Horace in *Satire* I.4.73–8, where he complains of people offering literary recitations in the middle of the Forum or in the baths.

[43] Plutarch, *De ad. et am.* 71a; see this chapter, n. 94. Temple of Peace at Galen, *Lib.Prop.* XIX.21; although Tucci (2017), 193–215 has convincingly argued against the identification by Palombi (2007), 71–2 and (2014), 338 of the specific auditorium in which Galen actually performed his dissections, there is general consensus that the temple was a location where the public might observe doctors grandstanding (cf. *Diff.Puls.* VIII.495).

Cogn. 9.19 (*CMG Suppl.Or.* IV, p. 112–14), though in that case it was Galen who was interested in his work rather than vice versa. For Galen's relationship to the Roman elite, see especially Schlange-Schöningen (2003), 137–221.

word.[44] The term ἀκροατήρια is the Greek equivalent of the Latin *auditoria*, which were venues dedicated to teaching and the giving of lectures.[45] In the Greek parts of the empire, ἀκροατήρια began to be associated with gymnasia.[46] Galen's own Pergamon, for example, provides the particularly grand example of a semicircular lecture hall that was added to the gymnasium in the second century AD, containing fourteen rows of seats and capable of seating up to a thousand people.[47] It was likely a more modest version of this type of structure that the doctor Asklepiades, who was honored by the double inscription from Perge and Seleucia, used when he performed his "lectures in the gymnasium."[48] In Rome, as Galen's remark indicates, the available *auditoria* varied in

[44] The term ἀκουστήριον appears twice in Galen (here and at *Ven.Sect.Er.Rom.* XI.194, where he contrasts treatises meant for written circulation with those written only for performance), once in Porphyry in the third century (*Vit.Plot.* 15.11), and once in Themistius in the fourth (*EisConstant.* 26c).

[45] The first attestation of ἀκροατήριον as a physical space (as opposed to an audience) does not occur until the Roman period, when Philo Judaeus (first century BC–first century AD) pairs it with θέατρον as two places full of philosophers delivering lectures (*Cong.* 64); compare the same pairing at Tacitus, *Dial.* 10.5 and, to polemical effect, at Tatian, *AdGr.* 22. The Latin equivalent, *auditoria*, was similarly not used to denote a physical space before the Augustan period; see Lewis and Short II.B and Tamm (1963), 17. Tamm (1963), 17–29 has analyzed the origins of these words and suggests that the Greek word arose first and the Latin followed as a translation of it, basing her claim in large part on the inscription at Chios (IGR IV.1703; McCabe Chios 15), which appears to contain the word and whose letter forms suggest a date as early as the first century BC; it is interesting to note, however, that the inscription describes the rights of a *Roman*, L. Nassius, to place statues "in whatever place in the ἀκροατήριον he prefers" (ἀναστῆ[σ]αι ἐν ᾧ ἂν βούληται τοῦ ἀκροατηρίου τόπῳ [ln. 14]) – the linguistic context is not purely Greek. Tamm does not take into account the evidence from Galen, which is essentially an alternative translation of the Latin term, suggesting that *auditorium* was the more culturally dominant word, at least in the second century AD; compare the early third-century AD inscription from Ephesus (IvE 3009) where the Latin term is transliterated, rather than translated, into Greek (αὐδειτωρίου) (cf. Engelmann [1993], 106, and Burrell [2009], 85). For the use of *auditorium* as a location, especially for teaching and lectures, see CIL VI.1017, Seneca, *Ep.* 52.11, Quintilian, *Inst.* 2.11.3, Tacitus, *Dial.* 10.7, 29.4, Suetonius, *Gram. et rhet.* 30.3, Pliny, *Ep.* 2.3.6, 5.3.11, 5.17.1, 6.17.1, 7.17.3, 7.17.13, Apuleius, *Apol.* 7.3. See also Ps.-Galen, *Part.phil.* 2 and Dio Chrysostom, *Or.* 32.8, which latter indicates both that the term was still fairly newfangled in Greek in the first century AD (ἐν τοῖς καλουμένοις ἀκροατηρίοις) and that it was a venue for public speaking in which comparative control could be exercised over the composition of the audience. For discussion of further textual evidence, see Tamm (1963), 8–23, and Rea (2014), 137–40, 147–9.

[46] See Robert (1970), 79–82, Rea (2014), 136, and Trümper (2015), 169. Two inscriptions, IGR IV.1703 (McCabe Chios 15) and Alt. von Aegae 43 (SEG 45.1656), attest to the link between this precise term and gymnasia.

[47] Robert (1970), 80–1, Trümper (2015), 178, 191–2. The gymnasium at Pergamon was one of the largest of the Hellenistic world, suggesting that this is the upper bound for the capacity of such *auditoria*. A variety of smaller multipurpose spaces were also available at the Pergamene gymnasium, allowing for various venues for lectures there; see Trümper (2015), 178. Less extravagant gymnasia would have deployed similar, less purpose-built spaces for lectures and related events; see Rea (2014), 136. Other extant archaeological examples of *auditoria* attached to gymnasia include Ephesus, Philippi, and Rhodes; see Tamm (1963), 7, n. 3.

[48] SEG 3.416 (IG IX, 1.104; Samama 051); see Chapter 2, "Medical Performance in the Hellenistic Period" at pp. 49–50. Indeed, this type of *auditorium* may have become a professional desideratum for physicians, if we can believe the claim that Severus Alexander granted salaries and *auditoria* to various professions, including doctors (Scriptores Historiae Augustae, *Alex. Sev.* 44.4).

size and grandeur. There were large, purpose-built *auditoria*, as well as a variety of private locations, including rooms in larger homes, no doubt including that of Boethus; indeed, literary evidence suggests that any room could have been transformed into an impromptu *auditorium* by the addition of tiered wooden platforms for seats.[49] Galen would likely have gravitated to the airier of these options in order to maximize natural light.[50] The capacity of all the venues would have varied considerably, but the larger ones would have been suitable to contain the flocking crowds attested for sophistic performances, suggesting that Galen's performance "in one of the large auditoria" and others like it had substantial audiences.[51]

In some instances, these larger events were linked to the smaller, private ones. A privileged few might get a private showing of a dissection that was also performed before a larger crowd on another occasion.[52] Some might even be invited to watch preliminary dissections made in preparation for a more public event.[53] On one often-cited occasion, what had been intended as a small, private gathering orchestrated by Boethus morphs into a largely attended multiday event. Boethus initially invited Galen to demonstrate to him privately the means by which breath and speech are produced. Whether this was his initial "test" or a subsequent demonstration is unclear, but it was never intended to be a completely one-on-one affair. Boethus' teacher of Peripatetic philosophy, Alexander of Damascus, who was in "constant attendance" at Boethus' anatomical events, was there, as were Adrian of Tyre, a rising rhetorical star who was also in Boethus' inner circle, and Demetrius of Alexandria, another public figure in the field of rhetoric.[54]

---

[49] For the public *auditoria* of Rome, see Tamm (1963), especially 7–23, and Rea (2014), 133–40, 145–8; a group of three examples in Rome from the Hadrianic period was recently discovered in the course of subway excavations (Egidi [2010], 107–116). Tucci (2017), 200–1 favors the idea that the auditorium Galen mentions was in Boethus' home; though it is highly likely that some of Galen's anatomical performances took place in a space there, it is not possible that the auditorium referenced by Galen at *Lib.Prop.* XIX.21 was located there, since, by the time of this dissection, which took place after the completion of *AA* and *UP*, Boethus had long since left Rome and died (*AA* II.215–16). For the transformation of rooms into *auditoria* by means of temporary tiered seating, see Juvenal 7.40–7, Tacitus, *Dial.* 9.3, and the discussions in Tamm (1963), 9–10, and Rea (2014), 139–40.

[50] For Galen's concern with lighting, see *AA* II.672, 721, S5, 192.

[51] Obviously, the size of the crowd would have dictated the content of the demonstration to a certain degree; demonstrations on vocal production or motor control, where the cessation and resumption of activity would have been easy to perceive even from a distance, would have been more practicable for large groups than, say, the vivisection of the ureters, where only the first row or two would have been able to see what was going on.

[52] *AA* S233; see also this chapter, n. 63, for Galen's frequent claim that he presents the same things both in private and in public.

[53] *AA* II.505.

[54] *Praen.* XIV.627; on these figures, see Nutton (1979), 189–91, and *AA* II.218 for Alexander's constant attendance (παρόντων ... ἀεί).

As appears to be his standard practice, Galen begins his demonstration with a speech describing what he is going to demonstrate.[55] He takes the extra, ingratiating step of inviting Alexander to lead the group in drawing conclusions from the things that become apparent during the dissection, perhaps hoping to ensure good behavior from this philosopher, whom he characterizes as notoriously contentious. Alexander, true to form, instead interjects very early on, questioning whether it is even logically sound to trust the evidence of one's own senses and thus scuttling the entire premise of the display. At this, Galen leaves in a theatrical huff.

In the wake of Galen's departure, the two rhetors begin to abuse Alexander and apparently spread the word in Roman intellectual circles about the interrupted display, with the result that "when this event was known to all the intellectuals in the city of Rome, including to Severus and Paulus and Barbarus, they all vehemently censured [Alexander] and thought it fit that the dissections take place in their very presence, gathering together into the same spot all the others who had a reputation for medicine and philosophy."[56] Galen's engagement with Alexander may not have turned out as he had originally planned, but the results of it ended up being far better than he could have hoped. The resulting gathering "lasted over several days," allowing Galen to perform for the large assembly numerous dissections related to the muscles and nerves controlling the thorax.[57]

These dissections were elaborate. In his *Anatomical Procedures*, Galen offers detailed directions for carrying out many of them, allowing us an authoritative picture of how they transpired. The first that he describes is the vivisection of the intercostal nerves, in which the vivisector compresses the nerves that run between the ribs in the back, causing the animal to lose the ability to exhale and therefore to phonate. As in his discussion of the dissection of the arm, he stresses the importance of timing in performance and the need to make certain preparations in advance in order to facilitate the best effect. He says that it is irrelevant precisely how you go about the operation if you are "examining it alone for yourself," but "if you are demonstrating" timing is everything.[58] One should open up the

---

[55] Debru (1995), 73–4 outlines the parameters of such a speech; see also von Staden (1997), 37–9.

[56] *Praen.* XIV.629 (ἐπεὶ δὲ καὶ τοῖς φιλολόγοις ἅπασιν, ὅσοι κατὰ τὴν τῶν Ῥωμαίων πόλιν ἦσαν, ἐγνώσθη τοῦτο καὶ τῷ Σεβήρῳ καὶ τῷ Παύλῳ καὶ τῷ Βαρβάρῳ, πάντες οὖν σφοδρῶς ἐπετίμησαν αὐτῷ καὶ παρόντων ἑαυτῶν ἠξίωσαν γενέσθαι τὰς ἀνατομάς, ἀθροίσαντες εἰς <τ>αὐτὸ τοὺς ἄλλους ἅπαντας, ὅσοι κατὰ τὴν ἰατρικήν τε καὶ φιλοσοφίαν ἦσαν ἔνδοξοι); following the text in Nutton (1979).

[57] *Praen.* XIV.629 (γινομένης δὲ πλείοσιν ἡμέραις τῆς συνουσίας).

[58] *AA* II.669 (κἂν μόνος ἐπὶ σαυτοῦ ποτ' ἐξετάζῃς … ἐπιδεικνυμένῳ δὲ).

area in advance, slip threads under all the nerves without tying them, and have "several assistants on hand for these sorts of demonstration" so that the threads can be tied as instantaneously as possible when the moment is right.[59] After giving the introductory lecture, we infer, which explains what is going to be shown and the theory behind it – the same kind of lecture that Alexander so rudely interrupted – one can then proceed:[60] "[the animal] bawls when struck, and then, immediately becoming mute upon the nerves being tied by the threads, it astounds the spectators. For it seems amazing that the voice is destroyed when small nerves along the back are ligatured."[61] Should the dissector want the spectators to be "still more amazed," he and his assistants can then loosen the threads "quickly," allowing the animal to regain its voice just as suddenly as it lost it.[62]

This is an overtly spectacle-oriented enterprise. Galen makes no secret of the fact that he is setting out to provide a good show. Indeed, it is later in his discussion of this same dissection that he offers the passage that began this chapter, contrasting how one ought to proceed when performing for small or large audiences, where he again underscores the need for a staff of assistants to make the demonstration a performative success. He tells us repeatedly that he has "often" performed this demonstration and a suite of related ones "both privately and in public," that these are things "often seen by many."[63] These dissections represent some of Galen's most advanced scientific knowledge, but they are also, and not unrelatedly, unabashedly for show.

Though the demonstrations on the voice were clearly Galen's signature performance, they were by no means the only ones in his repertoire. In another set, he demonstrates the leading role of the brain and spinal cord, rather than the heart, in sensory and cognitive activity. He describes these vivisections in great detail in the ninth book of *Anatomical Procedures*. The

---

[59] *AA* II.669 (ἔστωσαν δὲ πλείονες οἱ ὑπηρετούμενοί σοι κατὰ τὰς τοιαύτας ἐπιδείξεις).

[60] Debru (1995) walks through the general format that she believes Galen's anatomical demonstrations to have had. Owing to the nature of the evidence, she sometimes has to generalize widely from single anecdotes, but I think that there is enough evidence to be confident that the dissections were regularly preceded by a quite rhetorical introductory speech.

[61] *AA* II.669 (κέκραγε γὰρ οὕτω παιόμενον, εἶτ' ἐξαίφνης ἄφωνον γινόμενον ἐπὶ τῷ σφιγχθῆναι τοῖς λίνοις τὰ νεῦρα τοὺς θεατὰς ἐκπλήττει· θαυμαστὸν γὰρ εἶναι δοκεῖ, νεύρων μικρῶν κατὰ τὸ μετάφρενον βροχισθέντων, ἀπόλλυσθαι τὴν φωνήν).

[62] *AA* II.669 (μᾶλλον οἱ θεαταὶ θαυμάζουσι; τάχεως).

[63] *AA* II.665 (πολλάκις), 677 (δημοσίᾳ ἐθεάσασθε τοῦτο δεικνύμενον ... ἡμέραις ἐφεξῆς πολλαῖς), 690 (ὅπερ οὐ μόνον ἰδίᾳ πολλάκις ὑμῖν, ἀλλὰ καὶ δημοσίᾳ δεικνύντα με ἐθεάσασθε ... τὰ τοιαῦτα δεικνύντα με ἐθεάσασθε πολλάκις ἰδίᾳ τε καὶ δημοσίᾳ), 693 (θεασαμένῳ δέ τινι πολλάκις ἐμὲ τοῦτο πράττοντα); cf. *Lib.Prop.* XIX.13, 14, 15, 21.

dissector must open the skull and gently pull back the dura mater, leaving the top of the brain exposed. He can then either incise or compress various areas. Depending, in Galen's understanding, which ventricle is affected, the animal will be overcome by various levels of stupor; however, if the compression ceases or the incision is quickly closed, the stupor immediately lifts. In one particularly striking iteration, Galen points out where the two areas overlying the optic nerves are. Even with this area exposed to the air, the animal will blink if you bring something close to its eyes; however,

> should you go towards the animal while it is in this condition, and should you press upon … the place where I stated the root of the two optic nerves lies, thereupon the animal ceases to blink with its two eyes, even when you bring some object near to the pupils, and the whole appearance of the eye on the side on which lies the ventricle of the brain upon which you are pressing becomes like the eyes of a blind man.[64]

This particular display may even have encouraged some audience participation to ensure that Galen was not somehow duping his audience: Anyone in the crowd could get these results by pushing on the brain! In a less audience-reproducible, but equally striking move, Galen severs the spinal cord at various points, rendering everything below the point of incision devoid of both motion and sensation, "a result that is inevitable, clear, and intelligible."[65] Thus, much like the voice demonstrations, the vivisections on the brain involve the sudden incapacitation and, sometimes, equally sudden restoration of function to the animal – they, too, would have been amazing and astounding to spectators on a large scale.[66]

Were we only to have Galen's description of these brain vivisections in *Anatomical Procedures*, we would be forced to speculate that they would have been equally as suitable to performance as the vivisections related to the voice without being sure that he had ever used them performatively. However, we are fortunate to have confirmation of their performance in his text *On the Doctrines of Hippocrates and Plato*. There, he twice explains, more briefly, the same vivisectory compression or incision of the brain and how it results in the animal losing and regaining sensation and motion. On one of the occasions, he simply offers it as proof for his theories of brain function, again without any indication of performance.[67] On the

---

[64] *AA* S23.
[65] *AA* S27.
[66] Compare also the vivisection he describes in passing in *Hipp.Epid.IV* XVIIb.245, where he mentions the shouts evoked from the audience at the vivisection of a pregnant goat and the subsequent activities of the premature kid; cf. *Loc.Aff.* VIII.443 for a similar story, with similar shouting.
[67] *PHP* V.604–6 (VII.3.14–22 De Lacy).

other, however, he is explicit that "I often demonstrated [this] to not a few doubters," using it in tandem with his equally memorable proof that the heart does not have equivalent control over movement and sensation.[68] For this suite of performances, he starts by exposing the heart. He demonstrates that the left ventricle instantaneously gushes blood when pierced, disproving the Erasistratean claim that it was full of pneuma, which, in contemporary understanding, would have rendered it potentially capable of controlling thought and sensation. For an added element of spectacle, he sometimes uses things other than a lancet to pierce the heart, proving that, no matter how tiny the tool or swift its removal, it will always be stained by blood as soon as it enters the heart; he specifically mentions a needle and a writing reed, which latter would have added a nice crowd-pleasing touch, particularly if he took the logical next step and proved the presence of blood on the nib by writing with it. Should this fail to impress, his next move is to contrast the effects of damage or pressure to the brain and the heart. After demonstrating the immediate and dramatic effects of pressure to the brain, he then, sometimes even in the same animal, demonstrates the total lack of such effect when the heart is compressed. Not content to simply show this, he solicits audience involvement, like that I speculated for the vision display.[69] At first, he asks his volunteer to squeeze the heart with his fingers, but "when it leapt out of his fingers, throbbing violently, [Galen] ordered him to grasp it with bronze tongs and not even then was the animal affected, neither in sensation nor in voluntary movement, but rather it bawled greatly and breathed unhindered and moved all its limbs vigorously."[70] This, again, is clearly a memorable, audience-focused performance, which he tells us he performed repeatedly.

We are not lucky enough to have corroborating evidence for performance of all the dissections and vivisections that Galen describes in *Anatomical Procedures*. However, as I will explore in Chapter 9, he frequently frames the text as a tool for those learning to dissect, both to

---

[68] *PHP* V.185 (I.6.4 De Lacy) (πολλάκις ἐδείξαμεν οὐκ ὀλίγοις τῶν ἀπιστούντων).

[69] Another potential moment for audience involvement is at *PHP* V.624 (VII.5.28 De Lacy), where he explains that if you show an excised and dissected optic nerve to someone without telling them what it is, they will declare that it is from the brain. It is easy to imagine the ways in which Galen could have deployed this trick to humiliate a cardiocentric opponent.

[70] *PHP* V.186 (I.6.7 De Lacy) (πυράγρα ποτὲ χαλκέως ἐπιτρέψας τινὶ περιλαβεῖν αὐτήν, ἐπειδὴ καὶ τῶν δακτύλων ἐξεπήδα βιαίως παλλομένη· ἀλλ' οὐδὲν οὐδὲ τότε τὸ ζῷον ἔπασχεν οὔτε εἰς αἴσθησιν οὔτε εἰς κίνησιν τὴν καθ' ὁρμήν ἀλλ' ἐκεκράγει τε μεγάλα καὶ ἀκωλύτως ἀνέπνει καὶ πάντα ἐκίνει σφοδρῶς τὰ κῶλα). Compare *AA* II.635–6, where he says that he is accustomed to hold the heart with tongs since it leaps out of fingers.

explain how to do it and to explain *how to show it to others*. Performance is by no means the only, or even often the primary, goal of all of the procedures described there, but it is, through the very nature of the text, implicated for all of them. My own assumption is that, like the experiments to determine the control center of the body and of the voice, where we do have corroborating evidence, just about all of the vivisections and many of the dissections mentioned in *Anatomical Procedures* were performative to one degree or another once Galen had perfected them.[71] His own references confirm a busy performative schedule, further suggesting that he had many procedures in his public repertoire. Indeed, in *On My Own Books* he tells us that his public lecturing had become so widely popular and so productive of venom from his rivals that he foreswore it completely for a period – before eventually being pulled back into the fray by the devotion of his followers.[72]

Galen was by no means the only public dissector at work in the mid-second century. He is eager to highlight the frequency and popularity of his dissections and, indeed, to define himself as the best dissector of his time, with both the greatest skill and considerable social cachet. Whether or not we can trust his own evaluation that he was the best, we can be certain that he did have competition for the title. He makes it clear that there were other anatomists at work in Rome and beyond. In one episode, which I consider in greater detail in Chapter 4, a throng of "many doctors" communally dissect an elephant with the stated goal of ascertaining the structure of its heart, particularly whether it "had two apexes or one, and two chambers or three."[73] This seemingly simple research question was drawn upon the fault lines of the far more contentious debate between those following the cardiocentric Aristotle, who claims that the perfect heart has three chambers, though they are only all present (or visible, depending on which text you read) in large animals, and those following the cephalocentric discoveries of the Hellenistic anatomists, who saw only two chambers, namely the ventricles, counting the atria merely as antechambers. Galen tells us that he stakes out his anti-Aristotelian position prior to the dissection, presumably offering a predissection speech similar to those he gave in his own independent dissections. One must assume that the other doctors

---

[71] For a catalogue of Galen's vivisectory experiments, see Debru (1994), 1730–50.

[72] *Lib.Prop.* XIX.15, 21–22. For debate over the timing of this withdrawal from public life, see Debru (1995), 70, Boudon-Millot (2007), 188–9, n. 5, and Mattern (2013), 143–5. I agree with the modern trend in scholarship that has pushed this renunciation back to the period of his second stay in Rome.

[73] *AA* II.619; for the full text, see Chapter 4, "Anatomical Subjects: Other Animals" at pp. 108–9.

did not passively leave the floor to him, but rather that they took the opportunity to argue for their own positions as well. Galen prefers to paint himself as the only really competent participant in this dissection, calling his rivals "unpracticed," but, even despite this negative slant, his story clearly conveys their eagerness for and hands-on participation in the event.

Galen was certainly an active participant in that dissection, though there is no reason to think that he was its instigator, but his presence was not a necessary catalyst for all dissections in contemporary Rome. He describes dissections that he did not himself attend and implies many more left undescribed.[74] In one, the dissector in question, a doctor to whom Galen does not give a name, astonished not just his audience, but also, one assumes, himself when his dissection of a pregnant goat revealed that the uterus was empty and that the fetus was housed in the belly instead. This result was not a private one – it immediately gave rise to "considerable discussion and widespread reports."[75] A second doctor, whom Galen names as one Theophrastus, took it upon himself to quench this excitement by suggesting – whether with an illustrative dissection or not, he does not say – that the first doctor had begun by mistaking the urinary bladder for the uterus and thus thought that the actual uterus, where the fetus was safely and unremarkably ensconced, was the belly.[76] This story implies a fairly wide community of dissectors. Galen feels no reticence about calling out error by name, so his lack of identification of the first doctor gives the impression that he was just one of a crowd of dissectors, too otherwise unremarkable to bother singling out. Theophrastus, similarly, though he comes across as a key player in this story, a dominant authority in matters of anatomy, does not appear elsewhere in Galen's discussion of dissections; he seems to have run in a different circle.

Indeed, Galen enjoys denouncing other anatomists of his time, suggesting a heterogeneous group involved in the practice, comprising smaller circles of this kind. One favorite complaint was that some were more showy than practical. In the second book of his *Anatomical Procedures* he launches into an extended diatribe against such men in the process of explaining why he has chosen to foreground the anatomy of the limbs in the composition of his text. He underscores the medical usefulness of anatomical study and accuses other anatomists of being more interested in seeking

---

[74] For example, at *AA* S128 he addresses his readers, saying "I am acquainted with a large number of you who have already performed [the exposure of a nerve in the neck] excellently."
[75] *AA* S166.
[76] *AA* S167.

out glamorous new findings than in obtaining the most accurate possible knowledge of areas of the body most frequently subject to surgery.[77] He takes aim at "those skillful in anatomy" and "all the anatomists" who have only "carelessly" studied the anatomy of the limbs, favoring instead more contested and flashier questions such as "how many membranes (i.e., valves) the heart has in each of its mouths [and] how many veins nourish it and from where and how they are carried, and how a nerve, branching off from the pair that stem from the brain, arrives in it."[78]

Galen's immediately subsequent call upon "the young," that is, those just beginning the study of anatomy, to focus more on the medically useful and less on flashier topics such as "the dissection of the brain and the heart, and the tongue, and the lungs, and the liver and the spleen, and the kidneys, and the stomach, and the larynx, and embryos and the pregnant womb" gives further insight into the types of topics that anatomists found particularly attractive – and attracting.[79] On the one hand, these are organs whose functions were still very much up for debate in the second century; these are thus the open research questions of the time, suggesting that some anatomists were more interested to engage with theory than with professional practice. Additionally, they are organs that are easy to see, and many were also well suited to spectacular display. We saw already the frisson of interest created by the dissection of a pregnant uterus. The brain, the heart, the larynx, the lungs, and the kidneys all also feature in some of Galen's more audience-friendly experiments. Indeed, Galen emphasizes the popularity of this type of "flashy" anatomy:

> I see the doctors of today, all those who seem serious about anatomy, making small account of the more useful part of it and training in the part more suitable to sophists ... and with each passing day the enthusiasm for the part of anatomy of slight value is ever increasing, while just about everyone neglects the more useful part.[80]

---

[77] AA II.287–91.

[78] AA II.288 (οἱ περὶ τὰς ἀνατομὰς δεινοί), 290 (ἅπασι τοῖς ἀνατομικοῖς ὀλιγώρως τὰ τοιαῦτα ζητήσασιν), 288 (πόσους ἔχει καθ' ἕκαστον τῶν στομάτων ὑμένας ἡ καρδία ... πόσαι φλέβες αὐτὴν τρέφουσιν, ἢ πόθεν, ἢ πῶς φερόμεναι, καὶ πῶς τὸ τῶν ἀπ' ἐγκεφάλου συζυγιῶν ἀποσχιζόμενον εἰς αὐτὴν ἀφικνεῖται νεῦρον).

[79] AA II.290 (ἐγὼ τοίνυν παρακαλῶ τοὺς νέους, ἐάσαντας ἐν τῷ παρόντι τὰς ἐγκεφάλου τε καὶ καρδίας, καὶ γλώττης, καὶ πνεύμονος, ἥπατός τε καὶ σπληνός, καὶ νεφρῶν, καὶ στομάχου, καὶ λάρυγγος, ἐμβρύων τε καὶ μήτρας ἐγκύμονος ἀνατομάς...); cf. Loc.Aff. VIII.445.

[80] AA II.416–17 (ὁρῶ τοὺς νῦν ἰατρούς, ὅσοι γε δοκοῦσι περὶ τὴν ἀνατομὴν ἐσπουδακέναι, τοῦ χρησιμωτέρου μὲν αὐτῆς ὀλιγωροῦντας, ἀσκοῦντας δὲ τὸ σοφιστικώτερον ... καθ' ἑκάστην ἡμέραν ἀεὶ καὶ μᾶλλον ἐπιδίδωσιν ἡ περὶ τὸ φαυλότερον μέρος τῆς ἀνατομῆς σπουδή, τοῦ χρησιμωτέρου σχεδὸν ἁπάντων ἀμελούντων).

These passages are, of course, unabashedly polemical, but whatever perverse motives and professional shortcomings he may attribute to his contemporaries, his comments do indicate an active, diverse, and highly skilled group of anatomists at work in this period.

Interestingly enough, the root of Galen's displeasure here ties back to the Dio passage from the end of Chapter 2. Dio took aim at the pompous, sophistic doctor who holds forth on matters of obscure physiology rather than getting on with the business of curing patients. Though as I pointed out earlier, Dio's words-versus-deeds framework does not map onto the world of dissection that Galen is complaining about, Galen, too, is targeting arrogant, showy, detail-obsessed theorists who are unable to fulfill the most basic tasks of the practicing physician. He deplores the doctors who "greatly err in their phlebotomy" through ignorance of the anatomy of the arm, yet blithely spend their time "dissect[ing] bovine hearts and tongues, unaware that they are extremely unlike those of humans."[81] Again, he denounces the "daily" sight of

> doctors who are versed in how many and of what sort are the membranes in the heart or the muscles in the tongue and other such things, yet do not know the anatomy of the external parts, making the gravest errors in their prognosis and surgery of the diseases that affect those parts, while those doctors who know these things, though unversed in the others, daily proceed correctly.[82]

Galen, too, like Dio, compares these theory-focused incompetents with rhetorical grandstanders. He claims that anatomical details that lack immediate relevance to medical practice, such as the muscles in the tongue or the valves of the heart, are the province of "sophists," a favorite derogatory term in certain circles of this period.[83] Stripping away the value judgments inherent in these polemics, one sees the medical field divided into two spheres: those who emphasize patient practice and those who focus on research

---

[81] *AA* II.291 (ἐν ταῖς φλεβοτομίαις μέγιστα σφαλλόμενοι, καρδίαν ἀνατέμνουσι καὶ γλῶτταν βοείαν, οὐδ' αὐτὸ τοῦτο γιγνώσκοντες, ὡς εἰσιν ἀνομοιόταται ταῖς ἀνθρώπων); following the text in Garofalo (1986–2000).

[82] *AA* II.346 (θεωροῦντας ὁσημέραι τῶν ἰατρῶν τοὺς ἐπισταμένους μὲν, ὁπόσοι τέ εἰσι καὶ ὁποῖοι κατὰ τὴν καρδίαν ὑμένες, ἢ τῆς γλώττης οἱ μύες, ὅσα τ' ἄλλα τοιαῦτα, μὴ γινώσκοντας δὲ τὴν ἐκτὸς ἀνατομήν, ἐν προγνώσει τε καὶ χειρουργίᾳ τῶν κατὰ ταῦτα τὰ μέρη γινομένων παθῶν μέγιστα σφαλλομένους, τοὺς δὲ ταύτην μὲν γινώσκοντας, ἀγνοοῦντας δ' ἐκεῖνα, κατορθοῦντας ὁσημέραι). Compare II.419–20 for the ignorant damage inflicted by doctors who spend all their time enquiring into the cartilage of the pineal gland and the bones of the heart rather than learning basic anatomy; cf. II.341.

[83] *AA* II.284 (τὰ τοιαῦτα τῶν σοφιστῶν ἕνεκ' ἀναγκαζόμεθα πολυπραγμονεῖν); compare II.416 (σοφιστικώτερον). On the complexities of the use of the word sophist in this period, see, among others, Stanton (1973), 351–8, Brunt (1994), 48–50, and Swain (1996), 97–100.

questions. The latter group was particularly well served by dissection, and the popularity that both Dio and Galen attribute to them suggests that they were particularly likely to have practiced performative anatomy.

Galen's descriptions of his rivals' dissections are less numerous and less detailed than those of his own, but they nevertheless paint a picture of a spectacle- and performance-oriented world, geared towards the demonstration of showy and attention-grabbing new findings. Some, along the lines of the wordmongering doctors derided by Dio, appear to have simply described dissections or vivisectory experiments that they *could* do to prove the various points they were asserting.[84] As we will see later, Galen and his ilk took delight in the public shaming of such armchair anatomists. Others, however, actually did perform such dissections, though not always to Galen's approval:

> An instance of this [ignorance of anatomy] is what we have seen in this modern age, when a physician, influenced by his method of dissecting the eye, was led to state to those concerned with the study of anatomy who attended his lectures that the uveal 'tunic' is imperforate. Meanwhile another tried to show that the heart has three chambers, and yet another demonstrated that the fetus lies outside the uterus.[85]

This passage introduces three non-Galenic dissectors, the first demonstrating on the eye, the second on the heart, and the third on the uterus. We have already met the third of these dissectors, whose refutation Galen was happy to leave in the hands of his colleague Theophrastus. As for the second, with his decidedly Peripatetic take on cardiac structure, Galen tells us that he has "already described before how he ... deceived and misled those who attended his dissection"; this is a performative dissection in which this unnamed dissector controls the optics and the outcome and argues for a very different anatomy than Galen would have done.[86] The remaining dissector from the passage, the one demonstrating the tunics of the eye, fares particularly badly in Galen's hands: He describes the

---

[84] *AA* II.641–50.

[85] *AA* S53.

[86] *AA* S53. It is difficult to locate where exactly Galen thinks that he has told this story. The only instance that I could find of his describing someone attempting to prove a three-chambered heart was in his description of the elephant dissection discussed earlier (*AA* II.619), where "many physicians" were interested to see whether the heart had "two cavities or three." However, unfulfilled cross-references are by no means unknown in the Galenic corpus, and this does not sound at all like the scenario that Galen refers to here. While the elephant dissection was a group effort, the Arabic clearly indicates that this is "*his* dissection" (النشريحه) with a dedicated audience, whom he is directly addressing and, in Galen's view, deceiving.

procedural steps that would lead to this dissector being able to demonstrate convincingly, though erroneously, that the pupil is not a perforation in the membranes of the eye. If one does not completely separate all
the layers of the eye, then the hole in the uveal layer will be masked by
the unperforated layers above and below it. Though this sort of mistake
might easily be attributed to inexperience or incompetence, Galen offers
a darker interpretation, referring to it as a "pathway of illusion" designed
to "deceive and mislead" any "ignoramus" whom he might meet "in the
course of his professional work … who has not before seen the dissection
of the eye."[87] Anatomists, at least from Galen's view of his contemporary
world, had agendas. Both for this ocular illusionist and for the Aristotelian
anatomist who engineered a demonstration of a three-chambered heart,
dissection was a powerful tool by which to take over the narrative on a
subject and promote the views of one's own sect.

Dissection also, of course, had just as much potential for spectacle in
others' hands as it did in Galen's: We should not imagine that he was the
only anatomist drawing throngs to his shows. Though he is understandably less keen to describe the crowd-pleasing feats of his rivals, one can
nevertheless get a hint of them.[88] Consider, for example, his denunciation
of the practice of Quintus, a preeminent doctor and anatomist from about
a generation before him:

> I have heard it said of Quintus that he was accustomed to carry out [the
> dissection of the testicles] on a living he-goat, which he supported upright
> [erect] so that in this position it was similar to a man. But for my personal
> opinion I am of the view that it is superfluous to dissect the testicle of a liv-
> ing animal, since that is of no use either for the study of the constitution of
> the organs … or for the investigation of any particular functions. On the
> contrary, it makes the affair harder, more difficult and more troublesome as
> regards the comprehension of the organs upon which you can quickly and
> thoroughly instruct yourself. That is because blood must then necessarily
> burst out.[89]

Though Galen focuses on the problems attendant on hemorrhage, it is not
difficult to think of other reasons why Quintus had set himself up for an
unnecessarily troublesome task. The goat would surely not appreciate either

---

[87] *AA* S54.
[88] Not just Galen's rivals but also his students and followers performed dissections of their own; see,
for example, *Sem.* IV.595 and this chapter, "Performance to Discredit Rivals" at pp. 86–90.
[89] *AA* S155. For Quintus, see Chapter 7, "Quintus and His Students: Quintus" at pp. 237–9; there is
little doubt that he would have appreciated the potential for bawdy overtones in this experiment,
judging by the colorful anecdotes recounted of him by his students.

his initial trussing up or the subsequent operation; one cannot imagine that it submitted to it in stillness or in silence. Further, as Galen points out, there does not seem to have been any practical advantage to investigating testicles in this way – laying a live, or even dead, goat on its back would surely give you as close a parallel to human anatomy as was necessary. Rather, the main advantage would have been a performative one. The similarity of the genitals of the upright goat to those of a naked man would have been both striking and titillating. The ability to peek inside these intimately personal and myste-riously powerful organs, perhaps to wince jocularly at the pain of the animal without needing to feel any true compassion, and all the while to bask in the self-satisfaction that one was participating in science and philosophy not a raunchy, lowbrow pursuit – this surely would have drawn a crowd.

Performance for Advertisement

Though the public demonstrations discussed so far were more focused on scientific and performative skills than medical ones, they clearly also redounded to the benefit of the dissector's reputation as a doctor, and some doctors deliberately tapped into this potential. Galen tells us that his skill in public performance motivated audience members to seek him out for his professional medical services. In both cases that he mentions, the public performance convinced an audience member that Galen was the most competent doctor in the specific area on which they witnessed him present. In one case, the patient – the wife of a Roman in public office – was impressed by Galen's performance in a purely oral public lecture that she attended on the coughing up of blood.[90] Upon later developing these very symptoms, she summoned Galen and entrusted herself to him. In another case, the patient, already ill, witnessed Galen performing a dissec-tion that he immediately recognized as relevant to his own case:

> I know an intelligent and wise man who selected and honored me when he saw a single act of mine: I dissected an animal by which I demonstrated the organs of the voice and the organs of locomotion. Two months earlier, that man had happened to fall from a considerable height, thus rupturing many organs in his body, and losing his voice altogether, so that his voice became like a whisper. His organs were treated, became sound and recovered after several days; yet his voice did not return. When this man saw from me what he saw, he gained con-fidence in me and entrusted himself to me. I cured him in a few days because I knew where the affected place was and attended to it.[91]

[90] *MM* X.369.
[91] *Opt.Med.Cogn.* 9.9 (*CMG Suppl.Or.* IV, p. 107, trans. Iskandar).

In both of these instances, purely academic public performance on specific medical or physiological topics garnered Galen a reputation as the most knowledgeable doctor in relation to the specific areas he had addressed. Both of the performances here are consistent with the types of public performances that he describes elsewhere – we have already seen his description of the type of contexts in which he displayed the dissection of the organs of the voice – and there is no indication that he performed on these occasions specifically to attract business to his medical practice. Indeed, Galen's carefully crafted stance of disdain for the more entrepreneurial elements of the medical craft, most pointedly fee collection, suggests that he would not have framed any of his performances as advertising.[92] He rather paints attracting patients as a perquisite of display performance, valuable mostly in that it is a further testimony to his skill and reputation.

Galen's attitude to advertisement notwithstanding, most doctors would have viewed attracting patients as an important end in its own right.[93] In addition to the rhetorical self-promotion described in Chapter 2, doctors were happy to leverage the potential for spectacle in the practical aspects of their trade in order to increase business and establish a reputation. These sorts of activities could encompass the publicizing of interesting therapies that they would have performed anyway, such as surgeries, as well as the performance of animal dissections, which were done exclusively for show. Plutarch describes public surgery for advertisement as if it were a commonplace, though perhaps reproachably venal, occurrence in the second century. In a treatise of the *Moralia* rife with medical comparisons, he says that chastising a friend in public for an error is a species of self-promotion: "for it is not friendly but sophistic to gain glory from the faults of others, showing off before bystanders, like doctors doing surgery in the theaters in order to drum up business."[94] We see hints of this also in Christian authors, who find cause to mention witnessing surgery with surprising frequency. Though the Christian references are for the most part in significantly later sources, some pointedly link such scenes to "the ancient doctors" and to Jesus' lifetime.[95]

---

[92] On Galen's attitude toward financial gain, see particularly *Opt.Med.* I.57.

[93] Arrian, *Epict.diss.* III.23.27 reports, with disdain, that the doctors of Rome have taken to advertising, rather than just waiting to be summoned by patients in need.

[94] Plutarch, *De ad. et am.* 71a (οὐ γὰρ φιλικὸν ἀλλὰ σοφιστικὸν ἀλλοτρίοις ἐνευδοκιμεῖν σφάλμασι, καλλωπιζόμενον πρὸς τοὺς παρόντας, ὥσπερ οἱ χειρουργοῦντες ἐν τοῖς θεάτροις ἰατροὶ πρὸς ἔργ ολαβίαν).

[95] See [John Chrysostom], *Eclog.* 13 (PG 63.655), for ancient doctors, and John Chrysostom, *DeChrist. div.* PG 48.804, for Jesus' lifetime; cf. John Chrysostom, *In 2 Cor.*, PG 61.506 and *Hom. In Eph.*, PG 62.132, *Sacra Parallela*, PG 96.121, and the passages discussed later in this section, and in Bliquez (1984), 194, and Nutton (1995), 18.

Two citations in Arabic of a passage from Galen's lost work *On Difficult Diseases* also present a view of a medical professional working a crowd in Rome, in this case starting with a topical treatment, and only then escalating to some minor surgery. For this particular doctor, though, the attempt backfired considerably:

> [Galen] was passing through the city of Rome and came across a man around whom a circle of ignorant people had formed. The man was saying to them: "I am one of the inhabitants of Aleppo. I have encountered Galen, and he taught me all his sciences. This is a remedy that helps against worms in the teeth." This wicked man had [previously] prepared a ball made out of tar and cotton. He placed it onto amber and fumigated the mouth of the patient who believed that he suffered from worms in his teeth. The patient had to close his eyes. Once he had closed them, this man slipped a worm into his mouth, which he had at hand in a box. Then he extracted it from the mouth of the patient suffering from tooth[ache]. After he had done this, the fools threw the things they had to him [i.e., gave him their money]. He even did more than this: he used venesection in places other than the joints.[96]

Once the quack has dared to begin venesection (unsurprisingly, incorrectly), Galen comes forward, reveals his true identity, denounces the man as a fraud, and proceeds to report him to the authorities and suggest that he be whipped. Despite the unfortunate ending for the practitioner in this case, it would seem that, for the doctor in possession of a friendly audience, spilling some blood was the *pièce de résistance*.

This predilection for gory advertisement extended to the practice of dissection. Galen recounts the plight of one of his fellow-students in Smyrna: "I wrote the three books on the motion of the thorax and lungs a long time ago when I was still a young man. I did it to oblige a schoolfellow who was returning to his hometown for an extended stay and, though he wanted to demonstrate publicly, was not himself capable of producing the display speeches."[97] This friend was intending to start his new career in

---

[96] The same passage is relayed in two different Arabic sources; for bibliographical details, see Pormann (2005), 196, which is also the source of this translation.

[97] Galen, *AA* II.217 (τὰ μέντοι περὶ θώρακος καὶ πνεύμονος κινήσεως ὑπομνήματα τρία πάλαι ποτὲ ἔγραψα, μειράκιον ὢν ἔτι, συμφοιτητῇ χαριζόμενος εἰς τὴν ἑαυτοῦ πατρίδα πορευομένῳ διὰ χρόνου πλείονος, ἐπιδείξασθαι μὲν ἐφιεμένῳ δημοσίᾳ, μὴ δυναμένῳ δὲ αὐτῷ συντιθέναι λόγους ἐπιδεικτικούς). He describes the same circumstances again at *Lib.Prop.* XIX.17 in slightly different language: "The three other books on the motion of the lungs and thorax I wrote when I was living in Smyrna to oblige a schoolfellow, who was about to return to his home town after being abroad, so that, having studied them, he could perform an anatomical display" (τρία δ᾽ ἄλλα περὶ πνεύμονος καὶ θώρακος κινήσεως, ἡνίκα ἐν Σμύρνῃ διέτριβον, ἔγραψα συμφοιτητῇ χαρισάμενος μέλλοντι μετὰ τὴν ἀποδημίαν εἰς τὴν πατρίδα πορεύεσθαι χάριν τοῦ μελετήσαντα κατ᾽ αὐτὰ ποιήσασθαί τιν᾽ ἐπίδειξιν ἀνατομικήν); following the text in Boudon-Millot (2007).

his hometown with a memorable performance. Having honed his dissection skills while studying under Pelops in Smyrna, he plans to use them to establish a dazzling reputation and large clientele for himself. As we saw, however, public dissections were prefaced by performative speeches, which amplified and explicated the bloody scene to come for the spectators. Apparently, this young man lacks the eloquence of his loquacious friend but is nevertheless determined to harness this potentially lucrative form of advertisement.

The fascination with bloodshed, however, could also be used to opposite effect. A fourth century AD Christian author describes how the "ancient doctors" used to "make a public display of their various tools" in order to frighten the healthy into taking good care to remain so and thus avoid a more intimate acquaintance with the instruments.[98] He adds that a similar effect is obtained by witnessing surgery, which John Chrysostom (*c.* AD 350–407) elsewhere describes as a both populously attended and graphically unpleasant spectacle:

> [I]n the case of doctors, when they incise or cauterize or cut open (*lit.* dissect) a maimed or weakened part in another way, and when they cut off a limb, many men stand around the patient and the doctor doing these things.... And then it is possible to see the skin being cut and the bodily fluid flowing and the putrefaction being disturbed and to endure much unpleasantness springing from this spectacle and much pain and distress, not just from the sight of the trauma, but also from the agony of the one being cauterized and cut. For no one is so stone hearted that, standing beside those suffering such things and hearing them crying aloud, he does not lament and feel troubled and experience great distress in his soul.[99]

John Jejunator (d. AD 595) similarly links public surgery with public flogging as two activities designed to be so horrific to watch as to deter socially deviant or unhealthy behavior.[100] This perspective of the Christian sources suggests another reason why animal dissection may have been a

98 [John Chrysostom], *Eclog.* 13, PG 63.655 (τοὺς ἀρχαίους τῶν ἰατρῶν ... δημοσιεύεσθαι τὴν τῶν ποικίλων ἐργαλείων ἐπίδειξιν).

99 John Chrysostom, PG 51.55 (...ἐπὶ τῶν ἰατρῶν, ἐπειδὰν τέμνωσιν, ἢ καίωσιν, ἢ καὶ ἄλλῳ τρόπῳ πεπηρωμένον καὶ ἐξησθενηκότα ἀνατέμνωνται, καὶ κατατέμνωσι μέλος, πολλοὶ περιστοιχίζονται τόν τε ἄρρωστον καὶ τὸν ταῦτα ποιοῦντα ἰατρὸν ... κἀκεῖ μὲν καὶ δέρμα ἔστιν ἰδεῖν τεμνόμενον, καὶ ἰχῶρα ῥέοντα, καὶ σηπεδόνα κινουμένην, καὶ πολλὴν ἀηδίαν ἀπὸ τῆς θεωρίας ἐγγινομένην ὑπομεῖναι, καὶ πολλὴν ὀδύνην καὶ λύπην, οὐκ ἀπὸ τῆς ὄψεως τῶν τραυμάτων μόνον, ἀλλὰ καὶ ἀπὸ τῆς ἀλγηδόνος τῶν καιομένων καὶ τῶν τεμνομένων· οὐδεὶς γὰρ οὕτω λίθινος, ὡς παρεστὼς τοῖς ταῦτα πάσχουσι, καὶ ἀκούων ὀλολυζόντων, οὐχὶ κατακλᾶται, καὶ συγχεῖται, καὶ πολλῇ τῇ ψυχῇ δέχεται τὴν ἀθυμίαν); cf. *Eclog.* 13, PG 63.656.

100 John Jejunator, PG 88.1973.

popular form of advertisement: It allowed the doctor to highlight his skill without so vividly illustrating the pain that accompanied it.[101]

Performance for Formal Public Evaluation

In addition to pieces of showmanship initiated by the doctors, like the dissections and surgeries already noted, there were also more formalized moments of public evaluation, and dissection was sometimes an element of these events. No formal system of medical credentialing existed at this period, but that does not mean that some prospective patients and – in the case of salaried positions – prospective employers were not keenly interested in assessing the competence of self-avowed medical professionals.[102] Further, the highly competitive nature of the medical marketplace would naturally lend itself to organized competitions among doctors of the sort that were common in other intellectual pursuits, so it is not at all surprising to learn of formal medical contests in the Roman Empire.[103] We know concretely of two such events, in which a group of doctors competed and a winner was judged, both of which occurred in the second century AD, one attested in literature, the other epigraphically.[104]

In the first case, Galen recounts the circumstances around his landing the job of doctor to the gladiators in Pergamon, a role he held immediately after finishing his medical training:

> Once I attended a public gathering where men had met to test the knowledge of physicians. I performed many anatomical demonstrations before the spectators; I made an incision in the abdomen of a monkey and exposed

---

[101] On the general disregard for animal pain, see Chapter 5, "Animals in the Public Eye" at pp. 145–6.

[102] Galen's *Opt.Med.Cogn.* is predicated on the assumption that patients were anxious to have a way to ensure medical competency for themselves in the absence of any professional controls. In the more public sphere, it was also laymen who were responsible for hiring public physicians, though these decisions were not necessarily based on professional skill; the papyrological examples where physicians refer to themselves as "approved" (δεδοκιμασμένοι), for example, seem to indicate an evaluation relevant to fiscal obligations carried out by laymen more concerned with bureaucratic categories than technical competency; see Lewis (1965), 87–92, Hirt Raj (2006), 109, 229–30, Israelowich (2015), 40–1, and Nutton (2019), 137, but also the dissenting opinion in Zalateo (1957).

[103] On the prevalence of organized competitions in the Roman cultural scene, see Schmitz (1997), 110–12.

[104] Nutton (1995), 7, n. 23 has also cautiously proposed that we may have tenuous evidence for a third medical competition occurring in Smyrna in the form of a damaged inscription found there that appears to contain the suggestive terms *archiatros* and *agônothetês* (Le Bas and Waddington [1870], ins. 1523). While the existence of such an event in Smyrna would be plausible, this must remain a cautious suggestion: There are other ways of restoring the words in question (see the discussion at *I. Smyrna* 874) and, as Nutton himself points out, even the more medical reconstruction does not necessarily reference a medical competition.

its intestines: then I called upon the physicians who were present to replace
them back (in position) and to make the necessary abdominal sutures—but
none of them dared to do this. We ourselves then treated the monkey,
displaying our skill, manual training, and dexterity. Furthermore, we deliberately severed many large veins, thus allowing the blood to run freely, and
called upon the Elders of the physicians to provide treatment, but they
had nothing to offer. We then provided treatment, making it clear to the
intellectuals who were present that (physicians) who possess skills like mine
should be in charge of the wounded.... I have related these [details] in order
to indicate how examiners can distinguish between skillful and unskillful
physicians, [even] before trying to examine them in oral statements and
practice.[105]

It is unclear whether some element of vivisection or sample surgery was
intended to be a part of this competition or whether Galen introduced it (and
the ill-fated monkey) on his own initiative. The implication that the examiners
needed to be prompted to consider practical tests of surgical skill as a quality
control device suggests that oral examination had been all that was planned.

It is also ambiguous whether the gathering noted in this passage was
arranged expressly for the purpose of filling the position of physician to
the gladiators or whether it was a competition purely for the sake of competition, with Galen's job-offer as incidental to his successful performance.
Though some of the language in this passage would indicate the former, the
section that immediately precedes it suggests the latter. There, he first mentions that he was given the job and quotes the high priest who hired him:

When this man was asked about his method of examining me and his confidence in me which had led him to entrust me with their care, he replied, 'I
have seen that this man has devoted more time to learning this science than
any of the Elders of the physicians. I have seen them waste their time on
useless things; but I have never seen this man spend one idle day or night.
He never ceases on any day or at any hour to train himself in something
useful. Besides, we have recently seen his practical performance which more
correctly indicates skill in this art, than the many years of the Elders.'[106]

Nothing indicates whether the "practical performance" the high priest
alludes to here is the same as the performance Galen describes in the subsequent paragraph, but the narrative order suggests that it may not have
been. This would again imply, as I inferred from the Boethus passages
for Rome, that Galen was performing public or semipublic dissections or
treatments on his own initiative immediately after his arrival in Pergamon

---

[105] Galen, *Opt.Med.Cogn.* 9.6, 8 (*CMG Suppl.Or.* IV, p. 105, trans. Iskandar).
[106] Galen, *Opt.Med.Cogn.* 9.5 (*CMG Suppl.Or.* IV, pp. 103–5, trans. Iskandar).

as a fully fledged doctor – exactly the situation he describes in the case of his less confident friend whom we considered earlier.

In the second competition, attested in a series of inscriptions from Ephesus dated to AD 138–61, it is also ambiguous whether actual demonstrations of medical skill were an intrinsic part of the competition or whether it was a purely rhetorical event.[107] The inscriptions record the names of the winners of a "competition of doctors" (ἀγὼν τῶν ἰατρῶν), which had four categories: σύνταγμα, πρόβλημα, χειρουργία, and ὄργανον. Various scholars have proposed different solutions for how to envision what happened in each of these categories.[108] On my interpretation, they formed two parallel sets.[109] The first would have been purely rhetorical, requiring the contestants to deliver prepared speeches on themes set in advance (σύνταγμα) and improvised responses on topics proposed in the moment (πρόβλημα). The second pair of categories would then have offered a parallel set of prepared and impromptu events, but with a practical rather than rhetorical focus.

The first of these categories, ὄργανον ("tool"), has been puzzling to scholars. Some maintain that it consisted of displays of newly invented instruments, but it seems far more likely to me that it was a competition in the *use* of tools.[110] I propose that contestants in this event demonstrated set skills performed on dead animals with various surgical instruments – essentially dissection, but with an emphasis on process and technical skill – making for a predictable competition that could be prepared for in advance: the surgical equivalent of a prewritten speech. In contrast, the other category, χειρουργία ("surgery"), would present vivisectory challenges, of the sort that Galen thrust upon his rivals in Pergamon, leading to a more extemporaneous test of the participants' skills.[111] It is even possible that Galen, who traveled through Asia Minor for his medical education

---

[107] *I. Ephesos* 1161–9; the inscriptions are also collected and discussed in Keil (1905), Engelmann (1990), 89–92, Samama (2003), 70–71 and nos. 211–15, and Zimonyi (2014).

[108] In addition to the authors mentioned in the note above, see Horstmanshoff (1990), 182, Barton (1994), 148, Nutton (1995), 7–8, Mattern (2008), 69–70, Gleason (2009), 89, Bliquez (2014), 16, and Zimonyi (2014).

[109] I argue for this interpretation and the other claims here at greater length in Bubb (2022).

[110] This is the suggestion of Keil (1905), 133, which Nutton (1995), 7, and Bliquez (2014), 16 follow; Samama (2003), 70 shares my skepticism. It is also quite possible that a hybrid of these two opinions is true, namely that the event could have included deploying the manipulation of dead subjects to demonstrate and showcase the uses of newly modified or invented tools; my thanks to Vivian Nutton for pressing me on this issue.

[111] It is also plausible that the subjects of these trials were actual human patients, who may even have been solicited on the spot, adding to the unpredictability. At *Purg.Med.Fac.* XI.328 Galen imagines a competition of rival physicians in a stadium-like setting where jaundiced patients would be

during precisely the period in which these inscriptions were made, was inspired to pull his stunt with the monkey at the competition in Pergamon by witnessing these or similar events. Considering the contest as a whole, it seems, even more securely than in the parallel situation in Pergamon, that this is a case of competition purely for the sake of glory. There is no mention of a prize or position offered to the winners; however, the renown of successful public performance and the publishing of the names of the winners would have redounded to the benefit of the participants – several of whom had already attained the title of *archiatros* – and thus secured their medical credentials.[112]

Performance to Discredit Rivals

Over and above these formalized moments of competition, as in the Classical and Hellenistic periods, one of the most potent competitive events for doctors in Rome was simply treating patients. It was typical for multiple doctors to appear at a Roman sickbed, not to work as a cohesive medical team, but rather to argue and advocate for their own theories and vie with each other to be entrusted with the cure by the patient or his family.[113] Successful treatment of a patient, especially when coupled with the successful disproving of a rival's opposing diagnosis, could secure one reputation and ruin another.[114] Galen allows us an intimate glimpse into this high-stakes bedside world, in particular in his treatise *On Prognosis*, which details his rise to fame in Rome.

solicited from the crowd for treatment, perhaps modeling his dreams on an event like Ephesus'. More concretely, he recounts at *SMT* XI.432–3 ordering a drug-hawker who was selling a gout medicine to make a trial of it on a random passerby whom he noticed to be afflicted with the condition; the man happily volunteered as a patient, with unfortunate results. For more examples of impromptu medical interactions, see Mattern (2008), 53–5.

112 The suggestion in Keil (1905), 138 that the competition served as a sort of repeating proto-board exam for the continued holding of the post of public physician has not found much favor; see Wolters (1908), 295, Nutton (1977), 205, and Zimonyi (2014), 360–6; but also Shlange-Schöningen (2003), 107, n. 28, who believes "es ist naheliegend anzunehmen, daß diese Wettbewerbe dazu genutzt wurden, Kandidaten für die Stellung eines städtischen 'Oberarztes' oder eben auch eines 'Gladiatorenarztes' auszuwählen."

113 Galen colorfully describes such a scene at *MM* X.110–14 in which some of the disputants are "driven to tears" (ἀναγκαζομένοις δακρύειν) (114) and at *Diff.Puls.* VIII.495 affirms that he has even seen fights break out at patients' bedsides. For a more detailed discussion of this phenomenon, see Mattern (2008), 72–92. Even when a single doctor was called, that did not ensure that he came alone; Martial *Ep.* 5.9 humorously memorializes the retinues of students that could attend doctors.

114 Indeed, Galen suggests in *Opt.Med.Cogn.* (5.5, 8.2–3, 9.1, 9.24, 13.9–10 [*CMG Suppl.Or.* IV, pp. 70, 92, 100, 116, 132–4]) that a reliable and comparatively easy way to evaluate the skill of a physician is to observe his skill in prognosis and therapy by attending him on his rounds.

Galen begins *On Prognosis* by denouncing doctors who lavish their attention on the superficial means by which they might "be held in high repute by the general public," whether flattering and toadying or outfitting themselves with expensive tools and a lavish train of followers.[115] The subsequent stories make it clear, however, that garnering a reputation is the ultimate goal of every professional interaction of a doctor, avowedly or not. Galen prides himself that his reputation rests not on superficial qualities but on his skill, though he claims that there is danger even there: A doctor who can too accurately predict the outcomes of his patients risks being accused of sorcery or being driven out of the city – or even killed! – by a cabal of jealous and inferior physicians.[116] Despite these fears, hyperbolic or no, he lost no time upon his first arrival in Rome in setting about proving to bedside audiences wherever he found them that he was superior to all of his rivals.

Galen frequently mentions the crowded and contentious scene at the bedsides of prominent Romans in this text. Much of the crowd consisted of rival doctors. He describes how one husband – none other than the anatomy-loving Boethus – gathered together the "best-reputed doctors" to treat his wife, inviting them "separately and together" to come up with the best cure; he declines to engage in the "competition through speech" attendant on another patient who "gathered together the best of the doctors in the city."[117] The crowd was not always just a medical one, though. One embittered rival of Galen's, Antigenes, alternately addresses the doctors and the "layman" at his patient's bedside, predicting to them with relish that Galen's cure will fail spectacularly.[118] Antigenes is not alone in actively monitoring Galen's medical practice for mistakes; we repeatedly hear of doctors "praying openly that [he] would fail" and "rejoicing at the [supposed] failure of [his] prediction and therapy."[119] Nor was Galen completely immune to such *Schadenfreude*. He does not resist including in his narrative all the ways in which he bested competing doctors: He describes implementing a cure that "none of the doctors in the palace had been able

---

[115] *Praen.* XIV.600 (εὐδοκιμήσειεν παρὰ τοῖς πολλοῖς).

[116] *Praen.* XIV.601–2; cf. XIV.623–4 and *Opt.Med.Cogn.* 3.3, 8.8 (*CMG Suppl.Or.* IV, pp. 52, 98).

[117] *Praen.* XIV.641 (τοὺς ἀξιολόγους ἰατρούς), 646 (ἰδίᾳ τε καὶ κοινῇ), XIV.609 (ἀθροίσας τοὺς ἀρίστους τῶν κατὰ τὴν πόλιν ἰατρῶν ... οὐ βουλόμενος ἀμιλλᾶσθαι διὰ λόγων αὐτοῖς); cf. XIV.665–9.

[118] *Praen.* XIV.614 (ταῦτα λέγων πρὸς τοὺς παρόντας ἰδιώτας, ἀποστρέφων ἐνίοτε μὲν τὸν λόγον, ἀποβλέπων τε πρὸς τοὺς ἰατρούς); cf. XIV.619.

[119] *Praen.* XIV.656 (εὐχομένων φανερῶς ἀποτυχεῖν με) (cf. XIV.616), XIV.616 (ἐπιχαίρειν αὐτούς, ὡς ἀποτετευγμένης τῆς προρρήσεώς τε καὶ θεραπείας) (cf. XIV.615); compare *Opt Med Cog* 4.1 (*CMG Suppl.Or.* IV, p. 62).

to do," healing a patient whose illness had remained inscrutable to "the most famous of the palace doctors," and uncovering psychological problems that "earlier doctors had not noticed"; and he patently rejoices that "Antigenes well-nigh disappeared into the earth on account of his reckless defamation of me and Martianus, too, just like him."[120] By the end of his first summer in residence, he tells us,

> I performed on the premier citizens of Rome predictions and therapies worthy of great praise and I had a mighty reputation with everyone, as you know, and great was the name of Galen. But jealousy grew together with my reputation among those who thought themselves to be something and those who had been bested by me in every part of the art.[121]

Renown, it would seem, was won at the expense of one's rivals.

Surgeries, as we saw in passages from Plutarch and the Christian writers in the section on advertising, were particularly suited to performative contexts and thus offered a potentially quite public form of this rivalry. Galen often mentions the results of specific surgeries as being the stuff of public knowledge and discussion, and he describes several surgeries being attended by a crowd. In one example, of which he was particularly proud, he describes how he excised the fractured sternum of a slave, revealing his beating heart. This slave had been injured in the chest several months earlier. When pus began to accumulate at the site of the injury, the slave's owner called in a doctor who operated twice but was unable to get the pus to stop or his own incisions to heal. After the failure of this first attempt, the owner cast a wider net:

> [G]athering together many doctors, in whose number I was one, he ordered us to deliberate about a cure. When it was clear to all that the problem was a suppuration of the sternum, and there appeared to also be movement of the heart in the parts to the left of it, no one dared to cut out the affected bone. For they thought that they would necessarily make a perforation in the thorax when they did it. But I said that I would do it without causing what the doctors technically call a perforation. Concerning a complete cure,

---

[120] *Praen.* XIV.625 (μηδενὸς τῶν κατὰ τὴν αὐλὴν ἰατρῶν δυναμένου τοῦτο ποιῆσαι … μηδ᾽ αὐτοῦ τῶν ἐκ τῆς αὐλῆς οἱ εὐδοκιμώτατοι τὴν διάθεσιν τοῦ νοσήματος εὕρισκον), XIV.634 (ἐλάνθανε τοὺς ἔμπροσθεν ἰατρούς), XIV.614 (ὁ οὖν Ἀντιγένης μονον οὐ κατὰ γῆς ἐδύετο διὰ τὰς προπετῶς αὐτῷ γενομένας εἰς ἐμὲ βλασφημίας· ὁμοίως δ᾽ αὐτῷ καὶ Μαρτιανὸς); compare the numerous stories in this text in which Galen advocates for a different cure than the other doctors on the case and is proved right.

[121] *Praen.* XIV.625 (καὶ τοῦ θέρους ἐπιστάντος ἐπὶ τῶν πρωτευόντων ἐν τῇ Ῥώμῃ προρρήσεις τε καὶ θεραπείας ἐποιησάμην ἀξίας ἐπαίνου μεγάλου καὶ πολλὴ δόξα παρὰ πᾶσιν ἦν, ὡς οἶσθα, καὶ μέγα τοὔνομα Γαληνοῦ. συνηυξάνετό τε τῇ δόξῃ φθόνος ἐκ τῶν οἰομένων εἶναί τι καὶ αὐτῶν ὡς ἂν ἐν παντὶ μέρει τῆς τέχνης ὑπ᾽ ἐμοῦ νικωμένων); following the text in Nutton (1979).

however, I did not promise anything, since it was unclear whether any of the parts lying under the sternum were affected and to what extent.[122]

Galen does indeed successfully excise the sternum, in the process temporarily revealing the beating heart: "the heart was as clearly visible, as in the dissection of animals when we purposefully lay it bare."[123] The borderline between performative surgery and performative dissection could be slight. The reputation at risk here, however, was far greater. Galen was careful to hedge his bets and not promise anything about the outcome for the patient, but, even with such an insurance policy available, no other doctor is confident enough in his surgical skills or the resiliency of his reputation to be willing to risk his professional name. In the event, the slave, almost unbelievably, made a full recovery, explaining why Galen is so keen to work this story into his writings, even in locations where, he admits, "it is not strictly relevant to the topic at hand."[124]

On another occasion, he mentions a doctor who had operated on the neck of a child, accidentally rendering him half-mute. This surgeon's work, however, was not his own private concern: "it seemed astonishing to everyone that, although neither the trachea nor the larynx had suffered anything, the voice had been harmed. But when the nerves associated with speech had been demonstrated by me, they ceased to be astonished."[125] Here, the surgery does not take the place of an animal dissection, but actually leads into one. Galen takes advantage of a rival's failure in order to secure a stage for an anatomical display of his own.

Indeed, using impromptu dissections to prove others wrong appears to have been something of a hobby for Galen and at least some of his contemporaries. Galen encourages his readers to use demonstrations as tools in their arguments with rivals. In the context of attacking a belief held by earlier doctors,

---

[122] *AA* II.632–3 (... πλείονας ἀθροίσας ἰατρούς, ἐν οἷς ἦν κἀγώ, σκοπεῖσθαι περὶ τῆς ἰάσεως ἐκέλευσεν. ὡς δὲ πᾶσιν ἐδόκει σφάκελος εἶναι τοῦ στέρνου τὸ πάθος, ἐφαίνετο δὲ καὶ ἡ τῆς καρδίας κίνησις ἐκ τῶν ἀριστερῶν αὐτοῦ μερῶν, οὐδεὶς ἐκκόπτειν ἐτόλμα τὸ πεπονθὸς ὀστοῦν· ᾤοντο γὰρ, ἐξ ἀνάγκης ἐπ᾽ αὐτῷ σύντρησιν ἔσεσθαι τοῦ θώρακος. ἐγὼ δ᾽ ἐκκόψειν μὲν ἔφην αὐτὸ χωρὶς τοῦ τὴν καλουμένην ἰδίως ὑπὸ τῶν ἰατρῶν σύντρησιν ἐργάσασθαι· περὶ μέντοι τῆς παντελοῦς ἰάσεως οὐδὲν ἐπηγγελλόμην, ἀδήλου ὄντος, εἰ πέπονθε καὶ μέχρι πόσου πέπονθε τῶν ὑποκειμένων τι τῷ στέρνῳ); see also another version of the same story, which is fragmentary in the Greek (*PHP* V.181–2) but survives in full in two different Arabic versions (De Lacy [1978–84] 73–7).

[123] *PHP* V.181 (I.5.1 De Lacy) (ἦν οὕτω σαφῶς θεάσασθαι τὴν καρδίαν ὡς κἂν ταῖς τῶν ζῴων ἀνατομαῖς, ἐπειδὰν ἑκόντες αὐτὴν γυμνώσωμεν).

[124] *AA* II.632 (μὴ τῆς παρούσης πραγματείας ἴδιόν ἐστι).

[125] *Loc.Aff.* VIII.55 (θαυμαστὸν ἐδόκει πᾶσιν, ὅτι μήτε τῆς τραχείας, μήτε τοῦ λάρυγγος παθόντων τι, τὴν φωνὴν βλαβῆναι συνέβη· δειχθέντων δ᾽ αὐτοῖς ὑπ᾽ ἐμοῦ τῶν φωνητικῶν νεύρων, ἐπαύσαντο θαυμάζοντες).

he admonishes his readers to "be sure to expose the erroneous character of this belief and overcome its supporters, refuting and confounding their arguments by the following demonstration."[126] This is precisely the sort of dissection-as-education or -argument tactic that he deployed in the previous anecdote about the botched larynx operation. It seems descriptive, too, of his demonstrations "to naysayers" on the heart and brain and his perhaps not completely welcomed demonstrations on the presence of urine in the ureters.[127]

This urge to publicly outperform and humiliate rivals was completely in keeping with the times. We hear of similar antics among intellectual circles of the period, where impromptu public ordeals and subsequent mockery were a matter of course, and we know that it was an unremarkable practice in medical circles as well.[128] Galen tells us, for example, that he once was the victim of such behavior.[129] Innocently stumbling upon the disquisition of a gymnastic trainer who was criticizing Hippocrates' opinions on massage, he was asked by the doctors and philosophers in the audience to offer a Hippocratic rebuttal. After Galen had got well on his eulogistic way, the gymnast, by now apparently foaming at the mouth with rage, dragged forward a young slave, stripped him naked, and demanded that Galen offer an impromptu massage demonstration or else hold his tongue on the subject. Not to be outmaneuvered, Galen manages to gracefully demur, observing cuttingly that no one would ever be so idiotic as to ask Hippocrates to go into the kitchen and cook a sauce before agreeing to trust his advice on dietetics. The gymnast had not appreciated that he was taking on a master of aggressive, impromptu challenges.

Galen's hackles are particularly raised by speculative or "armchair" anatomists and by those who claim results without following up with a demonstrated proof. He describes "a certain very grand seventy-year-old man" who claimed that he had a method of proving that the arteries are naturally empty of blood, a central Erasistratean claim.[130] Though

---

[126] *AA* S264.

[127] This may also have been the case with Theophrastus' refutation of the supposedly extra-uterine fetus (discussed earlier in this chapter in "Performance for Public Display" at p. 71), though Galen does not say whether he used his own dissection or not in his refutation.

[128] Compare, for example, Gellius, *NA* XV.9 (cf. XIII.31) in which Gellius gets into a public argument with a deprecating grammarian; when challenged to bolster his side of the debate with linguistic theory, he turns the tables and challenges the grammarian in turn to say a word that breaks the paradigm Gellius has championed. The grammarian, while attempting to laugh the matter off, is patently stumped and put to shame before the crowd.

[129] *Thras.* V.894–5.

[130] *AA* II.644 (γέρων τις ἑβδομηκοντούτης πάνυ σεμνός). The degree of sarcasm to be read into the phrase "very grand" (πάνυ σεμνός) is unclear, but probably fairly high. Garofalo (1991*b*), 699

he described the necessary vivisection in great detail, Galen claims that "that man, despite having been around for seventy years, never dared to actually put this procedure to the test."[131] As soon as he hears of the proposed experiment, however, Galen immediately carries out the preparatory steps, both on a goat and a cow, and brings the prepared animals to the old man. He then appears to have done the final, conclusive, step of the vivisection in front of him, forcing him (and no doubt a crowd eager for the humiliation that would follow one way or another) to witness that his claims were false.[132]

Aggressive as that episode might seem, it turns out that Galen was being comparatively nice. More humiliating by far were the occasions when boastful anatomists were forced to themselves attempt dissections on the spot. Galen was particularly relentless in this practice. Criticizing doctors who assert the effects of ligating the pulmonary vein, a procedure that he declares to be impossible, he says that these men were incapable of even exposing the heart without killing the animal – and he knows, because he publicly forced them to try. And when they failed to expose the heart of the first animal, he then got another animal, "easily" exposed the heart for them, and "compelled" them to proceed with the ligation.[133] When they failed again, making a further perforation in their attempts, they tried to get out of the ordeal, saying it was not necessary to try it again. Galen, however, was inexorable: "But I swiftly again, on another animal, laying bare the heart presented it to them, and forced them to try again until they should have disgraced themselves over the things they had falsely bragged about."[134] Nor was he the only doctor travelling to arguments with a small herd of future vivisectory subjects in tow.[135]

translates it straightforwardly as "assai serio" and identifies the man as the Erasistratean Martianus, whom Galen mentions as a rival in *Praen.* (see this chapter, n. 120); while the advanced age in both cases makes this identification plausible, it is not necessary to believe that there was only one Erasistratean with an interest in anatomy at the time (see Chapter 7, "Anatomy in the Roman Intellectual Scene"at pp. 265–6). Singer (1956), 198, however, follows the more negative meaning (*LSJ* III) and renders it as "pompous." Given that this paragraph immediately follows one about a man who invented, for the same purpose, a device that Galen dismisses as fodder for comic writers, I am more sympathetic to Singer's interpretation.

[131] *AA* II.645 (ἐκεῖνος μὲν οὖν, ἑβδομήκοντα γεγονὼς ἐτῶν, τὴν ἐγχείρησιν ταύτην οὐδέποτ᾽ ἐτόλμησεν ἔργῳ βασανίσαι).

[132] For the outcome going the other way, compare *AA* S266 where the man who introduces the argument is the one proved wrong through dissection before a large crowd.

[133] *AA* II.637 (ῥᾳδίως; βιάζονται).

[134] *AA* II.637 (ἀλλ᾽ ἡμεῖς τε ἐν τάχει πάλιν ἐφ᾽ ἑτέρου ζῴου γυμνώσαντες αὐτοῖς τὴν καρδίαν παρέχομεν, ἀναγκάζομέν τε πάλιν ἐγχειρεῖν, ἄχρι περ ἂν ἀσχημονήσωσιν ἐφ᾽ οἷς ἠλαζονεύσαντο).

[135] Immediately after this passage in *AA* II.637, he mentions that "one of [his] companions" refuted another doctor in a similar way "in front of many witnesses."

Galen recounts, with evident pride, the similarly aggressive antics of some of his students.[136] The target here was another group of boastful Erasistrateans. Apparently, they had been for some time publicly proclaiming that they could demonstrate a great artery (i.e., aorta) empty of blood, without ever following through on the promise and performing the demonstration. Galen's students decided to humiliate them and they came prepared, furnishing themselves in advance with several animals and a large amount of money. The young men approach the ringleader of the group and provide him with an animal, demanding that he make good his promise. The man refuses them, saying that he only performs for a fee. They "immediately" whip out their purse of money – the adverb suggesting a certain glee at having so cannily foreseen this objection – and offer one thousand drachmas as a prize if he succeeds.[137] One can imagine the buzz of excitement among the "people thronged to the spectacle" as the stakes are thus raised.[138] Cornered, the erstwhile boaster does his best to wiggle out of the situation, but, "being forced by all those present," he eventually picks up the knife.[139] He botches the job immediately. Another of his companions steps up to have a try and meets with equal failure, with the result that he is mocked by the Galenic youths, who then proceed to deftly vivisect another animal, exposing the artery and ligaturing it on either side so that its *in vivo* contents can be accurately exposed. They cut the vessel, proving that it is full of blood, leaving their opponents sputtering that the experiment – which, the Galenists point out, they themselves had proposed – was flawed.

Another group of people who had seen some of Galen's work engaged in a similar, though more impromptu, exercise. Upon hearing someone expound incorrectly on one of Galen's own experiments, these better-informed audience members question his credentials:

> Those who had seen me do the procedure were astonished at his audacity and asked him if he himself had done [the procedure] or if he was trusting someone whom he had heard describe it. He said that he had done it very often indeed. So then, escorting in a goat, they forced him to show it. When he did not want to (because he did not know how), they showed to those

---

[136] The episode occurs at *AA* II.642–3. Galen refers to the actors only as "ambitious youths" (φιλοτιμοτέρων νεανίσκων), but he mentions later in the passage that they are performing the operation "as they had seen it at my side" (ὡς ἑωράκεισαν παρ᾽ ἐμοί), making their identification as students reasonable.

[137] *AA* II.642 (αὐτίκα).

[138] *AA* II.643 (τοῖς ἠθροισμένοις ἐπὶ τὴν θέαν).

[139] *AA* II.642 (πολλὰς μὲν ἀπορῶν ἐστρέφετο στροφάς· ἀναγκαζόμενος δ᾽ ὑπὸ πάντων τῶν παρόντων, ἐτόλμησε λαβὼν σμίλην τέμνειν).

present that the facts held in the opposite way and thus stopped his false pretentions from then on.[140]

In this case, the goat had to be found. This humiliation, unlike the previous one, was not premeditated and is framed much less aggressively than the others. The skilled dissectors gave the impostor a chance to back away from his claim, but, once he compounded his lies, they had no choice but to let the facts speak for themselves. The particularly striking thing here is that this rhetorically minded doctor had already drawn to himself a crowd of listeners as he expounded on anatomical topics – the content alone, even without the illustrative dissection, was a popular draw. That some of those he attracted were more competent in the subject than he is testifies still more to the popularity of anatomy. In any given scientifically minded crowd some might, unbeknownst to the others, be skilled anatomists. And those who were not saw it in their best interests to pretend to be.

---

[140] *AA* II.645–6 (θαυμάζοντες οὖν αὐτοῦ τὴν τόλμαν οἱ τεθεαμένοι παρ' ἐμοὶ τὴν ἐγχείρησιν ἠρώτων, εἴποτ' αὐτὸς ἐποίησεν αὐτήν, ἢ διηγουμένου τινὸς ἀκούσας ἐπίστευσεν. ὁ δὲ καὶ πάνυ πολλάκις ἔφη πεποιηκέναι. κομίσαντες οὖν αἶγα αὐτῷ δεικνύειν ἠνάγκαζον. ὡς δ' οὐκ ἐβούλετο, διότι μηδ' ἠπίστατο, δείξαντες τοῖς παροῦσιν ἐναντίως ἔχον τὸ φαινόμενον, ἔπαυσαν οὕτως τῆς εἰς τὸ λοιπὸν ἀλαζονείας).

CHAPTER 4

Practical Considerations of the Dissector

The dissection of the dead, although not cruel, is nevertheless nasty.
Celsus, *On Medicine*[1]

Reading accounts of dissection from centuries past, it is easy to gloss over the intense sensory impact they would have had on the participants. Dissectors of the ancient world would not have had recourse to refrigeration, anesthetics, or adequate artificial light: Displays of dissection would have been bloody, malodorous, and, no doubt, flyridden events to observe, and vivisections would have had the added elements of sound and struggle, as the animals protested their fate.[2] The dissector himself would have had further distasteful sensations as he manipulated the bodies and accomplished his tasks. Galen, the author to whom we owe the most details on the topic, is matter of fact and allows only the slightest hints of this reality to impinge on his descriptions, but it is not difficult to read the gore and stench between the lines.

In the first place, the dissector had to become comfortable with repeatedly killing animals. In a predominantly agrarian society with a robust and long-ingrained custom of animal sacrifice this would hardly be an outlandish requirement – certainly far less so than to the modern reader.[3] However, the deaths here are neither ritualized nor quick. For many dissections, Galen recommends that the animals be suffocated, either by strangulation or by drowning, which allows the vascular system to retain all of its blood for observation.[4] Though no doubt much of this preparatory slaughter was

---

[1] Celsus, *DM* proem.44 (mortuorum … [laceratio] etsi non crudelis, tamen foeda sit).

[2] Anesthetic drugs did exist (cf. Galen, *Comp.Med.Loc.* XIII.93; Dioscorides, IV.75.7), but evidence for their use is conflicting; see Bliquez (2014), 20–22 for a recent discussion. Given the prevalent views on animal treatment (see Chapter 5, "Animals in the Public Eye" at pp. 145–6), however, and the attested practice of human surgery without analgesics, it is very difficult to imagine that they would ever have been administered to animals. Further, the vivisections often require activity of some sort on the part of the subject, making the use of anesthetic as impractical as improbable.

[3] See Chapter 5, "Animals in the Public Eye" at pp. 145–7 and "Religious Practices" at pp. 152–3.

[4] See *AA* II.233, 423, S46; he canvasses several different ways to kill animals at *AA* II.701.

behind the scenes and left to underlings, Galen does advocate involvement on the part of the dissector – "you yourself should at some time choke an animal to death, either by using a noose or by immersing it in water."[5] Death by suffocation is a longer and more physically brutal affair than the swift and precise cut of the butcher or priest.

Far more brutal, however, is death by vivisection, a death in which both dissector and audience are implicated. It is in this area that Galen's few concessions to the potential squeamishness of his audience are to be found. In the most explicit of these, he instructs the reader engaged in the vivisection of the brain that "the cut should without pity or compassion penetrate the deep tissues … with this incision it frequently happens that the outflow of blood is such that the operator can be disheartened from renewing and finishing his dissection. But that need not make you timid."[6] The reluctance of a novice vivisector is easily understandable. The animals were typically strapped down to wooden boards with ropes or restrained by the hands of assistants, but they were not sedated in any way and, especially for the larger animals, immobilizing them and keeping them immobilized was no doubt a fairly difficult and even dangerous task.[7] Beyond these practical considerations, it was clearly also emotionally distasteful. Galen, hardened as he must have been to such scenes, mentions the screams of pain and "transient agony" of the animals, some of which were partially skinned alive in the process of their vivisection.[8] Though he discusses these elements without any emotion, even he was clearly shaken by the vivisection of monkeys. Their close resemblance to humans, which is elsewhere such a benefit, here becomes intolerable. He warns his readers on four occasions that the vivisection of monkeys should not be attempted – it is "a hideous spectacle," "loathsome" and "unpleasing."[9]

In addition to the evident suffering of the animals, as the quote about cutting without pity makes clear, there was an enormous amount of blood to contend with. Hemorrhaging, and the resulting loss of life or consciousness, was a procedurally undesirable outcome in vivisections, where the animal needed to be alive and properly functioning so that its physiology

---

[5] *AA* S46. For the outsourcing of menial tasks, see *AA* II.233.
[6] *AA* S19.
[7] See *AA* II.627, S24.
[8] Screams of pain at *AA* II.680; agony at S129; skinning alive at II.678; see also S81, where he described starving the animal prior to vivisection so it will be motivated to eat or drink after the operation, "though at first it can scarcely do either."
[9] *AA* II.690 (εἰδεχθές τ' εἶναι τὸ θέαμα), S18, 107, 109 ("leave the live apes [*sic*] alone").

could be observed. It is therefore unsurprising that Galen frequently offers advice or caution in areas where hemorrhage is particularly likely.[10] These warnings serve to underscore the goriness of the task at hand. He repeatedly describes consequences of an ill-placed cut, whether in the living animal or the newly dead: Blood will "spurt over," "bespatter," and "pour over" the hapless dissector, sometimes in "great quantity."[11] Even when less volatile, it lies in wait ready to "stream out," "gush out," and otherwise obstruct orderly dissection.[12]

The presence of flowing blood, however, was likely a welcome alternative to the cloying putrefaction that accompanied older, drier bodies. Especially in the summer heat of Rome, the stench must have been powerful. Galen mentions that he typically dissected the soft internal organs of his specimens immediately after killing them since they could not remain uncorrupted more than a day – though even the uncorrupted intestines of a freshly killed monkey, which he suggests you remove and "manipulate" extensively, would have been a putrid handful.[13] Despite this awareness, older specimens found themselves under the knife; Galen criticizes the practice, but also offers tips, including kneading stiffened muscles and pouring hot water over them to make them more pliable.[14]

Finally, the act of dissection did not consist merely in delicate cuts and dispassionate observation. Physical violence was sometimes required, especially in the opening of the thoracic cavity or in the breaking of bones. Though the "bone-breaker" was no doubt a merciless tool, Galen's instructions to rip open various parts of the rib cage with one's bare hands have a more brutal quality.[15] Indeed, he recognizes that it will likely take some time before a novice gains sufficient confidence in his manual strength to "tear away the clavicle in its entirety."[16] Beyond feats of strength, he expects the dissector to have no compunction about putting his hands to use, ripping apart muscles with his nails and pinching off hemorrhages with his fingers.[17] Dissection, in short, whether in execution or observation, was not for the faint of heart.

---

[10] *AA* II.599, 628, 639–40, 681, S24, 128.
[11] *AA* S128, 183, 197; cf. S155 where it "burst[s] out" during the vivisection of goat testicles.
[12] *AA* S191, 302–3, 316.
[13] *AA* II.505; II.567 (μεταχειριζομένῳ).
[14] Criticism at *AA* II.243; advice at II.251–2, 427–8.
[15] Bone breaker at *AA* S24; forcing open by hand at II.604, 608.
[16] *AA* S199; compare II.608 where he describes having bent open the rib cage "so violently" (βιαίως οὕτως) that some bones were broken.
[17] *AA* II.696; II.629.

For those who chose to engage in this bloody pursuit, some preparation was necessary. I will discuss the pedagogical guidance and background knowledge required for the practice in Chapter 9; here, I focus on the more concrete, physical requirements. The most detailed and explicit source for the practicalities of ancient dissection is Galen's *Anatomical Procedures*, and the following discussion will therefore focus specifically on how to dissect according to the program that he lays out there. What remains to us of the work of his predecessors and contemporaries is basically silent on the topic of *how* to dissect, and Galen's discussion of their practices is too limited to allow for a systematic look at the details of dissection outside of Galen. At most, his comments suggest that simian subjects were less common with other anatomists, but he certainly does not tout his basic procedures as materially different from standard practice.[18] He is never shy about highlighting improvements he has developed, so it seems comparatively safe to infer that his silence in this case means that the practices we have insight into here are grossly representative.[19]

At fifteen books, *Anatomical Procedures* is a comprehensive practical guide to the process of dissection, but, despite this procedural slant, it does not offer an introductory discussion of the materials required, but rather addresses each item (or not) as it comes up in the course of the book. Nevertheless, the text allows the reader to gather or infer a great deal about the practical necessities of dissection. For the purposes of discussion in this chapter, I have divided these prerequisites into two groups. The first and most important group consists of the anatomical subjects. Without a body to work on, dissection cannot occur, but Galen is flexible, though opinionated, about the species his readers can use. I consider first his discussion of monkeys, his preferred subjects, followed by that of other animals; in each case, I describe his guidelines and then offer social context for the acquisition of the animals he describes, including their price. Finally, I consider the controversial question of the use of human subjects. The second group of desiderata is more mixed and, for the most part, less

---

[18] Rufus, *Nom.Part.* 127, however, confirms that monkeys were already widely regarded as the ideal subjects in his day, and the half of the text that it introduces is linked to a concurrent dissection of a monkey (though no directions for dissection are given); however, the same passage does also include some discussion of alternative animals. See Chapter 7, "Rufus of Ephesus" at p. 223.

[19] Webster (forthcoming) makes the fascinating claim that development in the technology of medical instruments directly fed into the burgeoning of dissection as a heuristic methodology in the Roman period. It is certainly the case that evidence for medical tools is much richer for the late Hellenistic and Roman periods than for earlier times – a fact that further informs my choice to focus on Galenic evidence for this discussion of the practicalities of dissection.

essential. I begin with tools, highlighting the bare necessities, but covering the entire rage of implements he describes as useful; as with the animals, I include some discussion of how such tools might be acquired. Next, I discuss the books that he assumes his readers must have, focusing here on their accessibility and price, rather than their contents, which I will address in Part II. Finally, I consider the human assistants that Galen employs, and the ways in which such help might have been useful or necessary for other, less spectacle-oriented dissectors.

Anatomical Subjects

Monkeys

Galen repeatedly tells his readers that monkeys are the best subjects of dissection for a person wishing to gain insight into human anatomy.[20] The vast majority of the dissections he includes are described in terms of the simian body. As a result, he gives some care to issuing instructions for identifying which monkeys are the best for dissection. Certainly, it is clear that Galen expects his readers to purchase the monkeys live, since he repeatedly gives instructions on how to kill them. Different methods of slaughter are required for different types of dissection. Strangling and drowning have the advantage that they leave the animal's blood supply intact, which makes the arteries and veins easier to study.[21] Often he requires that the reader perform his dissection immediately after the death of the animal while its joints and membranes are still supple, but sometimes he specifies that the reader should choke the monkey in the evening and let it sit all night before dissecting it in the morning.[22] If the blood vessels will not be under consideration, however, it is usually preferable to kill the animal in such a way that the blood can be allowed to drain out so that it will not obscure the subsequent observations; this results in a "bloodless" animal as opposed to the "full-blooded" animals that have been suffocated in some way.[23] It is understandable, then, that there is considerable importance attached to the dissector's ability to control the method of killing.

---

[20] *AA* II.219, 430, 535, 548.

[21] See *AA* II.233, 423, S46. For the advantages of drowning, see II.233, 423.

[22] For examples of immediate dissection, see *AA* II.243, 251–2, 352–3, 473, 584, 623, S182, 183. For animals required to be left overnight, see S191, S207, S316.

[23] For example, at *AA* II.604. The distinction between full-blooded (πολύαιμος) and bloodless (ὀλίγαιμος) is made repeatedly, as for example at II.353.

There are some instances, however, where Galen acknowledges that his readers might not have total control over the state of their monkey. At one point he speaks of "procuring" a "newly-dead monkey," suggesting that they could be bought, found, or otherwise acquired already dead.[24] Again, he later seems to imply that the dissector is working at the whim of outside factors; he says "you must *try to arrange* that the animal which you dissect has already been dead for one day in advance. But *should it happen that* it has only just died on the self-same day [take the following measures]."[25] He is usually explicit about his expectation that dissections will take place within a few hours of the animal's death while it is still supple, but, as we saw earlier, he does offer suggestions for how to make the best of an animal that has already stiffened from rigor mortis.[26] All this implies that the monkey supply in Rome was not always as constant or reliable as Galen would have wished it to be.[27]

Despite these hints of dissatisfaction, Galen generally anticipates a fair amount of choice to be available to his readers in their simian purchases. He expects a variety of species to be for sale and therefore gives thorough advice on how to identify the monkeys most like man and therefore most appropriate for dissection, explaining how to differentiate them from other species, particularly the baboon.[28] He also expects his readers to have some choice in the physical characteristics of the monkeys they buy, beyond simply their species. At various times he specifies the ideal weight, size, age, and prominence of veins for specific dissections.[29] Though he does make concessions to the possibility that his readers might not have access to every variety along these lines that he wishes, he still expects them to be able to command some sort of choice. He says, for example: "Therefore, one should perhaps avoid [newborns] for this inquiry. Those [monkeys] that are thin from old age are the most suitable of all.... But if it should be necessary to choose between a pair of unsuitable animals, another not being available, it is better to choose the newborn than the large and fat one."[30]

---

[24] *AA* S13.

[25] *AA* S207; my emphasis.

[26] Expectation that the animal will be supple: *AA* II.243, 251–2, 352–3, 473, 584, 623, S182, 183; suggestions for softening at II.251–2, 427–8.

[27] In at least one case, though, it was Galen's busy schedule rather than the supply of monkeys that was at fault: At *Loc.Aff.* VIII.303 he explains that he was only able to get around to dissecting a progressively emaciating monkey after it died, "on account of unavoidable professional engagements" (δι' ἀσχολίας ἡμῶν ἀναγκαίας).

[28] *AA* II.222–3, 533–4, S13.

[29] Weight: *AA* II.353, 381, 500, S94; size: II.375, 500, S94; age: II. 425–6, 500, S16; prominence of veins: II.381.

[30] *AA* II.426 (διόπερ ἄν τις εἰκότως φεύγοι τὰ τοιαῦτα κατὰ τὴν προκειμένην ἐγχείρησιν· ὅσα δ' ὑπὸ γήρως ἰσχνά, πάντων ἐπιτηδειότατα ... εἰ δὲ καὶ ἐκ δυοῖν ζῴων ἀνεπιτηδείων αἱρεῖσθαι

Indeed, though Galen implies, and common sense corroborates, that monkeys were more expensive and more difficult to procure than general livestock, they may not have been as expensive or elusive as the modern reader imagines.[31]

There were several species of monkey available in imperial Rome, though the most popular by far was the tailless Barbary macaque (*Macaca sylvanus*), which was Galen's top pick for dissection.[32] Monkeys in general, and the Barbary macaque in particular, were quite popular as pets, and therefore must have been obtainable by the general public.[33] One of Martial's epigram gift-tags, for example describes a tailless monkey, which would very likely have belonged to this species.[34] Indeed, a passage in Pliny the Elder may suggest that monkeys were actually bred in Italy. He describes the fierce affection that they feel for their young and says, "they carry about the infants, to which tamed and domesticated females have given birth, and show them to

---

δεήσειεν, ἑτέρου μὴ παρόντος, ἄμεινον αἱρεῖσθαι τὸ νεογενὲς τοῦ μεγάλου καὶ πιμελώδους); following the text in Garofalo (1986–2000).

[31] At *AA* II.226–27 Galen acknowledges that his readers might have to use other animals than monkeys out of necessity. Scholars generally consider monkeys rare commodities and perhaps available to Galen only because of his wealth and social position; see Garofalo (1994), 1808, Grmek (1996), 103, Rocca (2002), 90 and (2003), 71–2, and Mattern (2013), 150–1. The notable exception is Eichholz (1951), 66–7, who says that in Galen's discussion of his expenditure he does not mention "equipment for experimental research, possibly because the materials required, animals and instruments, were not unduly expensive." This reasoning, however, is flawed, given that the passage he is referencing (*Aff.Pecc.Dig.* V.48) is advice that Galen gives to a nonmedical friend, with some autobiographical details, on what the uses of a gentleman's excess income ought to be, not a description of his own spending.

[32] Singer (1956), xxi suggests that much of Galen's work was actually done on the Rhesus monkey, on the grounds that the Barbary macaque was "never as common or as widespread as the Rhesus monkey, which is smaller and much easier to handle." Jennison (1937), 20, McDermott (1938), 28–29, 55, 97, and Toynbee (1973), 56, however, all agree that the Barbary macaque was the most common species available in the western Mediterranean. Singer also supports his claim with the weightier reason that he finds some of the anatomy Galen describes to accord better with Rhesus monkeys than Barbary macaques. This, too, should perhaps be taken with a grain of salt, since Singer himself used Rhesus monkeys, more readily available to modern dissectors, for his recreations of Galen's dissections, but it would not be surprising if some of Galen's descriptions were of Rhesus monkeys, since he used a variety of species. Older scholarship often uses the outdated classifications *Macaca inuus* or *Inuus ecaudatus* for the Barbary macaque and refers to it as the Barbary ape. This terminology is misleading, as the animal is in the monkey family (*Cercopithecidae*). In fact, when Galen uses his all-purpose word πίθηκος, he is almost certainly always referring to monkeys rather than apes. Though earlier scholars were seduced by Galen's descriptions of his specimens' tight homology with humans into claiming that Galen used anthropoid apes such as the chimpanzee at least occasionally, there is no reason to believe that Galen ever had any contact with a true ape; see McDermott (1938), 97 for a more detailed discussion.

[33] See generally Jennison (1937), 127–9, McDermott (1938), 131–6, Toynbee (1973), 55–7, and Lewis and Llewellyn-Jones (2018), 462–71.

[34] Martial, XIV.202.

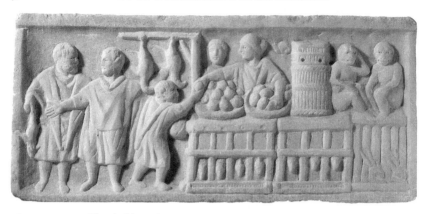

Figure 4.1   Marble relief from the Via della Foce at Ostia, late second century AD, Museo Ostiense (inv. 134). Image: © Archivio Fotografico del Parco Archeologico di Ostia Antica.

everyone."[35] Though it remains ambiguous whether he is discussing monkeys domesticated in Italy specifically, if that were the case, it would certainly have brought down their price. Regardless, people of all stations appear to have owned monkeys as pets, including butchers, sailors, merchants, and shopkeepers.[36] The sign for a shop at Ostia selling fruit, poultry, and small game (Figure 4.1), for example, includes two unrestrained, tailless monkeys sitting on the shop counter, seemingly there as store mascots: Given their inclusion on the shop sign, not to mention the engaging way that the artist has depicted them staring directly at the onlooker, one imagines that they were purchased as something of a marketing investment. Zooarchaeological evidence, too, confirms that simian pets are not merely a literary fiction – the juvenile Barbary macaque whose skeleton was found among human remains

---

[35] Pliny, *NH* VIII.80(54).216 (gestant catulos quae mansuefactae intra domos peperere. omnibus demonstrant...). Jennison (1937), 128 feels it likely that Pliny is giving an eyewitness account of monkeys he saw in Italy; Rocca (2002), 90, n. 29, however, dismisses the claim that domesticated monkeys were bred at all. Compare Plutarch, *Per.* 1.1, where Augustus objects to seeing "wealthy women in Rome carrying around the offspring of dogs and monkeys at their breasts and caressing them" (ξένους τινὰς ἐν Ῥώμῃ πλουσίους κυνῶν ἔκγονα καὶ πιθήκων ἐν τοῖς κόλποις περιφέροντας καὶ ἀγαπῶντας), indicating the availability and popularity of infant monkeys in the city.

[36] See Phaedrus, *Fab.* III.4 for the butcher, *Fabulae Aesopicae Collectus* 363 (Halm) for the sailor, and Timotheus, *Anim.* 51 for the merchant (cited, among others, in McDermott [1938], 134); for the shopkeeper, see Toynbee (1973), 56–7. Though we know nothing specific about the workings of the monkey trade in Rome, Galen implies that groups of monkeys were at least sometimes displayed in areas that were fairly large; he expects it to be possible for prospective buyers to be able to see monkeys "running swiftly" (τοῦ δρόμου τὸ τάχος) and says that seeing one running upright is a reliable indication that it would be a good subject for dissection (*AA* II.533).

at Pompeii was likely a pet of some kind, as were those whose traces remain at multiple different sites in Roman Britain, France, Germany, and Spain.[37]

A dedicated dissector would have quickly attained a privileged relationship with his purveyor of monkeys, given the rate at which Galen expects his readers to buy them. At various points in the text it becomes clear that Galen requires the reader to have switched to a new specimen, either because he gives instructions for how to kill it immediately before beginning the dissection, or because he assumes that the reader will have a fresh start on an area that had been cut up previously.[38] Occasionally he does say that he wants the reader to do several operations in a row on the same animal, but he makes it clear that this is a deviation from the norm.[39] In fact, for one investigation he requires the dissector to have two monkeys at once in order to use one as a guide.[40] Further, given the climate and lack of refrigeration in the Mediterranean, any one carcass would only have been fresh enough to use for a short time. As a result of these factors, not to mention Galen's frequent exhortations to practice and repeat, it would take dozens of monkeys to complete the course set out in *Anatomical Procedures*.[41]

In addition to this stream of live monkeys, Galen suggests having some monkey skeletons and skulls on hand to serve as guides for the underlying structure of the more recently killed animal that is being dissected. He says that he keeps "many skulls in [a fleshless] condition, some of them intact, others having had the upper parts of the cranium removed," and that he has "always at hand a large number of specially prepared bones of monkeys."[42] He prepares these bones himself by burying the bodies of monkeys in moist earth for four months and allowing all the tissues to decompose; he suggests that his readers do the same in order to gain a deeper understanding of bone structures, in particular for the skull and vertebrae.[43] This implies that Galen

---

[37] On Pompeii, see Bailey et al. (1999); on Britain, see Armour-Chelu (1997), 358 for a jawbone found in Wroxeter, and Hodgson (1990) for a piece of skull found at Catterick and reference to other finds, including a skull found at Dunstable; on the remains from Spain, which derive from the complete burial of what seems to have been a military mascot in Iulia Libica, see Lewis and Llewellyn-Jones (2018), 470, where they also mention remains found in France (Poitiers) and Germany (Rainau-Buch).

[38] For example, at *AA* II.308, 348.

[39] *AA* II.520, S297.

[40] *AA* S85–6.

[41] For examples of exhortations to practice and repeat, see *AA* II.289–90, 384–5, S16, 146, 159–60. As for the number of animals required, Galen makes it clear that he has dissected countless animals over the course of his career (II.278), even saying that not one in a thousand animals display a particular variation that he reports (II.652). Though that is probably a hyperbolic statement, it does point to the order of magnitude of animals that he dealt with.

[42] *AA* S33 and 230, respectively.

[43] *AA* S229–30.

expected the best-equipped dissector to have some land available to be specifically dedicated to the burial and exhumation of monkeys.

Other Animals

For those who cannot afford or cannot get access to monkeys, Galen offers
alternatives. He says that if for some reason the reader is lacking in monkeys he can use other animals, as long as he is aware of the differences
they present.[44] He explains that there is a clear and established hierarchy
of six classes of animals that are suitable for this kind of dissection based
on their similarities to human anatomy.[45] Macaques and other simian animals, including baboons and smaller tree monkeys, are the best in all circumstances, but the remaining five categories are bears, pigs, saw-toothed
animals (which roughly equate to carnivores), horned ruminants (particularly goats and bovines), and unhorned animals with an undivided hoof,
such as horses. For the most part he tacitly assumes that his reader is using
a monkey, but he will occasionally reiterate this assumption or explain the
differences between monkeys and other animals.[46] These explanations are
not frequent, thorough, or universal enough, though, to make the whole
of the directions easily adaptable for someone not using a monkey.[47]

There are some dissections, however, for which Galen affirmatively prefers other animals. The most common reason is that the organ under consideration is too small to be adequately inspected in a monkey.[48] In some
of these cases, the dissection of a larger animal should act as training for
the dissection of the area in the monkey, rather than as a replacement for
it, doubling the expense and effort; he is particularly insistent on this point

---

[44] *AA* II.226–7. At II.535–6 he gives more specific instructions for animals to try if you cannot get a
good monkey, starting with those monkeys which look less like man. At II.291 he condemns the
practice of dissecting ox parts without understanding their differences from human parts.

[45] *AA* II.375, 422–3, 430–1, 535–6, 547–8, S34, 90, with some variations of order among them; see
Garofalo (1991c) and Salas (2020), 111–18 for discussion of this classification system.

[46] See *AA* II.526 for an example of reiterating the expectation of a monkey and S248 where he explicitly
addresses the fact that his reader might have been working with another animal, such as a goat.

[47] He explains differences between monkeys and other animals at *AA* II.422, 428–30, 445, 495, 530, 556,
560, 570, 573, 655, 692, S66, 72, 109–10, 120, 143–4, 196. At other times (e.g., II.573, S90, 174), he
promises to explain structures in other animals after he has gone through the monkey, but he does
not deliver on this promise. Towards the end (S135–6, 193), however, he explains that he intends to
write a separate work on the anatomy of the lower animals.

[48] Galen recommends the use of larger animals in investigating parts of the kidney (*AA* II.580), the
heart (II.623), the brain (specifically the pineal gland) (S3), the testicles (S154, 157, 159), certain arteries (S214, 296) and nerves (S257, 261), the first two vertebrae (S286–7), and certain muscles (S292).
Salas (2020), 103–9 explores the ways that Galen navigates this need for magnification in a world
seemingly without it.

with respect to the testicles, since he feels that there is a medical advantage to be gained from doing the dissection on animals as close to humans as possible in appearance.[49] He also suggests using other animals as practice in situations where size is not a factor, presumably since monkeys were more difficult to come by and more expensive than the average farm animal. When discussing the dissection of the lower jaw, for example, he suggests that one begin by practicing on other animals where the operation is easier, but he does follow that advice with instructions on how to proceed if the reader wants to begin with a monkey right away.[50]

Galen also recommends that his readers use other animals in cases where the nonmonetary costs of using monkeys outweigh the advantages. Most notably, in vivisections of the thorax or larynx he repeatedly advises using pigs or goats rather than monkeys, both because of the disquietingly hideous spectacle of a monkey being vivisected and because monkeys offer no material advantage since they do not cry out in a loud enough voice for an impressive demonstration.[51] In some cases, using a monkey will cause problems that are not encountered with other animals. He explains that the blood of monkeys is thinner than that of many other animals and therefore that, in cases where an outrush of blood from the cadaver will obscure the veins the dissector is supposed to be locating, it can be advantageous to use a dog, lion, or other carnivore, since their blood is thicker and will be less obstructive.[52] Finally, in the case of dissections and vivisections of pregnant animals and their fetuses, he usually uses goats; he does not explain why, but presumably, in addition to the goat's greater size, it was much easier and less expensive to purchase a pregnant goat than a pregnant monkey.[53]

Galen mentions a wide number of animals that he has dissected. In addition to specifying general classes of animals, for example, large animals and the carnivorous saw-toothed animals, he specifically discusses oxen, horses, donkeys, mules, pigs, goats, sheep, roosters, dogs, cats, weasels, mice, bears, wolves, lions, elephants, camels, and hippopotami.[54] Purchasing the

---

[49] *AA* S257, 287; testicles at S157.

[50] *AA* II.440. For more suggestions that you should practice on other animals, see II.617–8, S109.

[51] *AA* II.690, S18–19, 107.

[52] *AA* S182, 191. He also explains ways to mitigate the flow of blood from the dead monkey so that the operation can be performed on it.

[53] Pregnant animals: *AA* S146, 151. He also indicates at *Loc.Aff.* VIII.443 that goats were the normal subjects for embryological work among anatomists generally.

[54] Oxen: *AA* II.291, 352, 623, 708, S3, 143–4, 154, 214, 259, 296; horses: II.352, 572, 623, S3, 45, 154, 214, 296; donkeys: II.352, S3, 154, 214; mules: II.352, S214, 296; pigs: II.495, 572, 573, S18–19, 107, 121, 143–4, 196, 260; goats: S18–19, 107, 143–4, 146, 151, 154, 248; sheep: S143–4, 154; roosters: II.623; dogs: II.440, 495, 573, S68, 143–4, 182, 287; cats: II.535; weasels: II.535; mice: II.535, 547; bears: II.495,

more common of these animals would no doubt have been more straight-forward than purchasing monkeys, but it, too, required a selection of live animals and a discerning and choosy buyer. He gives instructions as to the appropriate age and condition of the specimens, explaining the differences between dissecting a large pig and a few-days-old piglet, for example, or advocating the use of the brain of an extremely thin animal, such as one that has become emaciated by starvation, exhaustion, or disease.[55] He sometimes indicates that he expects his readers to have access to these animals immediately after their death, implying that the dissector or someone working for him would be responsible for the slaughter; however, he is not as insistent about this as he is in the case of the monkeys, and even offers suggestions for a few parts of the body that are most easily obtained piecemeal from butchers.[56]

The few instances where Galen suggests visiting the butcher offer rare glimpses into the practicalities behind dissection:

> For the most part, in large cities, prepared ox brains, stripped of most of the cranial parts, are available. And if it should seem to you that more bone than necessary remains on the parts to the side, order the butcher selling it to remove them; if he is not there, you will do it yourself in this way…[57]

He elsewhere advises, "you will succeed in the discovery and the study of this nerve most easily if you go to the butchers who slaughter cattle and sell separately every portion of them, and get them to produce for you the tongue complete with the larynx."[58] Similarly, he asserts that examining the trachea of the pig is "an easy and far from troublesome task for you" because "there are sometimes cut out [from the animal] the larynx and with it the whole of the lungs and the heart, and … together with these, the trachea."[59] He also assumes that the reader will generally be familiar

---

535, 547, S287; wolves: S287; lions: II.535, 573, S182, 191, 261, 287, 292; elephants: II.548–9, 572, 623, S214, 296; camels: II.548–9, 623, S296; hippopotami: II.548–9. At *UP* II.444 (I.324H) he also implies some familiarity with fish and aquatic mammals, namely dolphins, seals, and whales, and confirms his dissection of them at *PHP* V.540 (VI.5.7–13 De Lacy).

[55] Pigs: *AA* II.682; see also S19 where he suggests doing a vivisection experiment on a young animal and then an old, decrepit one for the sake of comparison; emaciated animals: S3.

[56] For immediacy, see for example *AA* II.580.

[57] *AA* II.708 (ἕτοιμοι δὲ τοὐπίπαν ἐν ταῖς μεγάλαις πόλεσιν ἐγκέφαλοι βόειοι πεπράσκονται τῶν πλείστων τοῦ κρανίου μερῶν γυμνοί. καὶ εἰ προσκεῖσθαί σοί ποτε δόξειεν ἐν τοῖς πλαγίοις μέρεσι πλείω τοῦ δέοντος ὀστᾶ, κελεύσεις τῷ πιπράσκοντι μαγείρῳ περιελεῖν αὐτά· μὴ παρόντος δ' ἐκείνου, πράξεις οὕτως αὐτός…).

[58] *AA* S259.

[59] *AA* S260, where Galen also mentions that this group of organs was so commonly kept together by butchers that it had a collective nickname, "the pluck" (see Fig. 5.2 for its depiction in the funerary relief of a butcher).

with the practices of butchers, as when he references their method for removing the intestines.[60] These repeated directions are not only unique in a work where Galen does not habitually give his readers any indication of how or where they should acquire any of the necessary materials for dissection, but they are also among the few textual sources that we have on the workings of butchers in Rome.[61]

The meat trade in Rome appears to have been quite organized. Some substantial fraction of animal slaughter and consumption was tied to the practice of sacrifice, but there was also a secular meat market in which the butchers slaughtered the animals on their own premises, as Galen implies.[62] Among the butchers, there appears to have been a distinction between the *lanii* and the *macellarii*, perhaps that the former both slaughtered and butchered, while the latter only butchered.[63] Galen's reference to "butchers who slaughter cattle" likely refers to another subgroup, the *bubularii*, or butchers specializing in beef.[64] While meat was a comparatively expensive food, a general consensus has emerged over the past few decades that it did form a typical part of the Roman diet across social strata, and that different cuts and varieties were available at different price points.[65] Certainly, both live and freshly slaughtered animals were readily sold in Rome. As we saw in Chapter 3, Galen describes a scene where an anatomist who was boasting at his leisure of his anatomical prowess on a Roman street corner was forced by the crowd to prove his claims with an impromptu dissection of a goat, which they were able to procure seemingly both spontaneously and immediately.[66] Wholesalers auctioned off animals in the several *fora* devoted to the different species (*forum boarium, forum pecuarium, forum suarium*), and it is presumably there that

---

[60] *AA* S278.

[61] For the Roman meat trade, see Frayn (1995) and MacKinnon (2004), 163–87.

[62] For sacrificial meat, see Corbier (1989), 225, Frayn (1995), 112–13, Garnsey (1999), 124, and MacKinnon (2004), 226; for the secular meat business, see Frayn (1995), 107–11, MacKinnon (2004), 175, 183–4, Gilhus (2006), 115, and De Ruyt (2007). Scheid (2007), 20, 26, however, believes that "toute viande était sacrifiée, quel que soit le contexte de l'abattage," and that those who slaughtered animals at home or in the markets did so after a simplified sacrificial ceremony; see also Belayche (2007), 31–2. The urban poor likely got most of their meat precooked from cook shops because of their limited kitchen facilities (Garnsey [1999], 126; Holleran [2012], 9), but Kyle (1995) has argued that the meat resulting from the *venationes* in the arenas was also given over for public consumption, affording an alternative avenue.

[63] Frayn (1993), 156–7 and (1995), 107–8.

[64] For discussions of the epigraphic evidence for *bubularii*, see Guarducci (1989–90), Priuli (1991), 294–7, and Williams (2002).

[65] See Corbier (1989), 224, Garnsey (1999), 123, MacKinnon (2004), 204–11, 225–6, Krön (2008), 79–86, Ikeguchi (2017), 36–7, and Hollander (2018), 64–5.

[66] *AA* II.646.

dissectors sought out the more common animals, along with butchers and those seeking sacrificial animals.[67]

Evidence for the cost of purchasing these animals is difficult to pin down. Several literary sources, whose reliability should be taken with caution, indicate that the price of meat was generally high – at times exorbitantly so. Suetonius reports that Caligula chose to feed the wild animals for the arena on convicts rather than on butchers' meat to save costs, and the Scriptores Historiae Augustae claim that Severus Alexander took a personal interest in lowering butcher prices.[68] The Price Edict of Diocletian of AD 301, which consists of lowered, ideal prices after a century of spectacular inflation and can therefore offer only the haziest of insights into the prices that would have been current in Galen's Rome, lists a pound of pork at 12 denarii and a pound of beef or goat at 8 denarii. To put this in context, it lists the wage of a farm laborer at 25 denarii per day, plus a wheat allowance, meaning that a pork chop would have cost him almost a quarter of his daily income.[69] As today, the cut and type of meat would dictate its price – sausages would have been within the reach of most, but a roasted whole animal was something more extravagant and reserved for special events.[70] It is reasonable to assume, then, that purchasing a whole animal suitable for dissection would have been expensive. For example, though goats were a common sacrificial animal and probably at the more affordable end, Galen does take the time to note in a description of one of his public demonstrations that its patron, the consul Boethus, "provided many kids and pigs," suggesting that the cost would have been nonnegligible even to a wealthy man like Galen.[71] In fact, it is possible that the rich imported their own animals to Rome on the hoof from their country estates to save money.[72] Galen himself had a villa in Campania and, though it would have been a bit of

---

[67] See Frayn (1993), 145–57, who argues that by the second century AD the cattle market in Rome had moved closer to the outskirts of the city and out of the *forum boarium*, which became appropriated for other more urban activities, but also Holleran (2012), 93–5, who counters that the cattle auctions continued to occur in the *forum boarium* at intervals, allowing for the attested noncattle activity to occur in the interims.

[68] Suetonius, *Calig.* 27.1 and Scriptores Historiae Augustae, *Alex. Sev.* 39.3.

[69] Diocletian Edict, III.IV.4; for farm wages, see Duncan-Jones (1982), 11.

[70] On the popularity and extravagance of whole roasted animals, see Frayn (1995), 110–11; cf. the whole calf served at Trimalchio's feast in Petronius, *Sat.* 59 and the recipes for whole roasted boar, kid, and lamb in Apicius, VIII.1.1–2, 6.4–11.

[71] *Praen.* XIV.627 (παρεσκεύασεν ἐρίφους τε καὶ χοίρους πλείονας); on the price of goats, see Toynbee (1973), 166. On Galen's wealth, including a house in Rome and a country villa, see Mattern (2013), 28.

[72] For this suggestion, see Garnsey (1999), 123, and MacKinnon (2004), 183.

a trek when he needed them in Rome, he could well have kept a herd of future anatomical subjects there.[73]

Indeed, the fact that Galen requests such specific subjects as animals that have become emaciated by starvation or disease, a category unlikely to have been met with in a standard meat market, argues against his always proceeding through normal livestock channels to acquire his specimens.[74] Thus, if he did not have his own private source, he must have put his name around as someone who was willing to take otherwise undesirable animals.[75] He expects his readers to be able to find similar sources. One particularly enlightening passage suggests that he was accustomed to pick up dead horses from the races at the circus; he explains a procedure that the reader can best employ "should it so happen that a horse, free from disease, collapses because of much racing (and this occurs quite frequently)," implying that the dissector should either be there on the spot or have an arrangement by which dead horses are delivered to him.[76] Indeed, such arrangements could extend to higher channels.

As we saw earlier, Galen seems to have had access to a variety of exotic animals and frequently suggests that his readers perform dissections on bears, lions, and other animals foreign to Italy, without any hint that these would, prima facie, be even harder to come by than monkeys.[77] Despite their far-flung origins, there was actually a plentiful supply of exotic animals coming through Rome every year for public entertainment, providing a potential source for a dissector in search of zoological variety. Indeed, this local supply of exotica was probably also used for medical purposes beyond just dissection. Galen frequently mentions by-products, such as fat and bile, of lions, leopards, hyenas, and bears as useful medical commodities.[78] The earlier Roman doctor Scribonius Largus (*c.* AD 1–50) even

---

[73] The main character of Juvenal's third satire, for example, walks his cattle from Rome to Cumae, a journey of comparable distance.

[74] Emaciated animal: *AA* S3.

[75] Apuleius tells us that he does something similar at *Apol.* 33, where he explains that he has asked fishermen and friends to bring or describe to him any strange fish they come across so that he can record them in his anatomical writings.

[76] *AA* S45.

[77] For example, bears (*AA* II.495, 535, 547, S287), lions (II.535, 573, S182, 191, 261, 287, 292), elephants (II.548–9, 572, 623, S214, 296; see also *UP* IV.348–49), camels (II.548–9, 623, S296), and perhaps hippopotami (II.548–9). *Pace* Scarborough (1985), who expresses skepticism that he had any real experience with such animals and suggests that he exaggerated passing glimpses of them for sensational value.

[78] For example, at *MM* X.957, *MMG* XI.105, 115, *SMT* XI.734, XII.277, 279, 368, 392, 619, 724, 949, *Comp.Med.Loc.* XII.394, 631, 724, 739, 782, 800, 932, 949, 955, 1008, 1038, *Comp.Med.Gen.* XIII.532, 619, 631. Compare Pliny, who similarly draws on the parts of a variety of exotic animals, including the urine of monkeys (*NH* XXVIII.29 [117]).

tells us that, upon hearing of a promising remedy containing hyena skin, he is able to go out and "immediately," though with some effort, procure a piece.[79] Galen almost certainly tapped into this pool of animals, and he may have done so with some degree of imperial sanction.

Galen's composition of *Anatomical Procedures* spanned well over a decade, beginning under the reign of Marcus Aurelius and stretching through that of Commodus to that of Septimius Severus.[80] He received an imperial salary from each of these emperors and served them as physician and pharmacist.[81] He proudly describes a few personal conversations with Marcus Aurelius and had relationships with various members of the imperial household, including Peitholaus, the imperial chamberlain.[82] We know that he was not loath to take advantage of the opportunities presented by his position. He reports helping himself from the imperial storerooms, presumably with permission, to some cinnamon – at the time an extremely rare pharmaceutical ingredient.[83] It is not at all difficult to imagine, then, that he also used his connections to gain access to the imperially owned wild animals.

By the time of Galen's arrival in Rome, the emperors had a fully established network of beast suppliers, handlers, and vivaria to import, train, and hold the astonishing number of animals used in public spectacles every year.[84] Plutarch (b. before AD 50–d. after AD 120), in searching out instances of the docility and cleverness of animals, claims that the steady and enormous flow of animals for the imperial spectacles in Rome allows one to draw up examples "by the bucket- and basin-ful."[85] To give a more concrete example of the scale: During the festival to celebrate Septimius Severus' tenth year of power in AD 203 – about five or ten years after Galen finished writing *AA* – a model ship was constructed in the amphitheater that disgorged one hundred animals a day, resulting in the slaughter of hundreds of bears, lions, lionesses, leopards, ostriches, wild asses, and bison over the course of a single week.[86] And that was but one of the animal attractions. We know a great deal about these events through detailed accounts in the textual record as well as artistic depictions; zooarchaeological finds

[79] Scribonius Largus, *Comp.Med.* 172 (*protinus*); cf. 38, where hyena gall is called for.
[80] See Chapter 9, "The Composition of Anatomical Procedures" at pp. 325–6.
[81] *Ant.* XIV.4; cf. Mattern (2013), 215.
[82] Conversations with Marcus Aurelius at *Ant.* XIV.4 and *Praen.* XIV.658–60; relationship with Peitholaus at *Praen.* XIV.650–57, 661–64.
[83] *Ant.* XIV.64; cf. Mattern (2013), 219.
[84] Rea (2001*b*) and Lindberg (2019) examine the logistics of the imperial animal supply.
[85] Plutarch, *De soll. an.* 963C (ἄμαις καὶ σκάφαις).
[86] Dio, LXXVI.1.

confirm both their scale and their scope: Excavations in and around the Colosseum have unearthed large quantities of animal bones, including a variety of wild and exotic species.[87] In order to acquire these creatures, the emperors deployed Roman soldiers, in conjunction with native experts, to hunt and import them, and we have epigraphic references to numerous imperial freedmen involved in the trade of these animals, including a supplier of wild beasts, a supplier of herbivorous animals, and the keeper of the imperial herd of elephants at Laurentum.[88] This herd was well established and well known: Juvenal refers to it, saying that elephants are not for sale in Italy and that the imperial herd is for Caesar alone.[89]

As Juvenal suggests, imperial control dominated this flow of wild animals. Though there were some private vivaria and wild pets among the senatorial class, the scale and variety would not have been comparable to those maintained by the emperors for public and private use.[90] In fact, imperial permission appears to have been required for the capture of elephants and for the hunting and capture of lions, so the supply of these animals in Rome outside the control of the emperors would have been limited.[91] As a result, any dissector interested in expanding his horizon beyond farm animals would likely have needed some level of official permission to gain access to the bears, lions, elephants, and camels that Galen frequently mentions.[92] Indeed, it seems most probable that they came to Galen dead after appearances in the arena, and some may actually have been lent for dissection on their way to other fates.[93] Donald Kyle has suggested that the animal remains of the *venationes* in the arena were sold

---

[87] For a summary view of the textual and material sources, see Rea (2001*a*); for the zooarchaeological perspective specifically, see De Grossi Mazzorin and Minniti (2019), who detail the animal remains, which include bear, wolf, giraffe, hyena, camel, ostrich, lion, leopard, and tiger bones.

[88] CIL 6.10208, CIL 6.10209, and CIL 6.8583 respectively. For the involvement of soldiers, see Bomgardner (2000), 24 and 212, Rea (2001*b*), 253–62, Epplett (2001), and Lindberg (2019).

[89] Juvenal XII.102–10. Though he describes the herd in terms of military use, it would seem that by AD 193 they were trained only for entertainment; Julianus considered using the imperial herd against Severus, but the animals were not willing to carry armed men (Dio, LXXIV.16.3.).

[90] Jennison (1937), 132–33, Rea (2001*b*), 269–74, and Epplett (2003), 88. In addition to the vivaria kept stocked for the games, both Marcus Aurelius and Commodus kept private enclosures for their own amusement; see Fronto, 3.20, Pliny, *Ep.* 6.31, and Epplett (2003), 86–7.

[91] Aelian, *NA* X.1 refers to obtaining permission from the emperor for elephant hunting; *Cod. Theod.* XV.11.1, dated to AD 414, clarifies that the killing of lions for self-defense is permissible, but affirms that permission to hunt or sell them remains restricted; see also the discussion of legal limitations on nonimperial use and ownership of animals in Lindberg (2019), 260–2.

[92] See Jennison (1937), 174–6, Bomgardner (2000), 23–5, Epplett (2003), 78–84, and MacKinnon (2006), 151.

[93] It is also possible that a dissector might have taken advantage of the many animals that died of natural causes prior even to appearing in a show; see Lindberg (2019), 258–9 for evidence of this attrition en route and in the vivaria.

or distributed for use as meat.[94] The more run-of-the-mill animals seem
to have been distributed to the masses by means of tokens, but Michael
MacKinnon has added the hypothesis that the exotic ones were kept for
the tables of the wealthy, a theory supported by the recent discovery of
what appears to be an ancient butchered giraffe leg in Pompeii.[95] Given the
extreme expense of these animals, an arrangement whereby the carcasses
were simply lent to the anatomist in this way between uses would have
been very advantageous.[96]

A striking example in support of this theory is Galen's description of an
elephant dissection, which is worth quoting in full:

> When an elephant of enormous size indeed was killed in Rome recently
> many doctors thronged to its dissection in order to find out whether the
> heart had two apexes or one, and two chambers or three. And I, even before
> its dissection, maintained that the same arrangement of the heart would be
> discovered as in all other animals that breathe air. These things were evident
> when it had been dissected. I easily discovered the bone in it also, insert-
> ing my fingers along with my colleagues. But those who were unpracticed,
> expecting to discover, since it was a large animal, that which is not evident
> in others, <after having searched a long time did not find it and>[97] believed
> that the heart of the elephant had no bone. I was going to show it to them,
> but since my companions were laughing at them, seeing that they were
> unobservant on account of their ignorance of the location, and were exhort-
> ing me not to show it, I held back my disclosure. However, when the heart
> was carried off by Caesar's cooks, I sent one of my companions, who was
> well practiced in these sorts of demands, to persuade the cooks to remove
> the bone in it; and thus it was done. It is even now in my possession, being

---

[94] See Kyle (1995), 181–205 and (1998), 184–94.

[95] MacKinnon (2006), 155–6. For the giraffe bone, see Ellis and Devore (2010), 5 and the forthcoming publication of their work at the site, which will address the bone's somewhat vexed dating (my
thanks to Steven Ellis for this advanced communication). At *Alim.Fac.* VI.664, Galen mentions
that, though he cannot recommend it for any health benefits, some people eat horses, camels,
donkeys, dogs, bears, lions, leopards, and panthers; while it is clear from the discussion there that
some of these people, for example those that eat old donkeys, presumably at the end of their working life, are driven to do so out of necessity, at *At.Bil.* V.134 he indicates that some people eat lions,
lionesses, panthers, leopards, bears, and wolves "for pleasure" (ἡδέως). Similarly, note that in the
elephant anecdote discussed later on this page the animal was being carved up by imperial cooks,
undoubtedly in order to supply a prestige dish for the imperial table.

[96] The little evidence we have suggests that animals for the arena were spectacularly expensive.
Bomgardner (2000), 211 has collected relevant figures, including 1,000 denarii for a leopard in early
third-century North Africa (inscribed on the Magerius Mosaic), 600,000 sesterces for top-quality
lion, and 400,000 sesterces for a second-class lioness in late third-century Rome (both from the
Price Edict of Diocletian; see this section, p. 104). Compare the price of 10 aurei (1,000 sesterces)
for a bear, albeit an overpriced one, given in a more contemporary source (Apuleius, *Met.* 4.16).

[97] After the conjecture in Garofalo (1991*b*), 665.

not small in size and producing a wondrous disbelief in those who see it that a bone of such size escaped the notice of doctors.[98]

There are several points to consider here. First of all, the elephant did not simply die, but rather was killed, making it extremely likely that this animal was a victim of one of the events in the arena.[99] It seems to have then been turned over to the medical community generally for dissection: Galen does not mention any doctor specifically being in charge and says that they all had hands-on access to the proceedings. Further, there were at least two schools of medical thought present; we have Galen and his companions pitted against another group, whom he refers to disparagingly as "unpracticed." The emperor's cooks also appear to have been present for the dissection, since they take away the heart at the conclusion, presumably for use in the emperor's dinner that evening. In fact, it is not unlikely that the doctors were cutting up the animal in concert with the cooks as they removed choice morsels of the carcass for the kitchen.

Given the great bulk of an elephant, it seems most likely that the doctors have come to it, rather than vice versa. This, coupled with Galen's comment, which I will explore in the following section, that doctors

---

[98] *AA* II.619–20 (μεγίστου γοῦν ἐλέφαντος ἔναγχος ἐν Ῥώμῃ σφαγέντος, ἠθροίσθησαν μὲν ἐπὶ τὴν ἀνατομὴν αὐτοῦ πολλοὶ τῶν ἰατρῶν ἕνεκα τοῦ γνῶναι πότερον ἔχει δύο κορυφὰς ἢ μίαν ἡ καρδία, καὶ δύο κοιλίας ἢ τρεῖς. ἐγὼ δὲ καὶ πρὸ τῆς ἀνατομῆς αὐτοῦ διετεινόμην εὑρεθήσεσθαι τὴν αὐτὴν κατασκευὴν τῆς καρδίας ταῖς ἄλλαις πάσαις τῶν ἐξ ἀέρος ἀναπνεόντων ζῴων· ἅπερ ἐφάνη καὶ διαιρεθείσης. εὗρον δὲ ῥᾳδίως καὶ τὸ κατ' αὐτὴν ὀστοῦν, ἅμα τοῖς ἑταίροις ἐπιβαλὼν τοὺς δακτύλους. οἱ δ' ἀγύμναστοι μέν, ἐλπίζοντες δὲ εὑρίσκειν, ὡς ἐν μεγάλῳ ζῴῳ, τὸ μὴ φαινόμενον ἐπὶ τῶν ἄλλων, ⟨…⟩ ὑπέλαβον οὐδὲ τὴν ἐλέφαντος καρδίαν ἔχειν ὀστοῦν. ἐγὼ δ' ἐμέλλησα μὲν αὐτοῖς δεικνύειν, τῶν δ' ἑταίρων γελώντων ἐφ' οἷς ἑώρων ἀναισθήτους ἐκείνους διὰ τὴν ἄγνοιαν τοῦ τόπου, παρακαλεσάντων δὲ μὴ δεικνύειν, ἐπέσχον τὴν δεῖξιν. ἀρθείσης μέντοι τῆς καρδίας ὑπὸ τῶν τοῦ Καίσαρος μαγείρων, ἔπεμψά τινα τῶν γεγυμνασμένων ἑταίρων περὶ τὰ τοιαῦτα παρακαλέσοντα τοὺς μαγείρους ἐπιτρέψαι τὸ κατ' αὐτὴν ὀστοῦν ἐξελεῖν· καὶ οὕτως ἐγένετο. καὶ παρ' ἡμῖν ἐστι νῦν, οὐ σμικρὸν μὲν ὑπάρχον τῷ μεγέθει, θαυμαστὴν δὲ παρέχον ἀπιστίαν τοῖς ὁρῶσιν, εἰ τηλικοῦτον ὀστοῦν ἐλάνθανε τοὺς ἰατρούς); following the text in Garofalo (1986–2000). It turns out that the last laugh is on Galen since elephants do not in fact have a heart bone (*os cordis*), though the structure is present in other large animals, such as cattle; there are, however, conditions that could lead to the presence of a bonelike structure in a given elephant, and there is a fibrous skeleton around the elephant's heart, which is what Mattern (2013), 152 suggests that Galen was feeling. See the extensive discussion of this passage in Salas (2020), 144–68.

[99] Though elephants are very trainable and were used for a variety of charming acts such as dancing and tightrope walking, not to mention their long history in the military, they were also frequently killed in the arena in various ways; see Toynbee (1973), 32–49. Commodus himself is credited with killing at least two elephants, in addition to hippopotami, rhinoceroses, lions, leopards, a giraffe, a tiger, and many bears (Dio, LXXII.10.3; 18.1; 19.1, Herodian, I.15.3–6); see Jennison (1937), 87, and Rea (2001*a*), 230–1. It is conceivable that this elephant was killed because it was sick or injured, but given the value of these animals such circumstances must have accounted for a tiny fraction of elephant slaughters: The death of such an animal would almost certainly have done double duty as entertainment.

were frequently granted a brief time with the corpses of convicts con-demned to death in the arena, suggests an arrangement whereby doctors were sometimes allowed access to the various remains of the amphithe-ater, on location, in the interval between slaughter and disposal.[100] Galen appears to have availed himself of these chances, and was apparently accustomed to seek still further favors. He tells us that the man whom he sent to ask the imperial cooks for the heart-bone was one of several companions who were well practiced in these sorts of demands, imply-ing that Galen was in the habit of frequently sending his subordinates to beg various anatomical desiderata from the imperial kitchens. A dis-sector's ability to take similar advantage would have lessened the burden of acquiring specimens. Though Galen's connections were high up the ladder in the imperial household, it is conceivable that the connections of a man of lower social standing could also have been efficacious. The actual handling of the animals was, after all, mostly in the hands of slaves and freedmen.

Humans

The question of human subjects has long dominated scholarship on the topic of dissection. There is now general consensus that human dissec-tion occurred during the early Hellenistic period, when Herophilus and Erasistratus made their famous investigations, but there has been – and continues to be – debate about whether humans were acceptable ana-tomical subjects during the remainder of antiquity. Edelstein conceived of human dissection as spanning the period from Hellenistic Alexandria to the first century AD, but Kudlien and von Staden influentially argued for a curtailment of the window to just the short period around the *floruit* of Herophilus and Erasistratus.[101] Most recently, Dean-Jones has pushed back on this position, arguing for a reevaluation of the evidence in Celsus and Galen, and suggesting that human dissection remained a live option

---

[100] *AA* II.385; see this chapter, "Anatomical Subjects: Humans" at pp. 115–18 for more discussion. Human corpses from the arena were taken to the *spoliarium*, a kind of waystation before disposal where their necks were slit to ensure that they were dead and their bodies were stripped of gear; see Kyle (1998), 158–9. It was presumably there that the doctors Galen mentions could have been allowed their surrep-titious investigations of corpses. Indeed, we have an inscription commissioned by a doctor who acted as *curator spoliarii* at Rome (CIL 6.10171); see Kyle (1998), 159, but also Sabbatini Tumolesi (1988), 17, who believes it to be a fake. It is conceivable that the animal carcasses were taken to a similar, or perhaps identical, location where the anatomists could have had access to them.

[101] Edelstein (1932) and (1935), Kudlien (1969), von Staden (1992*a*); see also Chapter 2, n. 118 and the further scholarship mentioned there.

all the way through the Roman period into Galen's day.[102] In keeping with this diversity of scholarly opinion, there is variation in the degree to which scholars have distanced Galen and his peers from the practice.[103] My own opinion is that, while sporadic human dissections of one kind or another no doubt occurred over the course of the roughly seven centuries considered in this book, aside from the brief window of state-condoned acceptability in the Hellenistic period, it was a largely clandestine and unsystematic activity that was not considered to be a viable avenue of medical research. Apart from the one notable asterisk, dissection in antiquity meant animal dissection.

Our first potential window into the question of human dissection after Herophilus and Erasistratus is Celsus.[104] In his discussion of the development of the medical art and the differences between the sects, he broaches the topic – which he says "has been often treated by doctors in many volumes and in large and contentious disputes" – of the utility and necessity of dissection and of its more flamboyant cousin, human vivisection.[105] Celsus first summarizes and then weighs in on this argument, which had clearly become a standard talking point in medical circles after the rise of the Empiricist sect. However, the historical debate was not about *human dissection* specifically, but rather about the epistemological value of dissection *tout court*. There is, therefore, no reason that we have to assume that the references to dissection of the dead in Celsus' account refer to anything but the unmarked practice of animal dissection, which, as we have seen,

---

[102] Dean-Jones (2018).

[103] Simon (1906), vol. 2, xxvi–xxix, Edelstein (1932), 53–4, Kudlien (1969), 79–81, French (1978), 157–8, Longrigg (1981), 161, and Grmek (1996), 102 come down against it completely. Others, such as Garofalo (1991*a*) 106–8, Rocca (2003), 67–8, Cosans (1998), 73–4, and Dean-Jones (2018) suggest that it was a viable possibility (to varying degrees) in the Roman period, but that Galen himself did not take advantage of it, offering various reasons why. Singer (1956), xxi–xxiii alone suggests without qualification that Galen dissected human cadavers and "knew more about human anatomy than he cared to have written down."

[104] Claims for human dissection prior to Herophilus and Erasistratus rest on tenuous evidence and have generally not met with much scholarly support (see Chapter 2, nn. 3, 23, 42); I think it is safe to assume that there was no systematic human dissection before them. The one most plausible exception would be the investigation of aborted, still born, or exposed infants (see Chapter 2, "Hippocratic Doctors" at pp. 19–22 and "Aristotle" at pp. 29–31 for the possibility of this practice by those authors); these infant bodies seem to have occupied a more liminal space in ancient thought than adult corpses. Exposed infants in particular were recognized as vulnerable to predatory intentions, usually by those desiring to rear them into slavery, but more grisly fates were equally present in the public imagination; see Harris (1994) and Moss (2021). Galen indicates that he is aware of their use as anatomical subjects, presumably in the Roman period, though he does not associate himself with the practice directly, as I will discuss later on in this section.

[105] Celsus, *DM* proem.45 (per multa uolumina perque magnas contentionis [disputationes] a medicis saepe tractata sint).

was the standard even for Herophilus and Erasistratus. Indeed, Celsus only actually mentions humans when discussing the obviously outré (but nevertheless ethically and rhetorically fascinating) case of human vivisection – and in each instance he explicitly emphasizes that the doctors are dealing there with *homines*, though it would be grammatically unnecessary to include the word if humans were meant throughout:

> Therefore [the Dogmatists say] that it is necessary to cut into the bodies of the dead and to investigate their organs and that Herophilus and Erasistratus did this in the best way by far, when they cut into guilty *humans*, granted alive out of prison by the kings, and, while breath even still remained in them, considered what nature had before concealed.... [The Empiricists say] that it is not only superfluous, but even actually cruel to cut into the belly and internal organs of living *humans*.... [I think that] to cut into the bodies of the living is both cruel and superfluous, but that it is necessary for students to do it to those of the dead: for they ought to know the position and the sequence [of the organs], which a corpse can show better than a live and wounded *human*.[106]

Clearly, the specific example of human vivisection was the most exciting flashpoint in this debate, even though Celsus acknowledges that it was only actually attested to have happened in Hellenistic Alexandria. Further, even if we were to suppose that humans are meant to be the objects of dissections of the dead in these passages, the debate would still remain a purely rhetorical one. Rufus, who, unlike Celsus, was unambiguously a practicing doctor and likely spent time in Alexandria itself, explicitly tells us that human dissection is not a viable option for him and that it was only used "long ago": It is therefore difficult to believe that Celsus is witness to human dissection as a routine element of medical education, of which Rufus, a mere generation or so later, is completely unaware.[107] Rather, Celsus is staking out his own stance on a long-standing moral chestnut that continued to delight into the following century, when the subject of

---

[106] Celsus, *DM* proem.23–4, 40, 74 (necessarium esse incidere corpora mortuorum, eorumque uiscera atque intestina scrutari; longeque optime fecisse Herophilum et Erasistratum, qui nocentes *homines* a regibus ex carcere acceptos uiuos inciderint, considerarintque etiamnum spiritu remanente ea, quae natura ante clausisset ... superuacua esse tantummodo: id uero, quod restat, etiam crudele, uiuorum *hominum* aluum atque praecordia incidi.... Incidere autem uiuorum corpora et crudele et superuacuum est, mortuorum discentibus necessarium: nam positum et ordinem nosse debent, quae cadauer melius quam uiuus et uulneratus homo repraesenta[n]t); my emphasis. Note that "corpse" (cadaver) is applicable to animals as well as humans (*TLL* cadaver, 2).

[107] Rufus, *Nom.Part.* 10 (πάλαι); on Rufus' career, see Chapter 7, "Rufus of Ephesus" at pp. 218–20. On Celsus: Schulze (1999) reopened the question of his being a practicing doctor, but scholarship has remained cautiously skeptical, as, for example, Nutton (2013a), 169 and 376 n. 67, and Gautherie (2017), 42–5.

human vivisection appears again (alongside such outlandish peers as cannibalism and mother–son incest) as fodder for rhetorical gymnastics.[108]
   Galen obviously offers the most scope for insight into the acceptability of
human dissection in the Roman period. Because he intends the dissection of
monkeys to be practically applied to the understanding of the human body,
he does mention disparities between the two species, which might imply a
detailed first-hand knowledge of human anatomy. However, none of these
insights would have involved invasive investigation into human bodies.[109]
For the most part, his references to human anatomy point the reader to
muscles or veins that are visible to the naked eye on the naked body. Because
their muscles are clearly defined and often on public display, athletes are the
main group to which he refers his readers for observation.[110] For observations of the internal parts, Galen does not advocate seeking out corpses for
dissection, but he certainly does encourage learning from any serendipitous
encounters with them. As we shall see, however, this encouragement is not
uniformly enthusiastic: He is much more comfortable discussing the examination of skeletons than of undecomposed cadavers.
   There are three places in *Anatomical Procedures* where Galen encourages the reader to take advantage of any chance encounter with a human
skeleton. In one, he simply tells the reader that the features he is discussing
can be seen "in such human cadavers as you happen to look at," and he
makes it clear in what follows that he expects such cadavers to have undergone enough decomposition so as to basically be skeletons.[111] In another,
he says that "it is necessary to learn the nature of all of the bones, as I said,
either from the bodies of men, or of monkeys, and, even better, if you are
able, from both."[112] In the third, he is speaking specifically of bones and

---

[108] Ps.-Quintilian, *Dec.Maj.* VIII. Compare, at a much later date, Ibn al-Nafis, who extensively affirms
his loyalty to the idea that dissection is fundamental to medical education, despite having previously said that religious precepts and his own moral objections have prevented him from practicing
dissection for himself; see the passages cited in Savage-Smith (1995), 99–101.

[109] *AA* II.322 discusses differences in toe size; II.323 explains that there is a tendon in human feet not
found in monkeys' feet; S196 describes a vein that takes a different route in the monkey from all
other animals including man. The most elaborate example is his explanation at S328 of how to map
an understanding of the nerves and vertebrae of a monkey onto those of a human being given that
the two species have a different number of vertebrae, upsetting the correlation of the numbering
system.

[110] *AA* II.274, 374, 392, 450, 480. All but II.392 refer specifically to athletes. At S63 he mentions the
parts of the eye that can be easily observed in humans.

[111] *AA* S229, where he continues by saying, "all these foramina you will see with your own eyes in a
cadaver in which all that overlies the bones is decayed and the bones alone remain, in their connections with one another, without separating from each other."

[112] *AA* II.226 (ἀπάντων, ὡς ἔφην, τῶν ὀστῶν κατανοῆσαι χρὴ τὴν φύσιν, εἴτ'ἐπὶ ἀνθρώπου σώματι,
εἴτ'ἐπὶ πιθήκων, εἰ δυνηθείης, ἄμεινον δ' ἐπ'ἀμφοῖν).

mentions his own experiences with stray bodies – clarifying for us under what circumstances one might "happen to look at" a human skeleton. After explaining that the easiest way to study the human skeleton is to go to Alexandria where the physicians have specimens that they use for teaching, Galen adds that even if you cannot travel there, as he did, it is still possible to get first-hand experience:

> I for one have seen [skeletons] very often, whenever some grave or tomb has opened up. But further, a river once, rising up to a grave made haphazardly a few months previously, easily washed it away and, in the force of its rush, dragging the body of the dead man whole (the flesh already having rotted away and the bones still connecting accurately with one another) washed it back up, having been dragged as far as a stade downhill. And since the ground that received it there was marshy and had steep banks, the body of the dead man was stranded against it, and it was possible to observe it in just such a way as a doctor might have arranged it on purpose for the instruction of young men. And I also observed once the skeleton of a thief lying on a mountain a little bit beyond the road. A traveler, coming upon him, had killed him after he attacked first, and none of the local inhabitants had any intention of burying him, but from their hatred of him they rejoiced in his body being food for the birds, which, eating his flesh, in two days left a skeleton for those who desired to look at it, as if for the purpose of teaching.[113]

It is noteworthy that, though learning from human skeletons is evidently acceptable, Galen considers it a stroke of luck to have the chance to examine one.[114] They appear to only have been preserved and kept on hand in Alexandria, a city that had a unique history of permissiveness for anatomical research on humans.[115] Though Galen feels no qualms about describing

---

[113] *AA* II.221–2 (ἐγώ γε οὖν ἐθεασάμην πάνυ πολλάκις, ἤτοι τάφων τινῶν ἢ μνημάτων διαλυθέντων. ἀλλὰ καὶ ποταμὸς ἐπαναβάς ποτε τάφῳ πρὸ μηνῶν ὀλίγων αὐτοσχεδίως γεγενημένῳ διέλυσέ τε ῥαδίως αὐτόν, ἐπισυράμενός τε τῇ ῥύμῃ τῆς φορᾶς ὅλον τοῦ νεκροῦ τὸ σῶμα, τῶν μὲν σαρκῶν ἤδη σεσηπυιῶν, ἀκριβῶς δ᾽ ἀλλήλοις ἔτι συνεχομένων τῶν ὀστῶν, ἄχρι μὲν σταδίου κατάντη συρόμενον ἐπηνέγκατο· λιμνώδους δὲ αὐτὸ ἐκδεξαμένου χωρίου, τοῖς χείλεσιν ὑπτίου, πρὸς τοῦτο ἀπεκρούσθη τὸ τοῦ νεκροῦ σῶμα, καὶ ἦν ἰδεῖν καὶ τοῦτο τοιοῦτον οἷόν περ ἂν ἐπίτηδες αὐτὸ παρεκεύασεν ἰατρὸς εἰς διδασκαλίαν μειρακίων. ἐθεασάμεθα δέ ποτε καὶ λῃστοῦ σκελετὸν ἐν ὄρει κείμενον ὀλίγον ἐξωτέρω τῆς ὁδοῦ, ὃν ἀπέκτεινε μέν τις ὁδοιπόρος ἐπεγχειροῦντα πρότερον ὁμόσε χωρήσας, οὐκ ἔμελλε δὲ θάψειν οὐδεὶς τῶν οἰκητόρων τῆς χώρας ἐκείνης, ἀλλ᾽ ὑπὸ μίσους ἐπέχαιρον ἐσθιομένῳ τῷ σώματι πρὸς τῶν οἰωνῶν, οἵτινες ἐν δυσὶν ἡμέραις αὐτοῦ καταφαγόντες τὰς σάρκας ἀπέλιπον ὡς εἰς διδασκαλίαν τῷ βουληθέντι θεάσασθαι τὸν σκελετόν); text following Garofalo (1986–2000).

[114] At *AA* II.222 Galen tells his readers that if they are not lucky enough (εὐτύχησας) to see a human skeleton, they should rely on monkeys instead.

[115] Galen says at *AA* II.220–21 that studying human skeletons "is very easy in Alexandria" and "for this reason alone, if for no other, you should make an effort to spend time in Alexandria" (ἔστι δ᾽ ἐν Ἀλεξανδρείᾳ μὲν τοῦτο πάνυ ῥάδιον ... πειρατέον ἐστί σοι, κἂν μὴ δι᾽ ἄλλο τι, διὰ τοῦτο γοῦν αὐτὸ μόνον ἐν Ἀλεξανδρείᾳ γενέσθαι).

his investigation of chance-found skeletons and encouraging others to take similar advantage, he makes no move to *keep* the two skeletons he found and use them for his own teaching, even though he finds keeping a wide variety of animal bones to be perfectly normal.[116] We can infer that the study of human skeletons was acceptable, but only tenuously so – the anatomist here would be beginning to navigate the murky waters between the condoned and the taboo.

Galen also broaches the more controversial subject of wholly preserved corpses. One passage in particular is central to this question and worth citing in full, despite its length:

> All these [externally visible] veins which you see in men without dissection, you will see in dissected monkeys. Therefore, it is clear that these animals also have the deeper veins arranged in a similar way to humans. Therefore, I want you to train yourself on them in advance frequently so that, if ever you should chance upon the dissection of a human body, you would be *readily* able to lay bare each of the parts. This is not a common happening, nor one a man untrained in this work can achieve *in the moment*. Indeed, *even at great leisure*, the most anatomical of doctors investigating the parts of the body reveal themselves to be in error on many points. Wherefore those who desired to dissect the body of a German enemy who died in their war against Marcus Antoninus, were unable to learn anything except the position of the organs. Someone who was trained in advance on other animals and especially on the monkey would have *most readily* laid bare each of the dissected parts. It is easier for a diligent man practiced in anatomy to learn something looking at a human body *quickly* than for one of those untrained men to accurately find an obvious thing *at great leisure*. For many have frequently observed whatever they wished in the bodies of those condemned to death and thrown to the animals, *briefly on each occasion*, as well as on unburied robbers lying in the mountains. And large wounds and deep-reaching areas of decay have laid bare many of the parts, which became known to those who were trained as having the same arrangement as in simian bodies, while to the untrained they were no help at all. And the many who frequently dissected dead exposed children were persuaded that humans are the same as monkeys in their arrangement. And through surgeries themselves, each time we do them, both when cutting out decaying flesh and when cutting off bones, the similarity becomes obvious to those who have trained in advance.[117]

---

[116] See *AA* S33, 229–30.

[117] *AA* II.384–6 (ταύτας οὖν ἁπάσας τὰς φλέβας, ἃς ἐπ᾽ ἀνθρώπων ὁρᾷς πρὸ τῆς ἀνατομῆς, ἐπὶ τῶν πιθήκων ἀνατεμνομένων ὄψει. δῆλον οὖν ὅτι καὶ τὰς διὰ τοῦ βάθους ὡσαύτως ἔχει τὰ ζῷα ταῦτα τοῖς ἀνθρώποις. ἐπ᾽ αὐτῶν οὖν προγεγυμνάσθαι σε βούλομαι πολλάκις, ἵνα, κἂν ἀνθρωπίνου ποτὲ σώματος ἀνατομῆς ἐπιτύχῃς, ἑτοίμως δυνηθῇς γυμνοῦν ἕκαστον τῶν μορίων· ὅπερ οὐ τὸ τυχόν ἐστιν, οὐδὲ ἀγυμνάστῳ περὶ τοὔργον ἀνθρώπῳ δυνάμενον ἐξαίφνης ἐπιτυγχάνεσθαι. κατὰ γοῦν

The purpose of this paragraph is to affirm that the study of simian anatomy is an accurate window into human anatomy. This affirmation goes two ways: On the one hand, his readers can be assured that the study of monkeys will give them reliable insight into the anatomy of humans and that, thus, the dissection of humans is basically superfluous; on the other hand, he points out that a fluency with simian dissection will allow a doctor to make the most of any opportunity to dissect a human, suggesting that he sees some value in doing so, were it possible. However, the passage sends mixed messages about the acceptability of such activity.

First of all, Galen goes out of his way to make the dissection of humans seem almost routine with his repeated polyptoton of πολύς – "many have frequently" (πολλοὶ πολλάκις) peeked into the bodies of the condemned and "many have frequently" (πολλοὶ πολλάκις) opened up exposed infants.[118] Nevertheless, he places all of this activity in the past tense: He does not portray this as ongoing activity, but rather as accumulated anonymous experience. Further, he deliberately distances himself from it by not claiming personal involvement – and thus the authoritative position he usually covets – in any of these practices, though he was eager to do so in the case of the chance-discovered human skeletons. He switches to the first person and the present tense only when discussing the unexceptionable practice of observing human organs during surgery.

πολλὴν σχολὴν οἱ ἀνατομικώτατοι τῶν ἰατρῶν ἐπισκοπούμενοι τὰ μόρια τοῦ σώματος, ἐν πολλοῖς ἐσφαλμένοι φαίνονται. διόπερ οὐδ᾽ οἱ βουληθέντες ἀνατέμνειν σῶμα πολεμίου Γερμανοῦ τεθνεῶτος ἐπὶ τοῦ κατὰ Μάρκον Ἀντωνῖνον πολέμου πλέον ἠδυνήθησάν τι μαθεῖν τῆς τῶν σπλάγχνων θέσεως. ὁ δ᾽ ἐπὶ τῶν ἄλλων ζώων καὶ μάλιστα πιθήκου προγεγυμνασμένος ἑτοιμότατα τῶν ἀνατεμνομένων μορίων ἕκαστον γυμνοῖ· καὶ ῥᾷόν ἐστιν ἀνδρὶ φιλοπόνῳ προγεγυμνασμένῳ κατὰ τὰς ἀνατομὰς ἐπισκεψαμένῳ τι διὰ ταχέων ἐν ἀνθρωπίνῳ σώματι νεκρῷ μαθεῖν, ἢ φανερὸν ἑτέρῳ τῶν ἀγυμνάστων ἐπὶ πολλῆς σχολῆς ἐξευρεῖν ἀκριβῶς. τῶν τε γὰρ ἐπὶ θανάτῳ κατακριθέντων καὶ θηρίοις παραβληθέντων ἐθεάσαντο πολλοὶ πολλάκις ἐν τοῖς σώμασιν ὅπερ ἐβουλήθησαν ἑκάστοτε διὰ ταχέων, ἐπί τε λῃστῶν ἐν ὄρει κειμένων ἀτάφων. καὶ τραύματα δὲ μεγάλα καὶ σηπεδόνες εἰς βάθος ἐξικνούμεναι πολλὰ τῶν μορίων ἐγύμνωσαν,ἃ τοῖς μὲν προγεγυμνασμένοις ἐγνωρίσθη τὴν αὐτὴν ἔχοντα κατασκευὴν τοῖς πιθηκείοις σώμασιν, τοὺς δ᾽ ἀγυμνάστους οὐδὲν ὠφέλησε. καὶ παιδία δὲ τῶν ἐκτιθεμένων νεκρὰ πολλοὶ πολλάκις ἀνατέμνοντες ἐπείσθησαν, ὡσαύτως ἔχειν κατ ἀσκευῆς ἄνθρωπον πιθήκῳ. καὶ κατ᾽ αὐτὰς δὲ τὰς χειρουργίας, ὅσας ἑκάστοτε ποιούμεθα, ποτὲ μὲν ἐκτέμνοντες σεσηπυίας σάρκας, ποτὲ δ᾽ ἐκκόπτοντες ὀστᾶ, καταφανὴς ἡ ὁμοιότης γίγνεται τῷ προγεγυμνασμένῳ); following the text in Garofalo (1986–2000); my emphasis.

[118] Kudlien (1969), 80 contends that this expression of frequency may well be an exaggeration and adds that, even if it is not, "dürften es bestenfalls Skelette gewesen sein, die man so inspizieren konnte." I agree that Galen is likely exaggerating the frequency, but, given his separate and personally endorsed instructions for investigating skeletons, it seems impossible that the bodies he is discussing in this passage are only skeletal remains. In addition to his emphasis on the fleeting nature of these chances – and he has already told us that it is perfectly acceptable to examine a skeleton at leisure – he explicitly states that, owing to their lack of experience with dissection, the doctors who had the chance to examine a dead German soldier were only able to ascertain the location of the viscera. The body in question there was therefore certainly nowhere near a skeletal state, so I see no reason to assume that the ones in the other examples would have been either.

Further, as my italicization highlights, Galen is concerned with the question of speed, which strikes me as very telling. While Galen can conceive of moments when access to the viscera of human corpses might be possible, he repeatedly underscores that they would be brief. He indicates that any chance to dissect a human corpse will come upon you suddenly and be fleeting: A dissector must prepare himself so that he can seize the opportunity "readily" (ἑτοίμως/ἑτοιμότατα) and "in the moment" (ἐξαίφνης). Those who had the chance to take a peek into the viscera of the condemned did so "briefly on each occasion" (ἑκάστοτε διὰ ταχέων). In his discussion of the dissection of the German foe, he underscores this point still more.[119] He points out first that even the very best anatomists are liable to make mistakes when proceeding in the best conditions and without time constraints, which is an idea that he repeatedly deploys for various purposes.[120] He presents it as no surprise therefore that the doctors in Germania – who were, in implicit contrast, neither the best anatomists nor working "at great leisure" – basically achieved nothing at all. He drives home the point by saying that even if granted "great leisure" these hapless doctors would still barely have been able to identify the major organs, whereas a trained dissector would have made the most of the fleeting opportunity to learn something while looking "quickly" at a human body.[121] Even when at the edge of civilization and with the permission of the emperor, all of these occasions have a furtive feel.[122]

---

[119] This seems to have been a memorable – and, one might therefore infer, isolated – event; Galen mentions it again at *Comp. Med. Gen.* XIII.604, where there is once again emphasis that access to a human body is an unexpected and fortuitous event (κἂν ἀνθρώπου ποτὲ) that must be taken advantage of *quickly* (ταχέως).

[120] See, most similarly, his excusing the mistakes of Aristotle at *AA* II.621 by pointing out that even Marinus, the epitome of the anatomical doctor, made many errors.

[121] Dean-Jones (2018), 239 interprets this sentence very differently and views it not as an abstract comparative, but rather as an assertion that some doctors did indeed "have the opportunity to examine a human body 'at their considerable leisure.'" It seems to me more in keeping with the context and style of the paragraph as whole to interpret this as a hypothetical extreme case that Galen is using to prove his point than as a description of what actually happened in Germania. I am similarly skeptical of her further deployment (pp. 243–5) of these doctors as the likely performers of public human dissections in Rome, including in the arena – while any argument from silence must be somewhat fraught, it is extremely difficult to believe that this activity could have been going on without being mentioned by Galen, who discusses the Roman anatomical scene at some length, or by the historians and other contemporary sources, who chronicled the types of events that occurred in the arena in some detail. Further (as Dean-Jones herself points out at p. 242), the minute scale and obscured sightlines of the dissection of viscera do not seem like promising fodder for an arena-sized event.

[122] In a final reference to human corpses at *AA* S107, the surviving text seems to actually require the practice of human dissection with the statement "you must, then, dissect a dead man and a monkey and other animals furnished with a voice which have, besides the voice, the vocal apparatus, the larynx." However, in reaction to the incongruity of such a statement, Garofalo (1991a) 110, n. 74 has suggested that the Arabic might be a mistranslation of something like ἀνατέμνων νεκρὸν πίθηκον ἢ ἄλλον τι ζῷον ("dissecting a dead monkey or some other animal").

Galen's remarks on the subject seem to imply not that human dissection was never practiced, but rather that it was not openly or routinely practiced.[123] His repeated insistence on the brief time allowed for the investigation of human corpses underscores the illicitness of the endeavor, as does his unusual reluctance to directly connect himself with any of the methods of human dissection that he mentions as occurring. Indeed, despite these hints that human subjects were not completely inaccessible to anatomists of the Roman period, there is no passage where Galen reveals knowledge of the human body that could only be obtained via dissection, and there are instances of marked ignorance in areas to which he would almost certainly have given first priority had he been able to dissect a human cadaver, for example the formation of the human larynx.[124] As a result, despite his repeated statements about the practices of the nameless "many" – which could be construed as a straightforward support for the validity of the comparative anatomy upon which he relies; or as a malicious attempt to throw suspicion on the more dubious activities of his colleagues; or even as an optimistic gambit to normalize a practice he would value – it is highly improbable that Galen ever dissected a human corpse, and, what is more, I believe that his expectation of his fellow anatomists' experience with the interior of the human body was that it would be limited to living subjects, unless luck threw a human skeleton in their way.

Observation of living human subjects, however, was clearly more involved than simply inspecting the muscles of well-developed athletes.[125] Galen mentions that in thin subjects with strong pulses the femoral artery – located in the groin, hardly an area subject to casual contact – is perceptible to the touch.[126] He also recommends that to see a certain vein more clearly, the reader should constrict the arm with a bandage or compress it with his hand after the person in question has had a bath, and he exhorts him to do this often and in many different subjects.[127]

---

[123] On the social contexts surrounding this taboo, see Chapter 5, "Anatomy in the Popular Imagination" at pp. 162–3.

[124] For a discussion of the larynx question, see Simon (1906), xxviii–xxix. He similarly has no knowledge of the vermiform appendix in humans, which is not present in monkeys; see Singer (1956), 249, n. 134.

[125] Though one might think that it would go without saying that human vivisection would be out of bounds for a society that did not countenance human dissection, Galen actually does say it somewhat ironically at *Temp.* I.632, in the context of explaining how one might ascertain the existence in a human patient of an anatomical variation he has observed in animals: "obviously I am not suggesting that you *dissect* a living human" (οὐ γὰρ δὴ ἀνατεμεῖν γε ζῶντας τοὺς ἀνθρώπους ἀξιῶ) (emphasis in the Greek).

[126] *AA* II.410.

[127] Bandage: *AA* II.376; hand: II.383–4.

Obviously both feeling the femoral artery and compressing the arms of many recently bathed men would most easily be worked into daily life by a doctor. Yet, given the high level of interest that Romans of this period took in their friends' health and bodily functions, it would not have been at all out of place for a dilettante dissector to solicit volunteers for this kind of endeavor.[128]

It is clear, though, that Galen does believe that doctors have a material advantage in their ability to use various operations to gain insight into the internal organs of humans. In general terms, he anticipates that the student of anatomy who also practices medicine will become convinced over the course of many surgical operations that the homology he relies on between monkeys and men does in fact exist.[129] Further, he explains that surgery can offer the same sorts of insight that are achieved by dissections of animals, for example in the case of hernia operations.[130] Indeed, the Empiricist sect believed that this sort of "chance anatomy" was sufficient to teach a doctor all that was necessary (and knowable) about the interior of the body.[131] Galen, however, is adamant that these surgical glimpses into the human body cannot substitute for animal dissection, since the operations are so brief that it is impossible to gauge what you are seeing unless you are already familiar with what you are looking for.[132] He demonstrates this opinion vividly with the anecdote from his student days under Satyrus in Pergamon about an epidemic of a necrotizing skin disease, which caused body parts to be "stripped of the skin, and some even of the flesh itself":

> Whichever of us had watched Satyrus, as we cut into any of the exposed parts easily recognized them and made an articulate diagnosis, ordering the patients to make certain movements, which we knew to be brought about by a certain muscle, drawing the muscles aside by a little bit and sometimes turning them away in order to see an adjacent large artery or nerve or vein. But we saw that all the others were seemingly blind and ignorant of the exposed parts and necessarily acting in one of two ways: either they caused distress in vain, lifting up and turning aside many sections of the exposed muscles, as a result of which they became hurtful to the patients, or else they did not even lift a finger to this kind of investigation. For those who were habituated better understood how to order a patient to move a part with

---

[128] See Mattern (2008), 84–7 and the correspondence of M. Cornelius Fronto, which routinely discusses details of his own and others' health (e.g., *Ad amicos* I.13, *Ad Antoninum Imp.* I.1, I.2.6–8, *Ad M. Caes.* III.8.3, V.29[44]).

[129] *AA* II.386.

[130] *AA* S157, 159. He discusses the general utility of open wounds for the study of anatomy at II.386.

[131] On the Empiricist position and Galen's condemnation of it, see *AA* II.288–89 and Chapter 7, "Anatomy in the Roman Intellectual Scene" at pp. 267–9.

[132] *AA* II.225–6, 385, S157.

an appropriate movement. Therefore, I learned clearly from this that, for those who have already learned something, investigation of wounds confirms what they have learned, but it is entirely unable to teach those who were in no way skilled beforehand.[133]

In addition to illustrating Galen's point that a chance glimpse into the human body is useless to those who have not previously trained themselves, this story implies that it was so acceptable for doctors to use patients as teaching tools that the patients were even complicit in this instruction and obligingly moved their limbs at the behest of both teachers and students. The patients here were perhaps exceptionally cooperative and the doctors exceptionally bold owing to the severe nature of the disease, but the anecdote demonstrates that, despite Galen's doubt as to its efficacy, a certain amount of anatomical learning could in theory be achieved through medical practice on human beings.[134]

Other Requirements

Tools

In addition to anatomical subjects, the dissector also had to equip himself with a selection of tools, of varying degrees of specialization. Galen does not lay out a set of required equipment at the beginning of *Anatomical Procedures* or anywhere else, but throughout the work, as they come up, he mentions or describes the various items that the reader will need to perform the dissections. By far the most common tool in his armory is the scalpel or lancet.[135] He requires it for skinning animals as well as for performing the

---

[133] *AA* II.224–6 (ἐψιλώθη μόρια τοῦ δέρματος, τινῶν δὲ καὶ τῆς σαρκὸς αὐτῆς ... ὅσοι μὲν οὖν ἡμῶν ἐτεθέαντο Σάτυρον, ἀνατέμνοντες τῶν ἐψιλωμένων τι μορίων ἑτοίμως τ᾽ ἐγνωρίζομεν αὐτὰ καὶ διηρθρωμένην ἐποιούμεθα τὴν διάγνωσιν, ἐπιτάττοντες τοῖς κάμνουσι κινεῖσθαί τινα κίνησιν, ἣν ἠπιστάμεθα διὰ τοῦδέ τινος ἐπιτελεῖσθαι μυός, ὀλίγον τι παραστέλλοντες καὶ παρατρέποντες ἐνίοτε τοὺς μῦς ὑπὲρ τοῦ θεάσασθαι παρακειμένην ἀρτηρίαν μεγάλην ἢ νεῦρον ἢ φλέβα. τοὺς δ᾽ ἄλλους ἅπαντας ἑωρῶμεν οἷον τυφλοὺς ἀγνοοῦντάς τε τὰ γεγυμνωμένα μόρια, καὶ πάσχοντας ἐξ ἀνάγκης δυοῖν θάτερον, ἢ πολλὰ μέρη τῶν ἐψιλωμένων μυῶν ἐπαίροντάς τε καὶ παρατρεπόντας, ἐξ ὧν ἀνιαροὶ τοῖς κάμνουσιν ἐγίγνοντο, μάτην ἐνοχλοῦντας, ἢ μηδὲ τὴν ἀρχὴν ἐπιχειροῦντας θέᾳ τοιαύτῃ· τὸ μὲν γὰρ προστάξαι τῷ κάμνοντι τὴν προσήκουσαν κίνησιν κινῆσαι τὸ μόριον οἱ †ἐν ἔθει† μᾶλλον ἠπίσταντο. ἔγνων οὖν ἐναργῶς ἐκ τουτωνὶ τὴν τραυματικὴν θέαν τοῖς μὲν ἤδη τι προδεδιδαγμένοις βεβαιοῦσαν ἃ μεμαθήκασι, τοῖς δ᾽ οὐδὲν προεπισταμένοις ἀδυνατοῦσαν διδάσκειν τὸ πᾶν); following the text in Garofalo (1986–2000).

[134] On the nature and severity of the disease, see Mattern (2013), 21, 41–2.

[135] The scalpel (σμίλη) appears to have been the most common medical tool in antiquity in general as well; Bliquez (2014), 72–83 discusses the various names and types available in the Roman period and adds "virtually every surgical set of any consequence come upon by archaeologists contains at least one specimen" (72).

vast majority of the internal operations. He expects the dissector to have several of these with a variety of blades, since he often specifies whether the scalpel should be sharp or blunt, depending on the purpose.[136] He sometimes also specifically requires that the scalpels be strong, usually when they will be used for severing bones, indicating variation on that front as well.[137] There were also a variety of models to choose from: He will occasionally specify that his readers should use myrtle-leaf shaped blades, for example, which had symmetrical convex cutting edges on either side of the knife.[138] He also describes a blade with two cutting edges that is convex on one side and concave on the other to use in demonstrations on the thorax.[139]

Though Galen prefers to use the smaller and more dexterous scalpel, there are occasions when he calls for larger knives instead.[140] In all but a few instances these are used to cut through large bones.[141] Galen's general term for knives is ἐκκοπεῖς – a word with a similar semantic force to cleaver – which, though not common, must have been a standard term, since he once refers to them as "the so-called cleavers."[142] He also mentions other large cutting devices, such as the carpenter's adze, which can be used to remove excess bone from an ox skull, the cutting block for excising ribs, a tool of his own invention for operating on pigs that he calls the elongated knife, and a group of presumably similar tools called the perforator, the lens (which he glosses as an "ossifrageous instrument"), the "bone-breaker," and the osteoclast.[143]

---

[136] *AA* II. 244, 247, 267, 310, 348, 423, 607, 673, S41. At II.607 he is explicit about the need for multiple scalpels of each kind.

[137] *AA* II. 314, 606, 607.

[138] *AA* II. 477, 674, 686, S19, 41 (αἱ μύρσιναι). See Garofalo (1994), 1812; four particularly fine silver-bladed examples from archaeological finds are pictured in Künzl (1983), 58, pl. 26, no. 1, 2, 6, 7.

[139] *AA* II.673. Pictured in Künzl (1983), 52, pl. 20, no. 24, 28; cf. Garofalo (1994), 1812.

[140] He makes this preference explicit at *AA* II.627: "use an animal that is still young so that you may cut with a scalpel rather than with knives" (ἔστω τοιγαροῦν ἔτι νέον τὸ ζῷον, ὅπως ἀνύτηταί σοι διὰ σμίλης ἡ τομὴ χωρὶς ἐκκοπέων).

[141] *AA* II.440, 592, 708–9, S24. Exceptions include II.574 where knives are used to cut up the abdominal organs and S27 where a "long, strong 'palm-leaf knife'" is used to sever the spinal marrow. Note that in the sections that survive only in Arabic it is more difficult to be certain about the exact terminology. I assume that the knife described in S27 is distinct from and bigger than the myrtle-leaf scalpel; though palm leaves and myrtle leaves have the same basic shape, palm leaves are much longer (emphasized by the inclusion of the adjective "long") and the term myrtle-leaf is accurately relayed elsewhere (e.g., S19, 41).

[142] *AA* II.592 (τοὺς καλουμένους ἐκκοπεῖς). Künzl (1983), 20 mistakenly identifies this term with chisels (Lat. *scalprum planum*), but Garofalo's (1994), 1811 reading of the Arabic confirms that it is a "bone-breaking knife" (Lat. *culter excissorius*).

[143] Carpenter's adze: *AA* II.709; cutting block: II.685; "long knife": II.682; perforator: S14; lens: S14, glossed at S15 and mentioned again at *MM* X.449 as the φακωτὸς ἐκκοπεύς (Garofalo [1991*b*], 838); "bone-breaker": S24; osteoclast: S15, 33.

Another tool that Galen makes frequent use of is the hook.[144] He instructs his readers to use hooks to raise areas of interest out of their surroundings for examination, to pull such areas out of the way when examining other structures, and to hold open or pull apart various incisions.[145] Many of these tasks require more than one hook, for example when pulling open both sides of an incision. The hooks can range from sharp to blunt, the former being employed to pierce things and hold them back and the latter to fish things out without injuring them. For the most part, Galen leaves this distinction up to the reader, only specifying in a handful of places the degree of sharpness required for a particular task.[146] In addition to the standard hooks, anyone working on vivisection of the nerves needs at least one hook with an eye bored into the end to allow a thread to pass through – once the demonstrator has secured a nerve with such a hook, he can then easily tie the thread around the nerve to ligature it. These hooks, which Galen tells us were known as "blind" or "one-eyed," were usually blunt, distinguishing them from curved needles, and were standard enough that he speaks of needing to modify them when it is necessary for them to have a bit of a point.[147]

Galen also requires the occasional use of needles and thread. In some of the live experiments the vivisector can use thread to secure foreign bodies inside the animal or to suture a wound closed so that the effects of experiments can be observed while the animal proceeds with normal activities.[148] One can also use a thin threaded needle in place of a hook to pull small fibers out of the way of the main investigation.[149] Galen can be quite specific about the kind of thread that is appropriate for various uses, mentioning linen thread, fine flaxen thread, and "stout thread, such as is suitable for sewing, or a thread such as is used for ligatures."[150] He is particularly concerned that the thread in nerve-ligature experiments not

---

[144] Like the scalpel, the hook (ἄγκιστρον) is almost universally present in surviving *instrumentaria*; see Bliquez (2014), 173.

[145] Raising: *AA* II.247, 254, 477, 487, 515, 668, S26, 132, 262, 263; retracting: II.435, 603, S19; holding open: II.349, S21, 41, 54.

[146] *AA* II.667, S41, 132, 262, 263.

[147] *AA* II.668, S132, 262, 263. See S263 for the need for modifications. At II.668 Galen distinguishes between a curved needle (βελόνην καμπύλην) and a pierced hook (ἀγκίστρῳ διατρήτῳ). Bliquez (2014), 177–80 discusses the "blind" hook, but his treatment suggests that outside of Galen the term seems to have designated bluntness rather than perforation; the Galenic passage naming the term is from the Arabic section (S262), so it is conceivable that something has been lost in translation here.

[148] For foreign bodies, in this case a reed, see *AA* II.646; for suturing, see S81, 129.

[149] *AA* S427.

[150] *AA* S132. For linen thread: II.646; for flaxen thread: S183.

be such as to damage the nerve in any way; he stipulates that it be neither too thin, so as to cut into the nerve, nor too coarse, so as to saw on the nerve, adding that he uses woven threads of yarn or wool in order to avoid these outcomes.[151]

Another frequent though less standardized tool is the probe or sound, used for insertion into tubes and cavities, for other exploratory activities where no damage is intended, and to provide a barrier to stop a knife from cutting deeper than desired.[152] Probes came in a variety of sizes, and it was important to have a range available in order to ensure having one suitable for any orifice in question.[153] Galen tells us that there were a variety of tools that were made specifically for this function.[154] These could be found in several materials, including bronze, iron, silver, copper, gold, and wood, but he seems to have favored wood, particularly boxwood because it is very hard.[155] However, he is not very particular about exactly what his readers use as a probe as long as it fits. In fact, he encourages his readers to use less technical objects if that is what they can find of the appropriate size, frequently recommending using a hair or pig's bristle for very small openings, and saying that when he has nothing else around he sometimes uses the back end of a writing reed as an all-purpose sound.[156]

The trio of scalpel, hook, and probe are the essential tools without which a reader could not perform the tasks described in this work, but Galen does mention a few others in passing as desirable for specific operations. He repeatedly instructs that shaving an area of a monkey makes it easier to cut into the skin, implying the need for some kind of razor, although some of the knives and scalpels already discussed may have done just as well.[157] For live experiments it is critical to have boards of various sizes suitable to variously sized animals, equipped with ropes or straps passed through

---

[151] *AA* II.670, S263–4.

[152] Insertion: *AA* II.713, S38, 75, 235; exploration: II.724, S1, 14, 76; barrier: II.574–5, 711.

[153] *AA* II.575; cf. S1, 75.

[154] Lists of terms: *AA* II.574, 581, 711, 724, S163. According to his descriptions there, ἔλασμα is the general term that anatomists apply to this class of instrument, but more precise terms include the διπύρηνον, a thin probe, the μηλωτίς, which is still thinner, and the interrelated μήλη, ἀμφιμήλη, which has two heads, and σπαθομήλη or σπαθίον, which has a flat area. See Bliquez (2014), 96–7, 108–47 for the ways in which Galen's definitions of these terms map onto other authors' uses and onto the reality of the archaeological record.

[155] For materials, see *AA* II.574, S1, 76. For his preference for boxwood, see II.574, 711, S1.

[156] *AA* II.713, S1, 38, 235. For the writing reed, see S1; similarly, Bliquez (2014), 111 suspects that the back end of other tools often did double duty in this way, accounting for the dearth of simple metal probes in the archaeological record.

[157] *AA* II.348, 423, S132. Bliquez (2014), 107 is inclined to believe that scalpels were used for shaving areas in surgery, based on the absence of razors in archaeological finds from surgical contexts.

holes to bind the animal down.[158] Also helpful in vivisectory experiments is a sponge to control hemorrhaging.[159] For some of his more advanced experiments, he requires a tube, whether a reed or a pipe, to be inserted into narrow passages to hold them open.[160] Beyond these he mentions once each a forceps, for clamping the beating heart, a pair of chisels, for excising ribs, a goldsmith's bellows, for blowing air into deflated cavities of the brain, a hammer, used along with one of the bone-breaking knives, and a spatula, which he seems to use simply as a large probe.[161]

Finally, the least technical but perhaps most employed "tools" are the dissector's own hands. Fingers can replace all three of the basic tools – scalpel, hook, and probe – in some contexts, and it is clear that for Galen they often do. He repeatedly gives his readers the choice of using a tool or their fingers, but often just assumes the use of fingers.[162] As I explored at the beginning of the chapter, these operations were not for the squeamish. Galen has his readers using their fingers to strip away flesh, to pull off skin, to hold the pulsating heart, and to pinch off an artery gushing blood.[163] He does concede, however, that, although he prefers to use his fingers for certain operations, others might prefer to use a tool, saying that "it is not necessary to use only the fingers for this task," and that "we do not have to use a scalpel *unless we want to*; for the fingers alone are sufficient."[164] In only one instance does he advocate the use of a tool over that of the hands, and that is a case where the fingers will obstruct the view in a way that a thinner scalpel will not.[165]

Both textual sources and archaeological finds confirm that the majority of the tools that Galen requires his readers to use were standard surgical tools and thus would not have been hard to come by (Figure 4.2).[166] For many, he mentions that there are different variations available as well as a

---

[158] *AA* II.627, S24. Even when not mentioned specifically, the board can be assumed to be present in all vivisectory experiments unless otherwise indicated.

[159] *AA* S24, 129.

[160] *AA* II.646, S2.

[161] Forceps: *AA* II.635–6; chisels: II.686; bellows: II.717; hammer: S16; spatula: S25.

[162] Fingers or scalpel: *AA* II.247, 349–50, 476, 516, 517, 696; fingers or hook: II.247, 515, 516, 603, S19; fingers only: II.516, 576, 628–9, 635–6, 715, S2, 19, 21, 132, 147.

[163] See the previous note generally and also *AA* II.628–9 for the artery and II.635–6 for the heart.

[164] *AA* II.349 (μόνοις δ' οὐ χρὴ τοῖς δακτύλοις ἄνευ σμίλης ἐπιτρέπειν τοὔργον) and II.350 (οὐδὲν δεομένων ἡμῶν, εἰ μὴ βουληθείημεν, εἰς τοῦτο σμίλης· ἱκανοὶ γὰρ καὶ οἱ δάκτυλοι μόνοι); my emphasis.

[165] *AA* II.476–7; he implies, however, that, though in this instance "*you* would do better to use a scalpel when you dissect" (σοὶ μέντοι βέλτιον ἀνατέμνοντι χρῆσθαι σμίλη), he is skilled enough to use his hands here; my emphasis.

[166] Many of the tools had likely been standard for centuries. The Hippocratic *Medic.* 2–9 – which has been dated to anywhere between about 350 BC and AD 50 (see Craik [2015], 165) – describes the equipment needed by a doctor and includes mention of sharp, broad, and curved scalpels, though the term

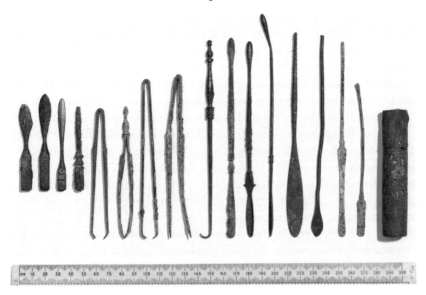

Figure 4.2   Leaded bronze surgical instruments, Roman, AD 1–400, British Museum, London (1867,0508.119). Image: © The Trustees of the British Museum. Note the three scalpel handles (first three from the left), the hook (ninth from the left), and the spatulas, which Bliquez (2014), 108 includes under the broad classification of probes (tenth through sixteenth from the left).

range of materials, from wood to precious metals, indicating that there was a thriving and diverse market in medical equipment.[167] In an unfortunately corrupt passage, he advises the use of scalpels such as have been found in

used is μαχαιρίον; on tools in the Hippocratic texts more generally, see Bliquez (2014), 23–50. Celsus' description of surgical tools available in the first century AD, which includes, for example, hooks differentiated by bluntness, offers an insight into the updates of the Hellenistic era; see Jackson (1994) and Bliquez (2014), 51–5. In general, archaeological finds confirm the literary reports; Künzl (1983) offers a catalogue of the numerous medical tools found in funerary contexts from across the Roman empire (cf. Bliquez [2014]), revealing a widespread uniformity and many specimens that correlate to Galen's descriptions. We also have a few assemblages of tools that were preserved *in situ* by disasters, including those found in various locations in Pompeii (Künzl [1998]), in Marcianopolis in modern Bulgaria (Kirova [2002]), and in Allianoi near Pergamon (Baykan [2012] and Nutton [2014]). One of the more remarkable of these assemblages is that found in the Domus "del chirurgo" at Rimini, where destruction by fire preserved over 150 metal tools in one house, though unfortunately fusing many of them together into puzzle-like clumps; see Jackson (2003) and (2009). The doctor who operated from this house owned "more than 40 scalpels and surgical knives, 19 spring forceps, and a range of sharp and blunt hooks, surgical needles and probes" (Jackson [2003], 314), a collection strikingly similar to the set of tools Galen describes using for dissection.

[167] *AA* II.574, SI, 24. Lucian mockingly mentions decadently produced medical equipment, such as silver cupping-glasses, gold-handled scalpels, and ivory instrument cases (*Ind.* 29), and Galen similarly expresses scorn for doctors with "silver implements" (*Praen.* XIV.600 [σκευῶν ἀργυρῶν]).

a certain type of case for medical instruments since early times.[168] Though the specifics here are in question, it is clear that this type of case has been standard for years and that Galen expects his readers to know what it is. It is therefore safe to assume that these scalpels were recognizable and easily attainable tools, all the more so since he says that horse doctors also use them.[169] In addition to equipment standard for surgery, he also mentions tools normally used by other trades, such as carpentry and goldsmithing.[170]

Some of the tools were less standard. Galen explains that the myrtle-leaf scalpel, one of his favorite kinds, is designed especially for the purpose of delicate cuts in the eye.[171] He also says that there are a variety of instruments that are prepared specifically for opening the skull, particularly for the purpose of cranial surgeries.[172] When a tool with specific and non-standard attributes was required, the customer could adjust it himself or order it specially.[173] In *On Avoidance of Grief*, Galen explains that the fire that burned his warehouse by the Temple of Peace also destroyed several instruments that he had designed, as well as the wax molds that he made for the smiths to create them, and adds that it will not be possible for him to replace them without "much time and a great deal of work."[174] He also says that the reader should use a tool that he designed himself, which he

---

Bliquez (2014), 16–20 points out that the majority of the surviving *instrumentaria* contain tools and containers of bronze or brass, with the exception of the cutting or puncturing implements, which are predominantly steel or iron, but he does mention some pieces with artistic flourishes and inlays of precious metals and adds that "one is struck by the aesthetic care expended on Greco-Roman instruments as opposed to those produced in modern times" (19).

[168] The text (*AA* II.607) reads †αἱ ἐν ταῖς κεφαλικαῖς ὀνομαζομέναις δέλτοις ταῖς ἀρχαίαις†; following the text in Garofalo (1986–2000). I have seen no conjectures as to the significance of the adjective κεφαλικός, which Garofalo (1994), 1811 calls "misteriose." Fischer (1997) argues that δέλτος/δελτάριον is simply the standard term for a rectangular case for surgical instruments; however, he does not discuss this passage in connection with his argument. For an overview of extant cases for medical instruments, see Künzl (1983), 28–9.

[169] *AA* II.607.

[170] Surgeons: *AA* II.685–6, S15; carpenters: II.708; goldsmiths: II.717.

[171] *AA* S41.

[172] *AA* S15.

[173] *AA* II.627, 646, 667, S146, 263. The latter two passages specifically say that the modifications can be done by the reader himself. For the suspicion that some of the tools in the assemblage from the Domus "del chirurgo" at Rimini had been custom ordered by their owner, see Jackson (2009), 74/86.

[174] *Indol.* 5 (οὐκ ἔτ' οἷόν τε σχεῖν ἄνευ χρόνου πο<λ>λοῦ καὶ ἀσχολίας μεγάλης); text according to Boudon-Millot et al. (2010). The idea of inventing a tool was not restricted to Galen. He mentions a boastful doctor who claimed to have invented a tool that would prove the absence of blood in the arteries (*AA* II.643–4) – in this case, however, the tool was never commissioned. See also Bliquez (2014), 7, 14–16 on what he calls "virtuoso" instruments, that is "fancy devices invented by a surgeon of renown for a particular purpose" (7), of which he gives several non-Galenic examples. Bliquez and Jackson (1994), 83–4 discusses an establishment in Pompeii where metal surgical tools were likely both manufactured and sold.

calls the "long knife," to excise the vertebrae of small animals; it is similar to a standard tool, the "so-called stake-knife," but it is thicker and must be made of the best quality steel, such as that from Noricum.[175] Thus if a dissector were intent on doing everything that Galen describes with equal precision, he would need to invest a significant amount of time and money in hunting down and/or creating all of his tools. However, a dissector of more modest ambitions could put together a sufficient toolkit through fairly straightforward purchases.[176] Even in the latter case, though, the cost would not have been negligible; Galen mentions that one of his acts of charity is to give tools to poorer doctors who cannot afford them.[177]

Books

Depending on his profession, location, and predilections, the dissector may also have required some books. Most of the time, the art of dissection, like that of medicine generally, was taught in person, by means of close observation and hands-on practice with a skilled teacher, such as Galen himself. The genre of the anatomical handbook, however, which rapidly burgeoned in popularity in the first two centuries of the Common Era, suggests that this in-person training was, at a minimum, supplemented by textual study. The second half of this book will explore the role of the text in the study of anatomy; here, I will simply consider the implications of the book rolls themselves as an element of the dissector's potential equipment.

Certainly, to follow the instructions outlined in *Anatomical Procedures*, which have so far been our guide in this chapter, the dissector would

[175] *AA* II.682 (τὸ πρόμηκες μαχαίριον, οὕτω γὰρ αὐτὸ καλῶ; τῷ καλουμένῳ σκολοπομαχαιρίῳ); Jackson (2009), 78/88 believes that one of the blades recovered in the Domus "del chirurgo" at Rimini might be an example of this variety. Galen is generally a proponent of high-quality tools; at *AA* S24 he says, "my advice is that this knife should be manufactured from exceptionally good steel, because I prefer that all such instruments with which you provide yourself should be of excellent steel." Noricum is located between the Danube and the Alps and was famous for its quality steel; see also Petronius, *Sat.* 70, Pliny, *NH* XXXIV.145, Ovid, *Met.* 14.712, Suda, *Lexicon* n. 561, and Scamon, *Hist. Frag.* 5.40.

[176] It was no doubt the case, however, that tools were easier to acquire in Rome and other large urban settings than in more provincial locations. Galen explains at *MM* X.942 that his preferred kind of suturing material, a Celtic import, is "very easy" (ῥᾷστον) to obtain in Rome, where it is "very cheap" (εὐωνότατα), but he acknowledges that those practicing elsewhere will likely have to make shift with something else (cf. X.958).

[177] Meyerhof (1929), 84 provides this passage, preserved in an Arabic fragment. For the full passage, see this chapter, "Other Requirements: Books" at p. 133. Bliquez (2014), 20 also notes that some tools appear to have had a centuries-long active life, consistent with being passed on from doctor to doctor.

have needed a selection of books, most obviously including *Anatomical Procedures*, which would itself have required multiple book rolls. There is a great deal of cross-referencing among the books, both forwards and backwards, strongly suggesting that Galen anticipated that his readers would own the entire work. In addition, he mentions a variety of other books that would be helpful, two of which are unequivocally required reading. He says that approaching *Anatomical Procedures* without having studied *On Bones* is like trying to build a house on sand, and also that anyone who wants to follow this course must have thoroughly learned everything in *On the Movement of the Muscles*.[178] Additionally, he several times refers his readers to others of his works, in particular to *On the Causes of Respiration* and *On the Voice*, but on each occasion he offers enough information on what is to be found there that everything essential could be gathered from *Anatomical Procedures*.[179]

Further, Galen conceives of *Anatomical Procedures* as a sequel or companion to *On the Usefulness of the Parts*, his more philosophically driven treatise in seventeen books on the functions of the parts of the body.[180] That said, he does not necessarily expect the readers of the former to have already read the latter. The focus of *Anatomical Procedures* is different – structure rather than function – and he therefore expects the audience to be different, though overlapping.[181] He does, however, anticipate that a reader might be using the two books in tandem. He has organized the two works so that they will follow the same order and is punctilious about excusing and explaining a two-book digression that interrupts this correlation.[182] Not only did he consider the order of *On the Usefulness of the Parts* generally worthy of repetition, but he also availed himself of the fact that keeping the topics in the same order would facilitate cross-reference.

---

[178] For *Oss.*, see *AA* II.460; he also expresses the need to be familiar with it at II.227 and 267 and refers the reader to it at S64. For *Mot.Musc.*, see II.458 and especially II.473; he elsewhere asks the reader to recall things they learned from it, as at S234 and 272.

[179] These references include *Caus.Resp.* (*AA* II.499, 661–2, S29), *Voc.* (S29, 108, 134, 270), *PHP* (II.615), *Controversies in Anatomy* (II.625), and unnamed works at II.664 and S255. The tendency to refer readers to his other works is characteristic of the entire Galenic corpus, as explored in Johnson (2010), 81. He almost never directs readers to the writings of other authors in this text, a referral to the physician Theophrastus's work at S167 being a rare exception. He does sometimes seem to expect that his readers are familiar with earlier writers such as Marinus and Herophilus (especially at S12), but he does not require this or directly refer his readers to their writing.

[180] He says this explicitly at *AA* S18 and implies it elsewhere, as at II.571. For more on the relationship between the two texts, see Chapter 8, "Dissection Elsewhere in the Galenic Corpus" at pp. 310–11.

[181] He specifically says at *AA* S156 that a surgeon will find sufficient information on the testicles here, whereas an anatomist should look at *UP* for a more holistic understanding.

[182] He explains his digression at its beginning (*AA* II.420) and again at its close (II.532), where he says that he is now reverting to the order of *UP*.

Galen frequently sends his readers to *On the Usefulness of the Parts* for more information on topics that he finds irrelevant to or too detailed for *Anatomical Procedures*, sometimes specifying which book the information can be found in, but more often not.[183]

Galen's assumption of access to multiple books – and, in some cases, a repeated access suggestive of ownership – offers some insight into the wealth and social connections expected of a student or practitioner of dissection. The prevalent view is that book-ownership was the province of the elite.[184] Phillips, however, has marshaled evidence to argue that buying a standard edition of a book would not have been out of reach for a skilled artisan or other person earning above the salary of a paid laborer.[185] Certainly it would be reasonable to suppose that a practicing doctor would have owned at least a few book rolls, though the typical collection would perhaps have been more along the lines of handbooks and summaries rather than multivolume treatises like *Anatomical Procedures*.[186]

Independent of their affordability, books beyond the level of popular literature were not always easy to find, even in Rome. Indeed, Galen says, in the context of describing his own skillful and public use of therapeutic lotions, that "the majority of physicians who saw these (performances) did not know where to find written material on this or on other subjects."[187] Though a book

---

[183] *AA* II.271, 285, 420, 443, 474, 568, 590, 616, S108, 156, 270. He gives a specific book at II.271, 420, 590.

[184] See Starr (1987), 221 and Johnson (2010), 21, where he argues that the bookroll was "an egregiously elite product," and 92–3, for an illustration of "the elitism that underlies Galen's repeated insistence on careful reading of the best treatises." See also Marshall (1976), 254, though he is discussing the "sizeable cash investment" needed to create a large working library, rather than the purchase of a few individual books, and Wiseman (1982), 39, where he claims that "the reproduction and distribution of written work ... was a rich man's luxury, and so was buying books." Similarly, Harris (1989), 225 (and n. 254) concludes that "for most people's pockets, though needless to say not for senators', [books] were likely quite expensive."

[185] Phillips (1985), 36–8. Furthermore, though he does not take an explicit position on affordability, White (2009), 284, credits grammarians – common frequenters of bookshops and hardly members of the moneyed elite – with a "more than ordinary appetite for the acquisition of books." He also concludes that "book buyers ... presented a profile indistinguishable from the rest of the reading public" (273).

[186] Nutton (2009), 21 reaches this conclusion from a survey of Galen's comments on the topic, which also imply that his less fortunate colleagues "owned a mere handful of books." Boudon (1994), 1428–9 notes that the price of books would have been prohibitive to medical students and that they relied primarily on oral teaching, perhaps with the occasional handbook as an aide-memoire; see also André (1987), 53 for a similar opinion. For evidence that a doctor would have had at least a small library, see *P. Ross. Georg.* 3.1, a papyrus from the third century AD containing a letter in which an army doctor asks his mother to air out the medical papyri that he left at home; cf. Marganne (2004), 83 and Hanson (2010), 191.

[187] *Opt.Med.Cogn.* 3.17 (*CMG Suppl.Or.* IV, p. 61, trans. Iskandar). There were also instances where Galen was actually unable to locate copies of his own works, for example *Comp.Med.Gen.*, which he tells us he was forced to rewrite after his copy burned (XIII.362–3); cf. Johnson (2010), 87–8. *Praen.* is an even more interesting case: Galen considered this latter work irretrievably lost, to the

of medical concoctions might seem legitimately recondite, literary books too could be difficult to find or exist in only a single copy in Rome.[188] Even the wealthy and well connected like Cicero and Aulus Gellius mention their difficulties in finding texts, the former in complaint, the latter as a source of some pride.[189] A reader looking for the books Galen recommends would have had recourse to booksellers, public libraries, and private collections.[190] Though booksellers traded mainly in current poetry, literature, and political speeches, they do seem to have offered a wide range of authors of various vintages; however, they did not necessarily offer guarantees of authenticity or accuracy.[191] Galen opens his *On My Own Books* with a scene he overheard in the *Sandalarium*, the booksellers' quarter of the day, of a man buying a book attributed to Galen that turned out to be no such thing. Rather it was so poor an imitation that a learned reader who happened to be on-hand discovered it was a forgery after reading a mere two lines.[192] Though their quality and selection may have left something to be desired, bookshops did have the merit of being open to any prospective book reader who could pay.[193]

Public libraries would have been a more reliable source, though perhaps a less egalitarian one. Galen frequently availed himself of the excellent collections in the various libraries in Rome, and we know that his own books would have been available to at least some library patrons, since he tells us that friends requested copies of all his works in order

---

point of not even mentioning it in *Lib.Prop.*, but the text actually survives to the present day, presumably deriving from a copy that had wandered so far from Galen's immediate circle that he was unable to locate it; cf. Nutton (1979), 48–51.

[188] See Starr (1987) for the circulation and purchase of books in Rome, especially p. 218 for their scarcity. See also Marshall (1976), 253–6.

[189] See, for example, Cicero, *Brutus* 129, *Ad Quint.* 3.4.5, 3.5.6, and *Att.* 13.32.2. For a survey of Aulus Gellius' comments and views on access to texts see Johnson (2010), 131–6.

[190] See *Loc.Aff.* VIII.148, where Galen lists precisely these three avenues in his search for a book by his predecessor Archigenes.

[191] See Kenney (1982), 22, Starr (1987), 220–3, and White (2009), 278–80 on the prevalence of current works. White (2009), 272–3 lists as a sampling of things we know to have been bought at bookshops "scientific treatises by Aristotle and Galen, the poetry of Horace, Lucan, and Martial, Pliny's speeches, and Quintilian's opus on the training of the orator" and he adds (p. 278) that there was no concept of older works going "out of print" since "a hundred-year-old title was no more or less complicated to copy and market than a modern author's newest work."

[192] *Lib.Prop.* XIX.8–9. Unreliability was by no means confined to technical works: Gellius mentions as commonplace a *grammaticus* being brought in to inspect a book before purchase (*NA* 5.4.2). See White (2009), 278, n. 30 for long list of complaints about the quality of bookshops' books by various authors.

[193] As far as the social implications of visiting such a shop, White (2009), 274 opines that Cicero was "hardly more likely to set foot in a bookshop than in a butcher's shop," but it should be pointed out that this fastidiousness did not stretch to Catullus, Galen, and Gellius, all of whom enjoyed frequenting bookshops as part of a day's entertainment (Catullus, 55.4, Galen, XIV.620, Gellius, V.4.1, XIII.31.1).

to put them into provincial public libraries.[194] How much of the public was actually admitted to public libraries, however, is open to debate. Dix has collected the relevant passages on access to public libraries in Rome, and, though none of them explicitly rule out the admission of those not connected to the emperor's circle, none of them confirm it either, which leads him to conclude that "given the economic, social, and cultural restrictions which bound most individuals in the ancient world, it seems safe to say that only a very small number are likely ever to have availed themselves of the opportunity to peruse the volumes in a public library."[195]

Perhaps the easiest way to acquire a book was to borrow it from a private owner and make a copy – or, more probably, have a copy made – but access to private collections was obviously predicated on social connections.[196] Galen considers the libraries of friends to be the equal of the public libraries as a source for the types of books he reads. On a hunt for variant readings in a treatise of Hippocrates, he says that he deliberately looked at "all the copies in the public libraries and all those in the hands of my friends."[197] In fact, his expectation that "many hands of men will pass it along," suggests that he anticipates *Anatomical Procedures* itself being

---

[194] For Galen's use of public libraries, see *Indol.*, especially as discussed by Nicholls (2011). For Galen's writings being requested for provincial libraries, see *Indol.* 21 (Boudon-Millot et al [2010]). Sadly, the copies destined for his friends in Pergamon were lost in the massive fire that destroyed Galen's warehouse, but there were already many other copies of his works in libraries in other cities.

[195] Dix (1994), 290. The main evidence for library access for the nonconnected is the reference in the *Historia Augusta* to libraries in the public baths, but the reliability of the author is suspect and, even if such libraries existed, they were more likely to have contained "light reading" than texts on anatomy (see Dix [1994], 286, 288, 290). Marshall (1976), 261 states without qualification that the public libraries were "not so much Carnegie-style institutions, 'public' in the modern sense, as the Emperor's libraries generously thrown open to his *amici* and urban *clientes* as a form of patronage." Nicholls (2011), 129–30 argues that the public libraries in Rome by the late second century AD were as powerful a draw to scholars as private collections and (p. 136) that "the imperial libraries seem to have been accessible to serious 'scholarly' readers," but he does not go into who would have been considered a suitable "scholar." Harris (1989), 228–9 believes that the public libraries "must to some degree have helped to make texts available to the learned and the respectable. It would however be crudely anachronistic to suppose that the sum of these efforts had any large-scale effect on the diffusion of the written word." Blanck (1992), 160, however, takes Suetonius at his word that Caesar created the first public library with open access to all.

[196] There is a great deal of evidence for peers sharing books in this way, for example, Cicero, *Att.* 2.20.6, 2.22.7, 4.14.1, 8.11.7. See Johnson (2010), 155, 167, and especially 180–5, which considers a letter from Oxyrhynchus (*P.Oxy.* 2192) requesting that several books be copied from the libraries of friends and sent to the writer. For the difficulties and expenses of copying and hiring copyists, see Marshall (1976), 254.

[197] *Hipp.Ep.* XVIIb.194–5 (ἅπαντα μὲν ἰδόντες τὰ κατὰ τὰς δημοσίας βιβλιοθήκας, ἅπαντα δὲ τὰ παρὰ τοῖς φίλοις). He also looks among his friends' libraries to replace his own writings when he loses them to fire (*Comp.Med.Gen.* XIII.362–3).

circulated through widening circles of friends and acquaintances in this manner.[198] So a reader of only modest wealth might acquire one or two books and then pool his holdings with like-minded friends in order to achieve a small collection, though the cost of copyists and papyrus would still have kept this method from being inexpensive.[199] For those without the means or friendships to allow this, owners of the larger private collections would also open their libraries to scholars.[200] Such a scholar, however, was presumably either a *cliens* of the wealthy book-owner or had a letter of introduction from a friend, once again requiring a reader to have the requisite social standing and connections.[201]

For the specific field of medical books, the connections required for access could be professional as well as social. Doctors and anatomists with successful schools of students were accustomed to present books containing their own works, or digests thereof, to students leaving to set up practices, and many would presumably also have had works by other medical writers available.[202] However, these books could be even more jealously guarded than the most elite private collection. Galen speaks of the frustration of trying to gain access to the writings of Numisianus, a preeminent anatomist of the previous generation who did not circulate his books widely.[203] He is critical of those who "conceal" their anatomical knowledge and "begrudge" it to others, a complaint that he also levels

---

[198] *AA* II.504 (πολλὰς δ᾽ ἀμείψειν ἀνθρώπων χεῖρας). Note that this is precisely the mode of dissemination proposed in Starr (1987) for literary texts.

[199] Johnson (2010), 94 believes that Galen envisioned just such a "culture of sharing" as the ideal core of the elite community. For evidence of small, specialized private book collections of this kind, see Houston (2009), especially Table 10.1, though he adds that "collections of even a few dozen volumes might well be considered, and in fact were, impressive" (246, n. 40). For the difficulties and expenses of copying and hiring copyists, see Marshall (1976), 254; however, see Skeat (1995) for a convincing refutation of the popular view that papyrus was prohibitively expensive.

[200] A famous early example is the library of Lucullus, which Plutarch describes as "open to all and … admitting Greeks without restriction" (*Luc.* 42.1–2) and which Cicero seems to have frequently (solebam) taken advantage of (*Fin.* 3.7–10; see *Att.* 4.10.1 for his similar use of the library of Sulla). For other examples of large private libraries, both for use and for show, see Blanck (1992), 157.

[201] Dix (1994), 282 specifically characterizes private libraries as "another benefit which a patron might bestow on a client" and "available only to the aristocracy and its dependents." Indeed, Marshall (1976), 257 expects that even Lucullus' famously open library "was not 'public' in any real sense and … an invitation to use its resources presupposed a social connection as an *amicus* or *cliens*."

[202] At *AA* S232 Galen explains that the anatomical works of Pelops in circulation are not his full treatise on anatomy, but "only such writings as he used to hand over to his pupils, and to which he appended the work on the *Introduction to Hippocrates*; these he would present when his pupils wished to return to their homes." The inclusion of his introduction to Hippocrates implies that Pelops' own library was large enough to include some Hippocratic references.

[203] See Chapter 7, "Quintus and His Students: Numisianus, Heracleianus, Pelops, and Aelianus" at pp. 243–5.

at some recipients of his own works who are too selfish to share them as he intended.[204]

To his credit, Galen practices as he preaches in regard to book sharing. By his own account, his book distribution was diffuse, with recipients ranging from wealthy patrons to poor students. Further, he chastises a wealthy friend for not choosing to spend his money on noble causes, "on the buying and preparation of books and the training of scribes either in speed-writing through signs or in beautiful and exact writing, just as also not on those who read aloud correctly," implying in the context that he spends his own wealth this way and shares the results liberally with his friends.[205] Indeed, Galen prides himself on his generosity to less fortunate doctors:

> I have struck up friendships with many of the doctors who flock to me and I have also presented numerous others to powerful men without having taken a bribe or gift from any of them. Rather, I gladly make a point of giving many of these men instruments or remedies of which they have need, and in certain cases I have not even constrained myself to this, but, over and above it, have given them monetary loans needed for their careers.[206]

Such self-avowed beneficence would surely have extended to making books available to the less fortunate.

Though Galen clearly did present the valuable gift of book rolls to some of his recipients, he seems to have more frequently allowed them to record his lectures at no cost and little inconvenience to himself.[207] However, the resulting texts would not have been edited treatises, like *Anatomical Procedures*, to which Galen would refer his readers from his other works; he considered them to be more akin to private notes than finished books.[208] Each mention that Galen makes of texts dictated by request in this manner is accompanied by astonishment that the text should have spread widely during the intervening years and a disclaimer that it was not meant for that purpose.[209] Indeed,

---

[204] *AA* S230–1. Criticism of his own students is at II.283 (see Chapter 9, "The Purpose of *Anatomical Procedures*" at p. 332). At *HNH*, XV.23–4 he goes so far as to accuse his contemporaries of purposely hiding or destroying the works of the ancients in order to have a monopoly on their ideas or even pass them off their own.

[205] *Aff.Pecc.Dig.* V.48 (μήτ'εἰς βιβλίων ὠνὴν καὶ κατασκευὴν καὶ τῶν γραφόντων ἄσκησιν ἤτοι γ'εἰς τάχος διὰ σημείων ἢ εἰς κάλλος <καὶ> ἀκρίβειαν, ὥσπερ γε οὐδὲ τῶν ἀναγινωσκόντων ὀρθῶς). In keeping with Galen's claims to allocate much of his wealth to his library, Nutton (2009), 21 believes that "it is very likely that [Galen's] was among the largest ancient collections of medical books."

[206] From the German translation of an Arabic source collected in Meyerhof (1929), 84.

[207] In some cases, he seems to have redelivered the speech privately to the shorthand writer, which would have cost him some time.

[208] See Cribiore (2019), 262–71 for the most recent discussion of the different levels of publication in Galen.

[209] See *Ven.Sect.Er.Rom.* XI.194, where a lecture dictated to a friend was circulated "without permission" (οὐ κατὰ τὴν γνώμην) even though it was "not composed as a written work, but as a

Galen did not even keep copies of these texts for himself. He highlights this rule with an exception – there were a few texts that he dictated to a friend's shorthand writer that he chose to finish properly and therefore retained copies of, considering them on a par with his other works for publication.[210] In fact, this method of composition would probably have differed hardly at all from his usual modus operandi; it is very likely that Galen composed the majority of his works, and especially those with an anatomical focus, by dictating to his own trained shorthand writer and then editing and polishing the results.[211] Though the shorthand writers Galen and his richer friends employed would have been able to produce extremely accurate transcripts of Galen's words, it is unlikely that the notes of the lectures he dictated to students would have been so complete or so accurate.[212] There would undoubtedly have been a substantial difference between the "bootlegged" copies of lectures dictated to students and the final versions that resulted from his collecting, editing, and releasing them for circulation at a later date with the subtitle "For Beginners." As a result of all of these considerations, I find it

---

lecture" (οὐ συγγράμματι πρεπόντως, ἀλλ'ἀκουστηρίῳ συνέκειτο), *Praen.* XIV.630, where he dictated a demonstration on the breath to Boethus' shorthand writer and "did not make provision for whether he was going to distribute them widely" (μὴ προοπώμενος εἰ μέλλοι δώσειν αὐτὰ πολλοῖς), *Lib.Prop.* XIX.10–11, where he gives a general overview of the books he did not intend for general circulation, including those dictated to young students, and XIX.14–15, where he is "baffled" (οὐκ οἶδ' ὅπως) to discover the wide circulation of a speech dictated for a friend. Galen's stance of naïve amazement at the popularity and distribution of any of his works should be considered with a healthy skepticism, but it is nevertheless a reliable indication that this category of text was not as meticulously monitored and therefore less cross-referenced than his more considered writings; cf. *MM* X.457, where he claims that he never even put his name on texts he wrote.

[210] At *Lib.Prop.* XIX.12–13 Galen explains that he possessed none of the works later designated "for beginners" until they were collected by friends and presented to him for editing. In contrast, he did have copies of other works written for friends because "they had been completely revised" (διὰ τὸ τελέως ἐξειργάσθαι).

[211] Dorandi (2000), 51–75 explains that though some authors certainly wrote by hand, it was also quite common to dictate (see especially p. 65, nn. 59–65) and that it may indeed have been "le procédé habituel de composition" for many, even including poets (p. 71). He concludes that those who most frequently used dictation were "les érudites et les auteurs techniques" (p. 68). For further evidence of the prevalence of composition by dictation, see Starr (1991), 337, n. 4 and also Marganne (2004), 85–6, specifically for the evidence of tachygraphy manuals with respect to medical writing. Galen almost certainly composed *AA* by dictation: He says at S136 that he composes his works on anatomy "with the animal placed in front of me, while I am looking at the things about which I am talking, especially when I am describing the method to be followed in their dissection," which strongly indicates dictation since his hands would have been occupied with the dissection.

[212] On the accuracy of professional tachygraphists, see Winter (1969) and White (2009), 279–80. Though Winter hypothesizes that "it is conceivable that stenography became a usual part of rhetorical education," since "there would have been no faster and cheaper way to obtain models" of oratory (p. 611), White believes (and I agree) that "the ability to transcribe a speech from oral delivery was a specialized skill possessed by a small subset even of the literate population. Few private persons would have commanded a clerical staff with the necessary training" (p. 280).

unlikely that direct transcription of lectures, personally or by hired stenographer, would have been a possible method of acquiring the books that Galen assumes the readers of *Anatomical Procedures* own.

In short, the possession of the minimum number of books Galen expects the reader of *Anatomical Procedures* to have – *Anatomical Procedures* itself, *On Bones*, *On the Movement of the Muscles*, and, optionally, *On the Usefulness of the Parts* – would have necessitated a significant outlay of money, though one not completely out of reach of the average aspiring practitioner.[213] In many cases the more restricting factor would probably have been the need for appropriate social connections. If the reader were lucky enough to be personally acquainted with Galen or one of his friends or students, he might be able to get a copy of one or all of the works at one or two removes from the source at relatively low cost – though Galen, unsurprisingly, seems to have been more generous with short beginner books such as *On Bones* and *On the Movement of the Muscles* than with grander multivolume books like *Anatomical Procedures*.[214] Readers who did not have access to Galen directly or indirectly, for example those living outside Rome, would have needed either the wealth and influence necessary to track down his books or the connections that would allow for access to public or private libraries.

As I will explore in Chapter 9, however, Galen was unusually insistent on the value of pedagogical texts for anatomists. His criticisms of the publishing practices of his colleagues and near predecessors point to a field dominated by oral instruction and close student–teacher relationships: One could reasonably take the position that many of those performing dissections in imperial Rome did not consider books an essential part of their equipment at all. These varying degrees of bookishness among dissectors in turn open up further uses to which books might be put by those who chose to employ them. Galen was not reticent about incorporating books into his public anatomical displays. In one extended, multiday demonstration described in *On My Own Books*, he opens the scene by laying out

---

[213] Without *UP* this would have come to a total of eighteen books, probably contained in roughly as many bookrolls. The addition of *UP*, which Galen does not present as "required reading" but constantly encourages his readers to reference, would have added a further seventeen for the fairly impressive total of thirty-five.

[214] At *Lib.Prop.* XIX.10–13 Galen describes his habit of giving casual copies of texts to friends and students "as a memorandum for those people, upon request, of the things they had heard" (αὐτοῖς ἐκείνοις γεγονότα δεηθεῖσιν ὧν ἤκουσαν ἔχειν ὑπομνήματα) (10), but he clarifies that these texts were later collected, organized, and edited into more official versions under the title "for beginners" (τοῖς εἰσαγομένοις) (13). Even these edited versions of the works for beginners are much shorter and less involved than his grand oeuvres like *AA* and *UP*.

treatises by all of his anatomical predecessors and promising to use dissection to prove that his understanding of anatomy was superior to them all.[215] This added element of scholarly erudition, not to mention extravagant book-ownership, no doubt set him and other like-minded dissectors apart from nonliterary rivals, all the more so in the second century, when scholarly achievement was considered by many circles to be the pinnacle of success.

Assistants

Finally, those engaged in high-profile public displays of dissection would absolutely have required assistants. Those contented with private anatomical study would have needed them less urgently but would likely still have employed them. Galen only occasionally suggests that his readers use the help of assistants, but he is probably tacitly assuming their presence quite often. These assistants could have been students, slaves, or servants. He himself was usually surrounded by a coterie of friends, students, and slaves, and often takes their presence for granted in a story.[216] He directly mentions the use of assistants in the context of menial tasks and in directions for vivisections and public demonstrations, but they were in the background much of the time, not only as aides to dissection, but also as lectors, since reading a book roll was a physically and intellectually more complicated feat than reading a modern book.

Galen occasionally assumes that his readers are in a position to have slaves or other servants to whom they can delegate menial – and domestically irrelevant – labor. Skinning an animal is a tedious, repugnant task and, unlike the numerous other repugnant tasks in *Anatomical Procedures*, not a particularly rewarding one. It seems to have been standard for anatomists to leave this job to underlings, either from distaste or from a sense of their own dignity; nevertheless, Galen repeatedly advocates that his readers do it themselves to ensure quality.[217] In this instance, then, the work does not necessitate an assistant, but Galen's haste to forestall the use of one

---

[215] *Lib.Prop.* XIX.22 (compare XIX.14); for the complete passage, see the epigraph to Chapter 6.

[216] The terms friend (φίλος) and companion (ἑταῖρος) are largely interchangeable and, the latter particularly, can refer to students as well; cf. Garofalo (2006), 64–5. He rarely refers to his own slaves directly; see Mattern (2008), 14–22 (friends and companions) and 139–40 (slaves).

[217] At *AA* II.233 Galen says that he originally had an assistant (τῶν ὑπηρετῶν τις) do his skinning for him out of "distaste, obviously, and a feeling that the task was beneath [him]" (ὀκνοῦντι δηλονότι καὶ μικρότερον ἢ κατ' ἐμὲ νομίζοντι τοὔργον), but he changed his mind upon discovering eight muscles that had previously been overlooked as a result of careless skinning. He indicates that entrusting this job to others for similar reasons is common among other anatomists at II.231–2 and instructs his readers to do it themselves both there and at II.351–2.

indicates his assumption of their common employment. These assistants would presumably have been servants or slaves, but, if the reader were a doctor with attendant students, he might have put them to work instead.[218]

Vivisections also required assistance, not so much for the avoidance of drudgery, but because restraining the struggling animal could be difficult and speed was often of the essence. Some of the tasks that Galen suggests using assistants for, such as shaving and tying or holding down live animals, would have required no anatomical skill.[219] Indeed, for all of the vivisections that he suggests the reader do for his own edification, a willing (and not squeamish) helper with no anatomical training would have been sufficient. In the vivisections of the brain, for example, he advises his reader to have an assistant so that he can act as an extra pair of hands to hold a vein out of the way and to compress areas to staunch bleeding.[220] Though he does not usually spell out the need for a helper, it often becomes clear from context that one would be necessary, as with the incision into the dura mater of the brain where he instructs the reader to be wielding three hooks, a scalpel, and his fingers almost simultaneously.[221] Skillful helpers are most necessary in large public dissections. Galen emphasizes this twice over the course of his discussion of the vivisection of the intercostal nerves: If you are working for yourself or for a few observers, you can work alone, but for a large crowd it is a necessity to have several assistants able to perform anatomical tasks.[222] He delegates difficult tasks to such assistants in his own demonstrations, and it is likely that they were either pupils or highly trained slaves or servants.[223]

---

[218] Galen describes entrusting skinning to a ὑπηρέτης (*AA* II.233) and a ἑταῖρος (II.351). The social status of the former is unclear, though, based on the use of the word in the Hippocratic Corpus, I would suspect a servant or slave (see Jouanna [2017], 131), but the latter is clearly of a higher social position. Previously in this passage he uses the same term, ἑταῖρος, to describe the person for whom his reader is doing a private dissection, which suggests that this reference is to a student.

[219] At *AA* II.627 he tells the reader to instruct "one of his assistants" (τις τῶν ὑπηρετῶν) to tie down and shave an animal; at S24 he says that the animal should be restrained either by straps or "by the hands of assistants."

[220] Vein at *AA* II.718; compression at S19.

[221] *AA* S21.

[222] At *AA* II.669, in contrast to what he expects "if you examine [it] alone for yourself" (κἂν μόνος ἐπὶ σαυτοῦ ποτ' ἐξετάζῃς), he suggests that when you demonstrate you use several assistants to put loops quickly around the intercostal nerves, a feat that requires a great deal of skill and practice, in order to be able to tie them all simultaneously and silence the animal in an immediate and spectacular fashion; at II.672–73 he goes so far as to say that in a large demonstration the entirety of the dissecting work should be left to others while you give the explanatory lecture. This is in contrast both to "private study" (γυμναζόμενον ἐπὶ σαυτοῦ) and to a demonstration "for a few diligent students" (ὀλίγοις τῶν φιλομαθῶν), in which one would work alone (κατὰ μόνας ... ἐπιδείκνυμεν).

[223] For medically trained servants in Galen's household, see Mattern (2013), 140; see also Jouanna (2017), 128–31 for the Hippocratic precedent.

The other main way in which assistants would have been useful to the reader of an anatomical guidebook like *Anatomical Procedures* is as lectors. Galen never actually mentions or suggests this; he does occasionally refer to his reader as a listener, but this could also be explained by the theory, which we will consider in Chapter 9, that *Anatomical Procedures* included material from a series of transcribed lectures.[224] Nevertheless, the use of lectors was extremely common in antiquity and would have been particularly helpful in the case of this text.[225] Both hands were required to read a book roll, and it could not be easily put down and then referenced in the way that a modern textbook can be; further, the text itself would have been unlikely to have punctuation or, indeed, word divisions, making it still more difficult to glance at or skim a set of instructions.[226] Galen indicates, as we saw earlier, that he invests his money in training or hiring "lectors who read well," and he would presumably have employed them, like his shorthand writers, in situations like dissections where his hands were otherwise occupied.[227]

Though employing a lector to read *Anatomical Procedures* would no doubt have been both convenient and unremarkable, Galen's directions do not presume it. On the contrary, he expects a great deal more from his own memory and the memories of his readers than is usual, or almost even credible, in the modern era.[228] In fact, there are numerous passages throughout the text that suggest that he expects his readers to read and internalize his instructions and only afterwards pick up the scalpel and dissect, a practice that does not particularly require the use of a lector. For example, when he discusses the results of damaging the intercostal nerves, he says that the readers will recognize the phenomena he is about to describe when they actually do the experiment.[229] He also sometimes describes dissections in a different order from that in which they are to be

---

[224] He tells the reader to "listen once now in order to remember forever" (ἀκούσας ἅπαξ νῦν εἰς ἀεὶ μεμνημένος ἔσο) at *AA* II.278 and refers to him as "listening" or a "listener" at II.550 and S83. Contrast II.353–54, S11, and 92 where he explicitly refers to his audience as readers.

[225] On the frequent use of lectors, see Harris (1989), 226 and especially Starr (1991), though he also indicates their high price (p. 339).

[226] On the physical and cognitive difficulties imposed by bookrolls, see Kenney (1982), 17–18, Starr (1991), 343, and Johnson (2010), 18–20, 22, 31, 192.

[227] *Aff.Pecc.Dig.* V.48; see this chapter, n. 205.

[228] Galen appears to have memorized a great deal of his predecessors' writings. He is able to reference Hippocratic commentators from memory, for example, even while his library remained in Pergamon (*Lib.Prop.* XIX.34). For examples of his frequent exhortation of his readers to memorize and remember, see *AA* II.278, 354, 364, 380, 393, 458, 589, 626, 680–81, S76, 88, 182, 192, 234–36, 248, 273, 290, 311.

[229] *AA* II.675.

done, requiring that the reader read ahead and internalize the directions so as to be able to apply them thoughtfully in the appropriate order.[230] He even goes so far as to engage the reader in imaginary or "verbal" dissections while they read before they set aside the book and do the actual dissections.[231] All of this suggests that, regardless of their preferences vis-à-vis lectors, Galen expects his readers to engage with the text thoroughly prior to dissection.

The final group of people required for dissections, at least the performative ones, was the audience. They certainly do not fall into the category of a material prerequisite, but their needs and expectations shaped the ways that anatomists performed their dissections. Accordingly, in Chapter 5, the final of Part I, I will offer a sketch of the contexts in which all of this anatomical activity was taking place, considering the social and cultural factors that informed not just the practice of the all dissections described so far, but also the ways in which they were received by their audiences.

---

[230] See *AA* S160 where he explains that "it can happen that what comes first in the description may come not first but second in the dissection." For example, at II.617, where he describes observations of the heart removed from the thorax but subsequently adds observations that should be made before its removal.

[231] Most particularly at *AA* II.444 (τῷ λόγῳ). See also II.550 and S101, where he tells the reader to "think of" (ἐννοήσας) or "picture in his mind" the animal he is describing in a certain way, and II.622 where he says that the reader should "learn the procedure in advance by words before turning to the dissection" (τῷ λόγῳ γε προδιδαχθεὶς ἐπὶ τὴν ἀνατομὴν ἦλθε).

CHAPTER 5

The Broader Social Contexts of Dissection

What enjoyment can there be for a cultured person when ... a magnificent beast is pierced through by a spear?

Cicero, *Letters to Friends*[1]

The answer to Cicero's question here is: a lot. The type of staged hunt that he describes was an enormously popular attraction in Rome – a popularity that highlights the fact that seeing an animal cut open for entertainment was a fairly routine matter in the ancient world. Indeed, the public dissections considered in Chapter 3 were by no means anomalous events; rather they were but one piece of a mosaic of interrelated phenomena. In this chapter, I will explore the practice of dissection within its broader cultural milieux. Many of the topics I touch on here were consistently relevant in fluctuating ways across the Mediterranean world over the centuries covered in this book, but there is also a notable concatenation of developments in the Roman period that dovetails with the emergence of performative dissection. In each period and place, social contexts informed the ways in which dissectors would have presented themselves and the ways in which their audience, if they welcomed one, would have received them.

I have broken the topic down into four parts. The first briefly covers parallels to the rhetorical and performative side of medicine generally and to public dissections in particular. Doctors promoted themselves within existing social frameworks, and they competed for public attention with contemporaries from a variety of spheres; their audiences overlapped with those of sophists, advocates, philosophers, and other public performers, and the similarities among all of these performances would have been salient to all involved. The second focuses on animals and the various circumstances outside scientific dissection in which their bodies were cut into and opened. While the public dissection or vivisection of an animal would be

---

[1] Cicero, *Fam.* 7.1.3 (quae potest homini esse polito delectatio cum ... praeclara bestia venabulo transverberatur?).

greeted today with protest from animal rights activists, it would not have raised any eyebrows in antiquity.[2] Indeed, people from across the ancient world were at home with animal viscera in a way that is foreign to modern society; they were familiar with the internal organs at a visual and tactile level that would have undergirded their reception of public dissection and their understanding of the anatomy it presented. However, this familiarity with the disemboweling of animals for different purposes would also have brought up associations that anatomists would have been keen to forestall; ancient doctors needed to distinguish themselves from butchers and those who practiced magic, both groups who also cut open animals for different ends. The third part of the chapter considers religious practices that involved the opening up of the body, whether actually or conceptually. Here, again, we find a direct parallel for dissection – namely the slaughter, inspection, and partitioning of animals for sacrifice and soothsaying – in a field that doctors vociferously differentiated themselves from. Here, too, we can find a glimpse of nonmedical conceptualizations of human anatomy, via religiously motivated ways of depicting and treating the body. The final section queries the Greeks' and Romans' general familiarity and comfort with viewing and imagining the insides of bodies, as well as the degree of popular interest in engaging with anatomical knowledge.

As these topics suggest, bodies – and, with them, conceptions about their structure and function – are implicated in just about every facet of life in antiquity. Further, the nuances, significance, and implications of these relationships change as we move across the moments and places encompassed by this book, from Classical Greece to Hellenistic Alexandria to Imperial Rome. A thorough evaluation of all of these topics would require a monograph of its own, yet they are essential to a holistic understanding of the development of dissection in antiquity. I have therefore attempted to thread the needle by offering here a summary and selective but, I hope, evocative survey of the wider world within which dissection in all its various guises was occurring.

Public Performances

As already explored in Chapters 2 and 3, the medical profession was a public one, and the Roman manifestation of performative dissection was but one aspect of this broader character. Public orations were an established part of elite medical practice. The epigraphic evidence for doctors like

---

[2] The public dissection of a euthanized giraffe at the Copenhagen Zoo in 2014, for example, attracted curious crowds, but also drew outraged condemnation from around the world.

Asklepiodorus of Elatea and Asklepiades of Perge and Seleucia attests to the popularity of such events in the Hellenistic period, and, in the Roman period, Galen indicates that both he and his peers lectured routinely.[3] These events, much like their rhetorical counterparts and like the forced dissections considered in Chapter 3, would sometimes get quite raucous – indeed, Galen evocatively likens the followers of the different medical sects to the notoriously rowdy fans of the different horse racing stables in Rome – and could devolve into debates between the lecturing doctor and his erstwhile audience.[4] More consensually arranged public debates were also popular. Galen reminisces about day-long – and multiday – debates among the doctors of his teachers' generation, including Pelops and Satyrus.[5] They remained a common reputational proving-ground in his own day: When Galen fantasizes about besting intellectual rivals, he imagines doing it "as if in a stadium."[6] Of course, doctors were by no means the only people seeking to attract public attention and accolades for their work and attainments; they would have been in competition with other public performers, all of whom adopted successful strategies from each other where they could. The connections between medical exhibitions, including those involving dissection, and the crowd-pleasing performances of the sophists have already been well documented.[7] Indeed, Aelius Aristides refers to this same Satyrus as both a doctor and a sophist.[8] The public activities of philosophers, too, exhibit interesting parallels with those of their medical counterparts, even

---

[3] On the epigraphic evidence, see Chapter 2, "Medical Performance in the Hellenistic Period" at pp. 48–50. In the Roman period, some lectures seem to have been primarily aimed at students and smaller groups (e.g., *Purg.Med.Fac.* XI.329, *Pecc.Dig.* V.64–5, *Ven.Sect.Er.Rom.* XI.191), others at a wider audience, though this can be ambiguous (e.g., *Lib.Prop.* XIX.13–15, *Loc.Aff.* VIII.142–3, *MM* X.10, 369, *Ven.Sect.Er.Rom.* XI.193–4, *Diff.Puls.* VIII.763–5, *Adv.Jul.* XVIIIa.247, 253).

[4] For audience behavior, see von Staden (1997), 47–51 and Mattern (2008), 9–11, 14–21. For Galen's comparison to race fans, see *Ord.Lib.Prop.* XIX.53; on the stables and their obstreperous fans, see Meijer (2010), 99–105. Galen himself is guilty of usurping someone else's lecture at *Thras.* V.894–5 and *Simp. Med.* XI.432–3; he is on the other side of the situation at *Praen.* XIV.627–8 and *Diff.Puls.* VIII.571.

[5] Debates involving Pelops and Satyrus at *Nom.Med.* 99v–101r (Meyerhof and Schacht [1931], 27–9) and *Lib.Prop.* XIX.16–17. Other debates: *Thras.* V.807, *Nat.Fac.* II.34, *Diff.Puls.* VIII.494–5, *MM* X.109–14, *Ven.Sect.Er.Rom.* XI.193.

[6] *Purg.Med.Fac.* XI.328 (ὥσπερ ἐν σταδίῳ).

[7] For a focus on anatomical exhibitions specifically, see Debru (1995), von Staden (1995) and (1997), and now Salas (2020), 27–35, 68–73; more generally, for parallels between doctors and sophists of the Classical period, see Lloyd (1987), 83–102 and, for parallels during the Second Sophistic, see Bowersock (1969), 59–75, Nutton (1979), 59–63, Kollesch (1981), Brunt (1994), 43–6, who provides a dissenting opinion, Swain (1996), 357–79, Mattern (2008), 7–11 and (2017), and Petit (2018), especially 1–8.

[8] Aristides, *Ier.Log.* III.8 (311 Jebb). It is ambiguous, however, whether or not the term *iatrosophist*, which appears in Late Antique authors, was prevalent in this period; see Bowersock (1969), 67, for an optimistic view, and Baldwin (1984), 16, Grilli (1988), and Brunt (1994), 43, n. 73 for more cautious analyses.

including some that are self-consciously drawn.[9] The trope of philosopher as doctor of the soul was a long-lived one, and Arrian's Epictetus carries it over to the performative sphere, explaining that philosophical lectures should not leave their audiences delighted by rhetorical prowess, but rather in great pain, as if having undergone a kind of public surgery.[10]

One intellectual sphere that has particular overlap with medicine generally and anatomy in particular is that of the law.[11] Unlike other comparable pursuits, these are both fields that require public performance for practical ends and operate at a high-stakes, sometimes even life-or-death, level. It is not a coincidence that the pivotal moment in both practices – the moment of judgment in a court case and the moment when a disease reaches its decisive turn for better or for worse – is called the crisis. Medical writers are aware of this metaphorical parallel, and Galen sometimes employs other jurisprudential language in his discourse as well, including likening medical debates to court procedures.[12] On the flip side, medical, and even specifically anatomical, quandaries served as fodder for forensic training; one of the major declamations attributed to Quintilian is a prosecutor's attack on a fictitious father who allowed one of his twin sons to be vivisected in order to cure the other of the mysterious ailment from which they were both suffering.[13] At a more visual and experiential level, court-mandated torture, even when not anatomically revealing, offers certain parallels to vivisection. In both Greece and Rome, the legal testimony of slaves was to be obtained under torture. This took a variety of forms, the most common of which were the rack and the wheel; in each case, the subject was stripped and tied with limbs outstretched – in a position highly evocative of Galen's vivisectory subjects – and pressure was exerted on the limbs to increasing levels of pain.[14] In some cases, the torturer partially flayed the victims or impaled their bodies with hooks, engaging with tools

---

[9] See Trapp (forthcoming). The term *iatrophilosopher* occurs in a graffito in Thebes by one Philagrios the Athenian, perhaps to be identified with the early fourth-century AD doctor Philagrios of Epeiros, who is cited by Oribasius and others; see Baillet (1926), lxii, 310–11 (no. 1298).

[10] Arrian, *Epict.diss.* III.23.27–32; cf. Dio Chrysostom, *Or.* 32.17–18, 77/78.43–5. The idea of the philosopher as doctor of the soul is visible already in Plato (*Grg.* 477e–80c, *Prt.* 313e; cf. *Tht.* 149a–150d).

[11] On the parallels between these two fields, see Bubb and Peachin (forthcoming).

[12] Galen explicitly notes at *Hipp.Prog.* XVIIIb.231 that the medical usage of the term crisis derives from the juridical: "the crisis relating to illnesses has been transferred metaphorically from those in the court" (ἡ κατὰ νοσήματα κρίσις ἀπὸ τῶν ἐν τοῖς δικαστηρίοις μετενήνεκται); he also compares the fear that an acutely ill patient feels to that experienced by someone being judged on a capital charge at *Di. Dec.* IX.772. For medical debates described in legalistic terms, see Galen, *Alim.Fac.* VI.454, *Dig.Puls.* VIII.718, 954–61, *Hipp.Prorrh.* XVI.689, *Adv.Lyc.* XVIIIa.196, *Mot.Dub.* 8.7 (Nutton [2011]).

[13] Ps.-Quintilian, *Dec.Maj.* VIII.

[14] Democritus, *Or.* XXIX.40, Aristophanes, *Plut.* 875, Cicero, *Tusc.* V.9 (23–4) and *Mil.* XXI (57), Seneca, *Ir.* III.19 and *Ep.* LXVII.3, Apuleius, *Met.* III.9, X.10, Ps.-Quintilian, *Dec.Maj.* VII.7, 13.

and outcomes similar to those arising in dissection.[15] Other common means
of torture, including whipping and burning, have less visual overlap with anatomical practices, but nevertheless subscribe to the same thesis: that invasive
manipulation of bodies can yield truths.[16] The dispassionate infliction of pain
for intellectual gain was not foreign to anatomists' audiences.

Happenings unrelated to medicine, rhetoric, philosophy, and the law
also filled ancient streetscapes, and would have been especially numerous and diverse on the densely populated streets of Rome. Impromptu
events of various sorts would inevitably arise, ranging from the type of she-
nanigans lampooned in the comedians and the satirists to more unusual
spectacles. Lucian, with his satirical eye, reports on a variety of events
that drew a crowd, from the self-immolation of Peregrinus at Elis to the
miraculous "birth" of Alexander's serpent god, Glycon, at Abonoteichus.[17]
Early Christian literature is another trove of interesting urban goings-on.
Tertullian describes a man in Rome who gained a popular platform for his
anti-Christian propaganda by allowing crowds to watch him be mauled
by animals for a fee.[18] The apocryphal *Acts of Peter* narrates a competitive
display of divine power across the streets of Rome in which bodies, both
human and animal, are silenced and compelled to speak, paralyzed and
reanimated, in both spontaneous and staged events.[19] The agonistic dissections that Galen describes would have been easily at home in this company.
Further, doctors attempting to drum up an audience would also have been
in quotidian competition with a variety of hawkers and street performers,
including jugglers, acrobats, conjurers, fire-eaters, and sword-swallowers.[20]

On the mechanics of the wheel, which was viewed as a particularly Greek device though also used in
Rome, see Faraone (1993), 11–14, and Syrkou (2021), 41–2; but see also Gagarin (1996), who argues
that torture was more of a concept than a reality in the Athenian courts.

[15] Aristophanes, *Ran.* 617–22, Teles, IV.16–17 (Hense); Ammianus Marcellinus XXIX.1.33. Gleason
(2009), 107 also points out that torture victims' mouths were sometimes held closed by means of
hooks and suggests that Galen may have done the same to his animal subjects to prevent undue
noise during his performances.

[16] Gleason (1999) and (2009) has already explored this idea extensively. For an ancient perspective, see
ps.-Quintilian, *Dec.Maj.* VII.3, where a poor man, begging to be tortured to add credence to his suit
against the rich murderer of his son, urges the jury to "open this breast and pull out the whole secret
of the brigand from my viscera" (aperite pectus istud et totum de visceribus meis latronis egerite
secretum); cf. VII.13 for a description of whipping and burning, including the anticipation of his
"bare vitals [being] burned by flames" (flammis urentur nuda vitalia).

[17] Lucian, *Peregr.* and *Alex.* 9–18.

[18] Tertullian, *Ad nat.* 14; cf. *Apol.* 16.

[19] Gleason (1999), 290–4 and (2009), 100–2 highlight this text and its parallels to Galen's vivisections.

[20] Jugglers and acrobats: Manilius, V.168–71, Seneca, *Ben.* VI.11.2; conjurers: Aristotle, *Oec.* 1346b23,
Tertullian, *Apol.* 23.1; fire-eaters: Diodorus, XXXIV.2.7, Athenaeus, IV.129d; sword-swallowers:
Apuleius, *Met.* I.4. On traveling performers and the bustling streetscape generally, see Blümner
(1918), Holleran (2011), 251–60, and Hartnett (2017), 64–5.

Some of these performers, just like Tertullian's masochistic entrepreneur and any doctor practicing – or imposing – dissection, employed animals to increase their appeal; there were snake charmers, tame bears, and performing pigs, as well as a variety of other trained animals, including the ever-popular monkey.[21] This brings us to the next aspect of ancient life in which dissection was inextricably embedded.

Animals in the Public Eye

Animals held a lively place in the public imagination throughout Classical antiquity. Greek and Roman art of all periods is rife with animal figures, both domestic and wild, acting as everything from decorative leitmotifs to central subjects; animals particularly dominate the decoration of everyday personal items, indicating their familiar popularity in the cultural sphere.[22] They are similarly prevalent in literature. Anecdotes about animal behavior were a perennial favorite: Aelian's seventeen-book treatise *On the Nature of Animals* is the most concentrated manifestation of this interest to survive, full of colorful stories and engaging facts, but, as his range of sources alone indicates, observations on the habits of animals had long been a source of pleasurable trivia stretching back to Herodotus.[23] Indeed, animals enliven Greek and Latin literature across genres, from Aristophanes' *Birds* and *Frogs* to Ovid's *Metamorphoses* to the exotic animals that sprinkle the pages of the Greek novels.[24] Beyond their intrinsic appeal, animals also offered a means of exploring humanity via the presumed revelatory capacity of animal characteristics for the understanding of human character; this capacity is exploited by texts like Aesop's fables and Lucian's *Golden Ass*, and manifests also in the entrenched popularity of zoomorphically inflected physiognomy.[25]

Despite this evident fondness for animals and even the penchant for anthropomorphizing them, there was little concern in antiquity for what we would today call animal rights. By and large, animals were considered a resource at the disposal of mankind and, while wanton cruelty towards

[21] Snake charmers: Martial, *Ep.* I.41.7, Celsus, *DM* V.27.3C, Aelian, *NA* IX.62, Paulus, *Dig.* 47.11.11; tame bears: Isocrates, *Or.* XV.213, Apuleius, *Met.* XI.8; pigs: Petronius, 47.8–9; monkeys: Lucian, *Apol.* 5 and *Pisc.* 36, Apuleius, *Met.* XI.8 (cf. the numerous examples collected in Toynbee [1973], 57–9); animal handlers generally: Plutarch, *Gryllus* 992A, Athenaeus, I.19d, and Blümner (1918), 21–2.

[22] For a broad overview of the place of animals in Classical art, see Harden (2014).

[23] On Aelian's *NA*, see Smith (2014).

[24] For the animals of the Greek novels, see Cioffi (2013), 62–103.

[25] On physiognomy, see Barton (1994), 95–132, especially 124–8, and Swain and Boys-Stones (2007).

them was frowned on and considered to be indicative of a poor moral character, there was no mainstream social objection to using and killing animals for the purpose of human profit and enjoyment, without much concern for their own happiness or comfort.[26] Indeed, the use of the body parts of animals in daily life was in every way unexceptional. Excepting a fringe of philosophical interest in vegetarianism, meat consumption was the norm and butchery was a routine activity.[27] Galen acknowledges that the preparation and consumption of animal flesh offers abundant opportunity for basic anatomical observations: He points out that it will be evident to his readers that the flesh of a baby animal is flabby and full of mucus whether they have cut it open for dissection or simply to eat it.[28] Similarly, he often refers to the anatomical knowledge available to butchers as a way of highlighting the inexcusability of his rivals' anatomical mistakes.[29] Rural life in an agrarian society would have engendered ample familiarity with animal innards – a fact cheerfully illustrated by the artistic motif of a peasant flaying and disemboweling a goat or deer (Figure 5.1), which is rigged up, incidentally, in an attitude not dissimilar to that Galen used for vivisection – but, even in the city, butcher stalls offered windows into the anatomical realia of animals.[30] A relief from Rome (Figure 5.2), for example, unmistakably displays not only several cuts of meat, but also the cluster of organs, including the trachea, lungs, and heart, that Galen describes as being a common find at butcher shops, where it was referred to as "the pluck."[31] Indeed, use of animal parts went well beyond just meat. Animal hides saw many uses, including some, like wineskins, where the original shape of the animal could be left unobscured.[32] Animal bones were

---

[26] See, for example, Aristotle's assertion at *Pol.* 1256b16–17 that "the other animals exist for the sake of man" (τὰ ἄλλα ζῷα τῶν ἀνθρώπων χάριν). On attitudes towards the treatment of animals in antiquity, see Sorabji (1993), Calder (2011), 99–115, and Newmyer (2011).

[27] On vegetarianism in antiquity, see Dombrowski (1984) and (2014), Sorabji (1993), 170–94, Calder (2011), 104–5, and Newmyer (2011), 97–111. On meat consumption, see Chapter 4, "Anatomical Subjects: Other Animals" at pp. 103–4.

[28] Galen, *Temp.* I.579; see also the comment in Singer and van der Eijk (2018), 109, n. 36. Galen also offers, at *MM* X.489, the same type of advice on the timing of slaughter for animals that will be fed to patients as he does for those that will be subjects of dissection.

[29] Galen, *Nat.Fac.* II.31, 72, 91, *PHP* V.645 (VII.8.6 De Lacy), *Comp.Med.Gen.* XIII.604, *HNH* XV.141, *Hipp.Epid.II* 4.1 (*CMG Suppl.Or.* V.2, p. 679); cf. *Alim.Fac.* VI.672.

[30] The same scene depicted in Figure 5.1 also appears on an early third-century Roman lamp; see Giroire and Roger (2007), 164 (no. 94).

[31] Galen, *AA* S260.

[32] Wineskins typically used an entire hide and retained the shape of the legs, which were tied shut; see Immerwahr (1992), 122. Aristophanes, *Thesm.* 733–4 plays on their zoomorphic shape and has a woman put booties on her wineskin's "feet" and pretend that it is her baby. My thanks to Kathleen Coleman for pointing me in this direction.

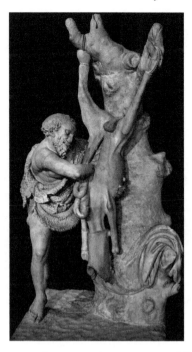

Figure 5.1   Marble statuette of a peasant skinning an animal ("Écorcheur rustique"),
second century AD Roman copy of Hellenistic original, Paris, Louvre (Cat. Ma 517).
Image: © Peter Horree / Alamy Stock Photo.

carved into all manner of useful and decorative objects but could also be
deployed in their unaltered form, as in the case of the knucklebones of
sheep and pigs, which were used as game pieces.[33] Even the internal organs
of animals were playthings: Galen describes a common game in which
children gradually coax an animal bladder into an inflated ball or balloon.[34]

Cutting into animal flesh for human purposes was accordingly not
given a second thought. In some instances, the animal itself was a patient:
The Roman agronomist authors, supplemented by the evidence from Late
Antique texts and compendia, offer a window into the veterinary practices

---

[33] On knucklebones, see May (1991) and Picaud (2004), 49–52; similarly, the vertebrae of the sheep
were so familiar that the author of the Hippocratic *Internal Affections* uses them as a unit of measure
(*Int.* 20 [VII.216 Littré]).

[34] Galen, *Nat.Fac.* II.17. See also the *Testamentum Porcelli,* a mock will of a pig, in which he leaves
his bladder "to the boys" (*pueris*); text available in Buecheler (1963) and commentary in Champlin
(1987).

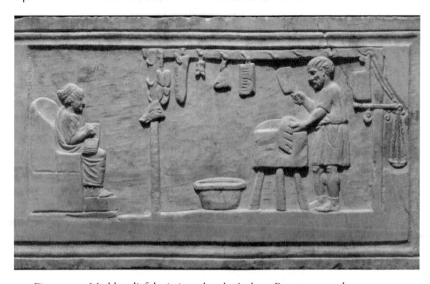

Figure 5.2   Marble relief depicting a butcher's shop, Roman, second century AD, Skulpturensammlung, Staatliche Kunstsammlungen Dresden (Inv. No. ZV 44). Image: © Azoor Photo / Alamy Stock Photo. The "pluck" is depicted just above the pig's head.

of antiquity, which include surgical procedures, some carried out by the farmers themselves.[35] Columella, for example, asserts that the owner of a flock of sheep ought to be "skilled in veterinary medicine" in order to perform emergency embryotomies, and his books on animal husbandry are full of simple operations to be carried out on various farm animals, including phlebotomy, lancing, and castration.[36] Galen, too, describes the neutering of female pigs by surgical removal of the ovaries, an operation that he says is quite common and is performed by "village folk," who have practiced sufficiently to learn the relevant anatomy.[37] In other cases, though, the animal was not the patient, but the remedy: The medical tradition is liberally populated with animal cures. As we have already seen, the Hippocratic *Diseases of Women* requires the doctor to remove and apply

---

[35] On ancient veterinarian medicine, see Fischer (1988), McCabe (2007), specifically on horse medicine, and the overview in Goebel and Peters (2014).

[36] Columella, *DA* VII.16 (veterinariae medicinae prudens).

[37] Galen, *AA* S137 (cf. *Sem.* IV.622); note that the translation in Duckworth, Lyons, and Towers (1962) misleadingly implies that this operation is magical rather than medical; see the more accurate Italian translation in Garofalo (1991*b*). At *Mot.Dub.* 11.24 (Nutton [2011]), Galen also recalls his own observations of horse doctors at work, indicating that such proceedings were open to the public gaze.

"the intestines, but not the liver and kidneys" of two mice.[38] Dioscorides' *Materia Medica* includes an entire section dedicated to the pharmacological use of animals and their by-products, including such choice anatomical morsels as the skin and liver of the hedgehog, the rennet of a hare, the belly of a weasel, the brain of a hen, the lungs of a pig, lamb, and fox, the livers of a donkey, she-goat, boar, lizard, and rabid dog, and the genitalia of a variety of animals, some, such as the testicles of the hippopotamus, no doubt sold already excised.[39] Celsus, Scribonius Largus, and Galen similarly describe various animal components for their medicaments, ranging from simple fats and suets to more specific organs, such as the liver of a wolf or the uterus of a sow.[40]

These medical uses were not far removed from their magical counterparts. Pliny's extensive treatment of remedies derived from animals knowingly walks the line between the medical and the magical, providing insight into another realm of practice for which animals were dismembered with anatomical precision.[41] His report on the uses of various parts of the hyena, for example, includes cures for eye conditions (using the gall), gastrointestinal troubles (the lungs), gout (the spine), and quartan fever (the liver), but also charms to ensure everything from good aim (the tooth) and success in legal actions (the rectum) to immunity from being barked at by dogs (the tongue) and universal hatred for one's foe (the eye).[42] Indeed, there seems to have been a sort of parallel anatomical literature in vogue in the field of magic: In addition to citing the magicians' piecemeal survey of the hyena, Pliny tells us that Democritus wrote an entire book on the magical uses of the chameleon, in which he proceeded "body part by body part."[43] Vivisection was also in the offing in these magical contexts; Pliny's

---

[38] *Mul. II* 76 (VIII.185 Littré) (κοιλίην, ἧπαρ δὲ καὶ νεφροὺς μή); cf. the disembowelment of puppies required at *Mul. III* 18 (VIII.440 Littré).

[39] Dioscorides, II.2, 19, 23–5, 38–41, 45–7, 49, 64; see Riddle (1985), 132–41. Indeed, where rarer or more expensive animals were concerned, their parts were likely purchased individually, rather than directly harvested by the practitioner, as in the case in Pliny of a treatment involving a calf's spleen, which he stipulates must be bought without haggling (*NH* XXVIII.57 [201]).

[40] Scribonius Largus, *Comp. Med.* 104 (sow), 123 (wolf); see generally the list of animal products in Jouanna-Bouchet (2016), 402–7.

[41] Pliny expresses his skepticism of the magical elements (especially in the dedicated discussion at *NH* XXX.1–6[1–18]), but nevertheless includes many; indeed, he clearly thinks that magic has some potential utility, *faute de mieux*, as in the case of quartan fever, for which he says the magical cures must be listed since there is no effectual medical remedy (XXX.30[98]). On animals in magic, see Ogden (2014) and Watson, P. (2019).

[42] Pliny, *NH* XXVIII.27(92–106); see Ogden (2014), 296–9.

[43] Pliny, *NH* XXVIII.29(112–19) (*per singula membra*); the modern consensus is that this is not actually the work of Democritus of Abdera, as Pliny asserts, but rather that of a pseudonymous author,

Democritus offers a truth-speaking charm that required the practitioner to "extract the tongue of a living frog with no other part of the body adhering to it" and place it over the heart of the woman suspected of mendacity while she sleeps, while another author describes the trickier proposition of removing the liver of a living lizard before eventually releasing it with a ritual statement meant to prevent liver disease.[44]

All things considered, it is thus in no way surprising that the mass slaughter of animals for public entertainment came to be looked on with not just equanimity but enthusiasm in the Roman period.[45] Hunting had long been a popular occupation, whether for sustenance, pest control, or elite amusement, but the staged hunts in Roman circuses and amphitheaters that evolved from these practices were less sportsmanlike affairs, offering no means of escape for the quarry.[46] Certainly, there were animal shows that did not involve any bloodshed, such as performing bears and tightrope-walking and dancing elephants, but in most cases animals were brought into the arena to kill or be killed in astonishing numbers.[47] Spectators delighted in watching the fates of these animals and particularly enjoyed anything unusual or astonishing; Martial, for example, offers not one but three epigrams commemorating the fortuitous anatomical exactitude of a spear-blow delivered to a pregnant sow in a staged hunt that allowed a piglet to escape her gravid uterus.[48] What little concern there was for the moral acceptability of these events focused largely on the effect on the audience members

probably the Hellenistic Bolus of Mendes, whose writing circulated under the name of the philosopher; see Gaillard-Seux (2009), 231–2.

[44] Pliny, *NH* XXXII.18 (49) (extrahat ranae viventi linguam, nulla alia corporis parte adhaerente); cf. XXVIII.29 (114) where both the eye and the tongue are removed from the living chameleon, XXX.7 (19), where the still beating heart must be removed from a mole, and XXX.30 (98–9), which requires the removal of the heart of a living viper, the right eye of a living lizard, and the ear tips and snout of a living mouse. The lizard liver is at Marcellus Empiricus, 22.41; see Watson, P. (2019), 130. Further, the Greek magical papyri include instructions to drown a cat prior to its manipulation (*PGM* 3.1–3), a magical practice that may have added uneasy undertones to Galen's advice that "you yourself should at some time choke an animal to death, either by using a noose or by immersing it in water" (*AA* S19); my thanks to Sean Coughlin, who brought this spell to my attention during a conference.

[45] On the popularity of the games of the arena, see Fagan (2011).

[46] On the history of hunting in antiquity, see Anderson (1985), Hughes (2007), and MacKinnon (2014). On the development of staged hunts, see Shelton (2014); some of the elite pleasure hunts were heavily rigged in favor of the hunters, but the outcome of the staged hunts was a still more manifestly foregone conclusion. On the hunts themselves, see also Chapter 4, "Anatomical Subjects: Other Animals" at pp. 106–7.

[47] Performing bears at Scriptores Historiae Augustae, *Carinus* XIX.2; elephants walking tightropes at Dio, LXII.17 and dancing at Aelian, *NA* II.11 (where they are also described as partaking, appropriately clothed, in a dainty dinner party); cf. Plutarch, *De soll.an.* 968b–d. On the numbers, see Chapter 4, "Anatomical Subjects: Other Animals" at p. 106.

[48] Martial, *Spect.* 14 (12)–16 (14) and the commentary in Coleman (2006), 126–30.

of observing the intense violence rather than the effect of the violence on the sufferers.[49] The animals typically only aroused pity when they appeared unusually human. Most famously, the crowd at the opening ceremony for Pompey's theater in 55 BC angrily objected to the slaughter of a group of elephants who had turned to the crowd to entreat mercy; it is no doubt in keeping with this emotional boundary that Galen recommends against the "hideous" vivisection of monkeys.[50] In general, however, this type of moral objection would not have been applicable to the anatomical displays by Galen and his peers, which promised both scientific enlightenment and general entertainment rather than gratuitous violence.

As should now be apparent, the practices of animal dissection and vivisection would have fit seamlessly into the broader world of animal usage. Dissectors benefited from this easy familiarity with the slaughter of animals and would not have had to justify or excuse their practices to the public at large. On the contrary, they would have been faced instead with the need to differentiate themselves from others with skillful knowledge of animal viscera and to prove that their anatomical knowledge was superior to and qualitatively different from that of their nonscientific peers. Galen takes care to paint butchers as having only a very basic, gross understanding of animal bodies – one at a level that an anatomist should be ashamed of – but his description of the elephant dissection has dissectors and butchers acting in concert, underscoring the superficial similarities in their activities.[51] The parallels with magic would have been even more troubling, as Apuleius could attest from firsthand experience.[52] Distinguishing medicine from magic was an early concern in the Hippocratic Corpus, and doctors throughout antiquity continued to need to defend their superiority in a crowded medical marketplace where magical cures never ceased to thrive.[53] Relatedly, doctors from the Hippocratic period

---

[49] For reactions to the violence of the arena, see Wistrand (1992), 15–29, Fagan (2011), and Newmyer (2011), 93–5. Seneca, *Ep.* 7 offers a particularly passionate warning about the moral dangers to the attendee of witnessing arena spectacles; cf. Augustine, *Conf.* VI.7–8 (11–13).

[50] On the emotional reaction to the elephant incident, see Cicero, *Fam.* 7.1, Pliny, *NH* VIII.7 (21–2), and Dio, XXXIX.38. For Galen on the vivisection of monkeys, see Chapter 4, n. 9. However, Galen also explicitly says at *AA* II.631–2 that he believes that brute animals suffer less from wounds than humans since they are less sensitive generally.

[51] On butchers, including the question of whether their practice fell into the secular or religious domain, and on the elephant dissection, see Chapter 4, "Anatomical Subjects: Other Animals" at p. 103. See also Tertullian's derogatory comparison of Herophilus' anatomical work to butchery (*An.* 10.4. and Chapter 6, "Herophilus" at p. 197).

[52] For Apuleius' differentiation of dissection from magic, see *Apol.* 29–41 and the discussion at the beginning of Chapter 1.

[53] *Morb.Sac.* 2–4 (VI.354–64 Littré); Galen, *Praen.* XIV.601–2 complains that a doctor who is too successful risks accusations of sorcery (cf. *Praen.* XIV.655, *Opt.Med.* I.55). On medicine versus magic generally, see Nutton (2013*a*), 272–7 and Gaillard-Seux (2015).

to the Roman one were intentional about defining themselves in opposition to religious practices that they viewed as superstitious.[54] Indeed, the dominant association when an ancient person saw someone open and examine an animal would have been with religious sacrifice and divination, practices to which we will turn next. A desire to avoid this association may well have been an element in dissuading doctors of the fifth and fourth centuries BC from publicizing their practice of dissection to a wide audience in the early days before it became a routine and recognized avenue of medical and philosophical research. Doctors of the Roman period – when dissection was a long-established practice and spectacles of animal death were public and diverse – could afford to be less self-conscious on this front.

Religious Practices

The final cluster of uses for animal bodies in antiquity to be considered – perhaps the most prominent of them all – falls into the realm of religion. Animal sacrifice was a cornerstone of both Greek and Roman religious practice. The specific details vary from place to place and cult to cult, but typically the animals were either stunned or immobilized and then killed before being laid prone (or hung) and eviscerated; the parts were then inspected and divvied up, with anatomically precise determination as to which parts were for human and which for divine consumption.[55] Doctors and anatomists had long seen the opportunities for anatomical and physiological observation represented by these practices.[56] The author of the Hippocratic *Fleshes* sees sacrifice as an excellent moment for studying the congealing of blood, while Galen notes that sacrificial practices offer evidence for his physiological theories: An ox that has been completely immobilized by the specific vertebral incision practiced by priests will still maintain certain functions, while another whose heart has been skillfully excised will even be able to run for a period despite its pulsating heart already lying on the altar.[57] In fact, when one of Galen's acquaintances

---

[54] Many of the objections in the *Morb. Sac.* passage in the previous note are to practices that fall on the line between magic and religion. Galen, *Praen.* XIV.615 specifically says that it would be insulting to accuse a doctor of any kind of divination, including extispicy.

[55] For an overview of sacrifice in antiquity with relevant bibliography, see Ekroth (2014). For the anatomical precision, visible in Greek inscriptions listing the specific cuts, organs, and parts of organs owed to various parties involved in sacrifices, see Carbon (2017).

[56] Annoni and Barras (1993), 191–6, 203–4 analyze early Greek sacrificial butchery from an anatomical perspective and draw parallels to medical and philosophical conceptualizations of the body.

[57] *Carn.* 8 (VIII.595 Littré). Galen, *PHP* V.238–9 (II.4.45–8 De Lacy); cf. *AA* S17, 30 for the vertebral incision and *MM* X.121 for the excised heart.

found an anatomical anomaly in the heart of a rooster he was sacrificing, he not only consulted the religious experts, but also informed Galen of what he had seen.[58]

The aspects of sacrifice most closely related to dissection were the divinatory practices of extispicy and particularly haruspicy. Extispicy involved the inspection of the entrails of a sacrificial victim either just to ensure generally auspicious normalcy or, more intently, to identify variations in the color, position, shape, or health of the important organs that could offer indications from the gods.[59] This search for the abnormal was obviously predicated on a familiarity with the usual appearance of the viscera of common sacrificial animals; indeed, Aristotle uses anomalous data from sacrifices to round out his understanding of variations and pathologies of the internal organs.[60] In the specific subfield of haruspicy, the liver – by far the most important organ for divination – was given detailed attention, requiring a keen awareness of hepatic anatomy.[61] Though his purpose was radically different, a haruspex drew on a similar level of expert knowledge as an anatomist, and the Etruscan specialists in the subject possessed texts dedicated to preserving and relaying their knowledge.[62] Beyond texts, there were even anatomical models available to the diviner, a particularly fine example of which has survived in the form of the so-called Piacenza liver; this bronze model represents a stylized but recognizable liver of a sheep, heavily annotated for divinatory use and recognizably depicting the gallbladder, lobes, and veinous openings.[63]

Unlike these haruspicy models, the most strikingly anatomical religious material to survive from antiquity does not purport to represent animal body parts, but human ones. There was an extensive tradition of anatomical votives throughout Greco-Roman antiquity.[64] From the late fifth and fourth centuries BC, Greek shrines, especially those related to Asclepius and other healing gods, began to be flooded with disembodied

---

[58] Galen, *AA* II.623; cf. *Loc.Aff.* VIII.304, where a similar context might be at play.

[59] See North (1990), Johnston (2008), 125–8, and Collins (2008), 338.

[60] Aristotle, *PA* 667a34–b2; cf. *HA* 496b19–29 and 559b20.

[61] On haruspicy, including its earlier Mesopotamian roots, see Jannot (1998), 34–9 and Collins (2008).

[62] For the texts, see Cicero, *Div.* II.50 and Jannot (1998), 20–33, 38–9.

[63] The Piacenza liver dates to around the end of the second century BC and is held in the Museo Civico Archeologico in Piacenza; a similar liver model can be seen in the hands of the haruspex Aule Lecu, as depicted on his cinerary urn (late second or early first century BC; Museo Guarnacci, Volterra). For interpretations of the model's use and meaning, see de Grummond (2013).

[64] See Draycott and Graham (2017*a*) and Hughes (2017). The practice is not just a Greco-Roman phenomenon, but is geographically and chronologically vast, continuing even to the present day; see Draycott and Graham (2017*b*), 1–4 and Hughes (2017), 1–2.

representations of eyes, ears, noses, mouths, arms, legs, buttocks, torsos, hands, breasts, genitalia, feet, knees, and other body parts; the surviving examples range from humble terracotta to precious metals and vary in size from miniature to life size to gigantic.[65] The meaning and purpose of these votives is open to debate, but their displays in the temple certainly would have confronted the viewer with an exploded, piecemeal vision of the body. A unifying element of this group, however, is that the body parts represented are overwhelmingly external.[66] Because of the lack of representation of the viscera here, some of the most anatomically interesting votives are not Greek but Italic.

The Italian peninsula has yielded abundant caches of anatomical votives, far outnumbering those found in Greece; the finds, mostly in terracotta, date from the fourth to first centuries BC and cluster particularly in the regions of Etruria, Latium, and Campania.[67] Many of the same types of figures appear here as among their Greek counterparts – feet, heads, hands, eyes, ears, genitalia – but, in notable contrast, these collections include a smaller but still significant number of representations of internal organs, offering a more concrete connection to anatomical knowledge and dissection.[68] There are two particular types of visceral votives unique to Italy that offer special points of interest here.[69] The first is the large collection of terracotta uteri (Figure 5.3).[70] What stands out particularly about these figurines is their anatomical shape: They are not bipartite and they thus seem to resemble the human simplex uterus more than that of any other mammal that the artisans responsible would realistically have been

---

[65] For a survey of the Greek votives, see Forsén (1996) and Hughes (2017), 26–39, who also points out that, though the dedication of anatomical votives became widespread in Greece for the first time in the Classical period, older Greek examples also survive (pp. 26–8) and the practice continued into the Roman Imperial period (p. 61). The useful catalogue in van Straten (1981), 105–51 includes the evidence from inventory inscriptions, which round out the picture of the extant votives.

[66] There were some representations of internal organs – the inventory inscriptions from the Athenian Asclepieion, for example, includes five hearts and a bladder (*IG* II² 1532–9) – but they are extremely rare; see van Straten (1981), 109, 111, and Hughes (2017), 81–2. One might possibly also include here the bronze skeleton dedicated to Apollo at Delphi, supposedly by Hippocrates himself (Pausanius, X.2.6); it seems to me likely, however, that this should be interpreted not as a skeleton, but as a statue of a severely emaciated patient similar to that described in Posidippus, *Epig.* 95, which was also dedicated as a votive offering to Apollo.

[67] See Decouflé (1964), Turfa (1994), Recke (2013), Flemming (2016), Haumesser (2017), and Hughes (2017), 62–105.

[68] Hughes (2017), 83–105 offers a discussion for why the Italian audience was more open to the display of internal organs than the Greeks, including the suggestion that the Romano-Etruscan emphasis on haruspicy and their related comfort with artistic depictions of animal viscera played a role.

[69] In addition to the uteri and polyvisceral votives considered here, there are also examples of individual hearts, intestines, testes, and, perhaps, a liver; see Turfa (1994), 226–7.

[70] On the uteri specifically, see Turfa (1994), Flemming (2017), and Bubb (forthcoming *a*).

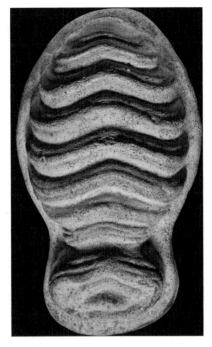

Figure 5.3   Terracotta votive of a womb, Roman, third century BC–first century BC, British Museum, London (1814,0704.881). Image: © The Trustees of the British Museum.

encountering.[71] It has been suggested, though not without controversy, that knowledge of human uterine anatomy may have arisen from postmortem surgical removal of uteri in the context of attempted fetal salvage – a process that Republican Roman law may actually have required in order to prevent the unwitting burial of viable infants.[72] If true, this claim

[71] The uteri of most mammals are bipartite (either fully duplex or bicornuate) and look completely different from the simplex uterus, which is present only in humans and some primates; see items A–C in Turfa (1994), Fig. 20.2. While, as we have seen, monkeys came to be common anatomical subjects, we have no evidence for their routine use before Rufus in the first century AD (Aristotle's brief mention of simian dissection at *HA* 502b25–6 does not include any resulting internal details). Further, while Herophilus' studies on the human female reproductive tract in the early third century BC may have highlighted the distinctive shape of the human uterus, it seems unlikely that these texts and ideas were yet circulating in the Italian peninsula in the period in which these votives are attested; cf. Flemming (2017), 124.

[72] Turfa (1994), 227–33. See also the skeptical responses in Dasen and Ducaté-Paarmann (2006), 247, and Flemming (2017), 125, who do not, however, fully tackle the anatomical singularity of the human uterus vis-à-vis the animal uteri that would have been routinely encountered during butchery and sacrifice. Indeed, Greco-Roman anatomical beliefs about the womb are plagued by the

would indicate a special form of anatomical intimacy with the human body specific to the Italian peninsula. I believe, however, that these votives are modeled not on human uteri, but on the pregnant bicornuate uteri of common farm animals, which, when carrying a fetus in a single horn, look remarkably like the votive representations.[73] While perhaps not as exciting as the suggestion of human anatomical data gleaned from fetal salvage, this theory nevertheless necessitates close observation of animal anatomy and a careful – sometimes extremely careful – replication of animal anatomical realia in terracotta form in order to depict a human internal organ.[74]

The second type are the equally fascinating polyvisceral votives. These represent multiple organs simultaneously and come in a few different types. Some present three-dimensional stacks of organs, with the intestines coiled on the bottom and the trachea projecting (or sometimes drooping) from the top; others represent the same organs on bas-relief plaques; finally, a small but remarkable subset depict the organs as if *in situ*, locating them within a lozenge-shaped opening in a torso, some clothed, some unclothed, some with heads and arms, others without (Figure 5.4).[75] The organs were carefully distinguished from each other – in some cases traces of different color paints survive – and were often arranged using strategic displacement and reorientation in order to maximize the visibility of each organ. The levels of detail and of realism are highly variable, but one can often pick out some subset of the trachea, the lungs, the heart, the stomach, the liver, and the intestines without too much hesitation.[76] The livers, when identifiable,

---

tenacious influence of animal comparison; even in the second century AD, Galen is still grappling with the mythical human cotyledon (*Ut.Diss.* II.905–6), a marked uterine feature in farm animals that humans do not share, and feels comfortable saying at *Ut.Diss.* II.891 that the goat and the cow (two animals with obviously bicornuate uteri) are "similar to woman in respect to their wombs" (γυναικὶ κατὰ τὴν μήτραν ἔοικεν). Flemming (2017), 126–7 raises the alternative point that the womb was analogically associated in some Hippocratic texts with cupping vessels and jugs; this certainly seems to be the visual cue at play in the Greco-Egyptian uterine amulet tradition, which emerged in the first centuries AD (see Hanson [1995] and Dasen and Ducaté-Paarmann [2006], 250–4), but does not, for me, adequately explain all of the features of the Italic votives.

[73] For a more detailed exposition of the evidence supporting this theory, see Bubb (forthcoming *a*).

[74] See Turfa (1994), 227–9 for the range of styles these votives display, including images of some of the more anatomically detailed.

[75] For examples of the "stack" type, see Decouflé (1964), Figs. 9 and 18, and Hughes (2017), Fig. 3.12; for plaques, see Decouflé (1964), Figs. 10 and 14, Gourevitch and Gourevitch (1965), Fig. 2, Recke (2013), Fig. 59.5, Haumesser (2017), Figs. 9.3 and 9.14, and Hughes (2017), Figs. 3.8 and 3.11; for further examples of the torso type, see Decouflé (1964), Fig. 7, Gourevitch and Gourevitch (1965), Fig. 1, Recke (2013), Figs. 59.13 and 59.15–16, Haumesser (2017), Figs. 9.4–6, 9.8–10, and 9.12–13, and Hughes (2017), Figs. 3.13–14.

[76] See the attempts at anatomical identification, probably more detailed than is realistic, in Decouflé (1964), plates IX, XII, and XVII, and Gourevitch and Gourevitch (1965), 2961.

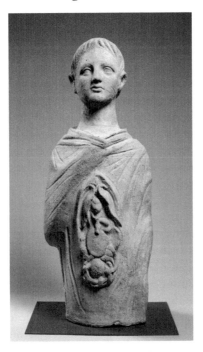

Figure 5.4   Anatomical votive, Vulci (Canino), third century BC–second century BC, Louvre, Paris (MNE 1341). Image: © Musée du Louvre, Dist. RMN-Grand Palais / Thierry Olliver / Art Resource, NY.

can be conspicuously multilobed, confirming – exactly as we would expect given the parallel practices in the scientific community – that these votives were modeled on animal viscera.[77] Further, in addition to the artistic license taken in the relative arrangement of the individual organs, it is clear that the lozenges embedded within torsos are not meant to open a realistic window into the underlying anatomy: There is little attempt to line them up correctly with the external anatomy, either in terms of scale or position, and the placid faces (at least in those models that have heads) show no perturbance about the disordered state of their abdomens.[78] Rather, instead of illustrating the exact interior of a specific body, these votives concretize

[77] See, for example, the plaque at Gourevitch and Gourevitch (1965), Fig. 2, which seems to be modeled on a canine liver (p. 2962) (compare the five-lobed liver in Decouflé [1964], Fig. 14); note that this plaque is also an example of a votive that retains its paint. Tabanelli (1962), 77–91 discusses the anatomical knowledge underlying these votives; cf. Haumesser (2017), 182, 191–2.

[78] Nevertheless, there are two examples that indicate a self-consciousness about the relationship between the internal and the external: One, in the Museo Nazionale Romano (Terme) in Rome,

the contemporary understanding of the interior of a generic body. In other words, we have evidence here for a group of people, distinct from their contemporaries in the scientific circles considered in Chapter 2, who are interested in conceptualizing internal human anatomy and who are using animal proxies to do so; further, they are working within a receptive broader community interested in purchasing and using their wares. Together with the uterine votives, these examples raise the possibility that the Roman context for the upsurge in anatomical interest in the first and second centuries AD was not a mere coincidence, but rather that the local history of interest in visualizing the inner workings of the body was particularly suited to foster public and performative anatomy.[79]

The final aspect of religion to consider here is the potential relevance of foreign influences. The Magna Mater cult, for example, adds another practice that would have made Galen's vivisections seem tame, namely the taurobolium, in which the priest stood in a pit underneath a platform on which a bull was sacrificed in order to be fully drenched in its blood.[80] Perhaps the most relevant religious culture for the question of dissection, though, is that of the Egyptians. There has long been curiosity about the degree to which the religious process of mummification influenced both Egyptian and Greek understandings of internal human anatomy. The author of *Doctor: Introduction* sees a tight connection, claiming that "from the opening up of the dead during embalming many aspects of surgery also seem to have been discovered by the first doctors."[81] Modern scholarship, though acknowledging that it was surely not a coincidence that Egypt was the site of the only moment when human dissection is known to have been openly practiced by the Greeks, has not uniformly endorsed the idea that the embalmers' free access to the human trunk translated into useful medical knowledge.[82] It is now increasingly clear that ancient Egyptian

---

depicts layers of incised skin and muscle, including sawn-off ribs, around the edge of the lozenge (see Haumesser [2017], Fig. 9.6), while another, in the Deutsches Medizinhistorisches Museum in Ingolstadt, is more accurately to scale than most and includes small holes around the edge of the lozenge that Recke (2013), 1078 (and Figs. 59.15–16) believes are meant to represent the stitches by which the imaginary torso would have been reclosed.

[79] Indeed, I suggest in Chapter 7, "Marinus" at p. 237 and "Quintus and His Students" at p. 239, that the city of Rome has just as strong a claim as Alexandria to be considered the epicenter of anatomical activity in the period.

[80] See Beard, North, and Price (1998), vol. 2, 160–2.

[81] Ps.-Galen, *Int.* XIV.675 (ἐκ δὲ τῆς ἐν ταῖς ταριχείαις ἀνασχίσεως τῶν νεκρῶν πολλὰ καὶ τῶν ἐν χειρουργίᾳ παρὰ τοῖς πρώτοις ἰατροῖς εὑρῆσθαι δοκεῖ); see also Gellius, *NA* X.10.

[82] See, for example, the range of opinions, mostly skeptical, in Lefebvre (1952), 58–9, Sigerist (1967), I.353–6, Leca (1971), 129–35, Ghalioungui (1973), 46–8 and (1983), 6–8, Majno (1975), 138–9, von Staden (1989), 29–30, 149–50, Nunn (1996), 42–4, Westendorf (1999), I.121, and Quack (2003), 10–11.

embalmers were indeed in dialogue with their medical contemporaries, but evidence for any substantial empirical foundation for ancient Egyptian anatomical knowledge remains elusive.[83] According to later Greek testimonies, there were Egyptian texts dedicated to anatomy, but none actually survives, and the extant medical texts do not offer sufficient details to give a conclusive picture of the state of anatomical knowledge.[84] While the descriptions of the skull and the surface of the brain that survive in the Egyptian medical papyri are evocatively accurate – though also not inconsistent with observation via the types of wounds whose treatment they are describing – the vascular system that underlies Egyptian nosological theories is heavily theoretical, and hieroglyphs representing internal parts of the body derive from animal anatomy.[85] Further, regardless of the situation on the Egyptian side, it is notoriously difficult to prove a transfer of knowledge of this sort from one culture to another.[86] It is certainly plausible, for example, that Herophilus' intense focus on the pulse was influenced by its centrality to the local medical tradition that surrounded him, but it is not possible to press the point much further than that.[87] Similarly,

---

[83] In addition to the suggestive case of Minemsehnet, a doctor whose grandfather was an embalmer (Ghalioungui [1983], 24–5, n. 59, and Nunn [1996], 44 and Appendix B, no. 70), there is now also the evidence of Papyrus Louvre-Carlsberg, which contains both medical and embalming texts; see Bardinet (2018) and Schiødt (2021). See also the interesting findings in Pahl and Parsche (1991), which suggest that dissection of the muscles and fascia may sometimes have been incorporated into the mummification process, though to what end is unclear.

[84] Julius Africanus (*fl. c.* AD 220), *Chron.* fr. 11, dyn1, and Eusebius (*c.* AD 260–339), *Chron.* I.45 – both excerpting the lost *Aegyptiaca* by the Egyptian Manetho (*fl.* 280 BC) – report that one of the Pharaohs of the First Dynasty wrote "anatomical books" (βίβλοι ἀνατομικαί); Clement of Alexandria (*c.* AD 150–216), *Strom.* VI.4.37 describes a collection of sacred Egyptian texts, including one dedicated to "the structure of the body" (τῆς τοῦ σώματος κατασκευῆς); see Nunn (1996), 42, 44. In addition to the medical papyri, there are a group of ritual texts that contain anatomical lists, associating each part of the body with a god, though each part is presented individually and simply by its name, making it difficult to glean much from them beyond vocabulary; see Walker (1996), 283–341. See also the Oracular Amuletic Decrees, collected in Edwards (1960), which contain similar anatomical lists entrusting various body parts to specific gods (with thanks to Amber Jacob for bringing them to my attention).

[85] The descriptions of the parts of the head are in the Edwin Smith Papyrus, especially Cases 4, 6, 7, 9, 18; see Nunn (1996), 49–52, Sanchez, Meltzer, and Smith (2012), and also Forshaw (2016), 126–31, which assesses the anatomical understanding indicated by surgical practices, both as described in the papyrus and as observed on mummies. For the vascular system, see Leca (1971), 153–65, Bardinet (1995), 60–120, and Ritner (2006). For the hieroglyphs, see Grapow (1954), 15, and Walker (1996), 259; in the context of the discussion of Italic uterine votives earlier in this section, it is interesting to note that the Egyptian hieroglyph for uterus is based on the bicornuate uterus of a heifer.

[86] See the discussion and bibliography in Bubb (forthcoming *b*).

[87] On the suggestion that Herophilus' pulse lore was influenced by local knowledge, see von Staden (1989), 9–13, and Ritner (2000), 115. Berrey (2017), 191–6, 202–6 does not discuss any possible Egyptian factor in the development of Herophilus' sphygmology, but he does argue for his adoption of an Egyptian type of water-clock technology in his measurements of the pulse.

it is an open question whether the Hellenistic Egyptian doctors maligned by Rufus as coining infelicitous anatomical terminology should be understood as native Egyptians or Greek Alexandrians; the terms in question are all skeletal, however, so this is not an area where privileged insights from embalmment would even have been at play.[88] In the cultural sphere, at any rate, the Greco-Roman attitude to the Egyptian practice was generally one of fascinated repugnance, suggesting that, even if possible, society at large did not consider this to be a desirable avenue for knowledge.[89]

Anatomy in the Popular Imagination

It is not the case, however, that ancient Greeks and Romans had no experience with the manipulation and display of human corpses. The attempted desecration of Hector's body is, of course, a central theme in the *Iliad*, and, though it functions there as a breach of acceptable conduct, there were circumstances outside fiction in which the meting out of postmortem punishment was condoned.[90] The Greeks, while generally diligent about the timely and proper burial of any and every body, endorsed the exposure of the corpses of those they deemed beneath contempt, such as temple robbers and perpetrators of other serious transgressions.[91] The Romans were still firmer believers in the deterrent power of the ill-treated criminal corpse: The bodies of the crucified were sometimes left on view along roads as they rotted, and the remains of particularly vilified people were even displayed in the very heart of Rome.[92] Decapitated heads and severed hands of the politically disgraced were mounted in the forum, and, in its northern corner, the *Scalae Gemoniae*, or Stairs of Mourning, were a notorious site for the display of – and even violence towards – the bodies of the high-ranking condemned after their execution.[93] Sejanus' body, for example, was left there for three days, during which it was abused by the populace before being dragged to the Tiber to be thrown in.[94]

---

[88] For the Egyptian doctors in Rufus, see *Nom.Part.* 133–4 and the discussion in Chapter 7, "Rufus of Ephesus" at pp. 221–2.

[89] Herodotus, II.85–90, 136; Diodorus, I.91.1–7; Teles, XXXI.9–10 (Hense); Cicero, *Tusc.* I.45; Lucian, *De luct.* 21.

[90] On the trope of corpse abuse in the *Iliad*, see McClellan (2019), 17, 27–41, and van der Plas (2020).

[91] Plato, *Leg.* 854e–855a, 873b, 909c, Diodorus Siculus, XVI.25; see also Parker (1983), 43–8.

[92] For the powerful messages embedded in the treatment of corpses, see Hope (2000); on deterrence specifically, with more examples, see Coleman (1990), 48–9. On crucifixion in antiquity, see Cook (2014), with examples of bodies being left to rot publicly after death at p. 429, n. 69; cf. Syrkou (2021), 51–2, 57–63.

[93] On severed heads and hands, which famously included those of Cicero, see Hope (2000), 113–14; on the *Scalae Gemoniae*, see Barry (2008).

[94] Dio, LVIII.11.5–6.

Other corpses were left on view not for punishment but from neglect. There were mass graves for the destitute, but their bodies did not always arrive there expeditiously; markers prohibiting the unceremonious dumping of bodies in inappropriate places had to be erected, and it was not a given that undertakers would get to a corpse before animals did.[95] While not subject to postmortem exposure, those condemned to death in the arena could be killed in such a way that their inner parts were revealed to the eager audience; victims mauled by bears, boars, and lions, for example, would surely sometimes have lost their viscera on the sands.[96] Soldiers' bodies, too, were subject to the unpredictability of battle, and during active campaigning they would have witnessed both the violent injuries of those wounded or killed in hand-to-hand combat and, in some cases, the rotting of corpses.[97] Indeed, it was precisely in this chaotic milieu, Galen tells us, that some doctors of his day were even able to hurriedly dissect the bodies of fallen enemies.[98]

The anatomical promiscuity of military conflict need not have been experienced only by its eyewitnesses. Classical literature abounds with gruesomely detailed moments of dismemberment and evisceration. The *Iliad* is full of descriptive battle scenes, including cleft-open and chopped-off heads, skewered eyeballs, spewing bowels, and a throbbing, excised heart.[99] The Greek tragedies, though less frequently engaging with martial themes, do not shy away from violent moments either; indeed, they have been described as "reek[ing] of blood and … strewn with corpses."[100] Latin authors particularly revel in gore. Seneca leans in to the bloody aspects of his tragedies to a greater extent than his Greek predecessors, from the savage butchery of Thyestes' sons – including a ghastly parody of extispicy – to Oedipus' clawing out of his eyes with his own hands.[101] Lucan takes things

---

95 For markers, see *CIL* I² 838, 839, 2981; for examples of animals interfering with, and sometimes dismembering, unburied corpses, see Hope (2000), 110–11. On the subject of exposed infants, another potential source of undisposed corpses, see Chapter 4, n. 104.

96 For capital punishment using animals, see Coleman (1990) and Kyle (1998). Galen confirms that the ravaged state of these bodies was an opportunity for speedy reconnaissance of human entrails at *AA* II.385 (see Chapter 4, "Anatomical Subjects: Humans" at pp. 115–17).

97 Bodies rotting on the battlefield: Suetonius, *Vitell.* 10; Tacitus, *Hist.* II.45.

98 Galen, *AA* II.385, *Comp.Med.Gen.* XIII.604, and the discussion in Chapter 4, "Anatomical Subjects: Humans" at pp. 115–17.

99 Homer, *Il.* 16.411–13, 10.454–7 (heads), 14.493–500 (eyeball), 17.314–15, 20.415–18 (bowels), and 13.441–4 (heart); see Lind (1978) for a longer catalogue.

100 Henrichs (2000), 173; though he also notes (pp. 176–7) that the violence is described, rather than occurring on stage.

101 Seneca, *Thy.* 720–75, *Oed.* 901–79; cf. *Pha.* 1085–1114 (the total dismemberment of Hippolytus' body), *Pho.* 155–65 (Oedipus' description of suicide without weapons), and *HF* 1002–9 (the splattered brains of Hercules' older child).

to the extreme, densely populating his work with bodies, both living and dead, undergoing explicit violence.[102] Pompey's inexpert decapitation and the subsequent embalming of his head offers a particularly gnarly example, while the early reminiscences from a veteran of the conflict between Sulla and Marius foreshadow the scale and frequency of violence to come: Limbs fly, severed tongues flop along the ground, eye-sockets ooze, intestines pool, and decapitated heads rot beyond recognition.[103] Lucan also includes a vivid example of the necromantic witch, a figure who loomed large in literature and the popular imagination; Erictho's ghoulish dismemberment of cadavers with her nails and teeth is rivaled only by her resurrection of a corpse, a process that plays out as a sort of travesty of medical treatment.[104] Finally, in one particularly nasty moment during his extensive catalogue of snakes, he describes the effects of the venom of the *seps*, which causes the flesh to rapidly melt off the body until "whatever man consists of is laid bare by the unholy nature of the pestilence: the bindings of the ligaments, the structure of the lungs, the hollow breast, and everything concealed by the vital entrails lies open in death."[105] Cato and his men – and Lucan's readers with them – are treated to a gruesome anatomy lesson as the flesh and organs of the living soldier dissolve.

Indeed, it might seem puzzling that amid this positive flood of human gore in the Roman period, both real and imagined, the dissection of human bodies remained a taboo, practiced only rarely, fleetingly, and discretely.[106] Here, again, the question of social context is informative. Roman dissectors were keenly aware of their reputations. Indeed, as we saw in Chapter 3, reputation building was a primary motivation for the majority of Roman dissections. Just as a dissector would be wise to differentiate himself from butchers, magicians, and priests, he could not be too cautious about disassociating his practice from cruelty, punishment, and death. Public dissections were meant to highlight cutting-edge scientific knowledge and impressive technical skills, and animals provided a familiar, disposable, and uncontroversial medium. The dissection of humans, in contrast,

---

[102] For a study of the maltreatment of corpses in Lucan and other Latin epics, including Statius' equally bloodthirsty *Thebaid*, see McClellan (2019); on Lucan's use of gore, see Bartsch (2001), 10–47.

[103] Pompey's head at Lucan, *BC* VIII.667–92; reminiscences at II.68–233.

[104] Lucan, *BC* VI.507–830. On the trope of the witch, including their frequent use of purloined body parts and the parallel practices attested in the *Papyri Graecae Magicae*, see Watson, L. C. (2019), 167–202.

[105] Lucan, *BC* IX.779–80 (quidquid homo est, aperit pestis natura profana: uincula neruorum et laterum textura cauumque pectus et abstrusum fibris uitalibus omne morte patet).

[106] On the question of human dissection, see Chapter 4, "Anatomical Subjects: Humans" at pp. 110–18.

whether done in public or in private, would have sullied the reputation of the doctors who performed it: Even if the exposure and maltreatment of human bodies was condoned in certain circumstances, it was in every case an intentional act of desecration.[107] Doctors, who worked tirelessly to promote themselves to potential clients as lifegivers and respectful stewards of the living body, simply could not have afforded to associate themselves with it. Even the vivisection of monkeys was too close to home.[108] In the deeply competitive world of Roman medicine, few would have risked the taint that human dissection would bring.

In contrast to the gore of politics and literature, anatomical knowledge manifests in the realm of fine arts primarily in the proportional beauty of the unviolated body. From an early stage, Greek sculpture demonstrates careful observation of muscular anatomy, with anatomical details becoming even more minutely attended to over time.[109] According to Pliny, Pythagoras of Rhegium (active *c.* 490–450 BC) first introduced the practice of representing sinews and veins, while a generation or so later Polycleitus' *Canon* – the name of both a text and an illustrative statue – laid out the exact proportional relationship of all of the parts of the body and was still hearkened back to by Galen as an exemplary study.[110] Once again, it is the Romans who show a penchant for the internal parts. The viscera themselves were not commonly depicted – though Roman audiences certainly did not balk at violent images of corporeal rupture – but human skeletons became a popular decorative motif in the late-Republican and early imperial periods, acting as anatomically recognizable memento mori on mosaics, lamps, gems, and cups (Figure 5.5).[111] They were particularly linked to the context of feasting, where the image of impending death was meant to encourage full enjoyment

---

[107] See Fagan (2011), 253 on the fact that, though arena audiences took pleasure in the suffering and death of the condemned, they were not favorably disposed towards the executioners who brought it about; indeed, the Latin word for executioner (*carnifex*) doubled as a general insult.

[108] See "Animals in the Public Eye" in this chapter at p. 151. Similarly, I suggest in Chapter 3, "Performance for Advertisement" at pp. 79–80, that animal dissections and vivisections may have served as a more palatable form of advertisement than public surgeries because they made the pain inflicted by the doctor less salient.

[109] Stewart (1990), 75–6 even suggests that Hellenistic artists benefited directly from the anatomical innovations in Alexandria. Kuriyama (1999), 112–16 demonstrates that this Greek emphasis on the depiction of muscles was an unusual and marked choice.

[110] Pliny, *NH* XXXIV.59; on Polycleitus' text, now lost, and statue, which is today identified with his *Doryphoros* and survives in numerous later copies, see Galen, *PHP* VI.449 (V.3.15–16 De Lacy) and *Temp.* I.566.

[111] On images of the viscera, Hughes (2017), 88, 91 points out multiple examples of depictions of animal organs in the context of sacrifice and haruspicy, as well as the depiction on a Laconian

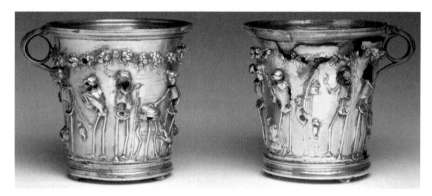

Figure 5.5   Two silver drinking cups, Boscoreale, *c.* 25 BC–AD 50, Louvre, Paris (BJ 1923, BJ 1924). Image: © Musée du Louvre, Dist. RMN-Grand Palais / Hervé Lewandowski / Art Resource, NY.

of the present moment; indeed, Trimalchio, in Petronius' famous dinner party, brings out an articulated silver skeleton, of a type that actually survives in numerous examples in the archaeological record, and positions it in various poses in a macabre entertainment for his guests.[112]

In addition to displaying his popular taste in trinkets, Petronius has Trimalchio partake in a final, more intellectual facet of social life in antiquity that would have been a backdrop for anatomical work: The persistent interest, even among those who were neither doctors nor philosophers, in the inner workings of the body. Trimalchio's foray into physiological theory is characteristically sophomoric, but it is symptomatic of a broader trend, visible across Greco-Roman literature.[113] Playwrights, both tragic and comic, often take special interest in the intricacies of bodies, whether whole or ruptured, functional or ailing.[114] Authors in other genres, both poetic and prose, also seem to have kept abreast of medical advancements

---

black-figure kylix of Prometheus' bloody, excised liver (Vatican Museum, inv. 16592). On the popularity of images of violence, see Lusnia (2020).

[112]   See Dunbabin (1986) and Garcia Barraco, M. E. (2020), which includes images of the extant model skeletons, or *larvae conviviales*, as well as depictions of skeletons in other media; Petronius, *Sat.* 34.8–9.

[113]   Trimalchio instructs his guests in the physiology and pathologies of digestion at Petronius, *Sat.* 47.2–7.

[114]   On medical language in Aristophanes, see Miller (1945) and Byl (1990) and (2006). Euripides is a particularly good example of this trend among the tragedians; see Craik (2001), Kosak (2004), and Holmes (2010), 228–74.

and depict up-to-date bodies in their texts.[115] It has long been observed that the Roman imperial period saw a markedly increased interest in – or, as some have characterized it, hypochondriacal obsession with – health and the body.[116] Aelius Aristides, with his cringingly detailed catalogue of ailments, is the poster child for the period's preoccupation with health, and his relationship to his body can be strikingly anatomical: In one vivid dream, he was sitting in the bath and, with the magical X-ray vision of a dreamer, saw that "the lower part of [his] bowels were disposed in a rather unusual way."[117] Aristides, though an extreme case, is not alone. Celsus and Plutarch urge their readers to stay abreast of their health and monitor their own bodies.[118] Aulus Gellius even finds studying books of anatomy to be a social desideratum: After observing an acquaintance lecturing his own doctor on the proper terminology for and distinctions between veins and arteries, he anxiously adds medical treatises to his list of leisure reading so as not to be caught out in any shameful ignorance.[119]

It is in the context of all of this that we must turn back to the passage from Apuleius that started the introduction to this book.[120] Apuleius presents it as unremarkable that a well-educated, philosophically inclined man of his day should concern himself with the anatomical details of sea creatures. Circumstances have forced him to explicitly distinguish his activities from magic, but he takes the condescending (and rhetorically effective) stance that his accusers are simply buffoons and that any intellectual would understand and appreciate the purpose and the value of his anatomical practices. Galen would have backed him up: It is a matter of no surprise to him that Roman government officials should interest themselves in the intricacies of nerves and arteries. Indeed, he considers doing so to be the prerogative of all self-respecting citizens, chastising those who "like beasts … are ignorant of their structure" and know how many slaves they possess but not how many organs.[121] In short, the cultural environment in which Galen and his peers and immediate predecessors found themselves, with its mix of Greek intellectualism and Roman social norms, was perfectly

---

[115] See Chapter 6, "Minor Hellenistic Authors" at pp. 207–8 and 214–15 for literary authors, both Greek and Latin, showing awareness of contemporary anatomical knowledge.

[116] See Dodds (1965), 29–36, Bowersock (1969), 71–5, and Foucault (1976), III, 121–6.

[117] Aristides, *Ier.Log.* I.8 (275 Jebb) (τὰ κάτω τῆς κοιλίας ἀτοπώτερον διακείμενα).

[118] Celsus, *DM* I; Plutarch, *San.Tu.* 127d–130a; similar solicitude is visible in the correspondence of Fronto, including with Marcus Aurelius (e.g., *Ad amicos* I.13, *Ad Antoninum Imp.* I.1, 2.6–8, *Ad M. Caes.* III.8.3, V.29[44]).

[119] Gellius, *NA* XVIII.10.

[120] Apuleius, *Apol.* 40.

[121] Galen, *Opt.Med.Cogn.* 9.15 (*CMG Suppl.Or.* IV, p. 111, trans. Iskandar).

suited to nurture an explosion of anatomical interest, in both its private, scientific manifestations and its public, performative ones.[122] Just as for the earlier efflorescence of interest in the Hellenistic period, however, the question of when and why this anatomical boom came to an end is vexed by a lack of evidence. Before attempting an answer, we must turn from social to medical history and follow the development of the anatomical literature that accompanied and underpinned all of the anatomical activities so far considered.

---

[122] Gleason (2009), 89 also suggests some performative developments in Roman politics that may have further contributed to making it an environment ripe for these sorts of displays.

PART II

Text

CHAPTER 6

Anatomical Texts of the Classical and Hellenistic Periods

Since I came forward in order to prove that nothing that I said in my anatomical writings was false, I set up in the middle [of the group] the books of all the anatomists, giving authority to each of those present who wished it to propose a part to be dissected, having announced that I would demonstrate that I wrote accurately in each area where I disagreed with those who came before. The thorax was proposed as a topic and, as I was making a beginning from the oldest sources and reaching for their books, some of the noteworthy doctors sitting in the front row thought it best that I not waste my time, but, since Lycus the Macedonian, being the student of Quintus, that most anatomical man, wrote about everything that had been discovered up to his day, I should, passing over the others, compare only the things he wrote to my own.

Galen, *On My Own Books*[1]

As this account vividly illustrates, an extensive library of anatomical texts had accumulated by the Roman imperial period. These texts transmitted wisdom about the interior of the body, drawing sometimes on the empirical observations of dissection, but in other cases on logical or theoretical deductions. Indeed, the writing of anatomical texts and the practice of dissection were never fully overlapping fields in antiquity, and the further back from Galen's day one goes, the less they overlap. In the earlier periods, as we saw in Chapter 2, dissection was neither a universal nor even a

---

[1] Galen, *Lib.Prop.* XIX.22 (ὁπότε προῆλθον ἐπιδείξων ἐμαυτὸν οὐδὲν ἐψευσμένον ἐν τοῖς ἀνατομικοῖς ὑπομνήμασιν, εἰς τὸ μέσον ἀνέθηκα τὰ τῶν ἀνατομικῶν ἁπάντων βιβλία τὴν ἐξουσίαν δοὺς ἑκάστῳ τῶν παρόντων ὃ βούλεται μόριον ἀνατμηθῆναι προβάλλειν ἐπαγγειλάμενος δείξειν, ὅσα διεφώνησαν τοῖς ἔμπροσθεν, ἀληθῶς ὑπ' ἐμοῦ γεγραμμένα. προβληθέντος δὲ ⟨τοῦ⟩ θώρακος ἐμοῦ τε τὴν ἀρχὴν ἀπὸ τῶν παλαιοτάτων ποιουμένου προχειριζομένου τε τὰς βίβλους αὐτῶν ἠξίωσάν τινες τῶν ἀξιολόγων ἰατρῶν ἐν προεδρίᾳ καθεζόμενοι μὴ κατατρίβειν με τὸν χρόνον, ἀλλ' ἐπειδὴ Λύκος ὁ Μακεδών, Κοΐντου μαθητὴς γεγονὼς ἀνδρὸς ἀνατομικωτάτου, τὰ μέχρι τῶν καθ' ἑαυτὸν εὑρημένα πάντα ἔγραψεν, ἐάσαντα τοὺς ἄλλους μόνα τὰ πρὸς ἐκείνου γεγραμμένα τοῖς ἐμοῖς ἀντεξετάσαι); following the text in Boudon-Millot (2007).

standard way of approaching the study of anatomy; anatomical texts from the Classical and even Hellenistic period are therefore more heterogeneous in content and, relatedly, tend to be less singularly focused on anatomy. Many of them nevertheless continued to exert influence on anatomists of later centuries; indeed, a substantial number of the texts to be considered in this chapter are completely lost to us, and what little we know about them is owing to the interest of subsequent authors, mostly from the Roman period. The goal of this chapter is therefore twofold. First, I will trace the development of anatomical texts in the Classical and Hellenistic periods, including the amount to which each relies on the practice of dissection; in addition, I will describe the degree of anatomical influence that each text or author still exerted in the Roman period, when dissection and anatomical writing became more fully integrated.

Galen is as aware as anyone of the developments in the genre of anatomical writing, and he provides a useful framework of three different categories of anatomical text, each of increasing specialization.[2] The most general class in his categorization consists of books that incorporate anatomy as an element rather than as a main focus; these tend to be of a medical or philosophical slant and to predominate among the older authors. His next category is that of the anatomical handbook; these began to circulate in the mid-fourth century BC and were consistently popular from then on.[3] Handbooks conveyed focused anatomical facts, offering lists and descriptions of bones, muscles, vessels and/or nerves, depending on the focus of the particular author. The simpler examples largely played the role of aide-mémoires, and it is easy to see how they would have supplemented an oral education; others appear to have delved deeper into physiology and may have been opportunities for the dissemination of their authors' broader theories. Galen's last and smallest category is that of anatomical "procedures"; these emerged in the Roman period and represented a new trend in anatomical writing. The text by Galen is the only surviving example of this type, and we know concretely of only two before it; they provide narrative instructions for the process of dissection rather than enumerating

---

[2] *AA* II.282–3.

[3] The word that Galen uses to describe the "handbooks" in this passage is συγγράμματα; however, this should not be taken as a direct Greek equivalent of the English word. Indeed, it is difficult to draw a meaningful and consistent difference between Galen's use of the words σύγγραμμα and ὑπόμνημα. Both can be used interchangeably to refer to unmarked "writing"; see, for example, *HNH* XV.1 where he calls the same text, his *Elements According to Hippocrates*, both terms in the same sentence (cf. *Ars Med.* I.411, where the terms are used quasi-synonymously, linked by τε καί). For further consideration of these terms, see von Staden (1998), 72–3, and Flemming (2008), 324–6.

the resulting anatomical data. Tracing this evolution of the genre limns a picture that mirrors the development of dissection, as outlined in Part I of this book. Anatomy did not operate as a separate subfield of medicine or philosophy until around the time of Aristotle, when Diocles purportedly wrote the first handbook; even then, it does not appear to have reached its apogee as a specialized area of study until Marinus published the first "procedures" in the Roman period.

In the epigraph to this chapter, Galen foregrounds this lengthy history of the anatomical text, but at the same time indicates that its very nature as a cumulative area of study rewards conflict between near contemporaries more than emulation of the great figures of the past. Unlike in the fields of rhetoric or philosophy, an anatomist in the Roman Empire could not automatically turn to the Classical period as the font of the greatest authorities on the subject: Even the most devoted Atticist had to admit that revolutionary discoveries had been made in the Hellenistic period and were still in the process of being argued, refined, and added to. Despite this, the contemporary social and academic mores imbued the most ancient voices, especially those of Hippocrates, Plato, and, to a somewhat lesser degree, Aristotle, with an amount of authority not necessarily commensurate to their quality in the field. This led to a delicate dance. On the one hand, aligning oneself with the authority of "the ancients" – in this context, authors working roughly from the fifth to the third centuries BC – lent a certain gravitas and irrefutability to one's claims; on the other, truly emerging victorious on a topic required detailed engagement with closer contemporaries. Accordingly, while they considered more modern generations of anatomists to be fair game for criticism, Roman anatomists, as we shall see, typically praised the ancients for their discoveries and elevated or even exaggerated their understanding, while forgiving them for their ignorance.

The "Pre-Socratics"

Despite the modern predilection for placing the beginning of the history of dissection among the so-called pre-Socratic philosophers, the surviving anatomical authors from the Roman period do not cite them as authoritative figures. Galen does not include them anywhere in his general lists of anatomists, though he does note that, among the ancients, philosophers studied anatomy just like physicians.[4] To take the examples considered in Chapter 2:

---

[4] *AA* II.280.

Alcmaeon, whose investigation of the eye seems to have included at least some degree of anatomical activity and has sometimes garnered him the title "father of dissection," does not feature in the surviving medical works of the second century other than Galen's, and there he appears only twice, both times in a general list of ancient natural philosophers.[5] While Anaxagoras does make a Roman-period appearance in Plutarch, using the dissection of the head of a goat to demonstrate that its malformed horns were the result of nature not of divine messaging, he does not surface among contemporary medical writers in any anatomical contexts.[6] Diogenes of Apollonia, whose description of the vessels Aristotle quotes in full as by far the longest of the three best accounts by earlier authors, receives only one citation, in which Galen explicitly says that he does not have access to his text, but is relying on Rufus.[7] Democritus of Abdera, who, as we saw, was credited with systematic dissection in the Hellenistic pseudepigraphic letters of Hippocrates, appears in Roman medical authors with some frequency, mostly for his atomist views, but not as an anatomical source; the results of his zoological inquiries appear only in Aelian.[8] There has been speculation, however, that the truncated *Anatomy* in the Hippocratic corpus derives from a longer Democritean source, suggesting a more robust, though still largely obscured, anatomical legacy.[9] Galen cites Empedocles, along with Democritus, as a natural philosopher of a stature comparable to Plato, Aristotle, and Theophrastus, but, like Democritus, he mentions him mostly for his foundational views on the composition of material things.[10] The area where Empedocles most closely impinges on anatomical topics is in the realm of embryology; Rufus cites him as the originator, perhaps, of the term amnion, but Galen only brings him up to criticize his theory of embryogenesis as absurd.[11] For authors of the Roman period, Hippocrates was the first substantial author of anatomy.

---

[5] For Alcmaeon's excision and possible dissection of the eye, see Calcidius, *In Tim.* 246 (DK 24A.10), Lloyd (1975*a*), and, as also for all the figures in this section, see the discussion in Chapter 2, "The 'Pre-Socratics'" at pp. 12–13. For Galen's two mentions of him, see *Hipp.Elem.* I.487 and *HNH* XV.5.

[6] Plutarch, *Per.* 6.2.

[7] Aristotle: quotation at *HA* 511b31–512b11 and judgment at *HA* 513a8–12; Galen: *Hipp.Epid. VI* XVIIa.1006; the citation in Rufus, unfortunately lost, seems to have provided a reference to Diogenes as the single dissonant voice on the topic of the comparative heat of males and females.

[8] See Chapter 2, n. 12. Interestingly, however, because of his prominent role as a dissector in the Hippocratic letters, Democritus would later get taken up as a key early figure in anatomy; already in the fourth century AD, he appears as the paradigmatic example of a dissector (see Chapter 10, n. 23) and, by the Renaissance and Early Modern periods, he is a foundational anatomical name (see French [1999], 239–43, and Lüthy [2000]).

[9] Craik (2006), 166–8.

[10] Galen, *Caus.Proc.* XV.193.

[11] Rufus, *Nom.Part.* 229; Galen, *Sem.* IV.616–20.

The Hippocratic Corpus

Confounding any discussion of anatomy in the Hippocratic Corpus is the fact that it is scattered piecemeal throughout texts focused on other subjects. The most promisingly entitled text, *Anatomy*, is a truncated work – indeed, the shortest in the corpus. It contains two head-to-toe lists of internal organs (1: trachea, lungs, heart, liver, kidneys, bladder; 2: esophagus, diaphragm, spleen, belly, intestines, colon, rectum) with some descriptions, but no theoretical or physiological framework. Given the brevity of the treatise, it is difficult to assign it a date with any great certainty, but it seems likely that it was circulating as early as the fourth century BC and that it was based on earlier, lengthier works, now lost.[12] Indeed, *On Joints* promises a dedicated work of anatomy that will describe

> the attachments of the veins and arteries, how many they are, of what sort, whence they arise, and in what sorts of ways they are capable of what sorts of things, and also the spinal cord itself, with what kind of coverings it is encased and from whence they arise, where they hold sway and to what they are connected, and what sorts of things they are capable of.[13]

Given that neither of these promised topics, which are quite advanced and combine both anatomy and physiology, appears in our *Anatomy*, it would be overconfident in the extreme to claim that *On Joints* here provides a trace of one of *Anatomy*'s direct antecedents; however, this reference does offer corroboration for the idea that texts with some anatomical focus were circulating – or at any rate conceived of – at an early date.[14] As for the purpose of the abbreviated work that has survived, Craik suggests that metrical elements in the composition might indicate that it was composed for memorization.[15] It thus seems likely that *Anatomy* is an epitome of more diffusely presented anatomical knowledge from lost Hippocratic works, and that it belongs to the emergence of anatomical handbooks in the fourth century.

---

[12] Craik (2006), 168 (and her preceding analysis).

[13] *Artic.* 45 (IV.190 Littré) (αἱ δὲ φλεβῶν καὶ ἀρτηριῶν κοινωνίαι ἐν ἑτέρῳ λόγῳ δεδηλώσονται, ὅσαι τε καὶ οἶαι, καὶ ὅθεν ὡρμημέναι, καὶ ἐν οἷοισιν οἷα δύνανται, αὐτὸς δὲ ὁ νωτιαῖος οἷσιν ἐλύτρωται ἐλύτροισι, καὶ ὅθεν ὡρμημένοισι, καὶ ὅπη κραίνουσιν, καὶ οἷσι κοινωνέουσι, καὶ οἷα δυναμένοισιν).

[14] Craik (1998), 11 suggests that there were pre-Hippocratic works on anatomy in the Doric dialect that have left traces in the Hippocratic Corpus, including *Fract.*, *Artic.*, *Mochl.*, and *Loc.*

[15] Craik (2006), 162.

The other texts in the corpus display variable levels of interest in – and various different approaches to – anatomy. Underlying all the Hippocratic texts is a basic understanding of and vocabulary for the major organs, but, as we saw in Chapter 2, only some authors of the Hippocratic Corpus were practicing dissection, while others were content to use other avenues for the conceptualization of internal anatomy. Indeed, many texts in the corpus offer scant mention of the structure of the body or none at all, but some authors did consider anatomy to be important, even fundamental, knowledge for the practicing physician. The authors of the surgical texts unsurprisingly fall into this category, given their evident interest in dissection. *On Joints* contains much discussion of anatomy and, though the received order of the text is too jumbled to be informative, two passages indicate than an understanding of underlying anatomy must be achieved "first of all."[16] *Leverage*, which is basically a summary of *On Joints* and preserves a much more logical order, confirms this primacy, opening with a fairly substantial anatomical section entitled "nature of bones."[17] *On Fractures*, too, while less explicit, contains criticism of the harm done by doctors who are not familiar with anatomy.[18] Beyond the surgical texts, *Epidemics VI* includes anatomical material at the beginning of what appears to be a list of things a doctor should know, and most of the more theoretical treatises include anatomy as something worth knowing, though only *Fleshes* and *Places in Man* particularly foreground it.[19]

Regardless of their opinion with respect to the fundamental position of anatomy in medical knowledge, many texts in the corpus do attempt some sort of anatomical overview. Some, like *Art* and *On Ancient Medicine*, do so quite vaguely. The former describes the body as being a series of cavities, the details of which are "known to those who trouble with such things"; the latter goes into a bit more detail, describing the basic shape or texture

---

[16] *Artic.* 45 (IV.190 Littré) and 79 (IV.316 Littré) (πρῶτον).

[17] *Mochl.* 1 (IV.340–4 Littré) (ὀστέων φύσις); compare *VC*, which also opens with two chapters on skeletal anatomy before broaching therapy.

[18] *Fract.* 3 (III.424–6 Littré).

[19] *Epid. VI* 6.14 (V.330 Littré). Anatomy appears as something worth knowing in: *Art.* 10 (VI.16 Littré), so as "not to be helpless before the more hidden diseases" (μηδὲ πρὸς τὰ ἧσσον φανερὰ ἀπορέειν); in *VM* 22 (I.626 Littré), as a final addition, so as to know which diseases are due to the shapes within the body, rather than to powers; in *Morb.Sacr.*, where it is appealed to repeatedly; in *Nat.Hom.* 11 (VI.58–60 Littré), which offers an abrupt – to the point of incongruous – anatomy of the vascular system. Anatomy is foregrounded in *Carn.* 1 (VIII.584 Littré), which opens with the idea that "how man and the other animals are naturally formed and come about" (ἄνθρωπον ... καὶ τὰ ἄλλα ζῶα, ὁκόσα ἔφυ καὶ ἐγένετο) is a central question to medicine, and in *Loc.Hom.* 2 (VI.278 Littré), which asserts in the second chapter that "the nature of the body is the beginning of the account of the medical art" (φύσις δὲ τοῦ σώματος, ἀρχὴ τοῦ ἐν ἰητρικῇ λόγου).

of each organ it considers, comparing them to everyday objects.[20] Others, such as *Nutriment, Sevens, Aphorisms,* and *Koan Prognoses,* do so very summarily, in keeping with their compressed styles.[21] A few offer more substantive observations. *Fleshes* begins by describing the generation of each part of the body, resulting in a catalogue of anatomical parts and their basic qualities, though rarely describing their structures; the author broaches, without real distinction, both what Aristotle would later categorize as the homoeomerous elements, like "cords" and "flesh," and the non-homoeomerous organs.[22] The author of *Places in Man* is generally very comfortable with anatomical terms and offers detailed accounts of the anatomy of the eyes and brain, the "cords," the vessels, and the bones.[23]

These latter two aspects of anatomy, the vascular and skeletal systems, get by far the most attention in the corpus. Descriptions of skeletal anatomy abound in *Fractures, Joints, Leverage,* and *Wounds in the Head,* though it is only in the first chapters of the latter two that it is consolidated into what one might consider an anatomical section.[24] *On Bones* is a compilatory work, which is, paradoxically, barely about the skeleton at all. The first chapter offers a broad anatomical overview of about the same brevity as that in *Anatomy,* fully half of which is dedicated to the skeletal system; the remaining sections are a collection of various anatomies of the vascular system, indicating that this was a subject that attracted considerable thought and not a great deal of consensus. One of these same accounts appears again in *Epidemics II* and another in *Nature of Man,* though in both cases seeming rather out of place.[25] Other texts, such as *Diseases IV* and *On the Sacred Disease,* also betray complex underlying vascular theories, though they do not lay them out in connected anatomical passages.

Anatomists of the Roman period were, of course, aware of the dearth of anatomically focused texts in the corpus.[26] Galen himself points out that in

---

[20] *Art.* 10 (VI.16–18 Littré) (ἃς ἴσασιν, οἷσι τουτέων ἐμέλησεν); *VM* 22–3 (I.626–34 Littré).

[21] *Alim.* 25 (IX.106 Littré), *Hebd.* 6–9 (West (1971), 369–70), *Aph.* 6.18 (IV.566–8 Littré), *Coac.* 499 (V.698 Littré); the latter two are simply lists of parts of the body that are mortal if wounded.

[22] *Carn.* 3–5, 7–12 (VIII.586–90, 594–8 Littré).

[23] *Loc.Hom.* 2 (VI.278–80 Littré) (eyes and brain), 3 (VI.280–2 Littré) (vessels), 4–5 (VI.282–4 Littré) (cords), and 6 (VI.284–90 Littré) (bones).

[24] *Mochl.* 1 (IV.340–4 Littré) and *VC* 1–2 (III.182–92 Littré).

[25] *Oss.* 10 (IX.178–80 Littré) appears at *Epid.II* 4.1–2 (V.120–6 Littré); *Oss.* 9 (IX.174–8 Littré) appears at *Nat.Hom.* 11 (VI.58–60 Littré) and also, in a somewhat shortened form, in Aristotle *HA* 512b11–13a7, attributed to Polybus, and immediately preceded there (*HA* 511b23–30) by *Oss.* 8 (IX.174 Littré), attributed to Syennesis of Cyprus.

[26] Modern scholarship considers the Hippocratic Corpus to be an amalgam of works by multiple authors gathered under one name, but authors of the Roman period considered all of texts in the corpus to either be the work of a single, historical Hippocrates, or to be to some degree spurious; see most recently the collection of articles in Dean-Jones and Rosen (2016), especially van der Eijk (2016).

Hippocrates "anatomical theory [is] mixed into medical books themselves, in which [he writes] about the diagnosis, prognosis, or cure of diseases."[27] Nevertheless, Hippocrates' position as the foundational authority in Greek medicine parlayed into a paramount importance in the field of anatomy.[28] For Galen, Hippocrates is a reliable source of wisdom on all topics, anatomy not least among them.[29] Like others before him, he frequently refers to him as "divine" and "most divine," casting him as an indisputable authority who knew no (or at least very little) wrong.[30] Any lack of complete explanation on Hippocrates' part Galen attributes to his innocence of the depths of ignorance, cynicism, and laziness that future generations would fall prey to; any seemingly erroneous statements, he often finds a way to explain in terms that reconcile them with more recent discoveries.[31] Galen routinely cites Hippocrates as *the* authority on anatomy. In fact, in the first four books of *Anatomical Procedures*, he is the only anatomical source whom Galen quotes directly. Similarly, Hippocrates, mentioned twice, is the only proper name found in his *On Bones for Beginners*, even though he uses terms directly coined by Herophilus and makes frequent anonymous references to "other" anatomists and doctors.[32]

Not all of Galen's contemporaries shared this opinion about Hippocrates, however. Martianus, an older doctor of wide repute whose anatomical writing was quite popular, disdains Galen's valuation of Hippocrates as an anatomist, claiming that "Hippocrates was, for him, not a subject of study in any aspect of anatomy" and that Erasistratus was his preeminent authority.[33] Galled by this blasphemy, Galen produces a text called *On the Anatomy*

---

[27] *AA* II.282 (αὐτοῖς τοῖς ἰατρικοῖς βιβλίοις, ἐν οἷς ἤτοι διαγνώσεις παθῶν, ἢ προγνώσεις, ἢ θεραπείας ἔγραψέ τις, ἀναμεμίχθαι τὴν ἀνατομικὴν θεωρίαν, ὅνπερ τρόπον Ἱπποκράτης φαίνεται διαπράττων).

[28] On the nuances and development of Hippocrates as a foundational authority, see King (2006) and Nelson (2016).

[29] On Galen's relationship to Hippocrates, see especially Smith (1979), as well as more recent contributions like Lloyd (1991), 403–16, and Boudon-Millot (2018).

[30] Galen describes Hippocrates as θεῖος at *QAM* IV.798 and *Caus.Puls.* IX.88 and θειότατος at *Nat. Fac.* II.189, *PHP* V.393 (IV.5.9 De Lacy), and *Di.Dec.* IX.775. See also his characterization of Hippocrates as the source "of all good things for us" (ὁ πάντων ἡμῖν τῶν καλῶν Ἱπποκράτης) at *MMG* XI.2 and his intention to treat a statement of Hippocrates "as if from the voice of god" (ὡς ἀπὸ θεοῦ φωνῆς) at *UP* III.22 (I.16H); cf. *Sem.* IV.542–3. For Hellenistic attributions of divinity to Hippocrates, see ps.-Hippocratic *Ep.* 2 (IX.314 Littré), Apollonius of Citium, *InHipp.Artic.* 1, and King (2006), 250–2.

[31] For case studies of the ways in which Galen deploys the Hippocratic Corpus, see Lloyd (1988), Potter (1993), Vallance (1999), Jouanna (2012), 313–33, and Curtis (2016).

[32] Hippocrates mentioned at II.735, 757; Herophilean term at II.745; references to "other" anatomists and doctors throughout, for example at II.748, 751, 753, 756, 771–2.

[33] Galen, *Lib.Prop.* XIX.14. The Greek here is lacunose, but Boudon-Millot (2007) was able to restore this section (her 1.9) based on the Arabic tradition; my translation here follows her French.

of Hippocrates in six books, as well as an *On the Anatomy of Erasistratus* in three.[34] Galen references the work on Hippocrates multiple times, indicating that it contained discussion of Hippocrates' approach to the "functions of the body and the soul," the vascular system, "the entire nature of the brain," the anatomy of generation and pregnancy, the genesis and composition of the nails, and the differences between the bladder and the gallbladder; at one point, he summarizes the contents of the text, saying that it served to prove that Hippocrates was interested in and familiar with "all the things made apparent by dissection."[35]

Indeed, Galen is confident that his Hippocrates was a practiced dissector. He frequently casts Hippocrates as the first competent anatomist, placing him at the beginning of lists of the best anatomists and generally insinuating that all later anatomists were simply following what he had already done.[36] He is most loquacious on the topic in his commentaries on various Hippocratic passages of anatomical tenor. In reference to the brief statement about the anatomy of intestines at *Epidemics VI* 4.6, he says "it is obvious that he wrote these things, too, as a memorandum for himself of things observed during dissection."[37] He held the same opinion of the most prominent of the anatomical passages, namely the extended passage in *Epidemics II* on the anatomy of the vascular system, which Galen repeatedly characterizes as a personal note not intended for larger circulation.[38] His extensive comments on this passage, which survive only in Arabic, paint Hippocrates as the most diligent of anatomists:

---

[34] On the latter, see this chapter, "Erasistratus" at pp. 202–3.

[35] Body and soul in *Ars Med.* I.409 (περὶ φυσικῶν ἢ ψυχικῶν ἐνεργειῶν) and *Hipp.Epid.II* 4.2 (*CMG Suppl.Or.* V.2, p. 707); vascular system in *PHP* V.528, 580 (VI.3.27, 8.67 De Lacy); brain in *PHP* V.610, 647 (VII.3.34, 8.14 De Lacy) and *Hipp.Aph.* XVIIIa.86; generation and pregnancy in *UP* IV.154 (II.293H), *Sem.* IV.537, 633, and *Gloss.* XIX.114; nails in *Plat.Tim.Comm.* at *Ti.* 76d3–e6 (*CMG Suppl.* I, p. 10) and *AA* II.337; bladder and gallbladder in *Nat.Fac.* II.15; complete familiarity with anatomy in *Hipp.Art.* XVIIIa.524 and *Hipp.Elem.* I.481 (ἐγίγνωσκεν ὁ Ἱπποκράτης ὑπὲρ ἁπάντων τῶν ἐξ ἀνατομῆς φαινομένων). It appears to have also included a section comparing Hippocrates' and Thucydides' accounts of plague (*Diff.Resp.* VII.851). Hunayn ibn Ishaq, who translated it into Syriac, summarizes the text's purpose at *Risala* 30: "to show that Hippocrates was thoroughly versed in anatomy ... adduc[ing as] proof texts from all of his books" (Lamoreaux [2016], 46).

[36] *PHP* V.650 (VIII.1.6 De Lacy), *AA* II.716, *Ven.Art.Diss.* II.780, *UP* III.468 (I.341H), *Loc.Aff.* VIII.212, *Foet.Form.* IV.652, *Hipp.Epid.II* 4.1 (*CMG Suppl.Or.* V.2, p. 645).

[37] *Hipp.Epid.VI* XVIIb.133 (εὔδηλον ὅτι καὶ ταῦτα ἔγραψεν εἰς ἀνάμνησιν ἑαυτῷ τῶν ἀνατομικῶν ὄντα θεωρημάτων). The "too" refers to the previous, nonanatomical lemma, which he also characterizes as a personal memorandum.

[38] Galen opines that this passage was a personal note that was later bundled with other such notes and circulated as *Epidemics II* at *Hipp.Epid.II* 4.1 (*CMG Suppl.Or.* V.2, pp. 617, 631–3) (cf. *Hipp. Art.*XVIIIa.529–30), though he also speculates there that it was intended to be read by members of his inner circle (pp. 663–5).

Hippocrates did not write what he wrote about this on the basis of reasoning or rational demonstration, nor because he believed it based on an inspiration granted to him by Asclepius while he was asleep or awake. Rather, he understood this by first cutting the lower abdomen along with the membrane that is spread over the belly and known as the peritoneum, then looking at what was underneath it and observing the intestines and viscera.… Just as Hippocrates discovered these things by cutting open the skin and observing what he saw underneath, so did Herophilus later on. He was not content to learn this from Hippocrates, but his aim was to learn it from the nature of things itself from which Hippocrates had learned everything he knew.[39]

Herophilus, thus, was a mere imitator of Hippocrates, who "was one of the most skillful and proficient observers of what appears during dissection."[40] He is not quite so explicit in his commentaries on *Fractures* and *On Joints*, but all of his anatomical comments there are also predicated on the assumption that Hippocrates was "extremely zealous about anatomy."[41] He particularly relishes the hypothetical dissection of the shoulder that occurs in the opening chapter of *On Joints*, which no doubt resonated with him on an autobiographical level, explaining that Hippocrates thought good "to teach the whole nature of [the head of the shoulder joint] through dissection"; he then recasts the Hippocratic instructions using language more reminiscent of *Anatomical Procedures* than of anything in the original text.[42] At a more subtle level, he repeatedly admonishes his readers that they cannot hope to understand Hippocrates' writing if they do not have a complete understanding of the underlying anatomy that he is describing, thus attributing a Galenic level of knowledge to Hippocrates.[43] Indeed, he considers the fact that one passage simply does not agree with observed anatomy to be grounds for suspecting scribal error.[44]

---

[39] *Hipp.Epid.II* 4.1 (*CMG Suppl.Or.* V.2, pp. 621–3, trans. Vagelpohl and Swain).

[40] *Hipp.Epid.II* 4.1 (*CMG Suppl.Or.* V.2, p. 633; trans. Vagelpohl and Swain); cf. p. 705, where he describes his "meticulous dissection of the nerves." Indeed, though it is unwise to read too much into the precise phrasing of the Arabic, it is possible that Galen conceived of Hippocrates, like Herophilus, as a dissector of humans. In explaining why ventral elements of the body are typically described as "above" those located more dorsally, he twice explains that this stems from the habit of "Hippocrates and other anatomists after him" of dissecting subjects lying on their backs; in the second instance he specifies that the subject of dissection was "human" at *Hipp.Epid.II* 4.1–2 (*CMG Suppl.Or.* V.2, pp. 653, 691) (الإنسان) (cf. p. 623, where others also wrote books on the vascular system in the manner of Hippocrates and Herophilus, having seen the vessels for themselves in the body of humans [الناس]). For a likely precedent for an Arabic translator falsely reading human dissection into a Galenic text, see Chapter 4, n. 122; the inclusion of Herophilus in the anecdote at p. 623, however, makes it more plausible to me that this could be an accurate rendering of the original Greek.

[41] *Hipp.Art.* XVIIIa.525 (ἀνατομήν τε μάλιστα σπουδάζων).

[42] *Hipp.Art.* XVIIIa.314 (διδάσκειν τὴν φύσιν αὐτῆς ὅλην ἐξ ἀνατομῆς ἀξιῶν); see also the discussion of this passage in Chapter 2, "Hippocratic Doctors" at p. 15.

[43] *Hipp.Art.* XVIIIa.303–4, 309–10, 425, 529, 531, 627; *Hipp.Fract.* XVIIIb.448.

[44] *Hipp.Art.* XVIIIa.538–41.

It is, in general, not lost on Galen that the flipside of his belief in Hippocrates' flawless anatomical knowledge is the need to explain anatomical passages in the corpus that are patently inaccurate. He achieves this with particular aplomb in his comments on *Nature of Man*. There he claims that, though the first half of the treatise is without doubt genuine – indeed, foundational – Hippocrates, the second part is a treatise on regimen by Polybus, Hippocrates' doctrinally faithful student, that was appended to it by means of a dubious bridge of spurious material, including the unfortunate interpolation of the completely inauthentic passage on the veins.[45] He excoriates the inaccurate anatomy that it contains, saying that it is not the result of poor dissection, but, rather, indicative of absolutely no attempt at dissection at all: Even a blind man, he complains, could have felt with his hands that the veins the author describes do not exist.[46] This very inaccuracy is his proof of inauthenticity, for he deems it impossible that Hippocrates, who "accurately writes not only about things clearly visible to everyone, but also about things difficult to observe," could so badly flub an anatomical description.[47]

Though we have seen that Martianus rejected Hippocrates as an anatomical authority, this is not grounds to believe that Galen was unique in his opinion of Hippocrates' anatomical prowess. Others also considered Hippocrates a fount of anatomical knowledge. In Rufus, Hippocrates edges out even Herophilus (that prolific discoverer of new things to be named) as the most cited author for anatomical nomenclature.[48] Galen's teacher, Pelops, included an anatomy of the entire body in the third book of his *Hippocratic Introductions*, indicating that he considered it to be a major element of Hippocrates' teaching.[49] The author of the second-century *Doctor: Introduction* also directly quotes Hippocrates in his section on the anatomy of the eye and, like Galen, takes pains to excuse a factual discrepancy in his description.[50] Some were even so wedded to

---

[45] *HNH* XV.11–12, 108–9, *PHP* V.528–9 (VI.3.29–30 De Lacy); see also Jouanna (2012), 319–24. Galen is here in tacit disagreement with Aristotle, who quotes this same passage on the blood vessels at *HA* 512b11–13a7 and attributes it to Polybus.

[46] *HNH* XV.133–48, particularly 142–3.

[47] *HNH* XV.147 (ἀκριβῶς φαίνεται γράψας οὐ μόνον τὰ σαφῶς ὁρώμενα πᾶσιν, ἀλλὰ καὶ τὰ δυσθεώρητα).

[48] In Rufus' *Nom.Part.* Hippocrates is named eight times and Herophilus six (and a further three times in the probably pseudonymous *Diss.Hum.*). After them, Homer comes in at four, as does Praxagoras (in three different passages, only two of which anatomical), Aristotle and Eudemus at three, Dionysius, son of Oxymachus, (who is unknown outside this reference; see the discussion of the various medical Dionysii at Tecusan [2004], 53–9, where he is number vi [p. 58]) at two (in one passage), and Mnesitheus, Euryphon, and Philistion each at one; Erasistratus appears only in *Diss. Hum.*, named twice in one passage.

[49] Galen, *Musc.Diss.* XVIIIb.926.

[50] Ps.-Galen, *Int.* XIV.711–12.

Hippocrates' accuracy that they defended readings that directly contradicted anatomical evidence. Galen laments that those who argue for the authenticity of the vascular passage in *Nature of Man* are maddeningly unconcerned with its divergence from visible anatomy and prefer the received text to the evidence of their own eyes: "Some of those who affirm this passage say that they trust Hippocrates, even if they are not themselves able to demonstrate [the reputed vessels], as if they were talking about a question subject to verbal argument, not perception, while others promise that they will demonstrate them, but never have demonstrated them."[51] These latter at least hope that the visible can be brought into line with the text. Others do not even bother to consider the results of dissection, like Sabinus, who blithely compliments Hippocrates on his "clear and plain" account of the nerves in a passage whose reconciliation with observed fact requires a great of deal of effort on Galen's part.[52] Hippocrates' anatomical authority was an entrenched fact in Hippocratic circles.[53]

From among the peri-Hippocratic authors, Galen singles out Euryphon as an anatomical expert. In *On the Dissection of the Uterus*, he places him in an exalted trio with Aristotle and Herophilus as the "best of the anatomists," putting Diocles, Praxagoras, Phylotimus, and "all the rest of the ancients" in a second tier.[54] Yet none of his references to Euryphon, though they include some direct quotations, pertain to anatomical subjects. He most often appears by virtue of his relationship with Hippocrates and for his views on the beneficial uses of breast milk.[55] Indeed, gynecology appears to have been the area where his writings exerted the strongest pull; Soranus cites him repeatedly for gynecological therapies, and the only mention of him in Rufus is to attribute to him an alternative name for part of the external female genitalia.[56] It is not surprising, then, that of Galen's two mentions of Euryphon as anatomist, the more strongly worded is in his juvenile work of gynecological anatomy. Even there, he seems to have been more a name to be admired than a source to be drawn on.

---

[51] *PHP* V.528 (VI.3.28 De Lacy) (ἔνιοι μὲν τῶν τιθεμένων αὐτὰ πιστεύειν Ἱπποκράτει φασί, κἄν αὐτοὶ μὴ δύνωνται δεικνύειν, ὡς περὶ λόγῳ θεωρητοῦ πράγματος, οὐκ αἰσθητοῦ διαλεγόμενοι, τινὲς δ' ἐπαγγέλλονται μὲν δείξειν, ἔδειξαν δ' οὐδέποτε.).

[52] *Hipp.Epid.II* 4.2 (*CMG Suppl.Or.* V.2, p. 681, trans. Vagelpohl and Swain).

[53] For the more difficult subject of Hippocrates outside Hippocratic circles, see Smith (1979), 222–46, and von Staden (1999a).

[54] *Ut.Diss.* II.900–1 (κάλλιστα ἀνατεμόντων ... τοὺς ἄλλους παλαιούς); he appears again at the end of the list of anatomists at *HNH* XV.136.

[55] Vis-à-vis Hippocrates: *Diff.Resp.* VII.891, 960, *HVA* XV.455, *Hipp.Epid.VI* XVIIa.886, *Hipp.Aph.* XVIIIa.149; on breast milk: *Bon.Mal.Suc.* VI.775, *Marc.* VII.701, *MM* X.474.

[56] Soranus, *Gyn.* I.35, IV.14, 36; Rufus, *Nom.Part.* 112.

Plato

Plato (*c.* 429–347 BC) does not seem an obvious figure to include in a catalogue of anatomical literature from antiquity, but his *Timaeus* carried significant weight in medical circles, despite some of its more allegorical elements. The second half of the treatise includes overviews of the parts of the body in the context of their creation by the gods; Plato's focus is more on physiology, but he offers anatomical descriptions as well, explaining the teleological rationale behind each structure.[57] Galen wrote a commentary on this treatise in four books – a substantial one given the amount of relevant material in the original text – which he describes as "concerning the things said in a medical way in the *Timaeus* of Plato."[58] He goes through the anatomical and physiological section of Plato's treatise in detail; though not completely uncritical, he is respectful, pointing out that "it is in no way surprising that Plato is unfamiliar with things related to anatomy, just like Homer."[59] Outside that commentary, he only refers to Plato's theories twice in his strictly anatomical texts – a reference to his explanation of the purpose of the diaphragm and a simultaneous excuse for and critique of his inexact way of referring to the spinal marrow – but he mentions him frequently in *On the Usefulness of the Parts*.[60] There he calls Plato "a zealous follower of Hippocrates, if anyone ever was" and cites the *Timaeus* repeatedly, usually on questions of physiology, including on the function of the flesh, the lung, the liver, the intestines, and the diaphragm, but also in a more anatomical way, claiming that he has a better (though still not sufficiently exact) term for the brain than Aristotle and other predecessors.[61] Nor was Galen alone in this high estimation of Plato's medical, if not directly anatomical, relevance. More than 10 percent of the surviving Anonymous London Papyrus is devoted to Plato's theory of the composition of the body in the *Timaeus* and its ramifications for disease theory.[62]

---

[57] Plato, *Ti.* 44d–46c, 69c–81e.

[58] *Lib.Prop.* XIX.46 (περὶ τῶν ἐν τῷ Πλάτωνος Τιμαίῳ ἰατρικῶς εἰρημένων ὑπομνήματα τέτταρα). The text survives only in fragments; see Schröder (1934), vii–xxviii.

[59] *Plat.Tim.Comm.* at *Ti.* 77d3–6 (*CMG Suppl.* I, p. 14) (οὐδὲν θαυμαστόν ἐστι τὰ κατὰ τὰς ἀνατομὰς ἀγνοῆσαι Πλάτωνα καθάπερ καὶ Ὅμηρον).

[60] *AA* II.503, S280.

[61] Flesh: *UP* III.37 (I.26H); lung: III.415, 621 (I.303, 450H); liver: III.309 (I.227H); intestines: III.327, 332 (I.240, 244H); diaphragm: III.314 (I.231H); brain: III.627 (I.454H). He also cites him as an authority on the origin of the red color in blood at III.272 (I.199H).

[62] Anonymous of London, XIV.11–XVIII.8 (4.5 columns out of 39).

Diocles of Carystus

It is with Diocles (mid-fourth century BC)[63] that we see a decisive move from anatomically relevant texts to more strictly anatomical texts. Galen assigns to him the dubious honor of having been the first to write an anatomical handbook after the fall from the golden age of Hippocratic medicine, when "children learned dissection at their fathers' knees":

> So then the art [of medicine], falling outside of the family of the Asclepiads and thenceforward becoming ever worse in the hands of many successors, required memoranda to preserve its theory. Earlier there was need neither for anatomical procedures nor for treatises of the sort that Diocles wrote first (as far as I know) and then, following him, some others of the ancient doctors and not a few of the more recent, whom I have mentioned.[64]

Galen's evaluation of Hippocrates as a consummate dissector unquestionably drives his narrative here; he presents dissection as an elementary and fundamental skill for the doctors of the sixth and fifth centuries BC and laments the deleterious consequences of its neglect in the generations after Hippocrates. In reality, however, the opposite is true: Diocles is witness to a growth, not a decline. He was a prominent figure in both the development of specialized anatomical texts – to whose enduring popularity Galen attests – and the popularization of dissection, two related phenomena that burgeoned simultaneously in the fourth century BC.

Diocles was a prolific author with many different areas of interest. In his collection of the surviving fragments, van der Eijk lists twenty different titles, which include treatises on therapeutics, prognosis, diet, and gynecology in addition to the text known as *Anatomy*.[65] It is thus not surprising that the majority of references to him by our sources from the imperial period, when at least some of his work seems to still have been circulating, are not anatomical in nature.[66] Of those that are, the most interesting

---

[63] On the question of his date, see Chapter 2, n. 64.

[64] *AA* II.280–1 (παρὰ τοῖς γονεῦσιν ἐκ παίδων ἀσκουμένοις … ἀνατέμνειν … ἐκπεσοῦσα τοίνυν ἔξω τοῦ γένους τῶν Ἀσκληπιαδῶν ἡ τέχνη, κᾆπειτα διαδοχαῖς πολλαῖς ἀεὶ χείρων γιγνομένη, τῶν διαφυλαξόντων αὐτῆς τὴν θεωρίαν ὑπομνημάτων ἐδεήθη. ἔμπροσθεν δ' οὐ μόνον ἐγχειρήσεων ἀνατομικῶν, ἀλλ' οὐδὲ συγγραμμάτων ἐδεῖτο τοιούτων, ὁποῖα Διοκλῆς μὲν ὧν οἶδα πρῶτος ἔγραψεν, ἐφεξῆς δ' αὐτῷ τῶν ἀρχαίων ἰατρῶν ἕτεροί τινες, οὐκ ὀλίγοι τε τῶν νεωτέρων, ὧν ἔμπροσθεν ἐμνημόνευσα); following the text in Garofalo (1986–2000).

[65] van der Eijk (2000–1), vol. I, xxxiii–iv.

[66] Galen implies that he had access to (at least some of) Diocles' writing at *Thras.* V.898: "Hippocrates and Diocles and Praxagoras and Phylotimus and Herophilus were knowledgeable about the entire art that concerns the body, as their writings make clear" (Ἱπποκράτης καὶ Διοκλῆς καὶ Πραξαγόρας καὶ Φυλότιμος καὶ Ἡρόφιλος ὅλης τῆς περὶ τὸ σῶμα τέχνης ἐπιστήμονες ἦσαν, ὡς δηλοῖ τὰ γράμματα αὐτῶν).

relate to gynecological topics, and they do not redound to his benefit.[67] Galen describes him, together with Praxagoras and Phylotimus, as having been ignorant of an element of uterine anatomy; he is not, however, surprised, "for, as a general rule they are similarly inexact on anatomical matters, for which reason they are of no concern to [him]."[68] Both Galen and Soranus also reproach him for his belief in uterine cotyledons in humans, the former with some clemency, since Hippocrates, too, is implicated in the error, the latter with more venom.[69] Thus, Diocles' lasting textual legacy in the field of anatomy seems to have been limited to the novelty of the genre he pioneered.

Our sources cite two other medical figures with anatomical interests who were roughly contemporary with Diocles. Mnesitheus and Dieuches were apparently also dissectors and anatomical authors, but the Roman authors who have preserved their names use them in a very limited fashion.[70] Dieuches appears in Galen as a name in lists with other doctors, with no indication that Galen had personally read him.[71] Mnesitheus, on the other hand, Galen does discuss individually about half a dozen times, but his only reference to his anatomical work is to point out that he erroneously (in Galen's opinion) denied that elephants have gallbladders.[72]

Aristotle

Aristotle's (384–322 BC) biological works contain the earliest substantial treatments of anatomy to survive to the present day in complete texts. The zoological texts, particularly *History of Animals*, but also *Parts of Animals*, *Generation of Animals*, and some of the shorter texts in the *Parva Naturalia*, offer evidence of Aristotle's extensive program of dissection. While none

---

[67] He appears, grouped with various other ancient authors, on topics of general anatomical nomenclature at *AA* II.716, *Ut.Diss.* II.890, and *Hipp.Art.* XVIIIa.736; on general theories of the vascular system at *HNH* XV.136; he is cited alone on basic theories of movement at *Hipp.Prog.* XVIIIb.124 and for his theory of adhesion at *Ut.Diss.* II.903.

[68] Galen, *Ut.Diss.* II.900–1 (ὁλοσχερέστερον γάρ πως καὶ οὐκ ἀκριβῶς περὶ τὰ ἀνατομικὰ ἔσχον· ὅθεν οὐδ᾽ ἐκείνων μοι μέλει).

[69] Galen, *Ut.Diss.* II.905; Soranus, *Gyn.* I.14. The Soranus passage is in keeping with his general opinion of Diocles; of his ten mentions of him only two lack some criticism or contradiction.

[70] Galen includes them both in his list of anatomists at *HNH* XV.136.

[71] See *MM* X.28, 462, *Ven.Sect.Er.* XI.163, *SMT* XI.795, and *HNH* XV.136.

[72] Galen discusses Mnesitheus alone at *Vict.Att.* 42 (*CMG* V.4.2, p. 440), *Alim.Fac.* VI.457, 479, 510–17, 645–8, and *MMG* XI.3; all but the final citation, which concerns his method of systemization, refer to his work on dietetics. Rufus' only mention of him (*Nom.Part.* 227) and Soranus' two (*Gyn.* 2.28, 48) are also in the context of diet. On the gallbladder, see *AA* II.569; it is interesting that Mnesitheus is Galen's scapegoat here, since Aristotle also held this opinion (*HA* 506b1–3), which is, in fact, the correct one.

of these is confined strictly to anatomy, the first four books of *History of Animals* systematically catalog both the external and the internal parts of every class of animal, while *Parts of Animals* reiterates much of this information in a more narrative structure, with the goal of explaining the purpose of the parts' construction and arrangement. Each of the texts, however, has a broader focus than just anatomy. Aristotle is also interested in physiology, in animal behavior, in procreation and generation, in sensation, and in motion; in short, his zoological agenda is noticeably influenced by his interest in the interplay between body and soul. Further, where he does focus directly on anatomy, his scope is far wider than in the other texts we have so far considered. Here, the dissection of animals is pursued for the sake of understanding the bodies of animals themselves, rather than as proxies for human anatomy. The vagaries of fish genitalia, the structure of insect antennae, and the folds of the pig's stomach are all given their due portion of intellectual weight. This zoocentric anatomy represents a new and distinct branch of the subject, which plays a role in the revival of dissection in the Roman period, as we saw with Apuleius in Chapter 1, but which leaves less of a mark on its anatomical literature.[73] Like his more medically focused colleagues, however, Aristotle does also recognize that animal anatomy is a window into that of humans, and humans, as the preeminent and most familiar member of the animal family, are a major focus of his interests.[74]

Of the surviving zoological works, *History of Animals* is the one that could most convincingly be classified as an anatomical text. The end of the first book contains a description of the external and internal parts of the human body, the internal section explicitly relying on comparison to animals whose organs have "a closely-resembling nature" to those of man.[75] The following three books cover in detail the external, internal, and generative parts of all manner of blooded animals, including vivipara, fish, reptiles, and birds, followed by those of the bloodless animals, namely hard- and soft-shelled creatures and insects. In addition to all of this descriptive anatomy, Aristotle offers here the first methodological statements that come down to us on the actual practice of dissection. He cautions against being misled by the effects that death, and dissection

---

[73] Kollesch (1997), 368 argues that Aristotle was the first to focus on the anatomy of animals for its own sake; Lennox (1994), argues that Aristotle was also the last author of antiquity to do so, though I feel that Galen and his peers, including Apuleius, present more of a challenge to this claim than he allows; cf. Chapter 7, "Anatomy in the Roman Intellectual Scene" at pp. 272–3.

[74] For the primacy and familiarity of humans, see for example *HA* 491a23–6, *PA* 656a9–14, 686a28–b20; for his study of animals as a proxy for humans, see *HA* 494b21–4.

[75] *HA* 494b24 (παραπλησίαν τὴν φύσιν).

itself, can have on the state of the body.[76] Further, he criticizes standard
practice in the field and offers his own improved method. He points out
that the vascular descriptions of his predecessors are extremely inaccurate,
and he attributes this to the fact that they based their theories either on
animals that were slaughtered and cut open – and whose vessels had thus
collapsed and become difficult to discern when the blood ran out – or
on extremely emaciated patients, whose superficial vessels would be quite
prominent, but whose interior ones would remain obscure.[77] His solution,
which Galen also champions for dissections related to the vascular system,
is to first starve an animal until it is extremely emaciated and then strangle
it, allowing the blood to congeal in the veins prior to dissection; this is his
advice to anyone who "makes it his business to learn about these sorts of
things."[78] For all this detail and instruction, however, the text still falls into
our first category of anatomically relevant medical and philosophical texts.
Though far closer to a dedicated anatomical book than Plato's *Timaeus*
or the works of the Hippocratic Corpus, where "anatomical theory [is]
mixed into medical books themselves," this is nevertheless not an anatomical "handbook," nor anything approaching an anatomical "procedure."[79]
Its scope and breadth make it something different: a compilation of observations of the natural world, many of which anatomical, in the service of
natural philosophy.

   In addition to these surviving texts, however, Aristotle repeatedly mentions another, which, though also distinctly zoological in character, should
more clearly be classified as a dedicated anatomical text: his *Anatomies*
(ἀνατομαί), which is now lost.[80] It was a lengthy, multivolume work that

---

[76] He describes the tendency of the heart to be displaced from its normal position during dissection
(*HA* 496a11) and the misleadingly bloodless state of the lungs in animal that has been cut into (*HA*
496b5–6).

[77] *HA* 511b10–23.

[78] *HA* 513a12–15 (εἴ τινι περὶ τῶν τοιούτων ἐπιμελές); for Galen's discussion of this method, see
Chapter 4, "Anatomical Subjects: Monkeys" at p. 95.

[79] For the citation, see this chapter, n. 27.

[80] References to this text are vexed by the ambiguity of the word ἀνατομαί, which could with equal
plausibility refer to a text called *Anatomies* or to performed dissections. Thus, a passage like the one
in *Somn.* 456b2, where he says, "what has been said is clear from the *Anatomies*/from dissections"
(φανερὸν δὲ τὸ λεχθὲν ἐκ τῶν ἀνατομῶν), could easily be referring to either; for a discussion of all
possible references, see Carbone (2011), 54–74. There are enough cases, however, where it is paired
with references to *HA* or to specific words for illustration to allay any doubts as to its existence as
a text; see Hellmann (2004), 67–71. Another, still more shadowy zoological text is the one referred
to as *On Animal Matters* (ζῳϊκά) and this, too, may have included some anatomical information;
indeed, two of the references potentially associated with this text include mention of dissection,
though it is possible that they derive from *Anatomies* instead (Athenaeus, VII.316c–d and 326c–d);
see Mayhew (2020), 131–2.

likely consisted of illustrations with some text.[81] Aristotle's own references indicate that the text was arranged in order to facilitate cross-species comparisons, as he repeatedly sends readers there to learn the differences in the same structure among various animals.[82] Indeed, it seems likely that the entire work was organized part by part, definitely including sections on both the male and female generative tracts, the digestive tract, the vascular system, and the respiratory system and its analogs.[83] Aristophanes of Byzantium may have still had access to some form of this text in the first century BC while writing his *Epitome* of Aristotle's zoological works.[84] He includes repeated anatomical observations that cannot be traced to elsewhere in the corpus.[85] Though we should be wary of pressing too hard on the evidence from the *Epitome*, it is noteworthy that Aristophanes frequently introduces discussion of the anatomy of specific animals in these passages with the participles "having been dissected" (ἀνατμηθείς) or "having been opened" (διοιχθείς). This rather suggests that the Aristotelian text did not offer directions for

[81] On the length, Chapter 2, n. 101; on the topic of its illustration, see Kádár (1978), 30–3, Stückelberger (1993), 139–42, (1994), 76 and (1998), 287–93, and Hellmann (2004), 67–9. There has been debate about the amount of text that accompanied these illustrations. Some, like Kádár (1978), 31, Stückelberger (1993), 140, and (1998), 288–9, and Louis (2002), xxxiii, assume that the work consisted exclusively of illustrations and acted as a kind of companion volume of plates or atlas for *HA*; recently Kullmann (1998), 134, and Hellmann (2004), 69, 76–7 and (2006), 337–40 have suggested that it was more of a stand-alone treatise, complete with short, quotable textual descriptions. This latter reading, which relies on what are likely direct citations of text from *Anatomies*, seems to me the more compelling.

[82] *HA* 509b21–4, 511a11–14, 565a12–13, *PA* 679b37–80a3, 684b1–5, 689a17–20, 696b14–16, *GA* 719a8–10, 746a14–15. The passages in Aristophanes' *Epitome* which may derive from this text (see Chapter 2, n. 99) also compare the internal organs of one animal to those of another at a striking rate, which could suggest that the text was grouped to facilitate this approach.

[83] For evidence of part-by-part organization, see *HA* 497a31–3, 509b21–4, 511a11–14, 565a12–13, *PA* 689a17–20, *GA* 719a8–10, and 746a14–15 (generative tracts), *PA* 674b15–17, 679b37–80a3, and 684b1–5 (digestive tract), *PA* 650a31–2, 668b28–30, and *GA* 740a23–4 (vascular system), *Resp.* 478a26, 478a34–b1, and *PA* 696b14–16 (lungs and gills). It is conceivable that it also contained a section organized animal by animal, since there are admonitions to look there to learn about specific animals' organs or general overall appearance (*HA* 525a7–9, 529b18–19, 566a13–15, and 530a30–1), though these specialized drawings could easily have been organized within a larger system-specific heading.

[84] For the complicated and uncertain transmission of Aristophanes' text, see this chapter, n. 208 For the traces of *Anatomies* in the epitome, see Düring (1950), 55–7, Kullmann (1998), 130, and Hellmann (2006), 332–3, who offers an argument for why the sections discussed here should be treated as genuine Aristophanes – and thus probably derived from genuine Aristotle.

[85] See Hellmann (2006), 337–45, for a detailed discussion of two specific examples. For details on the content of these passages, see Chapter 2, n. 99. Some have also raised the possibility that Aristophanes was pulling on material from a different collection of Aristotelian biological facts, referred to as *On Animal Matters* (ζωϊκά) (see Kullmann [1998], 128–9); others have suspected that *On Animal Matters* is identical to Aristophanes' *Epitome* (Kullmann [1998], 128, n. 19) or to Aristotle's *Anatomies* (Düring [1950], 55–7), but Mayhew (2020) now offers analysis suggesting that it was indeed a text in its own right.

dissection, but only the results of it, making it generically similar to, though broader in scope than, the handbook of Diocles.[86]

Aristotle's zoological texts were circulating in the Roman period.[87] Galen cites by name *Parts of Animals, History of Animals, Generation of Animals, On the Soul, On Sense and Sensible Objects, Problems,* which he considered a genuine work, and *On Sleep,* as well as *Physiognomy* and *Medical Things,* which latter he is aware is also attributed to Meno.[88] His direct, often extensive, quotations from – as well as numerous evident but unmarked references to – *Parts of Animals, History of Animals,* and *Generation of Animals* make it clear that he was intimately familiar with these texts.[89] Recent scholarship has also suggested that Aristotle's *Anatomies* was still available in the second century AD, based on the passage in Apuleius' *Apology* where he claims that his interest in dissection is in the service of "add[ing] to the books of anatomies (libros ἀνατομῶν) by Aristotle."[90] There is no other

---

[86] Nevertheless, Galen's assertion that Diocles' handbook was the first of its kind does little to settle the relative chronology of these two texts. While it is possible that Galen's evidence affirmatively places Diocles' work before that of Aristotle, it is also quite probable that the definition of the anatomical handbook used by Galen or his source relates strictly to discussions of human anatomy, thus disqualifying Aristotle's text from the category. It is further possible that Galen simply was not aware of this text's existence; he never mentions it, and it is not implausible that he could have interpreted the references to it within the Aristotelian corpus as referring to the practice of dissection, rather than a book called *Anatomies* (see this chapter, n. 80). Much ink has been spilled over the relationship between Diocles and Aristotle, with suggestions ranging from Diocles as member of the Lyceum (Jaeger [1940]) to Aristotle relying on Diocles' handbook for his description of human anatomy (Kollesch [1997], 370; cf. Byl [2011], 118); I am in most sympathy with the agnostic view expressed in van der Eijk (2000–1), vol. 2, xxxiv.

[87] Düring (1950), 61–2 traces a continuous line of familiarity with the biological texts from Theophrastus into the first century AD, though Lennox (1994), 15–17 argues that they were not available in the Hellenistic period.

[88] *PA: Temp.* I.566, *Sem.* IV.611, *QAM* IV.791–2, *PHP* V.200, 203 (I.8.2, 13 De Lacy), *MM* X.26; *HA: Nat.Fac.* II.173, *QAM* IV.795; *GA: Sem.* IV.516, 518, 557, 574–5; *DA* and *Sens.: Inst.Od.* II.871, *PHP* V.203 (I.8.13 De Lacy); *Prob.: Nat.Fac.* II.8, *QAM* IV.794, *PHP* V.641 (VII.7.15 De Lacy), *Hipp.Epid. VI* XVIIb.29; *Somn.: Caus.Symp.* VII.141; *Physiogn.: QAM* IV.797; *Iatr.: HNH* XV.26. In addition to these more biological texts, Galen also cites by name *Physics* (*Hipp.Elem.* I.448, 451), *On the Heavens* (*Hipp.Elem.* I.487), *On Generation and Decay* (*Hipp.Elem.* I.487, *Nat.Fac.* II.9, 167, *Diff.Puls.* VIII.687–8), *Meteorology* (*Nat.Fac.* II.9, 167, *Diff.Puls.* VIII.687–8), and *Metaphysics* (*Hipp.Epid.II* 2.13 [*CMG Suppl.Or.* V.2, p. 339]), as well as *Prior* and *Posterior Analytics* (*PHP* V.213 [II.2.4 De Lacy], *Diff.Puls.* VIII.706, 765), *Categories* (*Inst.Log.* 13.11.4, 16.1.4 [Kalbfleisch (1896)]), *Sophistical Refutations* (*Soph.* XIV.582, 593), and *On Interpretation,* for which he wrote commentaries (*Lib.Prop.* XIX.41–2, 47).

[89] Direct quotes of *PA* at *QAM* IV.791–4, *PHP* V.200–1 (I.8.3 De Lacy) (cf. *PHP* V.206 [I.10.2 De Lacy]); of *HA* at *QAM* IV.794–6; of *GA* at *Sem.* IV.516–18, 556–7, 574. He also directly quotes *DA* and *Sens.* at *Inst.Od.* II.871 and *Prob.* at *Hipp.Epid.VI* XVIIb.29. On Galen's relationship to *PA,* see Moraux (1985) and Lennox (1994), 18–22; cf. Moraux (1973–2001), 729–35 for his relationship to the biological works generally.

[90] Apuleius, *Apol.* 40 (libros ἀνατομῶν Aristoteli et explorare studio et augere). However, compare *Apol.* 36, where the text referred to as περὶ ζῴων ἀνατομῆς may refer to our *PA,* calling the reference at 40 into question; the idea of being able to "add to" (augere) Aristotle's texts, though, and the use

trace of it in the Roman period, however. Galen certainly makes no mention of the text, despite his not infrequent discussion of Aristotle's anatomical activity. This is a particularly notable omission because, in Galen's opinion, Aristotle is a significant and influential voice.

Galen had enormous respect for Aristotle. He appears frequently in the various lists of formidable ancients that Galen likes to deploy, especially when arguing that whichever claim he is in the midst of denouncing has no support from the authorities.[91] He is, together with Plato and Theophrastus, one of the "best philosophers" and he serves as an exemplar, with Plato, Hipparchus, and Archimedes, of the surpassing intelligence that is achievable by the human race.[92] Galen's references to him as a philosopher are overwhelmingly positive. He dedicated six treatises, totaling twenty-six books, to commenting on four of the six Aristotelian works on logic that came to be grouped as the *Organon*; though those texts have all been lost, his surviving works still convey his respect for Aristotle's more abstract philosophical work, various elements of which he refers to as "most marvelous of all" and "the best."[93] He also valued Aristotle as an authority in natural history, but it is here that a hint of tension arises. In *On the Powers of Simple Drugs*, he repeatedly praises Aristotle, Theophrastus, and their school as unquestioned authorities, deft in the study of nature.[94] He is also impressed by Aristotle's treatment of heat, which he refers to often, and especially by his innovative work with the elemental qualities, hot, cold, wet, and dry. However, while he acknowledges his importance in this line of inquiry, he is loath to grant him unqualified primacy. He opens *On Natural Faculties* with admiration for Aristotle's work on alteration and on the powers of the qualities, but he is quick to point out, almost in the same breath, that "Hippocrates, too, thought thus, being even earlier

---

of plural ἀνατομῶν in the passage at 40 – which is how Aristotle himself invariably refers to it – are both suggestive of the lost text, which was likely in a format more conducive to expansion than the more narrative texts that survive. For the availability of the text in the second century, see the positive assessments of Gigon (1987), 492, Stückelberger (1994), 77, and Hellmann (2004), 74, but also the doubts raised by Kullmann (1998), 130–1, who thinks that Apuleius had only Aristophanes' *Epitome*.

[91] For example, at *Hipp.Elem.* I.486, *Nat.Fac.* II.117, 140, 178, *PHP* V.450 (V.3.18 De Lacy), *MM* X.19, *SMT* XI.679, *Adv.Jul.* XVIIIa.269, 295, *CP* 15.193 (*CMG Suppl.* II, p. 52).

[92] *Nat.Fac.* II.110 (τῶν ἀρίστων φιλοσόφων); *UP* IV.359 (II.447H).

[93] On the commentaries, see *Lib.Prop.* XIX.41–2, 47, and Jouanna (2013). The cited praise in the surviving works occurs at *Diff.Puls.* VIII.688 (ὁ πάντων δεινότατος) and *PHP* V.213 (II.2.4 De Lacy) (ἄριστα). More generally, he often cites Aristotle as an obvious authority in matters of logic, for example in his repeated invocation of the idea that the that is prior to the why (*UP* III.496 [I.361H], *Hipp.Epid.VI* XVIIa.810, *Hipp.Epid.II* 6.5 [*CMG Suppl.Or.* V.2, p. 801]) and his evident sarcasm at the idea that anyone could surpass Plato and Aristotle on logic (*MM* X.28).

[94] *SMT* XI.467, 474, 629, 654, 657, 664, 690–1, 720, 731.

than Aristotle."[95] Indeed, both here and elsewhere, he casts Aristotle as writing "commentaries on Hippocrates' study of nature"; he asserts that many things were said "first by Hippocrates, second by Aristotle," though within this framework he is willing to admit that Aristotle furthered or completed ideas only sketched out by his medical predecessor.[96] While being thus classed with Hippocrates is undoubtedly a Galenic form of praise, it is also a pointed demotion of the philosopher's status. Neither Aristotle nor the Aristotelians would have considered this subordination much of a compliment.

In matters of anatomy and physiology this hint of tension blossoms into outright criticism.[97] Galen was naturally sympathetic to Aristotle's program of dissection and commitment to the discovery of *phainomena*; however, his resulting errors and inconsistencies cannot be covered up or otherwise explained as they might be for authors like Plato or Hippocrates, who are less explicit about their methodology. He frequently seems disheartened by Aristotle's anatomical mistakes, in part, paradoxically, because he is holding him to a higher standard. Festering at the root of this dissatisfaction is the fact that Aristotle is a strong defender of the centrality of the heart in all bodily functions, including thought and sensation – a position that Galen, rooted here in a Platonism bolstered by Hellenistic anatomical discoveries, cannot forgive him for. Indeed, to a greater degree than with any other ancient author except Erasistratus, Galen seems to feel an element of direct competition with Aristotle in the realm of anatomy, which speaks to Aristotle's influence in the field even as it seeks to diminish it. It is not idly that Galen mentions that some people think that his *On the Usefulness of the Parts* is "more profound and valuable than what Aristotle wrote."[98]

As a result, even his praise of Aristotle in anatomical or physiological contexts is, in the vast majority of cases, backhanded. In his juvenile work *On the Dissection of the Uterus*, the surrounding praise almost effaces the inner barb: Aristotle is linked with Herophilus and Euryphon as the "best anatomists,"

[95] *Nat.Fac.* II.4–9 (καὶ Ἱπποκράτης οὕτως ἐγίγνωσκεν Ἀριστοτέλους ἔτι πρότερος ὤν).

[96] *Nat.Fac.* II.88–9 (τῆς Ἱπποκράτους ... φυσιολογίας ὑπομνήματα; Ἱπποκράτους ... πρώτου, δευτέρου δ'Ἀριστοτέλους εἰπόντος); cf. *Nat.Fac.* II.90, 92, 125, *PHP* V.684–5 (VIII.5.24 De Lacy), *MM* X.15, 118, *Adv.Jul.* XVIIIa.264. He indicates that Aristotle went farther than Hippocrates at *Hipp.Elem.* I.489, *Nat.Fac.* II.90, *MM* X.15, 118. van der Eijk (2009), 272 suggests that this stance is a bit fluid in the Galenic corpus, with some texts being more willing to grant Aristotle primacy than others.

[97] van der Eijk (2009) explores this aspect of the relationship in detail.

[98] *Hipp.Epid.II* 4.2 (*CMG Suppl.Or.* V.2, p. 683, trans. Vagelpohl and Swain).

and the failure of all three to detect the fallopian tubes is really not blamable since they are so small that "anyone might miss them."[99] In *On the Usefulness of the Parts*, this very admiration is wielded as a source of dismay. In general, the text is full of praise of Aristotle, and his profound influence is often evident. Galen carefully articulates in the opening of the first book that, though he sometimes disagrees with his predecessors, he is not setting out to directly critique or replace them: They may have gotten a few things wrong, but in general they were a worthy group. He particularly singles out Aristotle as having written "much and well" on the subject of physiology and "being very skillful at describing both other things and the art of nature."[100] When it comes to the specific matter of anatomy, however, though he affords Aristotle the praise that he "is not careless of the things apparent from dissection or untrained in their usefulness," he does so only to underscore how appalling it is, therefore, that he erred so greatly in his discussion of the brain.[101] In *On the Doctrines of Hippocrates and Plato*, he takes a similar tack, but is even more aggressive. Aristotle, he points out, is "not a man to lie, nor altogether inexperienced in anatomy"; he must, therefore, be held accountable for what appears to be either blindness or deceit in his quest to support his cardiocentrism with the evidence of dissection.[102] Galen's proposed solution is that Aristotle observed the valves in the heart and that his preconceived desire to see the heart as origin of the nerves, combined with a loss of "patience to engage with the anatomy of the parts," led him to believe that they were the root of the nervous system and to walk away from the project before he had finished it in a manner befitting his own abilities.[103] Finally, in *Anatomical Procedures*, where only serious anatomists are allowed, Galen is openly dismissive of Aristotle. He is simply wrong about the anatomy of the heart – among many other anatomical points! – but he deserves to be forgiven because he was not a real anatomist; if an anatomical devotee like Galen's near predecessor Marinus is still liable to get things wrong, then it would be unfair to even criticize someone like Aristotle, who was "unpracticed in dissections."[104] This is a mighty comedown for the

---

[99] *Ut.Diss.* II.900–1 (κάλλιστα ἀνατεμόντων … ὥστε ἄν τινα λαθεῖν).

[100] *UP* III.21 (I.15H) (πολλῶν καὶ καλῶς εἰρημένων), 16–17 (I.11–12H) (δεινότατος ὢν τά τ' ἄλλα καὶ τέχνην φύσεως ἐξηγήσασθαι).

[101] *UP* III.620 (I.449H) (τῶν ἐξ ἀνατομῆς φαινομένων οὐκ ἀμελῶς ἔχων καὶ τῆς χρείας αὐτῶν οὐκ ἀμελέτητος ὤν), 623 (I.451H).

[102] *PHP* V.206 (I.10.2 De Lacy) (οὔτε γὰρ φιλοψευδὴς ὁ ἀνὴρ οὔτε παντάπασιν ἄπειρος τῆς ἀνατομῆς).

[103] *PHP* V.207–8 (I.10.7–9 De Lacy) (οὐκέθ' ὑπομεῖναι περὶ τὴν κατὰ μέρος ἀνατομὴν ἀσχοληθῆναι).

[104] *AA* II.621 (ἀγύμναστος ὢν ἐν ταῖς ἀνατομαῖς); cf. S216. Aristotle is not completely excluded from *AA*, however; Galen cites his discussion of waste products (*peritomma*) in a section clearly indebted to the zoological works (II.542).

erstwhile "best of anatomists": When the mature Galen has an anatomical point to prove he does not mince words.

In more purely zoological anatomy, however, where Galen does not feel so much of a need to defend his own theories, he is reliably deferential to Aristotle. He compliments him repeatedly for his overarching comparative work, saying that his views on teleology and on the classes of animals are "well-said" and "correct," as is his explanation of the differences between animals.[105] He is also quite happy to trust him on the anatomical details. He says that Aristotle's treatment of the stomachs in nonhuman animals is so well done that he himself does not need to broach the topic.[106] The general sense one gets is that Galen was simply not (yet?) interested in tackling zoological anatomy for its own sake.[107] The bulk of the Aristotelian biological corpus thus, though clearly familiar to him and valued by him, remains something largely apart from the anatomical works that he considers himself to be directly engaging with.

Despite these caveats and reservations, Aristotle is still an anatomical name to be reckoned with in Galen and in the Roman period more broadly. As with the example of the heart, Galen feels required to address Aristotle's opinions whenever they are relevant to the human anatomy that he is discussing. He is quite fed up, for example, that Aristotle had so much to say about testicles. He feels that the Aristotelian position – that they perform a similar steadying function to the weights on looms – is perversely uninformed by their interior anatomical complexity, and he laments that Aristotle tried to broach the tricky question of the physiology of their castration. But, since he did, he feels compelled to deal with what he said, and he does so by bringing to bear a litany of anatomical facts and counterfactuals.[108] In a less antagonistic vein, he also often takes the time to mention Aristotelian anatomical nomenclature when it differs from that of others.[109]

---

[105] Teleology: *UP* III.81 (I.59H) (καλῶς); classes of animals: *UP* III.848 (II.117H) (ὀρθῶς); difference of animals: *UP* III.177, IV.160 (I.130, II.298H), *PHP* V.464 (V.5.24 De Lacy).

[106] *UP* III.328 (I.241H); cf. *Sem.* IV.638–40, where Aristotle has "sufficiently" (ἱκανῶς) proven that some animals are by nature incomplete; other deferential citations of Aristotle's work on animals appear at *Nat.Fac.* II.173; *Inst.Od.* II.879; *UP* III.607, 896 (I.441, II.151H); *Hipp.Epid.II* 2.13 (*CMG Suppl.Or.* V.2, p. 339); *Caus.Symp.* VII.227.

[107] He does say, at *UP* IV.145 (II.286H), that someday he might "add to" (προστιθέντων) what Aristotle said about animals; cf. *UP* III.328 (I.241H), *AA* S193.

[108] *Sem.* IV.576–89, with the wish that Aristotle had not broached the topic at all at IV.582.

[109] Aristotle calling the great artery the aorta at *Ven.Art.Diss.* II.780, *Sem.* IV.541; his word for the diaphragm at *Loc.Aff.* VIII.328; his inconsistent terminology for the esophagus at *Loc.Aff.* VIII.333; his coining of the term homoeomerous at *QAM* IV.773–4, *PHP* V.673 (VIII.4.9 De Lacy), *San.Tu.* VI.384, 420, *MM* X.530, *HNH* XV.7, *CC* 1.1 (*CMG Suppl.Or.* II, p. 52).

It is in this same context of nomenclature that Aristotle makes his appearances in Rufus, who cites him three times. Once – in a discussion of the general nomenclature of the veins and arteries, which he frames with the observation that "in the oldest times" both types of vessel were just called veins – Rufus mentions Aristotle's particular name for the aorta, followed by the Praxagorean alternative.[110] Elsewhere, in his discussion of the uvula, he gently points out that Aristotle's term for it should properly only be applied to its diseased state, not to the organ itself.[111] Finally, he cites him on the ear, updating the Aristotelian assertion that, of the exterior parts of the ear, only the lobe has a designated name with the current, more detailed nomenclature of "the doctors."[112] For Rufus, then, Aristotle is still worth mentioning, but is somewhat hopelessly out of date. In the same vein, the author of *Doctor: Introduction* singles out Aristotle as having been the first to think of methodically writing down names for all the external parts of the human body.[113] However, doctors soon followed suit, and this is the last that we hear of him; Aristotle comes across as a founding rather than a currently influential figure for anatomy.[114]

Few of the Peripatetics working in the centuries after Aristotle appear to have merited notice in the Roman period for their anatomical views, in keeping with their general lack of enthusiasm for the topic. Clearchus, who worked in the generation following Aristotle, produced a text referred to as *On Skeletons*.[115] Three of the six citations attributed to this title discuss the various names for a single set of muscles; another engages in a bit of comparative anatomy, stating that man, bats, and elephants are the only creatures whose breasts are located at the sternum.[116] Though this suggests that the text went beyond a mere catalogue of bones, the only Roman

---

[110] Rufus, *Nom.Part.* 208–9 (τὸ ἀρχαιότατον).

[111] Rufus, *Nom.Part.* 61.

[112] Rufus, *Nom.Part.* 43–4 (οἱ δὲ ἰατροί).

[113] Ps.-Galen, *Int.* XIV.699.

[114] Aristotle's name does not come up in anatomical contexts in other Roman authors. Soranus mentions him only for his assertion, linked with that of Zenon the Epicurean, that the female is imperfect where the male is perfect (III.3). The Anonymous London Papyrus refers to his physiological theory of sleep-causation (XXIII.42, XXIV.6), but otherwise mentions him only as the author of the doxographic *Iatrika*.

[115] The title (Περὶ σκελετῶν) is preserved at Athenaeus, IX.399b (Wehrli v. 3, fr. 106a), where we also learn that the work was in at least two books; for discussion of the title, see Chapter 2, n. 156.

[116] For the muscles, see Athenaeus, IX.399b, Rufus, *Nom.Part.* 192, Pollux, II.146 (Wehrli v. 3, fr. 106a–107). For the comparative anatomy, see Pollux, II.164 (Wehrli, v. 3, fr. 110). This statement is slightly in tension with the similar remark in Aristotle (*HA* 497b34) that only man has breasts at the front of his chest, the elephant having them near but not on it. This variation is in keeping with the suggestion by Wehrli (1944–59), v. 3, 83 that Clearchus' anatomical work was influenced by non-Peripatetic, perhaps Hippocratic, sources.

medical author to cite it is Rufus, who disparages it in passing.[117] Eudemus of Rhodes, a contemporary of Clearchus, is mentioned by Apuleius as an important Peripatetic author of zoological treatises.[118] Galen, however, was familiar with his work in general – he wrote a commentary in three books on his treatise *On Style* – but does not see fit to mention his zoological interests; indeed, the citations of Eudemus in Aelian suggest that his interests lay in behavior rather than anatomy.[119] Finally, the Anonymous London Papyrus draws heavily on the Peripatetic *Iatrika*, which the author attributes to Aristotle himself, but which others, including Galen, attributed to his student Meno.[120] However, neither the author of the papyrus nor Galen consider that text, which was a doxography of fifth- and fourth-century doctors, as a source of anatomical insights.

Praxagoras

Praxagoras (fl. *c.* 300 BC)[121] is among the first doctors after Hippocrates to have a sect of followers that persisted into the Roman period.[122] Though the remaining fragments of his writings are few, and he has historically been overshadowed by the Alexandrians in allotment of scholarly interest, he was an important authority figure in ancient medicine.[123] Indeed, a medieval scholium to a line in the *Iliad* directly quotes Praxagoras on the internal anatomy of the throat, suggesting that at some point, likely during the scholarly heyday in the Hellenistic period, he had entered a lexicon or commentary as the preeminent authority on anatomy.[124] His writings were

[117] Rufus, *Nom.Part.* 192 (Wehrli v. 3, fr. 106b), where he accuses it of having incorrectly described the names of the muscles along the spine. The received text of Rufus lists the name here as Cleitarchus (Κλείταρχος) rather than Clearchus; however, citations of the exact same passage at Athenaeus, IX.399b (Wehrli v. 3, fr. 106a), and Pollux, II.185 (Wehrli v. 3, fr. 107) both attribute it to Clearchus; cf. Kowalski (1960), 87, 142, n. 38, and Sideras (1994), 1131.

[118] Apuleius, *Apol.* 36.

[119] Galen, *Lib.Prop.* XIX.42, 47; cf. *Indol.* 15 (Boudon-Milot et al. [2010]), where Galen mentions owning works by Eudemus, and *Adv.Jul.* XVIIIa.269, where he appears in a list of Peripatetic authorities for the four elements. Aelian, *NA* III.20, 21, IV.8, 45, 53, 56, V.7; see Chapter 2, n. 158.

[120] See Chapter 2, "The Later Hellenistic Period" at pp. 45–6. Plutarch also references this text, citing it for an unusual symptom of liver disease (*Quaest.conv.* 733c).

[121] On the question of his date, see Lewis (2017), 1–3.

[122] See Galen, *PHP* V.192 (I.7.17 De Lacy) (Steckerl 11; Lewis 3.68) and *UP* III.671 (I.487H) (Steckerl 15); see also the discussion in Lewis (2017), 29, 110–11.

[123] The complete fragments are collected, with an idiosyncratic interpretation, in Steckerl (1958) and a thematic subset in Lewis (2017); for the history of scholarship, see Lewis (2017), 6–8.

[124] Scholium to *Iliad* XXII.325 in the Venetus B manuscript (Marciana 453=821) (Steckerl 10). Erbse (1969), vol. 1, xvii–iii dates the manuscript to the eleventh century, but this particular scholium is in the hand of the latest scribe, dated to later than the thirteenth century and sourcing his information from the *Etymologicum Magnum*, the *Suda*, the *Epimerismi Homerici*, and similar texts.

still current in the Roman period; Galen seems to have had direct access to them, likely including the work known as *Anatomy*.[125]

Galen's evaluation of Praxagoras' reliability as a dissector is mixed. We saw earlier his scathing analysis of his anatomical abilities in conjunction with those of Diocles, but elsewhere he is more positive. For example, at one point he joins him with Aristotle as having proven through their treatises that they had "observed many other things accurately in dissections"; he includes this praise, however, only to come down particularly harshly on the unfortunate pair for having had the audacity to claim that the heart was the center of the nervous system, asserting that they need to either have been blind or addressing blind people in order to say such a thing.[126] Indeed, as for Aristotle, much of Galen's negativity on his value as a source no doubt stems from Galen's own disagreement with the basic tenets of Praxagorean physiological doctrine, especially as related to the cardiovascular system. Rufus is more impartial and cites Praxagoras' terminology for the "thick" artery (aorta) and "hollow" vein (portal vein), underscoring that the cardiovascular system was the anatomical area in which his writings continued to hold clout.[127]

In addition to Praxagoras' most famously attributed student, Herophilus, we know of two others who retained reputations for dissection in the Roman period: Pleistonikus and Phylotimus. Though he features in Galen's list of ancient anatomists, Pleistonikus' few appearances outside general lists relate mostly to digestion.[128] Phylotimus has a more robust presence generally, but also seems to have loomed larger in the field of dietetics than elsewhere.[129] The other minor figures in dissection whom Galen mentions from around this period, namely Chrysippus, the teacher of Erasistratus, and two of his other students, Aristogenes and Medius, are similarly uncited in this area.[130] Although all three appear in the list of "the less and the more accurate anatomizers" that Galen

---

[125] Galen cites him directly at *Ut.Diss.* II.906: "For Praxagoras basically says so in these very words" (ὁ γάρ τοι Πραξαγόρας ὧδέ πώς φησι αὐταῖς λέξεσι). See also the discussion at Lewis (2017), 28.

[126] Galen, *PHP* V.187–8 (I.6.14 De Lacy) (ἄλλα πολλὰ τῶν κατὰ τὰς ἀνατομὰς ἀκριβῶς ἑωράκασιν).

[127] Rufus, *Nom.Part.* 199, 209.

[128] For fragments of Pleistonikus, see Steckerl (1958), 124–6.

[129] The variant spelling Philotimus also occurs. Like his teacher, he also appears in the Homeric scholia, once for placing the controlling power of the body in the heart, which was a central Praxagorean doctrine (*Scholia in Homerum* 10.10a), and once in a series of different authorities' terms for the waist (*Scholia in Homerum* 11.424d). See Steckerl (1958), 2–4, 108–23 for brief comments and fragments.

[130] On distinguishing this Chrysippus from the several other doctors who shared his name, see Berrey (2014), which includes a provisional list of testimonia. For Aristogenes and Medius' relationship to him, see Galen, *Ven.Sect.Er.Rom.* XI.197.

marshals in order to condemn the system of veins as described in the Hippocratic *Nature of Man*, they do not come up again in any anatomical context.[131]

Herophilus

As explored in Chapter 2, Herophilus (*c.* 330–260)[132] was a major figure in the practice of dissection and in the development of ancient anatomy, as well as other areas of medicine. von Staden has identified six, or possibly eight, titles that are securely attributed to him, which include an *Anatomy* or *Anatomical Things* in at least four books.[133] This unremarkable title – the same as given to the comparable works of Diocles and Praxagoras – could perhaps indicate a handbook along the Dioclean model.[134] Certainly, the vast majority of the references to the text from the Roman period revolve around simple questions of nomenclature. On the other hand, these references to Herophilean nomenclature sometimes also include more descriptive comments or even references to physiological theory, suggesting that, compared with the simple litany of structures present in the surviving exemplars of anatomical handbooks, Herophilus' had a more verbose and detailed style, less concerned with establishing a codified nomenclature than its later role would suggest. In his discussion of the styloid process in the skull, for example, which continues to bear the name derived from his likening it to a writing implement, he apparently also offered a comparison to the famous Alexandrian lighthouse, the Pharos, which led to the alternate, equally Herophilean term, pharoid.[135] Similarly, his description of the parts of the eye appears to have been rife with similes – Celsus attributes the term "cobweb-like" for the retina to Herophilus, but Rufus, while acknowledging that that is the standard ancient term, adds that "since Herophilus compares it to a drawn-up casting-net, some also call it 'net-like'"; elsewhere, we learn that he compared the iris to the skin of a

---

[131] *HNH* XV.136 (οὔτε τῶν ἧττον οὔτε τῶν μᾶλλον ἀκριβῶς ἀνατεμνόντων). Indeed, Galen is concerned that Chrysippus' books generally are in danger of being completely lost (*Ven.Sect.Er.Rom.* XI.221).

[132] For the vexed question of Herophilus' dates, see von Staden (1989), 43–50.

[133] von Staden (1989), 72–8; Galen refers to the anatomical work as *Anatomy* (ἀνατομή) at *Sem.* IV.596 (von Staden T18; cf. T19) and *Anatomical Things* (ἀνατομικά) at *AA* II.571 (von Staden T17).

[134] von Staden (1989), 67 agrees that "the good physician … wrote his own handbooks for use by his students and followers. It is in this pedagogic context, too, and not only in the more obvious context of making public one's scientific views, that Herophilus' writings belong."

[135] Galen cites him as calling it styloid at *AA* S252 (von Staden T90) and pharoid at *AA* S70 (von Staden T92); cf. *AA* S84 (von Staden T91), where it is rendered "columnar" in the Arabic.

grape, smooth on one side, rough on the other.[136] In a different direction, several sources discuss not just his naming of the cerebrum and cerebellum, but his conviction that the seat of the control center for the body was located there, indicating that he may have included some physiological theory in his anatomical descriptions.[137] The three surviving fragments of the text confirm this general picture of a detail-oriented and thorough text that still fits within the general framework of an anatomical handbook, though any extrapolation from such a tiny sample is necessarily tenuous.[138]

Though Herophilus' *Anatomy* survives today only in these scattered glimpses, it appears to have been circulating up to and during the second century AD. Both Galen and Soranus frequently cite Herophilus, and Galen indicates that he had access to his writings and expected his contemporaries to as well.[139] Indeed, Herophilus' fame was tightly bound up with his reputation as dissector and expert on the body: A sizeable majority of all surviving references to him relate to either anatomy or physiology. Though Galen occasionally expresses criticism of his work in other areas, his valuation of Herophilus' worth as an anatomist is almost uniformly positive, a rarity in the contentious Galenic corpus.[140] He is, for Galen, "a man who is known by everyone to have surpassed the great majority of the ancients, not only in breadth of knowledge but in intellect, and to have advanced the art of medicine in many ways"; in his anatomical writing, he writes

---

[136] Celsus, *DM* 7 (von Staden T88) (archnoidem); Rufus, *Nom.Part.* 153 (von Staden T89) (ἐπειδὴ δὲ Ἡρόφιλος εἰκάζει αὐτὸν ἀμφιβλήστρῳ ἀνασπωμένῳ, ἔνιοι καὶ ἀμφιβληστροειδῆ καλοῦσιν); ps.-Rufus, *Diss.Hum.* 12–13 (von Staden T87, where he speculates that the iris is meant) (on the authorship of this text, Chapter 7, "Rufus of Ephesus" at p. 229). It is, of course, possible that these descriptions occurred in the treatise *On Eyes* and are thus not indicative of the style of the *Anatomy*.

[137] Galen, *UP* III.665–7 (I.482–4H) (von Staden T77–8) discusses Herophilus' naming of the structures as well as his conviction that the cerebellum exercises more control than any other part of the brain. Tertullian, *An.* 15.5 (von Staden T139) and Ps.-Plutarch, *Plac.* IV.5 (von Staden T137b; cf. T137e) also ascribe to him the view that the command center is located in the base of the brain.

[138] For these three fragments, see Chapter 2, "Herophilus and Erasistratus" at pp. 38–9.

[139] Galen, *Dig.Puls.* VIII.869: "Herophilus wrote clearly, at least for those who do not casually engage with his books" (σαφῶς Ἡροφίλου τοῖς τε μὴ παρέργως ἐντυγχάνουσιν αὐτοῦ τοῖς βιβλίοις ... γεγραφότος); he also on three occasions gives book numbers of the text, indicating both direct citation and a supposition that this would be useful information for others (*AA* II.571, *Sem.* IV.596–8 [von Staden T60a–61]; cf. *Hipp.Epid.II* 4.1 [von Staden T62] which also contains a reference to a book number according to the reading of Pfaff [*CMG* V.10.1, p. 318], but not according to that of Vagelpohl and Swain [*CMG Suppl.Or.* V.2, p. 645]). For further evidence that the works were still circulating in Roman times, see von Staden (1989), 70 and (1999a), 111.

[140] For examples of nonanatomical criticism, see *Trem.Palp.* VII.605–6 (von Staden T141), *Diff.Puls.* VIII.723–4 (von Staden T150), *Dig.Puls.* VIII.911–13 (von Staden T173), *Hipp.Prog.* XVIIIb.20 (von Staden T33), *Sem.* IV.582 (von Staden T189), where "even he" (καὶ αὐτός) was wrong about the role of the testicles in the generation of semen, and *Sem.* IV.596–8 (von Staden T61), where his mistaken theories provoke "astonishment" (θαυμάζειν) in contrast to his accurate dissection.

"correctly," "truly," "carefully," "accurately," "most accurately," and "with the highest degree of accuracy."[141] In a few places, Galen expresses a need to add to what Herophilus has written, but in only two instances does he criticize his work as an anatomist, once with a heavy sugar coating, once surprisingly bluntly.[142]

Herophilus' reputation as a dissector was current in the Roman period even outside scientific circles, though to less flattering effect. The Christian author Tertullian (*c.* AD 160–*c.* 240) singles him out for rebuke, calling him "that notorious Herophilus, the doctor or butcher, who cut up six hundred men."[143] Yet, despite his obvious feelings about the propriety of Herophilus' methods and the doubt he immediately after expresses – channeling his Methodist source, Soranus – about the reliability and thus the utility of dissection in general, Tertullian does cite him as the person who is in the best possible position to speak to the internal organs, indicating an enduringly high degree of authority.[144]

Anatomists of the Roman period seem to have both trusted Herophilus and actively relied on his tradition. Yet, though he is frequently cited as the discoverer or namer of a structure, his nomenclature was not so sacrosanct as to be universally followed. There are repeated instances where the term he uses is only one of those circulating, and it is sometimes explicitly different from the one a Roman author prefers or considers standard.[145] Galen gives some insight

---

[141] *Med.Exp.* 13.6 (Walzer [1944]) (von Staden T147); *AA* II.571 (von Staden T60) (ὀρθῶς; ἀληθῶς), *Loc. Aff.* VIII.212 (von Staden T80) (ἐπιμελῶς), *Sem.* IV.596–8 (von Staden T61) (ἀκριβῶς), *AA* II.570 (von Staden T60) (ἀκριβέστατα), and *Ut.Diss.* II.895 (von Staden T114) (ἐπὶ τὸ ἀκριβέστατον). In addition to these words of individual praise, Galen also frequently lists him in elite anatomical company, as at *PHP* V.650 (von Staden T68), *UP* III.21, 468 (I.15, 341H) (von Staden T136, 70), *Hipp.Epid.II* 4.1 (*CMG Suppl.Or.* V.2, p. 622) (von Staden T126), and *Us.Puls.* V.163–4 (von Staden T154).

[142] He proposes to expand on Herophilus' description of animal livers at *AA* II.571 (von Staden T60), to supplement his description of the nerves, which lacked an account of the beginnings of each one, at *Loc.Aff.* VIII.212 (von Staden T80), and to complete his (and others') list of the arteries with no veins beside them at *AA* S221–2 (von Staden 128). He criticizes Herophilus, along with Aristotle and Euryphon, for not noticing a structure in the anatomy of the uterus, though he avers that they usually dissect "most beautifully" (κάλλιστα ἀνατεμόντων) and with "accuracy" (ἀκρίβειαν), at *Ut. Diss.* II.900–1 (von Staden T107); however, he says quite abruptly that he described the valves of the heart "carelessly" (ἀμελῶς), in contrast to Erasistratus who did so "accurately" (ἀκριβῶς), at *PHP* V.206 (I.10.4 De Lacy) (von Staden T119).

[143] Tertullian, *An.* 10.4 (von Staden T66) (Herophilus ille medicus aut lanius, qui sexcentos exsecuit).

[144] For Soranus as Tertullian's source, see von Staden (1989), 236 and the bibliography there.

[145] For example, Rufus, *Nom.Part.* 155 (von Staden T93), where Herophilus' term for the hyoid bone is contrasted to the clearly victorious "Y-shaped" (ὑοειδὲς) attributed to "some people"; Galen, *AA* S173 (von Staden T99), where Galen indicates that Herophilus' famous christening of the duodenum as "twelve fingers long" is cast as an alternative, used by "some," to that used by "the anatomists," and *AA* II.719–20 (von Staden T124), where "those around Herophilus" (οἱ περὶ τὸν Ἡρόφιλον) have a different name for the "so-called choroid plexuses" (τὰ καλούμενα χοροειδῆ

into the flavor of Herophilean anatomy in the second century AD by saying that he follows Herophilus in lieu of the other options because he prefers the "old custom in the application of names."[146] Thus, Herophilus remained a reliable source in the areas that he had uncovered, but he was perhaps a bit musty.

Erasistratus

Though he was a productive author and a skilled dissector, Erasistratus (c. 330-255/50 BC)[147] did not write a text dedicated to anatomy.[148] Instead, he appears to have been content to fold his anatomical findings into his writing on other subjects. For example, Galen cites one of his most groundbreaking anatomical discoveries – a detailed description of the valves in the heart – as appearing in his work *On Fevers*.[149] He may have included a section on anatomy and physiology in his *General Writings*, but the lack of a truly dedicated anatomical text was striking enough that Galen, as he did for Hippocrates, felt justified in putting together an *Anatomy of Erasistratus* in three volumes.[150] Thus, surprisingly enough given his stature as a dissector, Erasistratus belongs back in Galen's first category of anatomical texts as an author of books that incorporate anatomy as an element rather than as a main focus. Because of this scattershot approach and the loss of his corpus, the only way to access Erasistratus' literary anatomical record is through his reception in Roman authors.

Unlike the school of Herophileans, which finally petered out in the middle of the first century AD, the Erasistrateans continued to be a vocal sect throughout the second century, ensuring that Erasistratus' writings were still circulating and influential in Rome.[151] Galen cites multiple titles on dozens of

---

πλέγματα). Similarly, Galen mentions him in regard to his numeration of the cranial nerves, but he appears there only to prove that, though different in appearance, his version is not fundamentally incompatible with Marinus' version, which Galen, at least, has adopted as superseding it; see *AA* S11–12 (von Staden T82)˙ and *Hipp.Epid.II* 4.2 (*CMG Suppl.Or.* V.2, p. 686) (von Staden T83).

[146] Galen, *AA* S164 (von Staden T101).

[147] On the question of his dates, see Chapter 2, n. 117.

[148] Garofalo (1988), 22 lists the known titles of Erasistratus' work as *General Writings* (Καθόλου λόγοι), *Health* (Ὑγιεινά), *On Fevers* (Περὶ πυρετῶν), *On the Bringing up of Blood* (Περὶ αἵματος ἀναγωγῆς), *On Paralysis* (Περὶ παραλύσεως), *On Hydropsy* (*De hydrope*), *On the Stomach* (Περὶ κοιλίας), *On Gout* (Περὶ ποδάγρος), *On Medicines and Poisons* (Περὶ δυνάμεων καὶ θανασίμων), *On Divisions* (or *On Sects*) (Περὶ διαιρέσεων), and *Cookery* (Ὀψαρτυτικόν). For a brief overview of the anatomical contents of the various works, see Garofalo (1988), 23.

[149] *PHP* V.548 (VI.6.4 De Lacy).

[150] Garofalo (1988), 23 speculates such a section; on Galen's *Anatomy of Erasistratus*, see later on in this section.

[151] On the Erasistrateans, see Garofalo (1988), 4–5. The idea, based on the passage at *Ven.Sect. Er.Rom.* XI.221, that the works of Erasistratus no longer survived in the time of Galen is clearly a

occasions, including some fairly lengthy direct quotations; Celsus and Aulus Gellius both also claim a direct familiarity with his writings.[152] The vitality of the Erasistratean sect also had significant ramifications for the reception of Erasistratus' ideas in the Roman period. Galen's pointed distaste for the contemporary sect often embitters his discussions of their ancient forebear. Particularly in contexts where he is arguing against one of the fundamental Erasistratean doctrines – for example, that the arteries are vessels for pneuma, devoid of blood, or that there are no natural faculties, like specific attraction, at work in the body – he can become scathingly and aggressively critical of Erasistratus. He calls him "careless," "contentious," "malicious," "not just ignorant, but lacking in intelligence," "silly and absurd," and "at the furthest limits of unintelligence," and accuses him of saying things that are "utterly false," "incredible," full of "the paltriest sort of reasoning" and "deceit and sophistry"; at various points he even rises to the pitch of comparing him to a thieving slave and of claiming that not only is he a bad physician, whose theories were developed without reference to any actual patients, he is also a terrible writer.[153]

While all this criticism would seem to indicate that Galen had the lowest possible opinion of Erasistratus' merits, this is far from the case. When not roused by his animosity for the modern Erasistrateans or by the particular Erasistratean theories that he views as misguided, he generally treats Erasistratus as a worthy and important member of his revered group of ancient authorities. He appears in his catalogues of eminent voices – particularly when Galen is setting out to prove a point to one of his many non-Erasistratean rivals.[154] Galen even pairs him with Hippocrates as "the most renowned of doctors."[155] Indeed, in his list of scholarly requirements to be expected of the best doctor, he distinguishes Erasistratus as the next most important author to study after Hippocrates, followed by all the rest of the ancients in a generic group.[156]

misinterpretation; for rebuttals of this assertion, which seems to stem from a statement in the index to Kühn (1821–33), XX.228, see Harris (1973), 195, Longrigg (1981), 177, and Garofalo (1988), 4, n. 9.

[152] Celsus, *DM* III.4.9 (idque apud Erasistratum quoque invenio); Gellius, *NA* XVI.3.5 (cum librum forte Erasistrati legeremus διαιρέσεων primum); for an analysis of Soranus' (and perhaps Caelius Aurelianus') likely access to his texts, see von Staden (1999*a*), 90–6.

[153] *Nat.Fac.* II.109 (ῥᾳθυμίας); *At.Bil.* V.132 (φιλονεικῶν); *HVA* XV.744 (κακοηθείας); *Nat.Fac.* II.115 (πρὸς τῷ μηδὲν τούτων γιγνώσκειν οὐδὲ ... σωφρονεῖ); *Nat.Fac.* II.166 (εὐηθέστερός ... καὶ γελοιότερος); *Ven.Sect.Er.* XI.159 (ἐσχάτως ἀνόητος); *Art.Sang.* IV.734 (ψευδῆ παντελῶς); *Loc. Aff.* VIII.311 (ἀπίθανα); *MM* X.377 (λογισμῷ φαυλοτάτῳ) (cf. *Nat.Fac.* II.92–3); *Nat.Fac.* II.141 (πανουργεῖν τι καὶ σοφίζεσθαι). The comparison to a slave is at *Nat.Fac.* II.66 and the suggestion that he is oblivious to the realities of patients and a bad writer at *Ven.Sect.Er.* XI.159.

[154] *Nat.Fac.* II.30, *Thras.* V.879, *MM* X.28, *Adv.Jul.* XVIIIa.270, *Cons.* 1 (*CMG Suppl.* III, p. 2).

[155] *Cons.* 1 (*CMG Suppl.* III, p. 14) (οἱ ἐνδοξότατοι τῶν ἰατρῶν, Ἐρασίστρατος καὶ Ἱπποκράτης).

[156] *Opt.Med.Cogn.* 5.2 (*CMG Suppl.Or.* IV, p. 69); cf. *Hipp.Epid.III* XVIIa.506 where he discusses proper methodology for exegetical work on the texts of Erasistratus.

Galen happily cites Erasistratus as an authority in areas where they do not disagree.[157] He will use him as an ally when it suits him, and feels quite at home characterizing his writing as "correct," "useful," "perfectly true," "clear and succinct," and "praise-worthy" when he feels it is warranted.[158] But even with this sometimes charitable outlook, the occasions when he praises Erasistratus are vastly outnumbered by those when he finds fault. Indeed, often his most comfortable stance vis-à-vis Erasistratus is one of qualified criticism. He opens *On Venesection Against Erasistratus* in characteristic style, querying why Erasistratus, being otherwise "competent in all the other aspects of the art ... and so careful with the smallest details," would fail to mention so popular a remedy as venesection.[159] He sometimes even speculates that his contentiousness got the better of his intelligence, arguing that he surely must have known his own position was wrong.[160] In fact, one of his favorite ploys is to pit Erasistratus against the modern Erasistrateans, not only suggesting that he has a privileged relationship with the ancient, but also that Erasistratus was more sensible than his misguided disciples make him out to be.[161]

This complicated relationship carries over to the field of anatomy, but with a striking reversal. Where in general Galen's praise of Erasistratus is far outweighed by his criticisms, on anatomical topics the balance is in equal disequilibrium but in the opposite direction: Erasistratus appears most often as a trusted anatomical authority. He joins Herophilus and Hippocrates as exemplars of famous names in

---

[157] *Thras.* V.880, 897, *San.Tu.* VI.77, *Loc.Aff.* VIII.34, *HVA* XV.698, *Hipp.Epid.VI* XVIIb.264, *Hipp. Off.Med.* XVIIIb.867 (cf. *CMG Suppl.Or.* I, p. 45), *Praen.* XIV.634, *Hipp.Epid.VI* XVIIb.198–9.

[158] Using Erasistratus as an ally at *Nat.Fac.* II.204, *Loc.Aff.* VIII.69; "correct" (ὀρθῶς, καλῶς) at *At.Bil.* V.139, *Alim.Fac.* VI.458, *HVA* XV.438, *Hipp.Epid.VI* XVIIb.10; "useful" (χρήσιμον) *At.Bil.* V.139; "perfectly true" (ἀληθέστατόν) at *Loc.Aff.* VIII.14; "clear and succinct" (διὰ ταχέων τε καὶ σαφῶς) at *HVA* XV.435; "praise–worthy" (ἐπαινεῖν ... χρή) at *HVA* XV.436; cf. *PHP* V.281 (II.8.38 De Lacy), where he offers Erasistratus as an example of the right way to support one's assertions with arguments. However, so convincingly vitriolic is Galen's abuse of Erasistratus in some passages that the Aldine edition of *Alim.Fac.* negates Galen's praise of him at VI.458 (changing ὀρθῶς for οὐκ ὀρθῶς) contrary to manuscript evidence (Grant [2000], 70 follows this reading); a fuller picture of the relationship shows this change to have been unwarranted, as acknowledged by the readings in Powell (2003), 31, and Wilkins (2013), 6.

[159] *Ven.Sect.Er.* XI.147 (τἆλλα τῆς τέχνης ἱκανὸς ὢν ... κἂν τοῖς σμικροτάτοις οὕτως ἐπιμελὴς...); Galen uses this seeming praise of Erasistratus' attention to detail as a frequent means of exploiting the gaps in his theories (e.g., *Loc.Aff.* VIII.317, *Ven.Sect.Er.* XI.170–1, *Ven.Sect.Er.Rom.* XI.203–4, 207, 214–16, 219).

[160] *Nat.Fac.* II.110–12, *At.Bil.* V.140.

[161] Particularly good examples of this tactic are to be found at *Nat.Fac.* II.68, 78, 101–2 and *Ven.Sect. Er.Rom.* XI.247–8.

the field, and his anatomy constituted at least a small direct component of Galen's education.[162] On repeated occasions, Galen endorses Erasistratus' anatomical authority, even directly allying himself with it. He views his anatomy of the heart as all but perfect; he aligns himself with the Erasistratean version, rather than the Herophilean one, saying outright that anyone who counts the orifices the of the heart the way Herophilus does "disagrees with Erasistratus and me."[163] In one text, he says that Erasistratus' description of the cardiac valves is so competent that for him to retread the subject would be superfluous, and he elsewhere points out that Erasistratean cardiac anatomy is so well accepted by the modern medical community that "anyone not familiar with [the valves] would seem to be truly ancient."[164] He is also a proponent of his work on the brain and the nerves, with some qualification; he explains that Erasistratus was initially incorrect about the precise origin of the nerves, but that "when he was an old man and had leisure to devote himself to the observations of the art, he made more accurate dissections and he, too, recognized that the pith-type substance of the nerves has sprung from the encephalon."[165] Even in contexts where he is generally out of charity with Erasistratus, his respect for his anatomical integrity endures, as when, in the midst of a text dedicated to discrediting the core Erasistratean tenet of naturally bloodless arteries, he grudgingly admits that "Erasistratus, with all his other follies, did not dare to tell lies about anatomy."[166]

---

[162] *UP* III.468 (I.341H), *PHP* V.650 (VIII.1.6 De Lacy), *HNH* XV.136. Garofalo (1988), 22 uses the last of these instances – where Erasistratus appears in a larger group, but Herophilus is singled out with Eudemus as the two most influential voices – to argue that Galen generally considered Erasistratus not to be "alla stessa altezza" as these two in dissection; his other pairings of Herophilus and Erasistratus, however, render his opinion of their relative merits less clear-cut (see particularly *AA* II.624 and *PHP* V.206 [I.10.4 De Lacy], where Erasistratus clearly comes out ahead). For the Erasistratean element of Galen's anatomical education, see *AA* II.660.

[163] *AA* II.624 (διαφωνεῖν Ἐρασιστράτῳ τε καὶ ἡμῖν). The main emendation that he would add is a largely hypothetical, physiologically necessitated one, namely the presence of minute interventricular pores to allow the passage of blood from the right ventricle to the left (he points out this flaw at *Nat.Fac.* II.77; his own argument for the pores in the septum is summed up at *Nat.Fac.* II.207–9); these structures are not visible in dissection, however, so the fault that Galen finds with Erasistratus here is fundamentally with his physiology, not his anatomy.

[164] *Us.Puls.* V.166 (cf. *PHP* V.206 [I.10.4 De Lacy]); *PHP* V.548–9 (VI.6.4–8 De Lacy) (ἀρχαῖος ὄντως εἶναι δόξειεν ἂν ὁ μὴ γινώσκων αὐτούς).

[165] *PHP* V.602 (VII.3.7 De Lacy) (ὅτε πρεσβύτης ὢν ἤδη καὶ σχολὴν ἄγων μόνοις τοῖς τῆς τέχνης θεωρήμασιν ἀκριβεστέρας ἐποιεῖτο τὰς ἀνατομάς, ἔγνω καὶ τὴν οἷον ἐντεριώνην τῶν νεύρων ἀπ' ἐγκεφάλου πεφυκυῖαν); cf. *PHP* V.646–7 (VII.8.12 De Lacy), *Hipp.Aph.* XVIIIa.86.

[166] *Art.Sang.* IV.735–6 (πρὸς <ταῖς ἄλλαις μωρίαις οὐκ ἐτόλμησεν Ἐρασίστρατος> τῶν φαινομένων ἐξ ἀνατομῆς καταψεύδεσθαι), following the restoration of the lacuna and the resulting translation suggested in Furley and Wilkie (1984), 182 in light of the Arabic version.

This praise becomes qualified, however, whenever questions of physiology intrude. Erasistratus' conception of the heart as a whole, while a paragon of anatomical work, is fundamentally at odds with Galen's views at the physiological level. Galen repeatedly puzzles at how the two of them could have such divergent understandings of the functional ramifications of the same anatomical phenomena.[167] Similarly, on the brain, though praising his basic observations as "correct," he argues that Erasistratus draws improper conclusions.[168] This skepticism bleeds over into his evaluation of his predecessor's accuracy in vivisectory experiments, which usually have more physiological than anatomical research goals. He repeats one of Erasistratus' experiments to determine the origins of the pulse, and reports that the outcome is the exact opposite of what Erasistratus wants it to be, adducing this discrepancy to a reproachable degree of "over-boldness" in hastily announcing things before having seen them; nevertheless, in the very next paragraph, he dismisses more recent attempts to demonstrate that arteries are devoid of blood, saying that, if there were any possible way to prove this through vivisection, Erasistratus would certainly have found it, being, as he was, a surpassingly clever and fine anatomist.[169]

Galen's respect for Erasistratus' anatomical skill, however, does not extend to the modern Erasistrateans. On the contrary, dissection and especially vivisection are tools that he frequently uses against them. This sometimes entails also using them against their founder, particularly in matters of physiology, such as the presence or absence of blood in the arteries.[170] Occasionally, though, he will instead take the position – at the same time sardonically impudent and rhetorically effective – of using Erasistratus' own anatomical work to support him against the Erasistrateans. He intimates, for example, that one group of Erasistrateans have deliberately ignored Erasistratus' accurate description of the heart valves and that they are incapable of understanding a difficult anatomical passage in his *General Principles*, though Galen, of course, could explain it if he wanted to.[171]

Though all of this yields a fairly robust picture, a concentrated portion of Galen's interaction with Erasistratus as an anatomical source would have been found in his lost *On the Anatomy of Erasistratus* in three books.

---

[167] *PHP* V.552 (VI.6.19 De Lacy), *Ut.Resp.* IV.477–8, *UP* III.492–4 (I.358H).
[168] *UP* III.673 (I.488H), *PHP* V.610 (VII.3.32 De Lacy); compare *Loc.Aff.* VIII.317, 323 and *Nat.Fac.* II.170 for similar rhetoric on other anatomical topics.
[169] *AA* II.648 (τοσαύτη τίς ... τόλμα); cf. *Art.Sang.* IV.715, 735–6.
[170] Galen uses dissection and vivisection against Erasistratean tenets repeatedly, as at *Nat.Fac.* II.175, *Art.Sang.* IV.715, 732, *PHP* V.184–5, 562 (I.6.1–3, VI.7.7 De Lacy).
[171] *Ut.Resp.* IV.476, *Nat.Fac.* II.93–5.

Galen explains the origin of this book, which he wrote as a sort of companion or counterpoint to *On the Anatomy of Hippocrates*, in his *On My Own Books*.[172] Both texts, it transpires, were written "with rather an eye towards ambition" in response to the cantankerous goading of a well-respected Erasistratean doctor many years his senior.[173] This doctor, Martianus, heard tell that Galen was passionate in praise of Hippocrates and declared in response that "Hippocrates was, for him, not a subject of study in any aspect of anatomy, while he regarded Erasistratus as marvelous, both in the other parts of the art and in that one."[174] Sensing an opportunity to make a name for himself, Galen responds to this implicit challenge by writing his books on the anatomy of each ancient. While he refers repeatedly to the contents of his *Anatomy of Hippocrates*, his only references to the companion work on Erasistratus relate to the fact of its composition.[175] The polemical circumstances of the work's origin suggest that it may not have been exactly a paean to Erasistratus' anatomical prowess, but it is also difficult to believe that he would have deviated too much from his general position on his predecessor's abilities.[176]

Outside of Galen, other evidence corroborates Erasistratus' continued importance in medical discourse in the Roman period, as well as the differing opinions prevalent as to the legitimacy of his views. The author of the Anonymous London Papyrus, for example, spends a good amount of time criticizing Erasistratean doctrine, while the author of its Parisian counterpart groups him with Hippocrates, Diocles, and Praxagoras as "the four" – the only ancients whose opinions he feels the need to record.[177] Despite this continued importance, his relevance on anatomical issues was shaped and diminished by his lack of dedicated anatomical writing: Though recognized as an important name in the field, he is only cited infrequently

---

[172] *Lib.Prop.* XIX.13–14; cf. *AA* II.216–17 and *Lib.Prop.* XIX.37–8.

[173] *Lib.Prop.* XIX.13 (φιλοτιμότερον).

[174] *Lib.Prop.* XIX.14 (1.9 Boudon-Millot [2007]) (<...> οὐδέν, θαυμάσιον δὲ τὸν Ἐρασίστρατον ἀποφαίνεται τὰ ἄλλα τῆς τέχνης καὶ ταῦτα); the text and my translation of the lacuna in the Greek follow Boudon-Millot's edition and restoration from the Arabic tradition.

[175] For his *Anatomy of Hippocrates*, see this chapter, "The Hippocratic Corpus" at pp. 176–7.

[176] Hunayn ibn Ishaq, who read this text and translated into Syriac, confirms this idea of a book balanced between praise and critique, telling us that "his purpose in it is to explain what Erasistratus said about anatomy in all his books, and then to show where he was correct and where he was wrong" (*Risala* 31) (Lamoreaux [2016], 46).

[177] Anonymous of London, XXI–XXXIII; Manetti (2011), ix dates the text to the first century AD. For Erasistratus and the other ancients in the Anonymous of Paris text, see van der Eijk (1999*b*); this text is difficult to date with precision, but it is generally assigned to the Roman period: perhaps after AD 40–60, per van der Eijk (1999*b*), 325–6, and "of the imperial age," per Garofalo and Fuchs (1997), vii. See also Plutarch, *De cur.* 518D, where Herophilus and Erasistratus are paired with Asclepius as quintessential doctors.

for anatomical data as such. Rufus, for instance, does not mention him at all in his *On the Names of the Parts of the Body*; he appears only once, in the discussion of the anatomy of the nerves, in *On the Anatomy of the Parts of Human Body*, which is attributed to Rufus, but more often considered pseudonymous.[178] Celsus describes the high esteem in which Erasistratus is held, together with Herophilus, for his superior anatomical knowledge, ascribed to the vivisection of condemned criminals, but his only direct references to his opinions are on questions of nosology and therapy.[179]

The bulk of Erasistratus' impact on the Roman anatomical world was, in keeping with his own literary output, on questions of anatomo-physiology. The author of the second-century *Doctor: Introduction*, who references his opinions on a variety of subjects, mentions him only once for his anatomy, and not favorably: He disagrees with Erasistratus' explanation for the composition of brain tissue, citing Hippocrates and Plato as witnesses. However, as so often in Galen – and as the inclusion of Plato here suggests – the author's problem with the Erasistratean position rests more on physiological than anatomical grounds.[180] Pliny, though overlaying some distinctly Erasistratean physiology on his description of anatomy, only actually cites him on therapeutic questions.[181] In a more general way, the author of the pseudo-Dioscoridian *Theriaca*, which dates perhaps to the first century AD, attributes Erasistratus' good understanding of nosology to his discoveries from dissection, placing the emphasis on postmortem analysis of diseased organs, rather than pure anatomical research.[182]

More playfully, Plutarch, in one of his *Table Talk* tableaux, offers two vastly different evaluations of Erasistratus' anatomical accuracy; while a doctor present at the meal contends that Erasistratus "rightly" contested Plato's claim of the transit of drink through the lungs by giving an accurate description of their texture, Plutarch staunchly defends Plato, asserting that, in fact, the tragedian Euripides "sees more sharply than Erasistratus"

---

[178] Ps.-Rufus, *Diss.Hum.* 72–3; for this text, see Chapter 7, "Rufus of Ephesus" at pp. 229–30.

[179] Celsus, *DM* proem.23 (cf. 47); see Chapter 2, "Herophilus and Erasistratus" at p. 37. To be fair, Celsus is generally reticent about offering specific sources in his anatomical sections; however, he does directly credit Herophilus with anatomical nomenclature at *DM* VII.7.13b. Overall, Celsus has quite a high opinion of Erasistratus, linking him with Hippocrates as an exemplar of the 'Rationalist' approach to medicine (*DM* proem.47); cf. von Staden (1994), 83–5.

[180] Ps.-Galen, *Int.* XIV.709. Similarly, Soranus' criticism of the triplokia should be characterized as theoretical rather than anatomical (*Gyn.* 3.4).

[181] On Pliny's use of Erasistratus, see this chapter, "Minor Hellenistic Authors" at pp. 213–14.

[182] Ps.-Dioscorides, *Ther.* 15.5; Sprengel (1829–30), vol. 25, xiv–xv discusses his reasons for considering this work spurious and suggests a tentative date in the first century AD. The same claim is repeated in Paul of Aegina, V.18.

and has a more accurate understanding of pulmonary anatomy![183] Aulus Gellius picks up on this passage in Plutarch and offers more details.[184] The Gellian version, which studiously avoids choosing sides, makes it clear that, despite any flourishes about Euripides, the question at stake is once again a physiological one: The alternative camp does not offer a different anatomy for the throat, simply a different understanding of its function. All of these instances are predicated on a general consensus that Erasistratus was a noteworthy, if controversial, authority on physiology, a subject to which his work on anatomy was largely ancillary.

Minor Hellenistic Authors

Galen attests to a gap in anatomical activity following the work of Herophilus and Erasistratus, and the evidence largely bears him out.[185] No sign of dissection between the mid-third century BC and the mid-first century AD survives, and activity surrounding anatomical texts is correspondingly thin. The text called *On the Heart* that became attached to the Hippocratic Corpus does contain detailed anatomical work, but its dating is difficult. As I explored in Chapter 2, it is almost certainly Hellenistic and probably within the same half-century as the productive period of the two famous Alexandrians.[186] It may still have been in current circulation in the Roman period, as the experiment it describes involving dissecting a pig whose throat has been dyed by drink seems to have captured the interest of Galen and perhaps also Plutarch; however, it is not at all clear whether it was already circulating under the name of Hippocrates at that point. Plutarch may provide evidence that it was, but his purported knowledge of the text rests on very shaky evidence. He does not directly cite the text at all, but merely includes Hippocrates as an example of a doctor who agrees with Plato's view on the transit of drink through the lungs.[187] While *On the Heart* does offer vivid support for this theory, it is not the only text potentially attributable to Hippocrates to do so. *On the Nature of Bones* contains two different passages that could easily be read this way and, unlike *On the Heart*, it is independently attested as an acknowledged part

---

[183] Plutarch, *Quaest. Conv.* 698B (ὀρθῶς), 699A (βλέπων τι ὀξύτερον).

[184] Gellius, *NA* 17.11.

[185] See Chapter 7, "Rufus of Ephesus" at pp. 226–8 and "Marinus" at p. 231.

[186] See Chapter 2, "Praxagoras and the Hippocratic *On the Heart*" at p. 35–6, especially n. 110 for the question of dating.

[187] Plutarch, *Quaest. Conv.* 699C, in the context discussed in the previous section.

of the Hippocratic Corpus in the Roman period.[188] Meanwhile, though Galen recounts the exact same porcine experiment found in *On the Heart*, using striking verbal parallels, he does not attribute it to anyone, nor does he mention this text elsewhere.[189] As Harris points out, Galen would have leapt at the chance to attribute the anatomically sophisticated description of the heart here to Hippocrates; the fact that he does not suggests either that he did have this text, but did not know it under that attribution, or that, as Duminil has it, the experiment was a commonplace, and he is citing it from somewhere else entirely.[190] Either way, this reference offers evidence for the continued influence of an independent strand of Hellenistic anatomy.[191]

After the period of Herophilus and Erasistratus, in which the Hippocratic *Heart*, too, was likely written, evidence for further Hellenistic anatomical literature becomes extremely hard to find. The Herophilean and Erasistratean schools seem to have precipitously lost interest not just in dissection but also in anatomical writing. From among the Herophileans, Eudemus has a very good reputation with Galen as a dissector, but left little footprint independent of Herophilus.[192] Galen usually mentions him in tandem with his more famous colleague, singling the pair out, for example, as examples of those particularly skilled in anatomy.[193] Nevertheless, he does seem to have left some of his own original work, since Galen and Soranus each cite his independent opinion once: Galen criticizes his rigid analogy of the bones of the thumb with those of the big toe, while Soranus contrasts his opinion of the umbilical vessels with that of Herophilus.[194] Among the Erasistrateans, the only sign of activity is the fact, reported by the author of *Doctor: Introduction*, that Erasistratus' immediate followers Apollonius of Memphis and Xenophon

---

[188] *Oss.* 1, 13. Duminil (2003), 140 (cf. p. 221, n. 6) decides to stretch the grammar at *Oss.* 1 in order to avoid the seeming relationship between drink and the lungs, but there does not seem good reason to do this, especially given the even clearer reference to the theory at 13, where the lungs are described as being troubled by any foreign object that enters them "either in the drink or in the passage of air" (ἢ ἐν τῷ ποτῷ ἢ ἐν τῇ τοῦ πνεύματός διόδῳ) (text as per Duminil [2003]), suggesting that both liquid and air are conceived of as normal entrants to the lungs. For knowledge of *On Bones* by Erotian and Galen, see Duminil (2003), 127–34.

[189] *PHP* V.719 (VIII.9.25 De Lacy); compare to the Hippocratic version at *Cord.* 2 (IX.80 Littré).

[190] Harris (1973), 95; Duminil (2003), 166.

[191] The striking cardiocentrism of the text (*Cord.* 10–11 [IX.88–90 Littré]) makes it more in keeping with an Aristotelian, Praxagorean, or even Stoic context than a Herophilean or Erasistratean one; however, the text is charmingly idiosyncratic and defies attribution to any one author or school, as discussed in Duminil (2003), 175–81.

[192] For disambiguation of the several figures in ancient medicine named Eudemus, see von Staden (1989), 62–3.

[193] Galen, *HNH* XV.134, 136; cf. *Sem.* IV.646, *Loc. Aff.* VIII.212, *Lib.Prop.* XIX.30, *PHP* V.650 (VIII.1.6 De Lacy).

[194] Galen, *UP* III.203 (cf. Rufus' mention of his opinion on the acromion at *Nom.Part.* 73); Soranus, *Gyn.* 1.57.

worked in the field of anatomical nomenclature, though neither is credited with actual substantive advances in anatomy.[195] While Xenophon, who may have been directly associated with Praxagoras as well as Erasistratus, does not come up elsewhere as an anatomical name, Apollonius appears to have written an *On Joints*, perhaps a Hippocratic commentary like that of the later and more famous Apollonius from Citium.[196]

Although the anatomical writings of Herophilus and Erasistratus do not appear to have inspired any significant amount of new anatomical research among later Hellenistic physicians, they did rapidly succeed in influencing the accepted knowledge in the field. As Galen reveals in his comments on the general consensus regarding the Erasistratean description of the cardiac valves, the discoveries of these two experts formed the foundation of subsequent anatomy.[197] The blossoming in the following centuries of surgery as a special medical subfield – one that Celsus indicates was especially associated with Alexandria – was a development of this enhanced understanding of the body.[198] More broadly, these new Hellenistic discoveries and theories can be found to constitute general knowledge about the body in the later Hellenistic and early Roman periods, even in not strictly medical or scientific texts. Callimachus (mid-third century BC), for example, seems to allude in his poetry to Herophilean developments both in the anatomy of the eye and in gynecology.[199] In prose, the twenty-third pseudepigraphic Hippocrates letter offers a poetically couched survey of the internal organs of the body. Although Craik has seen in it verbal echoes of the Hippocratic *Anatomy* and has posited a conscious Democritean influence as well, the substance of the anatomy and physiology is clearly from the early Hellenistic period.[200] Philo Judaeus of Alexandria (first century BC–first century AD) also appears to have been familiar with the discoveries and theories made in his own hometown, mentioning in his description of punishments meted out by God that some

---

[195] Ps.-Galen, *Int.* XIV.699 and notes in Petit (2009), *ad loc.*

[196] For Xenophon's affiliation with Praxagoras, see Oribasius, *Coll.Med.* XLIV.15 (extracted from Rufus) (cf. XLV.11 where he is cited for his work *On Cancers*); for Apollonius' text, see Erotian, *Gloss.* 52–3. For the limited engagement with anatomy in Apollonius of Citium's *InHipp.Artic.*, see Chapter 2, "The Later Hellenistic Period" at pp. 43–4.

[197] See this chapter, n. 164.

[198] Celsus, *DM* VII.proem.3. For discussion of the Hellenistic surgeons, with collected fragments, see Michler (1968), especially pp. 7–11 for the role of anatomy and pp. 136–7 for the dating of individual figures; cf. Mazzini (1999), 44–5, 359–65. For papyrological evidence from this period, see Marganne (1998), 1–34.

[199] See Oppermann (1925) and Most (1981). Similarly, Solmsen (1961), 195–6 suggests that Apollonius of Rhodes is alluding to Herophilus' discoveries at *Argon.* III.761–5.

[200] Craik (2006), 166–8; for Herophilean and Erasistratean elements, see Smith (1990), 33, where he points out that these are "used casually, not in a self-conscious display that it is modern," and Craik (2006), 167–8.

would affect "the blood in the veins and the air in the arteries," apparently envisioning an Erasistratean body as the subject of this divine retribution.[201] Anatomical writing impacted Hellenistic philosophers as well. The Stoics engaged peripherally with anatomy, through their doctrine, similar to that of the Peripatetics, that the heart was the seat of the soul and the ruling organ of the body. The sect's founder, Zeno of Citium (335–263 BC), who was a nearly exact contemporary of Herophilus, had propounded this view, arguing, according to Galen, that since reasoned discourse passes through the windpipe from the chest, the seat of reason must be in the chest rather than the brain.[202] His followers, including the one most influential for the development of the sect, Chrysippus of Soli (c. 280–207 BC), continued to uphold this teaching. Galen cites a variety of arguments that Chrysippus used to support this cardiocentric view of the soul, most of which were purely dialectic; for example, that one points to one's chest when referring to oneself, that one's chin naturally also points in that direction when saying "I" (egō), and that common opinion holds that the activities of the mind, such as anger, can be perceived in the chest.[203] Chrysippus was also aware of the anatomical dimension of this debate and its recent developments. However, he was not so convinced by dissection's indications that the brain was the source of the nerves to give up his own position as hopeless; rather, he referred to it as a question that had not yet reached resolution, citing Praxagoras as an authoritative voice on

---

[201] Philo, *Praem. et poen.* 144 (τοῦ μὲν ἐν φλεψὶν αἵματος … τοῦ δ᾽ ἐν ἀρτηρίαις πνεύματος). Philo's interest in Hippocratic medicine is evident from his writings, but Hogan (1992), 195–206 has also explored his more subtle familiarity with Hellenistic developments, including his use of Erasistratean language in his description of the stifling effect of close quarters on the respiratory system at *Leg. ad Gaium* 125–6, his belief that pulse lore, a particularly Herophilean development, was of first importance to practicing doctors at *Prov.* 2.17, and his sophisticated description of the function of the liver at *Spec. leg.* 216–18. While Hogan (1992), 200, like Colson (1939) in the Loeb edition, translates the passage here to be describing the air in the trachea (the older meaning of the word ἀρτηρία), this seems to me on the whole to be the less likely interpretation. Philo does elsewhere refer to the trachea as simply ἀρτηρία (*Vit. Mos.* I.84, *Decalogo* 32), but in each case as a member of what seems a linguistically fixed triad of "mouth, tongue, throat" (στόμα, γλῶττα, ἀρτηρία); when discussing it as an independent anatomical entity (*Post.Cain.* 104, *Quod deus sit immutabilis* 84), he uses the more modern term τραχεῖα ἀρτηρία, which was already standard in medical parlance in the first century BC in both Greek and Latin (cf. Cicero, *Nat.D.* 2.136, Lucretius, IV.528–9, and Langslow [2000], 36 and n. 100). Especially in the context of the other evidence for his familiarity with Hellenistic medicine, the μὲν-δὲ opposition so clearly set up in this passage between the veins and the arteries with their contrasting contents seems to me most likely to be a reference to the already popularly established Erasistratean theory.

[202] *PHP* V.241 (II.5.8 De Lacy).

[203] *PHP* V.213–16 (II.2.5–14 De Lacy) for the first two arguments; the argument by common opinion is handled at length across the second and third books of *PHP* (e.g., V.268–9 [II.7.7–13 De Lacy]).

the dissenting side.[204] Further, despite this engagement with the scientific tradition, he seems to have felt that anatomy, though potentially useful in the inquiry, was not, in fact, capable of providing final and incontrovertible proof; therefore, despite candidly admitting, according to Galen, that "the heart did not grace him with the knowledge that it was the source of the nerves" and that he was "inexperienced in anatomy," he nevertheless felt confident in arguing for his own position on different grounds.[205] This attitude seems to have been representative of early Stoic engagement with anatomy. Even the later Posidonius (*c.* 135–*c.* 51 BC), whom Galen refers to repeatedly as "the most scientific" of the Stoics for his interest in geometry, does not appear to have broached dissection as an avenue of proof.[206]

On the Peripatetic side of things, the focus was less on new anatomical developments and more on reformulation of Aristotle's own biological data; here, too, however, some familiarity with Hellenistic anatomical ideas is evident. Aristophanes of Byzantium, who succeeded Eratosthenes as the head of the library of Alexandria in around 194 BC, wrote an epitome of Aristotle's *History of Animals*, including a summary of the end of the first book, in which Aristotle goes through the external and internal parts of man part by part.[207] The original text is witnessed only by a single small papyrus fragment; however, a tenth-century AD compiler included significant portions of it in an extant work that also contains extracts from Aelian and others.[208] Albeit hardly at a conclusive scale, a comparison of the papyrus fragment with the Byzantine text suggests that the compiler transcribed Aristophanes' text in full, rather than epitomizing the epitome; thus, by cross-referencing the compilation with the texts of Aristotle and Aelian, it is possible to make some shrewd guesses about which parts of the tenth-century text derive directly from

---

[204] *PHP* V.189 (I.7.1 De Lacy); cf. *PHP* V.288–9 (III.1.12–15 De Lacy), where he refers to this as an unresolved problem among philosophers and physicians, and also the discussion in Tieleman (1996), 189–95.

[205] *PHP* V.187 (I.6.13 De Lacy) (μετρίως ἀποφηνάμενον ὡς μήθ' ὅτι τῶν νεύρων ἀρχὴ ἡ καρδία τὴν γνῶσιν αὐτῷ χαρίζεται ... ὁμολογεῖ γὰρ ἀπείρως ἔχειν τῶν ἀνατομῶν).

[206] *PHP* V.652 (VIII.1.14 De Lacy) (ὁ ἐπιστημονικώτατος τῶν Στωϊκῶν) and *QAM* IV.819 (ὁ πάντων ἐπιστημονικώτατος); cf. *PHP* V.390 (IV.4.38 De Lacy). The collected fragments of Posidonius in Edelstein and Kidd (1972) confirm a decided interest in scientific topics, but no real engagement with biological subjects, beyond the inclusion of some noteworthy fauna in his geographical writings (ff. 243–5).

[207] For discussion of Aristophanes' agenda in the writing of this epitome, see Chapter 2, "The Later Hellenistic Period" at pp. 47–8.

[208] *P.Lit.Lond.* 164; see Roselli (1979) and (1989). Lambros (1885) provides an edition of the Byzantine compilation.

Aristophanes.[209] Though significantly condensed, the majority of the Aristotelian material in the text is quite faithful to the original text in *History of Animals* as we have it today. Deviation from Aristotelian language and information occurs in two ways: Either an entire sentence or two containing non- (indeed, sometimes un-) Aristotelian material is interpolated or there are edits internal to the grammar of a largely Aristotelian sentence. While it must remain ambiguous whether the former were inserted by Aristophanes or by the Byzantine compiler, I think that it is reasonable to infer that the latter derive directly from the Aristophanic text.[210]

Working under these assumptions, the edits in the section addressing human anatomy are suggestive of the evolution of anatomical knowledge and norms in the roughly 150 years that intervened between Aristotle in the mid-fourth century and Aristophanes in the early second. For example, Aristophanes appears to have definite ideas of his own about the details of anatomical practice by various figures. Aristotle's description of the human brain is quite generic. His only differentiation of it from other species' is that it is "biggest and moistest," two superlatives that are easily in line with his theoretical framework of what *should* be true; otherwise, his description is applicable "to all animals."[211] Aristophanes, however, inserts language that implies a more active manipulation of humans on Aristotle's part. He begins the description of the human brain, which itself begins the entire section on human internal organs, with the participle "having been opened up," a word he elsewhere applies to dissection; further, in conveying the orthodox Aristotelian statement that the brain is bloodless and cold to the touch, he modifies the brain to be that "of a living human."[212] Is Aristophanes, perhaps, extending to Aristotle the norms – and resulting authority – of human dissection and vivisection that applied to Herophilus and Erasistratus, who lived and operated in his own city only a few generations before him? In contrast, where Aristotle discusses the erroneous deductions of earlier anatomists, who drew conclusions on

[209] See Roselli (1979), 14 and (1989), 339, and Hellmann (2006), 333. Lambros (1885) made an initial pass at this cross-referencing in his apparatus; from this, it is easy to see at a glance that the Aelian passages cluster at the end of the text, but there are some scattered through the more heavily Aristotelian sections as well.

[210] For Aristophanes' general willingness to edit Aristotle's zoology, even on factual matters, see Slater (1982), 341–2 and the response in Blank and Dyck (1984), 19–20.

[211] *HA* 494b28–9 (κατὰ μέγεθος ... πλεῖστον, ὑγρότατον), 34 (πᾶσιν).

[212] Aristophanes of Byzantium, *Ep.* II.12 (διοιχθείς; τοῦ ἀνθρώπου ζῶντος); cf. II.14 where he alters Aristotle's comment that the entrance of air into the chambers of heart is only visible in larger animals in order to make it clear that he thinks Aristotle learned this through dissection.

the state of the blood in the lungs based on lungs "removed from dissected animals," Aristophanes chooses to alter the text to read lungs "removed from sacrificial animals," denying intentionality to the pre-Aristotelian anatomists and exalting Aristotle's status from the opposite direction.[213]

Also strikingly, Aristophanes updates Aristotle's anatomy in a few places. Mostly he is glossing or marking outdated vocabulary; he repeatedly modifies Aristotle's term for the trachea (ἀρτηρία), which becomes the standard term for the arteries and would thus have had the potential to be very confusing for a naïve Hellenistic reader, and marks out his vascular terms as idiosyncratic.[214] He similarly alters, explicates, and adds to Aristotle's vocabulary for the digestive tract, which is quite vague, to bring it into conformity with his day's more precise terminology.[215] In addition to these more cosmetic changes, he on one occasion acknowledges that the actual substance of Aristotle's information may be outdated. When he gets to the description of the interior of the heart he writes, "it has in it, he says, three chambers, but not, like the majority of doctors say, two."[216] The insertion of the qualification "he says" and the inclusion of distinctly post-Aristotelian medical beliefs about the heart combine to politely indicate Aristophanes' doubt on the veracity of Aristotle's opinion and his reliance on more modern anatomical wisdom.[217] Further, some of the longer interpolations, if they are in fact the work of Aristophanes, would confirm that he is indeed consulting other, more medically focused anatomical books while creating his epitome. There are inserted sentences on the number and position of the vertebrae, the incurability of problems of the lungs, and a long passage on the wandering womb.[218] All told, given that the original texts of Aristotle were still in circulation during the Roman period, it

---

[213] Aristotle, *HA* 496b5–6 (ἐκ τῶν διαιρουμένων τῶν ζῴων); Aristophanes, *Ep.* II.24 (ἐκ τῶν ἱερείων).

[214] *Ep.* II.14 (ἡ λεγομένη *τραχεῖα* ἀρτηρία … τῆς *τραχείας* ἀρτηρίας), 16 (τῆς *τραχείας* ἀρτηρίας); *Ep.* II.21 (ἡ μεγάλη *λεγομένη* φλέψ … ἡ *καλουμένη ἀορτὴ* φλέψ); Aristophanes' additions are italicized.

[215] *Ep.* II.16 (εἰς τὴν κοιλίαν τὴν *λεγομένην* ἄνω), 17 (ἡ δὲ ἄνω κοιλία), 19–20 (ἡ δὲ *λεγομένη* κάτω κοιλία *ἐκπέφυκε μὲν ἐκ τοῦ ἐντέρου*, ὁμοία δέ ἐστι τῷ σχήματι τῇ ὑείᾳ· πλατεῖα γάρ ἐστι καὶ κοίλη. *τὸ δ' ἀπ' αὐτῆς πρὸς τὴν ἕδραν παχὺ καὶ βραχὺ ὑπάρχει, ὃ δὴ καὶ ἀρχόν καλοῦσι*. τὸ δὲ *λεγόμενον ἐπίπλοον* ἀπὸ μὲν τῆς ἄνω κοιλίας ἤρτηται, ἔστι δὲ τὴν φύσιν ὑμὴν πιμελώδης); Aristophanes' additions are italicized.

[216] *Ep.* II.21 (ἔχει δὲ ἐν αὐτῇ, φησί, κοιλίας τρεῖς, ἀλλ' οὐ καθάπερ οἱ πολλοὶ ἔφασαν τῶν ἰατρῶν δύο).

[217] After Erasistratus the heart was generally considered to be two chambered (i.e., the two ventricles – the atria were conceived of as ante-chamber extensions of the vessels that connect to them), although Herophilus had included the atria for a count of four; see Galen, *AA* II.624 and this chapter, "Erasistratus" at p. 201.

[218] Aristophanes of Byzantium, *Ep.* II.9, 23, 30. There is also a two-sentence interpolation asserting that humans and dogs are the only creatures that vomit and explaining why (II.17); there is a similar, but not quite identical, claim at Aelian *NA* IV.20.

is unlikely that this text had much impact on serious anatomical literature of that time, where it is not mentioned. Being far more approachable in size and arrangement than the original, however, it did contribute to a general knowledge on the subject.[219]

Latin authors from the Republican and early Imperial periods also exhibit an awareness of more recent developments in anatomo-physiology. The academic encyclopedism of the early Roman period saw an interest in bringing Greek medical thought into the domain of Latin literature, and both Aulus Cornelius Celsus (*fl. c.* AD 14–37) and Pliny the Elder (AD 23/4–79) offer fairly substantive anatomical information. Celsus opens the fourth book of his *On Medicine* with what he calls "a sort of survey, at the level necessary for a healer to know" of the internal parts of the body.[220] He provides a succinct outline of the internal organs, focusing largely on the digestive tract with only a very cursory mention of the vascular system and no mention of the nervous system. A similar survey of the bones and their articulation opens the eighth book. In both cases, he relies openly, though anonymously, on Greek sources, either transliterating or directly citing Greek terms, usually in cases where Latin vocabulary falls short.[221] In addition to these explicitly anatomical sections, moments of anatomical interest appear throughout the text, especially in the seventh book, which contains detailed and decidedly Greek anatomies of the eye and the male reproductive organs, the former attributing one term directly to Herophilus.[222] In general, he is extremely familiar with and interested in Hellenistic medical authors, and it is not surprising that his anatomical knowledge draws on

---

[219] The papyrus fragment dates to the second or third century AD, suggesting active interest in that period (Roselli [1989], 338, 40); for other evidence of the popularity of the text, which was a source for both Pliny and Aelian, see Düring (1950), 62–4, and Kullmann (1998), 132–9.

[220] Celsus, *DM* IV.2.1 (conspectum quendam, quatenus scire curanti necessarium est). Although there is debate about the degree to which Celsus' medical advice is based on personal experience (for a recent resume of the arguments for and against, see Langslow [2000], 45–8; cf. Gautherie [2017], 42–5), there is no suggestion that his anatomical knowledge relied on anything but textual research.

[221] Usually, but not invariably, as, for example, at VIII.15 and 19, where both the Latin and the Greek terms are given; for parallels with the Hippocratic *Anatomy*, see Craik (2006), 156. For an extensive analysis of the use of Greek terms in Celsus and other Latin medical authors, see Langslow (2000), 76–139. It is noteworthy that Latin had its own serviceable anatomical vocabulary: Langslow (2000), 118–21 counts only five Greek anatomical terms that Celsus implies to have been borrowed as the current, functional term in Latin medicine; the remaining 98 percent of anatomical terms in his text have a recognizable and functional Latin word or phrase.

[222] The eye at VII.7.13, with citation of Herophilus at VII.7.13B; the reproductive organs at VII.18.1–2.

them as well.[223] Further, Celsus' preface offers a detailed description of the history of and debate surrounding the practice of human dissection; it is to him that we owe the knowledge of Herophilus' and Erasistratus' vivisection of condemned criminals.[224]

Pliny ends the eleventh book of his *Natural Histories* with a piecemeal anatomical survey, taking into account many different animals as he moves from part to part. While the vast majority of his information is Aristotelian in nature, he is clearly drawing on other sources as well.[225] In his list of contents and sources, he includes Aristotle for this book, but also Hippocrates and the Hellenistic medical writers Herophilus, Erasistratus, Asclepiades, and Themison.[226] Pliny's description of the heart shows some influence of these other voices; he latches onto the statement in *Parts of Animals* that the number of chambers of the heart is variable depending on the size of the animal and claims that, while in large animals the number is three, "in no [other] is it not double."[227] Though technically rooted in Aristotelian doctrine, this emphasis on the two chambered heart is quite antithetical to Aristotle's overarching conception of three-chambered cardiac structure and is evocative of the Hellenistic context, where two, as we have seen, became the standardly accepted number.[228] The Hellenistic influence comes to the fore most forcefully in the passage on the vascular system. In good Erasistratean fashion, he glosses the arteries as "paths of the breath" and the

---

[223] von Staden (2010) examines the ways in which Celsus draws on (and diverges from) his Hellenistic sources when discussing anatomy and physiology, focusing in particular on his treatment of the brain and the vascular system. For Celsus' general familiarity with and interest in Hellenistic medical writing, see also von Staden (1994) and (1999*b*).

[224] Celsus, *DM* proem.23–4; see Chapter 2, "Herophilus and Erasistratus" at p. 37 and Chapter 4, "Anatomical Subjects: Humans" at pp. 111–12.

[225] As Capponi (1995) and Kullmann (1998), 132–5 have explored, it is likely that Pliny's source for Aristotelian information was not – or not solely, as Ernout and Pepin (2003), 5–23 would have it – Aristotle directly, but rather included an epitome or epitomes of some sort, almost certainly Aristophanes of Byzantium's among them (on which see earlier in this section).

[226] Pliny, *NH* I.11c.10.

[227] Pliny, *NH* XI.182 (in nullo non gemino).

[228] Aristotle's statement at *PA* 666b21–22 that the number of chambers varies according to the size of the animal is at odds with his teaching at *HA* 496a4, 19–20 and 513b27–30, where it is invariably three (though he concedes that in small animals sometimes only one or two of the three is visible). Even in the *PA* passage (666b22–35), however, he is clear that three chambers is ideal and two is acceptable only where there really is not room to accommodate three; further, in that passage he is also, unlike Pliny, willing to entertain the possibility that some animals have only one.

veins as "channels of the blood" and then segues immediately to a discussion of the pulse in which he directly pays tribute to the role of "Herophilus, master of medicine, with marvelous skill" in systemizing sphygmology; he may even allude here in a somewhat garbled way to vivisectory experimentation in his claim that "the arteries lack sensation ... when they are cut only that part of the body [in which they are located] grows numb."[229] This passage, however, seems to have been a conscious and largely discrete moment of modernization of his otherwise ubiquitous Aristotelian source – to which he indeed reverts immediately afterwards. Nor is he at all bothered by including elsewhere information that contradicts the very doctrines alluded to in this Hellenistic passage; he describes the liver as receiving blood from the heart, an Aristotelian rather than Erasistratean direction of flow, and repeatedly implies that veins are responsible for sensation, making no account of the nervous system at all.[230]

Just as in the Greek context, some familiarity with Hellenistic conceptions of anatomy penetrated into Latin discourse even outside scientific contexts. Cicero (106 BC–43 BC) includes a small anatomical passage in the second book of his *Nature of the Gods*, which contains a hodgepodge of physiological theories.[231] His description of digestion combines the two different theories that Celsus will later attribute to Hippocrateans and Erasistrateans respectively, while his use of the notoriously polyvalent word *nervus* leaves his level of familiarity with the nervous system ambiguous, but is at best suggestive of a Praxagorean rather than Herophilean/ Erasistratean model.[232] His understanding of the vascular system, however,

---

[229] Pliny, *NH* XI.219–20 (spiritus semitae; sanguinis rivi; discriptus ab Herophilo medicinae vate miranda arte; arteriae carent sensu ... praecisisque torpescit tantum pars ea corporis). Capponi (1995), 181–4 (cf. Ernout and Pepin [2003], 190–1) is puzzlingly hesitant to claim an Erasistratean influence in Pliny's description of the arteries in this paragraph; the direct mention of Herophilus in the same section, combined with the reference to air-filled arteries and the seeming allusion to vivisection, makes it overwhelmingly probable that the entire paragraph is reliant on Hellenistic information, for which Pliny himself names Erasistratus and Herophilus as his authorities.

[230] Indeed, if Erasistratus were not directly named in the list of sources for this material, one might be more tempted to see here the influence of Praxagoras, who is not named, but whose cardiocentric model and connection of sensation to the heart and vascular system are more compatible with Pliny's overall Aristotelian outlook. On the liver, XI.192 (cf. Capponi [1995], 130–1 for some interpretative challenges in this passage); on sensation through veins (and in one case also arteries), see XI.135, 149, 213.

[231] Cicero, *Nat.D.* II.133–9. van den Bruwaene (1978), 186 suggests that Cicero may have derived his information from consulting encyclopedic sources containing medical information while traveling in Asia Minor.

[232] Cicero, *Nat.D.* II.136, where digestion is achieved by a combination of heat, the Hippocratean model, and crushing, the Erasistratean one (cf. Celsus, *DM* proem.20 and the discussion in van den Bruwaene [1978], 188, n. 411). Cicero, *Nat.D.* II.139 describes "the *nervi*, by which the joints are held together/controlled and whose interweaving extends to the entire body" (nervos, a quibus

is a squarely Hellenistic dichotomy of the veins as pathways for blood and the arteries for air.[233] This familiarity with anatomical developments grows even more mainstream over time, with Horace (65 BC–8 BC) and Seneca the Younger (*c.* 4/1 BC–AD 65) each making comments suggestive of awareness that the nerves are associated with sensation.[234]

All told, anatomical literature prior to the revival of interest in the first centuries AD is a mixed group. Unsurprisingly, the figures who appeared in Chapter 2 as noteworthy practitioners of dissection reappear here as influential anatomical authors. However, skill in dissection did not automatically correlate with influential status as an anatomical author. Erasistratus, one of the most prominent of all pre-Roman dissectors, did not particularly privilege anatomical writing, and his footprint as an anatomical authority is therefore small. In contrast, the texts of the Hippocratic Corpus – and even Plato's *Timaeus* – maintained considerable influence as anatomical citations, even though their relationship to dissection is, at best, obscure and their approach to anatomy is in many instances openly theoretical. Indeed, the theoretical needs of later authors drove the reception of anatomical texts as much as anything: the cardiocentric anatomies of Praxagoras and Aristotle continued to hold sway in certain circles even after Herophilus and Erasistratus' further advancements in dissection had refuted them.

---

artus continentur eorumque inplicationem corpore toto pertinentem). The vocabulary surrounding the relationship of the *nervi* to the joints leaves it ambiguous whether he is using the word to describe tendons, ligaments, or nerves, all possible meanings for this word at this period; André (1991), 209 categorizes this instance under the meaning of ligament, citing similar but less ambiguous language at Pliny, *NH* XI.217. Either way, he chooses to attribute to them an origin in the heart, adopting an Aristotelian or Praxagorean cardiocentric outlook, which is perhaps not surprising given his interest in Stoicism (for the cardiocentric sympathies of which, see earlier in this section and Chapter 7, "Anatomy in the Roman Intellectual Scene" at p. 272).

[233] Cicero, *Nat.D.* II.138.

[234] Horace, *Sat.* 2.4.53 (odor nervis inimicus) and Seneca, *Epist.* 122.6 (quod libere penetrat ad nervos) indicate a belief that the nerves are operative in the sensation of smell and taste respectively; cf. André (1991), 209.

CHAPTER 7

Anatomical Texts of the Roman Period

One ought not to be unfamiliar with the modern authors and those
who lived a little before us ... for the powers of these men might
be helpful to us also in this respect: we would not approach them
enslaved in our opinion, as we do with the ancients. For the ability to
find fault with some of what has been said renders us bolder in making our own attempts, and one compares oneself with more pleasure
when convinced that, when compared, one does not appear lacking,
and sometimes might even appear better.

Dio Chrysostom, *Orations*[1]

Dio Chrysostom (*c.* AD 40/50–after 110) offers this advice in the context of
rhetoric, but his sentiments would have resonated perfectly with the anatomists among his peers. Reverence for the ancients was a typical feature of
intellectual life in this period, and the medical community was no exception. Galen boasts that in the course of his medical studies he has "gone
without sleep at night in order to examine the treasures left to us by the
ancients."[2] Hippocrates, as we have just seen, was endowed with a godlike
authority; even Hellenistic authors were sometimes put on the same ped-
estal – Galen refers to Herophilus' name as "revered" and chastises those
who would falsify his teaching.[3] In short, the ancients, for all their variable accuracy and influence, were collectively a formidable body, forming
the cornerstone of medicine generally and anatomy in particular. All the

---

[1] Dio Chrysostom, *Or.* XVIII.12 (δεῖν ... μηδὲ τῶν νεωτέρων καὶ ὀλίγον πρὸ ἡμῶν ἀπείρως ἔχειν ...
αἱ γὰρ τούτων δυνάμεις καὶ ταύτῃ ἂν εἶεν ἡμῖν ὠφέλιμοι, ᾖ οὐκ ἂν ἐντυγχάνοιμεν αὐτοῖς
δεδουλωμένοι τὴν γνώμην, ὥσπερ τοῖς παλαιοῖς. ὑπὸ γὰρ τοῦ δύνασθαί τι τῶν εἰρημένων
αἰτιάσασθαι μάλιστα θαρροῦμεν πρὸς τὸ τοῖς αὐτοῖς ἐπιχειρεῖν [ᾖ] καὶ ἥδιόν τις παραβάλλει αὐτὸν
ᾧ πείθεται συγκρινόμενος οὐ καταδεέστερος, ἐνίοτε δὲ καὶ βελτίων <ἂν> φαίνεσθαι).
[2] *Opt.Med.Cogn.* 9.3 (*CMG Suppl.Or.* IV, p. 103, trans. Iskandar).
[3] On the reverent attitude that was typical towards Hippocrates, see Chapter 6, "The Hippocratic
Corpus" at p. 176; for Herophilus, see Galen, *Dig.Puls.* VIII.954–6 (von Staden T162) (ὀνόματι
σεμνῷ).

surviving medical authors from the Roman period cite ancient authorities extensively.[4]

While it generally behooved a Roman anatomist to treat the ancients with this sort of overwrought diffidence, the moderns were available as a foil to his own brilliance. An excellent example of this dichotomy is the starkly different ways in which we saw Galen handle Erasistratus and the modern Erasistrateans: The former he sometimes quite forcefully disagrees with, but nevertheless treats with some respect and will cite as a reliable authority; the latter he mercilessly denounces in some of his ripest language across several pointed treatises. Already in Chapter 3 we saw dissection as a battleground for the fierce in-person competition between anatomists of different schools; here we will look to the texts, both those that survive and those whose contents need to be reconstructed, to further plumb the diversity and breadth of the anatomical scene in the century or so leading up to the height of Galen's fame as doctor, author, and dissector.

Chapter 6 traced the development of anatomical writing, from general texts of medicine or philosophy that included some anatomical topics to the emergence of dedicated anatomical handbooks. These handbooks did not eclipse the former variety of anatomical writing, but they grew steadily in popularity: In fact, our best examples of this genre date to the Roman period. Indeed, the renewal of interest in dissection at the end of the first century AD parallels a simultaneous explosion of activity in the textual record. This plethora of texts, only a small fraction of which survive, included both handbooks and general treatises with anatomical sections. Interestingly, we also see several examples of texts that form almost a hybrid of these two models: Rather than general texts that refer to anatomy in passing, these are lengthy texts constructed around anatomical scaffolding, but also include physiological, nosological, and therapeutic topics.[5] This period also welcomed a completely new genre. The first procedural anatomical text appears at the turn of the second century and represents, for the first time, a complete fusion in the practices of dissection and of writing anatomy.

---

[4] Galen paints the Methodists as rejecting the theories of the ancients and instead propounding a radically innovative form of medicine. The Methodist writing that survives to us, however, namely that of Soranus and Caelius Aurelianus, nevertheless makes liberal, albeit usually critical, mention of ancient authorities, especially Hellenistic authors; see the discussion in von Staden (1999a).

[5] The anatomical texts of Marinus and Lycus, both discussed later in this chapter, fall into this category, as, arguably, does Galen's own *On the Usefulness of the Parts.* Herophilus' *Anatomy* was perhaps also of this character (see Chapter 6, "Herophilus" at pp. 195–6).

Rufus of Ephesus

Rufus of Ephesus (*c.* AD 80–*c.* 150)[6] was a respected and prolific doctor of the early Roman empire. Galen does not mention him with great frequency, but when he does his good opinion is generally evident; he refers to his work on melancholy as the best in the field by a modern author, repeatedly cites him as an authority in pharmacology, and respects him as a careful and thoughtful editor of Hippocrates.[7] This good reputation continues into the fourth century, when Oribasius, to whom we owe significant extracts, refers to him as "Rufus the great."[8] Although only a handful of his works survive, anywhere from forty-six to one hundred and nine titles have been attributed to him.[9] Of this long list, only three relate to anatomy and, of those three, only one is universally agreed to be genuine: *On the Names of the Parts of the Body* is accepted to be a work of Rufus, while considerable doubt surrounds the authorship of *On the Anatomy of the Parts of the Human Body* and *On Bones*.[10] This proportionally tiny

---

[6] Dates according to Sideras (1994), 1086. However, the evidence is somewhat ambiguous, and it is also possible to make an argument for a *floruit* around AD 50 (as, e.g., Singer [1925], 42); see also Abou-Aly (1992), 22–8, who tentatively suggests an active period "at some time between the middle of the first century AD and its end" (p. 25), and Nutton (2008), 140–1, who explains the rationale for each dating, but refrains from endorsing either one (but cf. Nutton [2006], where he lands in the middle ground, suggesting a *floruit* "around AD 100").

[7] For his excellence on melancholy: *At.Bil.* V.105 (ἄριστα); for his pharmacology: *Simp.Med.* XI.796, *Comp.Med.Loc.* XII.425, *Ant.* XIV.7 (the name Rufus without a signifying place name also appears at *Comp.Med.Loc.* XIII.92, 1010 [Μήνιος Ῥοῦφος], and *Ant.* XIV.119, but the identity of these other Rufi with Rufus of Ephesus is subject to debate; cf. Abou Aly [1992], 26–9); for his exegetical work: *Hipp.Prorrh.* XVI.636–7, 735, *Hipp.Epid.VI* XVIIa.849, 956, 993, 1006, XVIIb.29–30, 93, 113, *Ord. Lib.Prop.* XIX.57–8.

[8] Oribasius, *Eun.* praef.1.6 (Ῥούφῳ τῷ μεγάλῳ).

[9] Sideras (1994), 1089–1102 counts forty-six (not including those he considers pseudepigraphic), significantly lowering the previous, more promiscuous, counts of ninety-six and one hundred and nine suggested by Ilberg (1930) and Daremberg and Ruelle (1879), xxxii–xxxix respectively. For the extant works, see Daremberg and Ruelle (1879), still the standard edition of Rufus' oeuvre as a whole, which includes a mixture of complete texts and fragments, as well as several that one or the other of the editors (the manuscript was completed by Ruelle after Daremberg's death) believed to be pseudepigraphic; Sideras (1994), 1089–1170 lists the genuine surviving Greek texts as *De renum et vesicae morbis*, *De corporis humani appellationibus*, *De satyriasmo et gonorrhoea*, and *Quaestiones medicinales*, adding to them *De podagra*, which survives in Latin, as well as a text on jaundice and, possibly, another consisting of case histories, both of which survive in Arabic. For more details on the Arabic tradition of Rufus, see Ullmann (1994) and Pormann (2008).

[10] On the latter two texts, which I do not consider to be the work of Rufus, see the end of this section. Daremberg appears to have doubted their legitimacy, but Ruelle is more enthusiastic about considering *Anatomy* to be genuine (Daremberg and Ruelle [1879], xxi–ii, xxviii–ix; Lloyd (1983), 151, n. 107, while skeptical of many of Ruelle's arguments, remains open to his suggestion that it was at least derived from original work by Rufus. Ilberg (1930), 9–12, on the other hand, offers a detailed explanation for why he believes that Rufus is not the author of these two texts; Sideras (1994), 1089, and Ullmann (1994), 1345 both accept his judgement, but Abou-Aly (1992) is less clear on the issue

fraction of attention paid to anatomy in Rufus' corpus may simply be in keeping with his general lack of emphasis on the topic; as far as the evidence we have suggests, it was not a crucial foundation to his therapeutics in the way it later would be for Galen.[11] Certainly, Galen never refers to him as an authority in an anatomical context. Yet, despite this, his anatomical writing was continuously influential, spawning epitomes, yielding extracts, and, seemingly, attracting other minor works of anatomy into the orbit of its reputational gravity.

Rufus opens *On the Names of the Parts of the Body* by positioning anatomical nomenclature as a fundamental set of data for a physician to know, in the same way that the names of the notes are for a musician or the names of the letters for a literate person or geometrical terms for a mathematician. As these examples indicate, his concern is not so much with heuristic or therapeutic benefits that might arise from the study of anatomy, but rather with developing a mutually intelligible way of talking about the body that allows physicians to learn and to teach without just "pointing as if [they were] mute."[12] He then goes on to provide an enormously valuable insight into how anatomy was taught in the late first or early second century AD: "Listening and looking at this slave, you will first thoroughly remember the external parts; then, when it is necessary to name the internal parts, we will attempt to teach you by dissecting some animal which is very similar to man."[13]

The remaining structure of the text is indeed divided into two sections, with the internal parts following the external ones. This textual arrangement reinforces the message of the prefatory paragraph; far from being a rhetorical introduction, this passage is describing different instructional needs for internal and external parts that meaningfully impacted the way that anatomical data were grouped and taught. This consistency suggests that animal dissection was an active instructional element for some doctors at this period – even for those who, like Rufus, do not emphasize it in their medical writing.

---

and mostly treats them as if genuine. Nickel (2009) has recently reexamined the question in detail and argues convincingly that *On the Anatomy of the Parts of the Human Body* and *On Bones*, though by the same author, were not written by Rufus.

[11] For the place of anatomy in Rufus' larger medical program, see Thomssen (1994), 1255–7, and Nutton (2008), 144–6, but also Abou-Aly (1992), 148–55, 249, who offers a handful of instances where anatomy is implicated in Rufus' discussion of treatment and diseases.

[12] *Nom.Part.* 6 (δεικνύντα ... ὥσπερ κωφόν).

[13] *Nom.Part.* 9 (ἀκούων δὴ καὶ ἀποβλέπων εἰς τὸν παῖδα τοῦτον διαμνημονεύσεις τὰ ἐπιφανῆ πρῶτον· εἶτα ὡς χρὴ καλεῖν τὰ ἔνδον, ζῷόν τι, ὃ μάλιστα ἀνθρώπῳ ἔοικε, διελόντες, διδάσκειν σε πειρασόμεθα· οὐδὲν γὰρ ἐμποδών, εἰ μὴ καὶ παντάπασιν ἐοίκασιν, τὸ γοῦν κεφάλαιον ἑκάστου διδάξαι).

The subsequent sentences raise the question of how long-standing the practice of dissection in medical education was. Rufus acknowledges that animal dissection is not a perfect window into human internal anatomy – though he asserts that it is good enough for the level of detail that concerns him – and he mentions that "long ago they learned these sorts of things in a much better way on humans."[14] While this is surely a reference to the time of Herophilus and Erasistratus, several centuries before Rufus was writing, it is unclear how tight a connection Rufus saw between their practices: Can we infer an unbroken tradition of dissection, sometimes of humans, sometimes of animals, as a basis for medical education? Or is Rufus describing a recent revival of a defunct practice, but with inferior subjects? First of all, the question of geographical continuity is surely pertinent here; while very little is known concretely about Rufus' biography, there are convincing indications that he spent some time in Egypt.[15] The natural assumption is that Rufus' reason for this Egyptian sojourn would have been to pursue his education in Alexandria, which Galen confirms was still a powerhouse of medical education in the Roman period.[16] Though not conclusive either way, this might support the idea that Rufus sees himself as participating in a continuous local chain of anatomical tradition. However, the evidence from Galen is not without complications. He tells us that in Alexandria osteology is taught using human skeletons and strongly implies that it is the only place where this is done, suggesting that the practice is a relic of the more permissive practices of the Hellenistic period and should therefore have been occurring continuously through Rufus' time as well.[17] Rufus' failure to mention human skeletons might conceivably be interpreted, therefore, as evidence that he was not familiar with the customs of Alexandrian education; however, first, his tract does not dilate at any length on bones, which seem to have often been relegated to their own dedicated texts, making the omission less noteworthy and, second, Rufus is clearly describing his teaching practices, not his own education – if he were teaching in Ephesus, for example, human skeletons would not have been to hand.[18]

---

[14] *Nom.Part.* 10 (πάλαι δὲ γενναιότερον ἐπὶ ἀνθρώπων ἐδίδασκον τὰ τοιαῦτα).

[15] Rufus mentions Egyptians and Egypt more frequently than any other people or place, including his hometown of Ephesus; see Ilberg (1930), 2–3, Abou-Aly (1992), 29–35, Sideras (1994), 1087, and Nutton (2008), 144. He also appears in Vindicianus' list of anatomists associated with Alexandria (*Gyn.* praef.), which is, however, of dubious utility; see von Staden (1989), 52.

[16] For Galen's references to Alexandria, see von Staden (2004).

[17] *AA* II.220.

[18] Galen himself separates osteology out from the rest of his anatomical writing, and he indicates that this was a common practice (*AA* II.220). For the tension between Rufus and Galen's evidence on this point, cf. Nutton (1993), 16.

The indications from within the text certainly uphold the goals and methodology that Rufus describes in his opening paragraph. As promised, his agenda is heavily inflected by linguistic concerns. The goal of the text, to which he largely adheres without adornment, is to document the multiple words that Greek has for any given area of the body, sometimes simply listing them as interchangeable synonyms, sometimes differentiating the mainstream from the less-so.[19] He also reports dialect variations, historical differences, and the quirks of individual authors, both medical and non-medical, occasionally offering etymological theories and only rarely adding physiological or nosological details.[20] Though he is usually content to list the alternatives in this way, in a few cases he adjudicates on correct usage. For example, he points out that, though there is a set phrase that can be used to describe carrying something tucked under your armpit, to extract the word for armpit out of that phrase and use it as an anatomical term is "not Greek."[21] He also several times opines that other terms are sometimes used "incorrectly."[22]

It is in this context that we must understand one of the more controversial passages in this treatise; here, Rufus is discussing the sutures of the skull and he adds:

> The names of these are not ancient but have now been instituted by certain Egyptian doctors who speak simple Greek: "crown-like" for the one on the front of the head, "lambda-shaped" for the one around the back, "yoked-up" for the one in the middle, and "scale-shaped" for the ones at the temples. These same men also named parts of other bones that were anonymous for the ancients, which I will not pass over for the sake of clarity in the current parlance of doctors.[23]

---

[19] In the former case, he offers lists of alternatives connected by καί or ἤ (*Nom.Part.* 13, 19, 20, 23, 32, 47, 55, 59, 60, 62, 64, 66–8, 91–2, 95, 97, 100–1, 103, 105, 111, 115–16, 125, 152, 157, 159, 166, 169–71, 193–5, 197, 225) (conversely, he also periodically mentions that the same word can refer to multiple things; cf. 144 for a particularly egregious example); in the latter, he begins by offering one word, but then adds alternatives used by "some people" or "others" (οἱ δέ: 30, 48, 79, 95, 101, 111, 114, 155, 199; ἔνιοι δέ: 51, 153, 185; ἄλλοι δέ: 16, 100, 110, 116, 139, 153, 189, 199, 222).

[20] Dialects: *Nom.Part.* 32–3, 79, 107, 201; temporal variation: 112, 133–4, 171, 199, 208, 210; individual authors: 33, 88, 120, 154, 193, 195, 202 (Hippocrates), 61, 209 (Aristotle), 63, 68, 113, 170 (Homer), 79 (Epicharmus), 112 (Euryphon), 123, 149, 153, 155, 203 (Herophilus), 192 (Clearchus), 199, 209, 226–7 (Praxagoras), 201 (Philistion), 205 (Eudemus), 205–7 (Dionysius, son of Oxymachus), 227 (Mnesitheus), 228 (Zenon), 229 (Empedocles); etymology: 27, 51, 99, 146, 153, 169–71, 195, 210, 229; physiology: 58, 136, 150, 160, 197, 210; nosology: 199.

[21] *Nom.Part.* 76 (οὐχ ἑλληνικὸν).

[22] *Nom.Part.* 124, 139, 192 (οὐκ ὀρθῶς); cf. 103, 200, 210.

[23] *Nom.Part.* 133–4 (ὀνόματα δὲ αὐτῶν παλαιὰ οὐκ ἔστιν, ἀλλὰ νῦν ἐτέθη ὑπό τινων Αἰγυπτίων ἰατρῶν φαύλως ἑλληνιζόντων· στεφανιαία μὲν τῇ πρὸς τὸ βρέγμα, λαμβδοειδὴς δὲ, τῇ περὶ τὸ ἰνίον,

This passage leaves ambiguous the precise identity of these "Egyptian doctors," namely whether we ought to understand them to be Greeks living in Egypt, presumably Alexandria, or to be native Egyptians who have learned the Greek language and contributed to Greek medical discourse.[24] The scorn that Rufus feels for these physicians and their upstart naming system is palpable but does little to resolve this issue. To some degree, the question hinges on how to translate the adverb he uses to describe their linguistic skill, which I translated as "simple": φαύλως. It can certainly carry the meaning of "badly," and could thus be a reasonable way of describing someone speaking Greek as a second language without complete fluency. In this case, these doctors would represent another layer of complexity in the question of the interactions between Greek and Egyptian medicine and add further evidence for the fluidity between these two cultures in Ptolemaic Egypt.[25] However, φαύλως can equally well mean "simple," "ordinary," or "indifferent," a more subtle criticism that could describe the sort of solecisms that less linguistically keen native speakers are apt to fall into – for example, erroneously extracting a word for armpit out of a fixed phrase, as Rufus earlier implied to be a sin some Greek speakers were prone to.[26] Indeed, the terms that cause him to take such umbrage here are not in any way bad Greek, just rather unimaginative neologisms. It would not at all be out of character for Rufus, a keen Hippocratean and stickler for linguistic purity, to take offense at the newfangled terms of recent contemporaries simply for their newfangledness.

Although this focus on linguistic questions is a uniform theme of the entire text, Rufus cleanly maintains the dichotomy between external anatomy based on a human subject and internal anatomy based on the dissection of animals. The first half of the text is decidedly human-focused, including comprehensive discussion of aspects with

---

ἐπιζευγνύουσα δέ, τῇ μέσῃ· λεπιδοειδεῖς δέ, ταῖς τῶν κροτάφων. οὗτοι δὲ καὶ τῶν ἄλλων ὀστῶν μόρια ὀνομάζουσιν ἀνώνυμα τοῖς πάλαι, ἃ ἐγὼ οὐ παραλείψω διὰ τὴν εἰς τὰ νῦν τῶν ἰατρῶν δήλωσιν). Note that three of these terms appear without comment in the discussion of the bones of the head at the beginning of the *On Bones* that circulated under Rufus' name (*Oss.* 3), indicating that they had indeed become the current standard nomenclature.

[24] Jouanna (2004), 20–1 takes it as certain that native Egyptians are meant, whereas Lloyd (1983), 158, and von Staden (1989), 481, n. 3 gloss the term as basically equivalent to Alexandrian (and thus, implicitly, Greek); Abou-Aly (1992), 31–2, and Nutton (2008), 144 weigh both options.

[25] On the general question of contact between the two traditions of medicine, see Jouanna (2004), Lang (2013), 100–38, and Andorlini (2016); for the fluidity between the two cultures in general, see, for example, Dieleman and Moyer (2010). For Egyptian knowledge of anatomy specifically, see Chapter 5, "Religious Practices" at pp. 158–60.

[26] Compare Galen's scorn for medical students who "cannot read well" at *Lib.Prop.* XIX.9 (οὐδ' ἀναγνῶναι καλῶς δυνάμενοι) (cf. Chapter 9, "The Audience of *Anatomical Procedures*" at p. 339).

less obvious medical relevance, such as names for the different areas of facial hair.[27] Even in this section, though, there is anticipation of the dissection to come; when discussing the eye in the context of the external anatomy of the head, Rufus begins to address the layers of the eye, but adds that further details will be forthcoming "a little later, in the dissection of the animal."[28] When he does pivot to the internal organs, he underscores that the discussion is linked to the dissection of a particular animal, using a pointedly deictic pronoun to indicate that the dissection should indeed be conceived of as concurrent: "we will attempt to name the internal parts while dissecting *this very* monkey."[29] Although we are meant to conceive of a specific dissection accompanying the composition of this text, Rufus is also keen to signal that the information conveyed is based on the cumulative evidence of multiple dissections. He discusses the comparative advantage of monkeys over other species, laying out a hierarchy of similarity to humans, and he twice indicates that some anatomical features are present only in some species or in some individuals.[30]

In addition, there are two moments when Rufus directly mentions his own anatomical experiences outside of routine teaching. At the very end of the treatise, he switches out of the present tense, which he uses consistently for the rest of the treatise, into the past, and describes the fetal membranes as he observed them to be on one particular occasion: "While dissecting, we saw this membrane [the amnion] to contain a liquid, one much purer than that in the chorion, and, to us, thinking it through, it seemed that this was like the sweat of the fetus, while the other, like urine, was emptied through the urachus into the chorion."[31] The passage continues, still in the past tense, to further describe the amnion and the chorion, as well as the umbilicus and its vasculature. Rufus' use of the first person plural here raises the question of whether he is referring to a personal or a group

---

[27] *Nom.Part.* 49.

[28] *Nom.Part.* 29 (ὀλίγον ὕστερον ἐν τῇ διαιρέσει τοῦ ζῴου).

[29] *Nom.Part.* 127 (τὰ δὲ ἔνδον τουτονὶ τὸν πίθηκον ἀνατέμνοντες, ὀνομάζειν πειρασόμεθα); emphasis in the Greek (τουτονὶ).

[30] *Nom.Part.* 127 for the comparison of animal types; Rufus articulates a four-fold hierarchy, with monkeys closest to humans, followed by animals with toes, then animals with a divided hoof, and finally solid-hoofed animals (compare with Galen's six-fold hierarchy, discussed in Chapter 4, "Anatomical Subjects: Other Animals" at p. 100). Rufus references variation among species or individuals at *Nom.Part.* 131, 168.

[31] *Nom.Part.* 230–2 (ἐωρῶμεν δὲ ἀνατέμνοντες τοῦτον τὸν χιτῶνα περιέχοντα ὑγρὸν, πολὺ δὴ καθαρώτερον τοῦ ἐν τῷ χορίῳ· καὶ λογιζομένοις μὲν ἐφαίνετο ὥσπερ ἱδρὼς εἶναι τοῦ βρέφους, τὸ δὲ διὰ τοῦ οὐράχου ὥσπερ οὖρον εἰς τὸ χορίον ἐκδιδόναι).

dissection: Although the authorial plural is certainly an uncontroversial way for an author to refer to himself individually, Rufus does not use it often.[32] Indeed, in this text his authorial comments are exclusively in the first person singular, except in contexts related to dissection, where, conversely, he always uses the plural and never the singular. This strongly suggests that the form in these contexts is functioning as a true plural – that dissections, including the one that accompanies the second half of the text, were a group undertaking for which Rufus did not take exclusive personal responsibility.[33] Even with this caveat, though, it is clear that he is recounting a firsthand experience, and that it involved not just rote dissection for illustrating preconceived anatomical terms, but acute observation and analysis of what was observed.

In the other instance, Rufus uses his own experience to directly gainsay Herophilus' opinion on the lack of complete homology between male and female reproductive anatomy:

> For to Herophilus it does not seem that the female possesses varicose assistants [like males have], but in the uterus of a sheep we have seen varicose vessels growing out of the ovaries on each side; and these perforated into the cavity of the uterus and, when they were squeezed, a somewhat mucus-like liquid came out. And there was great suspicion that they were seed-related and of the same type as the varicose ones [in males]. But how this question stands, the dissections will perhaps show.[34]

Again, we see that Rufus is recalling his own engagement with dissections, which included heuristic manipulation and data-based challenging of received anatomical wisdom. Again, however, his use of the plural and the somewhat awkwardly impersonal construction of the conclusions drawn – "there was great suspicion" – suggest that Rufus was not personally driving this research but was more of an observer or collaborator; certainly elsewhere, including in the sentence immediately preceding this passage, he is

---

[32] For an analysis of Rufus' use of the first person across his entire corpus, see Sideras (1994), 1217–25, especially 1219, where he remarks "den Plural ἡμεῖς δέ (wir aber) für die eigene Person verwendet Rufus viel seltener."

[33] First person plurals occur in the context of dissection at *Nom.Part.* 9, 127, 186, 230; the remaining uses of the first person plural elsewhere in the text unambiguously function as generic plurals, for example "the canal through which we hear" (43) (ὁ πόρος διὰ οὗ ἀκούομεν), "the buttocks on which we sit" (116) (ἐφέδρανα, ἐπὶ ὧν καθίζομεν), etc. (cf. 11, 15, 58, 67, 79, 82, 121).

[34] *Nom.Part.* 186–7 ('Ηροφίλῳ μὲν γὰρ οὐ δοκεῖ τὸ θῆλυ κιρσοειδεῖς ἔχειν παραστάτας· ἐν δὲ προβάτου ὑστέρᾳ εἴδομεν ἐκ τῶν διδύμων πεφυκότα τὰ ἀγγεῖα κεκιρσωμένα ἑκατέρωθεν· συνε τέτρητο δὲ ταῦτα εἰς τὸ κοίλωμα τῆς ὑστέρας, ἀπὸ ὧν ὑπόμυξον ὑγρὸν πιεζούντων ἀπεκρίνετο· καὶ ἦν πολλὴ δόκησις σπερματικὰ ταῦτα εἶναι, καὶ τοῦ γένους τῶν κιρσοειδῶν. τοῦτο μὲν δὴ οἷόν ἐστιν, αἱ ἀνατομαὶ τάχα δείξουσιν).

not shy about couching his conclusions in a decisive first person singular.[35] Regardless of how prominent his own role in the process, however, he is witness to a practice of anatomical inquiry, one that, as his forward looking final sentence indicates, is ongoing.

This final sentence raises further interesting questions of its own. As we have seen in earlier authors, referring one's readers to "dissections" (αἱ ἀνατομαί) is an ambiguous move, as this is both a standard way to refer to the practice of dissection and a standard title for anatomical texts. Is Rufus indicating that this is an open research question that future dissections will grapple with?[36] This would certainly be grounds for positing that Rufus is involved in or at least aware of an active program of heuristic dissection, which might therefore argue for widening the scope of the anatomical renaissance that Galen associates solely with Marinus and his school. Alternatively – though not necessarily inconsistent with that broader conclusion – is Rufus indicating an intention to write a more detailed anatomical text, addressing a question to which he already feels that he knows the answer?[37] There are two similar moments elsewhere in his corpus that might support this second interpretation. The first occurs earlier in *On Names*, when Rufus mentions some cranial nerves, and adds that "there will be discussion of these in the dissections (ἐν ταῖς διαιρέσεσιν)."[38] This promise is not followed through anywhere in this text and is phrased differently from the other, fulfilled, cross-reference.[39] In the fulfilled promise he clearly specifies which dissection he means – it is the dissection of the single animal that he has already signaled is soon going to accompany the second half of the text. In the sentence in question, in contrast, Rufus is already in the midst of that dissection and appears to be referring to future, unspecified dissections, or, as the verb more specifically suggests, to the discussion or text that will result from or accompany them. The second similar moment occurs in his *On the Pulse*, which survives only in what seems to be an abridgement and may not even be genuine, thus unfortunately weakening any interpretation that presses too hard on its contents or wording.[40] For what it

---

35 The first person singular appears at *Nom.Part.* 7–8, 88, 134, 155, 206, 229.
36 In this case, the adverb in the sentence (τάχα) should be translated as "perhaps," as I have done.
37 In this interpretation, τάχα might be more accurately rendered as "presently."
38 *Nom.Part.* 145 (ὑπὲρ ὧν ἐν ταῖς διαιρέσεσιν εἰρήσεται).
39 When he says at *Nom.Part.* 29 that he will discuss the membranes of the eye in the second half of the text, he is more concrete about both the timing and the circumstances, saying "it will be discussed a little later, in the dissection of the animal" (εἰρήσεται ὀλίγον ὕστερον ἐν τῇ διαιρέσει τοῦ ζῴου).
40 For this text, see Daremberg and Ruelle (1879), xxvii–xxxi, where Ruelle argues against Daremberg for its authenticity, and 219–32; Menetrier (1924), 97 believes it antedates Rufus, while Harris (1973),

is worth, however, the text as it stands has Rufus tell his readers, "I was planning to refer those desiring to learn [about the movements of the heart] to anatomy (ἐπὶ τὴν ἀνατομήν), but, lest I seem grudging and malicious, I will describe it briefly."[41] It is certainly plausible that this is a reference to the practice of anatomy and that he is suggesting that his readers observe the heart's movements through vivisection; however, the phrasing here is highly suggestive of reference to a book. Galen uses almost identical language for cross-references between his works.[42] All three of these moments might thus plausibly be interpreted to suggest that Rufus was planning to write a more detailed anatomical text; however, any attempt to coordinate the three instances into amalgamated support for such a theory immediately runs into the difficulty that each of them refers to this putative work by a different title. If Rufus does have a new project in mind, it is a nebulously conceived one, and there is no evidence that he ever carried it through.

Regardless of whether we interpret these three passages as references to dissections or to a text describing them, they certainly indicate that Rufus feels that anatomy is a subject actively in progress. Even in moments more strictly related to nomenclature, he indicates that the field is changing and continually updating; he calls out naming practices that he feels to have been proven wrong and suggests that some of the older names might be best retired – even his discussion of the neologisms of the Egyptian doctors, despite its scorn, conveys a sense that the field is burgeoning with activity.[43] However, this conclusion immediately runs up against Galen's assertion that there was a significant lull in anatomical activity that was broken only by the pioneering work of Marinus.[44] While there is uncertainty surrounding the precise dates of both Rufus and Marinus, the general consensus is that Rufus is the earlier figure.[45] This would make the idea

---

181–9, 262–6, though acknowledging the uncertainty, treats it as genuine since he is not aware that "any conclusive evidence has been adduced to show that it could not have been Rufus' work" (263).

[41] *Puls.* III.3 (ἐβουλόμην ἀναπέμπειν τοὺς βουλομένους μαθεῖν ἐπὶ τὴν ἀνατομήν· ἵνα δὲ μὴ δόξω φθονερὸς εἶναι καὶ βάσκανος, διὰ συντόμων παραστήσω).

[42] Galen, *UP* IV.328 (II.424H) (ἄμεινον οὖν μοι δοκεῖ ... ἐπὶ τὴν τῶν ἀνατομικῶν ἐγχειρήσεων ἀναπέμψαι πραγματείαν) and *Hipp.Off.Med.* XVIIIb.663 (ἐνόμισα πρὸς τὴν τοῦ κοινοῦ λόγου πραγματείαν ἀναπέμψαι τὸν βουλόμενον ἀκριβέστερον περὶ τούτων γνῶναι). Indeed, Ruelle (Daremberg and Ruelle [1879], xxviii–ix) latches on to this passage as a reference to *On the Anatomy of the Parts of the Human Body*, supporting his theory that that is a genuine text, even though nothing there corresponds to what is promised here; see Lloyd (1983), 151, n. 107.

[43] *Nom.Part.* 145, 200, 210.

[44] For Galen's description of the lull, see *PHP* V.650 (VIII.1.6 De Lacy).

[45] See, for example, Singer (1925), 42–5, May (1968), 31, Nutton (2013a), 140, 219; Grmek and Gourevitch (1994), 1493 group the two more tightly, but still suggest that Marinus' place is "entre [Rufus] et Galien."

that Rufus was witness to an active anatomical community troublingly at odds with our slender evidence for the period.

There is, however, vanishingly little support for the general assumption that Marinus is Rufus' junior – such a claim is found nowhere in the ancient sources and the chronological evidence does not necessarily enforce it. Adopting the most probable dating for each figure would, in fact, make them contemporaries; indeed, following the equally popular – though also tenuously supported – trend of locating both figures in Alexandria could make them colleagues.[46] This opens up the interesting possibility that the dissections Rufus describes were none other than those performed by Marinus and his school. This is far and away the tidiest solution to this dilemma, but by no means the only one – indeed, one might argue that its very tidiness tends to prejudice against its plausibility. Further, although the likeliest dating for Rufus is about the same as that for Marinus, there is a somewhat less convincing but still not implausible case for dating him to the middle of the first century, which would put him a solid generation or two earlier.

It is therefore necessary to account for three different scenarios: In one, Rufus is on the order of fifty years older than Marinus and thus represents the anatomical scene immediately prior to what Galen characterizes as Marinus' renaissance. In the others, Rufus is a contemporary of Marinus and thus either describes a parallel manifestation of this renewed interest in dissection or is a secondary witness to Marinus' activities. Squaring the first of these three scenarios with both Galen's claim of Marinus' exceptionalism and Rufus' evidence for engaged anatomical practice before him would imply that Galen found Marinus to be pioneering for the *way* he practiced or taught anatomy, rather than for the fact that he did. In other words, dissection had continued to be used for educational purposes during some or all of the "lull," with occasional pockets of deeper interest, but Marinus was the first to transform this into a thriving field of study. Alternatively, one could take Rufus' evidence as grounds to doubt the individuated narrative that Galen presents us with, suspecting that Marinus was simply the most famous outcropping of a movement that had broader and earlier roots.

If we instead turn to the scenarios in which they are more or less contemporaries, the tensions in the evidence are lessened. We could eliminate them altogether through the tidy dovetailing of both Rufus' and Galen's

---

[46] For Rufus' dates and location in Alexandria, see this chapter, nn. 6 and 15, respectively; for Marinus, see this chapter, n. 59 for his dating and n. 85 for the speculation that he, too, was in Alexandria.

evidence and believe that Rufus witnessed and described Marinus' teaching. Alternatively, we can take Rufus as amplifying the picture that Galen paints; in this – to me the most likely – scenario, Marinus would emerge as simply the most visible or the most famous name attached to a groundswell of renewed interest in dissection that took place several decades before Galen's birth. In short, however one arranges the dates, the most likely takeaway is that Marinus' anatomical interests did not spring up in a vacuum. While I suspect that dissection, though perhaps not a prominent or universal feature in the late Hellenistic period, never completely went away as a teaching tool, it seems that in the later first and early second centuries AD the sociopolitical and intellectual climate in the Roman empire was such as to nurture an increased interest in pursuing this art.[47] Marinus emerged as the most visible name by taking the most influential approach to this renewed wave of practice and, as we will shortly explore, by his notable innovation in developing a new genre of anatomical writing, which more deeply integrated texts into the study and teaching of anatomy and, no doubt, served to fix him as the premier name in the renaissance. Certainly, Rufus' text is not terribly innovative: It remains squarely a handbook of anatomical data, containing no instructions or encouragement to dissect and only very occasional information that moves beyond mere nomenclature.[48] No matter what broader experience with dissection or views on the state of the field of anatomy we might seem to descry in the background, *On Names* is very much a traditional, if quite linguistically focused, handbook.

Yet, although it did not strike Galen as an anatomical text worthy of any mention, *On Names* does seem to have resonated with its wider audience. The first half, on the external parts of the body, enjoyed particular popularity. Already in the second century, Pollux was freely plundering it to fill the second book of his *Onomasticon* on the parts of the body, and the author of the pseudo-Galenic *Doctor: Introduction* may also show familiarity with it, though the identity of their subject matter may be sufficient

---

[47] Celsus' endorsement (*DM* proem.74) of dissection as a teaching tool, though possibly to some degree rhetorical, also enforces the idea of a certain level of sustained interest in the practice prior to its resurgence, but it does not seem to have been deep or widespread; see also the discussion in Chapter 2, n. 178.

[48] This is not to say that the anatomical contents are not of interest for those tracing the development of anatomical knowledge. As May (1968), 29–31 enumerates, Rufus provides a valuable, non-Galenic window into the lost world of Hellenistic anatomy; clearly, however, I do not fully agree with her assessment that "his dissections were made in order to verify anatomical facts already a part of the tradition and demonstrate them to students, not in order to add further facts to that tradition" (29).

to explain the similarities.[49] In the fourth century, Oribasius generously excerpts the first half of the text in his collection of medical extracts, and these same sections circulated separately in an epitome of uncertain date.[50] In addition to launching these varied spin-offs, *On Names* cemented Rufus' name as an anatomical one, resulting in two further texts being attributed to him: *On the Anatomy of the Parts of the Human Body* and *On Bones*. These two brief treatises likely date to more or less the same era as Rufus and can plausibly be considered to be the work of the same author or even to be two parts of one original whole.[51] *Anatomy* offers a description of the internal parts of the body, not including the skeletal system, which is handled in *On Bones*. The introductory sentence of the latter frames the text as a sequel to a complete discussion of the internal parts, serving as a nice segue from the one to the other. The introductory paragraph of the former, however, has a noticeably different feel from the rest of the text, suggesting that its claim to follow on a complete discussion of the external parts was a later addition, perhaps added to smooth the transition from the epitome of the first half of *On Names*, with which it eventually circulated.[52]

The basic structure and genre of these texts is the same as that of Rufus' *On Names*, but their character is noticeably different.[53] Rufus sets out to catalogue anatomical nomenclature – to make it possible for all anatomical texts and conversations, past, present, and future, to be mutually intelligible. His is a pointedly scholarly undertaking. The two pseudonymous texts, in contrast, smell far less of the library. Where Rufus' work is peppered with references to specific authors and their names for things, these texts are almost completely devoid of this type of direct attribution. *On Bones* references no historical figures, and *Anatomy* does so only twice, each time to a different end than *On Names*. In the first instance, the author gives Herophilus' description of the internal anatomy of the eye, but not his actual terminology; in the second, at the very end of the

---

[49] For Pollux, the apparatus in Bethe (1900) signals the parallels to Rufus, many of which were also collected in Haupt (1869), 224–8; cf. Kowalski (1960), 12. For *Int.*, Sideras (1994), 1132 claims that in *Int.* "finden sich zum Teil wörtliche Zitate des Rufus"; however, Kowalski (1960), 11 is skeptical of direct influence, and Petit (2009), xxix (n. 34) and 133–43 treats Rufus as a parallel for the text rather than a source.

[50] Oribasius, *Coll.Med.* XXV.1; for the epitome, with cross-references to *Nom.Part.*, see Daremberg and Ruelle (1879), 233–6. For the relationship between these two very similar, but not completely identical texts, see Sideras (1994), 1132–3.

[51] Nickel (2009), 71, 74 (cf. this chapter, n. 10); *Anatomy* mentions Asclepiades, but not Galen, which suggests a date somewhere between the first century BC and the mid-second century AD.

[52] Nickel (2009), 65–7.

[53] For broader stylistic analyses of why this text ought not to be attributed to Rufus, see Ilberg (1930), 9–12, Lloyd (1983), 151, n. 107, and Nickel (2009).

treatise, he describes the contrasting views of Erasistratus, Herophilus, and Asclepiades on the differentiation (or not) of motor and sensory nerves.[54] This second moment reads much more as a medical than a linguistic history, which fits with the tenor of the text as a whole.

The pseudonymous works in general have a more practical medical focus than *On Names*. *Anatomy* repeatedly mentions the consequences when various parts of the body are injured and includes descriptions of the appearance and physiology of body parts along with their names.[55] *On Bones* even describes the clavicle by comparing it to a medical catheter, suggesting an audience of practicing doctors.[56] Notably, however, these texts have much less to offer on dissection than *On Names* does: There is no direct discussion of the practice. One would not expect to find anything of the sort in *On Bones* with its more desiccated subject matter, though there is some allusion there to the direct observation of bones.[57] *Anatomy*, however, has exactly the same scope for including dissection as *On Names*, but does not use it.[58] Because we are dealing with only two data points here, it is difficult to draw any really solid conclusions from this difference. One might try to argue that this absence of interest in dissection could be grounds to date the pseudonymous texts earlier than *On Names*, placing them before any beginning of a revival of interest in the practice. However, there are dissection-free anatomical handbooks circulating even in the anatomical heyday of Galen's lifetime, suggesting that it is more likely that the texts' different characters simply reflect the different agendas of the authors. To my mind, the most plausible inference – if it is permissible to extrapolate broadly from such small indications – is that the circles interested in anatomical research in this period overlapped with those taking a philological and academic approach to medicine. In other words, the exegesis of Hippocrates and the dissection of monkeys, disparate as they seem, were hallmarks of the same kind of medical thinking, and there were other, more workaday, circles less interested in both.

---

[54] *Diss.Hum.* 12, 72–4.

[55] Injury: *Diss.Hum.* 21, 30, 51, 55. For a sense of the more descriptive tenor, compare, for example, *Nom.Part.* 147 and *Diss.Hum.* 4–6 on the membranes of the brain or *Nom.Part.* 57 and *Diss.Hum.* 19 on the tongue.

[56] *Oss.* 12.

[57] *Oss.* 40.

[58] The single reference to cutting – that no loss of function occurs if the uvula is cut off (*Diss.Hum.* 21) – is far more likely to be a surgical comment than a vivisectory one, especially given the parallels at *Diss.Hum.* 51 and 55. The author also references animal anatomy comparatively (cf. *Diss.Hum.* 3), but, as we have seen, this is a standard feature in anatomical texts dating back to the Classical period and is not comparable to the explicit dissection described in *Nom.Part.*

Marinus

As we saw in the discussion of Rufus, Marinus (*fl.* early second century AD)[59] holds a place as a pivotal figure in the history of dissection and of anatomical texts. This reputation is entirely owing to Galen, who provides all of the extant references to this otherwise forgotten physician.[60] He says that it was Marinus "who reviv[ed] anatomical study after the ancients, as it had been neglected in the intervening time."[61] My analysis of Rufus' texts has already called into question the extent to which Marinus deserves unilateral credit for the renewal of interest in dissection; indeed, Galen himself introduces a larger cast of characters in his commentary on *Nature of Man*, closely grouping Marinus and his younger contemporary Numisianus, followed by the latter's son Heracleianus, as the successors to Herophilus and Erasistratus.[62] However, there is little doubt that he was a central figure in the new anatomical scene. Galen says that he was "well-versed in the knowledge of anatomy and had studied it thoroughly," calls him "the most skillful of all anatomists and the one with the most detailed knowledge," and offers him as an example of those "who dedicate the whole of their lives to this study [of anatomy]."[63]

The most detailed insight that we have into writing by Marinus is Galen's description of his "anatomical books in twenty parts," which, for clarity,

---

[59] This is my own estimate of his dating, based on Galen's comment that Marinus was of his grandparents' generation at *Hipp.Epid.II.* 4.1 (*CMG Suppl.Or.* V.2, p. 623); Galen was born in AD 129 and one might reasonably put the age of his grandfathers at between fifty and seventy at the time of his birth. This in turn suggests a generation born around AD 60–80 and therefore a possible range of professional activity from about AD 80 to AD 150, at which point it is clear from Galen's focus on learning from his students that Marinus himself was no longer living. Scholarship has been somewhat divided on the question of Marinus' dates. A common approach is to give the very narrow *floruit* of *c.* AD 129, based on Galen's birthday and his remarks about his grandparents, as Deichgräber (1930), Singer (1957), 45 (at *c.* AD 120), Grmek and Gourevitch (1994), 1494, Manetti and Roselli (1994), 1580, Boudon-Millot (2007), 201 and (2012), 50, Ross and Nutton (2016); others trend earlier, suggesting around AD 100 (Smith [1979], 66, Fig. I, Garofalo [1994], 1819) or the end of the first century AD and into the first decades of the second (Sarton [1927], I.281, von Staden [2004], 210, Nutton [2013*a*], 140, 219).

[60] The two references to Marinus in Oribasius (*Coll.Med.* XXV.57.23, 31) are themselves excerpted from Galen. Osen (2022), which appeared just as this book was going to press, offers a new study of Marinus, advocating for greater attention to his importance and exploring some of his anatomical discoveries; my thanks to Christopher Cosans for bringing it to my attention.

[61] Galen, *PHP* V.650 (VIII.1.6 De Lacy) (ὁ μετὰ τοὺς παλαιοὺς ἐν τῷ μεταξὺ χρόνῳ τὴν ἀνατομικὴν θεωρίαν ἠμελημένην ἀνακτησάμενος).

[62] Galen, *Hipp.Nat.Hom.* XV.136.

[63] Galen, *Hipp.Epid.II* 4.1 (*CMG Suppl.Or.* V.2, pp. 623, 675, trans. Vagelpohl and Swain); *AA* II.621 (οἱ τὸν ὅλον ἑαυτῶν βίον ἀναθέντες τῇ θεωρίᾳ ταύτῃ); cf. *AA* S233.

I will refer to as the large anatomy.[64] Galen was sufficiently impressed by this masterwork to create his own summary of it in four books and to rank this summary as a useful addition to his own anatomical output.[65] Although neither Marinus' original nor Galen's summary survive, Galen does take the trouble to enumerate the contents of both in his *On My Own Books*.[66] From this detailed table of contents, we can learn a good deal. First of all, it is apparent that Marinus was not operating with the internal/external dichotomy that is so central in Rufus and the texts attributed to him. He instead adopts Aristotle's more formal organizational principle, beginning his work with a discussion of the homoeomerous parts before moving on to the compound parts; it seems likely, indeed, that he was directly influenced by *Parts of Animals*, where Aristotle articulates the reasons for approaching the study of the body in this way.[67] His first six books, which Galen grouped into the first book of his summary, center on the homoeomerous parts, namely the skin, hair, nails, flesh, fat, and suet, followed by various internal membranes, then the veins and arteries, together with other vessels, like the ureters, and the liquids they contain, and finally the bones. He then pivots to the compound parts, turning, in books seven through ten, which comprise Galen's second grouping, to a head-to-toe look at what one might call the nonsystemic parts of the body; the major focus is on the musculature, but he also includes things like the teeth, the gums, the epiglottis, the ears, the tonsils and other assorted parts of the body that are neither homoeomerous nor central parts of the digestive or respiratory systems. The third group of books, the eleventh through the fifteenth, begin again at the top of the body, but this time deal with the major internal organs and with the vascular system, while the final five books address the brain and nervous system.

Galen's enumeration of these chapters not only gives us a good indication of the contents of the large anatomy, but also offers several insights

---

[64] Galen, *Lib.Prop.* XIX.25 (τῶν Μαρίνου βιβλίων ἀνατομικῶν εἴκοσιν ὄντων).

[65] Galen, *Lib.Prop.* XIX.25; Nutton (1993), 18, and Boudon-Millot (2012), 53 offer the plausible speculation that Galen's summary was the work of his student days.

[66] Galen, *Lib.Prop.* XIX.25–30 (4.9–33 Boudon-Millot [2007]); significant portions of this section are missing in Kühn and have been restored by Boudon-Millot.

[67] Aristotle, *PA* II.1 (646a13–b36), 2 (647b10–29); the organizational division between homoeomerous and compound parts is also active in *HA*, but it is less emphasized and the order of the two categories is inverted. Aristotle, of course, also used the internal/external dichotomy to organize his texts, especially *HA*, but I do not think that Rufus, who clearly articulates a different reason for his arrangement, was consciously hearkening back to this. To my knowledge, no one has noticed this Aristotelian organization of Marinus' text before; indeed, May (1968), latching on presumably to the repetition of the vascular system, criticizes the text as "rambling" (p. 40), "diffuse, poorly arranged, and repetitive" (p. 33).

into its broader character. First of all, the Aristotelian organizational scheme appears to have run deeper than just the ordering of topics, judging by the repetition of the vascular system in the third and fourth chapters and then again in the fourteenth and fifteenth. In the first pair of chapters, the veins and arteries are being handled as homoeomerous objects in and of themselves, as underscored by their juxtaposition with other tubular structures in the body, such as the ureters, spermatic vessels, and glandular ducts; Marinus handles here the character, contents, origins, and activities of the veins, arteries, and "vessels perceptible by reason," which last are likely the capillaries already hypothesized in the Hellenistic period.[68] The second appearance of the veins and arteries, in contrast, considers them in the broader context of the compound organs, and describes their paths and connections rather than their essence, beginning with the veins above the liver in the fourteenth book, followed in the fifteenth by the vein between the liver and heart (*inferior vena cava*), the veins below the diaphragm, and all of the arteries.[69] The whole text also appears to have vacillated between more strictly anatomical topics and more physiological ones. Galen indicates that Marinus systematically broached various historically contested questions of function, including the presence of blood in the arteries, the transit of drink through the lungs, the entrance of air into the stomach, and the pulsation of the brain and whether it participates directly in respiration.[70]

Galen's references to Marinus in other contexts can also help to round out our understanding of this text. We learn that he engaged in some discussion of earlier sources and historical nomenclature in his anatomical work, which is not at all surprising given that we know that he also, like Rufus and seemingly all of his own students, took an exegetical interest in Hippocrates.[71] Galen also makes clear what the highlights of Marinus'

---

[68] Galen, *Lib.Prop.* XIX.25–6 (τῶν λόγῳ θεωρητῶν ἀγγείων); it is conceivable that the hypothetical vessels might also refer to the microvessels contained in Erasistratus' *triplokia*, though the context and lack of comment to the effect make this less likely.

[69] Galen, *Lib.Prop.* XIX.29.

[70] Galen, *Lib.Prop.* XIX.26, 28–9; indeed, Boudon-Millot's restored text suggests that at least one of these debates may have been given its own subheading, at XIX.28 (4.23 Boudon-Millot [2007]); see her discussion Boudon-Millot (2007), 204, n. 1.

[71] For historical discussions in his anatomical text, see Galen, *AA* II.716 (cf. *Lib.Prop.* XIX.30, though it is unclear whether the reference to Hippocrates and Eudemus there originated with Marinus or with Galen); for his work on Hippocrates, see Galen *Hipp.Aph.* XVIIIa.123, 163–4, *Hipp. Epid.II* 4.2 (*CMG Suppl.Or.* V.2, p. 687), *Hipp.Epid.VI* 5.14 (*CMG* V.10.2.2, p. 287–8). Smith (1979), 67 expresses some doubt as to whether or not Marinus wrote full-fledged commentaries on Hippocrates; regardless, it is certainly clear that he took an interest in elucidating Hippocrates' writings and opinions, whether in dedicated treatises or within his own anatomical work.

anatomical contributions were. He repeatedly emphasizes his continued importance in the area of the nerves: Marinus made some new discoveries and established an updated system of numbering and labeling the nerves that had become standard by Galen's day.[72] He may even have written a dedicated treatise on the origins of the nerves; in the section of his *Anatomical Procedures* preserved in Arabic, Galen mentions Marinus' "work on the roots of the nerves," though the fact that fully a quarter of the large anatomy relates to the brain and nervous system makes it possible that it is to one of the books there that Galen is referring.[73] Certainly, the lengthy discussion in his large anatomy would have showcased his extensive and innovative work. Similarly, Galen singles out Marinus as being the most accurate of everyone who had written on the muscles prior to himself; he notes, however, that even he was not without error and, further, that he did not address the topic in a dedicated book, nor even in an uninterrupted fashion.[74] This criticism chimes nicely with the hodgepodge of topics present in the seventh through tenth books of the large anatomy, as Galen describes them, while indicating that the discussion of the muscles there was of a notably high standard. Galen also points out his description of the bones – which he explicitly situates as a part of the large anatomy – as having been particularly good.[75] Galen's praise of Marinus' work on glands, presumably referring to the contents of the second book, is especially interesting since it refers to the section of the work dealing with the homoeomerous parts; his extensive discussion of it confirms the different agenda of that part of the text.[76] This section did not contain merely a list of the different glands in the body or a description of their anatomical situations; Marinus begins, rather, by considering glands together as a class and dividing them, in good Aristotelian fashion, into two types – those that stabilize and those that produce fluids – and then describing the characteristic substance of each type. Finally, Galen reiterates that Marinus' writing was based on his own personal dissections and that "it was he himself who had set his hand to and had observed everything that he explained in his writings"; this is a point well worth mentioning.[77] With the complacent disinterest of the Herophileans on

---

[72] Discovery at *Nerv.Diss.* II.837; numbering and labeling at *Nerv.Diss.* II.837, 839, *UP* III.575, IV.294 (I.418, II.398H), *AA* SII–12, 246, *Hipp.Epid.II* 4.2 (*CMG Suppl.Or.* V.2, p. 687).

[73] *AA* SII.

[74] Galen, *Musc.Diss.* II.926.

[75] Galen, *AA* S233.

[76] Galen, *Sem.* IV.646–8.

[77] Galen, *AA* S233; cf. *Hipp.Epid.II* 4.1 (*CMG Suppl.Or.* V.2, p. 623).

one end and the secondhand observations of Rufus on the other, it had been, so far as we can tell, nearly four centuries since anyone had premised a book on observations from their own active manipulation of animal bodies. All told, then, Marinus' large anatomy must have been an ambitious, enormous, and cutting-edge anatomical treatise, combining Aristotelian structure and an early Hellenistic commitment to hands-on research.

There is one topic, however, that I think we can confidently believe to have been a book distinct from the large anatomy. Galen credits Marinus with being the first to write an *Anatomical Procedures*, the last and most detailed of the anatomical genres I laid out at the beginning of Chapter 6. Galen's story is romantic but, like most romanticized history, does not bear much scrutiny or offer much substantive information:

> I do not blame the ancients for not writing anatomical procedures, but I do praise Marinus for having written one. For the ancients it was superfluous to write memoranda, either for themselves or for others, since they trained with their fathers from childhood: just as they trained to read and write, so they trained to dissect. Indeed, the ancients were sufficiently zealous about anatomy, not just the doctors, but philosophers too. And there was certainly no danger for anyone who had learned in this way of forgetting the method of the procedures—no more than those who had trained since childhood would forget how to write the letters of the alphabet. But since, as time passed, it seemed to be wise to share the art, not just with family, but with outsiders as well, immediately from that moment this degraded the art.... Formerly, there was no need of anatomical procedures, nor of the type of handbooks, which Diocles, as far as I know, was first to write.[78]

According to this view of things, the purported decline of medicine must already have begun in the fourth century BC, necessitating Diocles' innovation. Yet, at that time, Marinus' contribution was still centuries in the future, and the Hellenistic golden age of anatomy was only just dawning. Galen offers here, then, no real catalyst for Marinus' work, only an elaborate excuse for his inability to find plausible Hippocratic antecedents for

---

[78] Galen, *AA* II.280–2 (οὔτε τοῖς παλαιοῖς μέμφομαι μὴ γράψασιν ἀνατομικὰς ἐγχειρήσεις, καὶ Μαρῖνον ἐπαινῶ γράψαντα. τοῖς μὲν γὰρ περιττὸν ἦν αὐτοῖς ἢ ἑτέροις ὑπομνήματα γράφεσθαι παρὰ τοῖς γονεῦσιν ἐκ παίδων ἀσκουμένοις, ὥσπερ ἀναγινώσκειν καὶ γράφειν, οὕτως ἀνατέμνειν. ἱκανῶς γὰρ ἐσπουδάκασιν οἱ παλαιοὶ τὴν ἀνατομήν, οὐκ ἰατροὶ μόνον, ἀλλὰ καὶ φιλόσοφοι. οὔκουν φόβος ἦν ἐπιλαθέσθαι τοῦ τρόπου τῶν ἐγχειρήσεων οὐδενὶ τῶν οὕτω μαθόντων, οὐ μᾶλλον ἢ τοῦ γράφειν τὰ περὶ φωνῆς στοιχεῖα τοῖς ἀσκηθεῖσιν ἐκ παίδων καὶ ταῦτα. ἐπεὶ δὲ, τοῦ χρόνου προϊόντος, οὐ τοῖς ἐγγόνοις μόνον, ἀλλὰ καὶ τοῖς ἔξω τοῦ γένους ἔδοξε καλὸν εἶναι μεταδιδόναι τῆς τέχνης, εὐθὺς μὲν τοῦτο πρῶτον ἀπολώλει, [τὸ μηκέτι ἐκ παίδων ἀσκεῖσθαι τὰς ἀνατομὰς αὐτούς] ... ἔμπροσθεν δ' οὐ μόνον ἐγχειρήσεων ἀνατομικῶν, ἀλλ' οὐδὲ συγγραμμάτων ἐδεῖτο τοιούτων· ὁποῖα Διοκλῆς μὲν ὧν οἶδα πρῶτος ἔγραψεν); following the text in Garofalo (1986–2000).

it; neither does he offer any description of Marinus' innovatory text. We are left to wonder at its length, its character, and its contents, being assured only that it was sufficiently "lacking and unclear" to warrant Galen writing one of his own.[79]

The most we can glean about Marinus' *Anatomical Procedures* is that it was "a single large book."[80] Galen also tells us that the initial two-book version of his own procedures followed the same order as Marinus' and that he subsequently changed the order in his rewrite to follow that of his own *Usefulness of the Parts*.[81] Together, these two pieces of information suggest that the character of Galen's first *Anatomical Procedures* was very similar to Marinus'. At two books, Galen's offering would likely not have been that different in length from Marinus' one long one; Galen's criticisms of the clarity and completeness of his predecessor's version suggest that his initial impetus was simply to write a more thorough and user-friendly version of a manual that he had found to be helpful.[82] As for the contents and purpose of the text, we must assume that they were the same as Galen's extant procedures – a series of instructions for how to dissect, rather than description of the anatomy made visible by dissection. It is this move to capture the instructions in writing that seems to have been Marinus' biggest innovation and to have initiated what Galen considers to be a new genre. All this effectively precludes any idea that Marinus' *Procedures* was identical to or a part of the large anatomy.[83] We are dealing with a self-contained, coherent, and novel unit, and there is nothing in Galen's enumeration of the twenty books of the large anatomy that would correspond to it.

The encyclopedic coverage and careful research of the large work on anatomy and the innovatory nature of the work on procedure cemented Marinus' name as an important one, and his books were apparently plentiful in Rome.[84] Yet in many ways his influence seems to have been

---

[79] Galen, *AA* II.283 (ἐλλιπεῖς τε ἅμα καὶ ἀσαφεῖς); cf. II.470 (ἀσαφὲς μὲν τὴν ἑρμηνείαν, ἐλλιπὲς δὲ τὴν θεωρίαν).

[80] Galen, *AA* II.470 (ἓν … μέγα βιβλίον).

[81] Galen, *AA* II.234. For the initial version of Galen's text, which is not extant, see Chapter 8, "The First *Anatomical Procedures* (*AA₁*)" at pp. 278–87, where I also suggest that Marinus' text may have followed the order of his large anatomy, in the same way that Galen's second *AA* is linked to his *UP*.

[82] For further comparison of the two works, including their possible lengths, see Chapter 8, "The First *Anatomical Procedures* (*AA₁*)" at pp. 279–81.

[83] Scholarship to date has generally assumed or implied that these two texts are the same; see May (1968), 33, Grmek and Gourevitch (1994), 1494–7, Boudon-Millot (2012), 50, Nutton (2013a), 219, and Osen (2022), 232.

[84] Galen complains that he is unable to track down a specific work by Marinus on Hippocrates and emphasizes that its scarcity is strange, given that "very many of Marinus' writings are to be found in Rome" at *Hipp.Epid.VI* 5.14 (*CMG* V.10.2.2, p. 288) (from Pfaff's German translation of the Arabic).

rapidly outdated by the success of his own school. Marinus' students and his students' students comprised the stars of the anatomical world during Galen's medical education, and the contemporary books with which Galen's work is most in dialogue are theirs. There has been some debate about the location and formality of Marinus' "school." The general tendency is to assume that Alexandria was the center of his and his students' activities and teaching; while there are various reasons that might make this a tempting solution, there is no evidence that directly supports it.[85] Indeed, there is just as much reason to link him with Rome.[86] What is clear, however, is that, wherever he expounded them, Marinus' twin legacies of anatomy and Hippocratic exegesis rapidly became widespread; his students and their disciples are associated, as we shall see, with Rome, Alexandria, Pergamon, Smyrna, Corinth, and beyond.[87] The wave of anatomical resurgence, far from being a localized concern, washed across the intellectual centers of the Eastern Mediterranean and, inevitably, their capital.

Quintus and His Students

Quintus

The one figure we can confidently list as a direct disciple of Marinus is Quintus (d. *c.* AD 145).[88] Galen tells us that he was the most distinguished of Marinus' students, who were many and varied; in fact, Quintus' reputation appears to have effectively overshadowed those of his peers, since we

---

[85] von Staden (2004) offers a survey of the prevalence of this assumption in scholarship (p. 210, n. 118) and queries its validity, pointing out the lack of supporting evidence for Marinus' location there, as well as for the idea that it was the main seat of anatomical study generally in this period (pp. 209–14); the assumption persists, however, as in Boudon-Millot (2012), 50 and Osen (2022), 225–6.

[86] See this chapter, n. 99.

[87] Hippocratic exegesis dated back to the Hellenistic period and was not exclusively Marinus' legacy, nor was anatomy, as I argue throughout this chapter, but they were the joint cornerstones of his teaching, and all of his students appear to have sustained his interest in them. Indeed, Gourevitch (1998), 117–20 dubs Marinus and his intellectual followers the "Anonymous Sect" and views these as two of their hallmarks.

[88] Galen tells us that "he was preeminent in the time of Hadrian" (*AA* S231) and that he died shortly before the period when Galen was studying with Satyrus at Pergamon in AD 146–7 (*AA* II.225); see Grmek and Gourevitch (1994), 1512. The Arabic tradition of *Hipp.Epid.VI* XVIIb.151 suggests that Quintus was of Galen's father's generation – something that his *floruit* under Hadrian and his status as the student of Marinus, who was of Galen's grandparents' generation, would already confirm; the Greek tradition of the same text, however, indicates instead that Quintus was from Galen's fatherland of Pergamon (κατὰ τὴν πατρίδα); see Grmek and Gourevitch (1994), 1505, n. 45.

cannot name any of these others with certainty.[89] It is clear that he carried on his master's emphasis in anatomy. Galen describes him as "a most anatomical man," who had "gained a not inconsiderable reputation through anatomical perspicacity," and recounts one of his apparently memorable vivisectory dissections.[90] Further, his students were adept dissectors, confirming that this formed a major part of his legacy. Like Marinus, he had other interests as well: We hear of his successful medical practice, his work on Hippocratic texts, and his opinions on the compounding of drugs.[91] Unlike Marinus, however, he did not leave behind any written works. Galen complains that "he composed no writings on anatomy such as Marinus did" and that it is therefore impossible to know whether or not Quintus had anticipated a discovery that Galen made, inferring grumpily that either he had not or he "concealed it from us and grudged it to us."[92] In a more charitable mood, he groups Quintus with no less than Socrates and Pythagoras as examples of people who "did not write any treatises," and consoles himself that, like those great figures, Quintus had students who were willing and able to witness to his teachings.[93]

What he lacked in literary output, Quintus made up for in personality. He was, by all accounts, a memorable character, and his students were not loath to recount either his teachings or his more colorful episodes. Galen tells us of his fame and success as a practitioner in Rome: He was "the best doctor of his generation" and one of "the famous doctors of our time."[94] Although this high standing brought him rich and important patients, he was not one to court wealth or curry favor. In a clearly much-enjoyed anecdote, he arrives one morning, stinking of wine, at the bedside of a "wealthy and very powerful man"; when the headache-ridden patient recoils and raises a polite objection, Quintus gauchely tells him to put up with it, retorting that he has had to endure

---

[89] Galen, *HNH* XV.136.

[90] Galen, *Lib.Prop.* XIX.22 (ἀνδρὸς ἀνατομικωτάτου), a comment that he puts in the mouth of another doctor; *AA* S231. For the vivisection, see *AA* S155 and the end of this section.

[91] Practice: *AA* S231, *HNH* XV.68, *Praen.* XIV.602; Hippocratic work: *Hipp.Prorrh.* XVI.751, *Hipp.Epid.I* XVIIa.6, 24–5, 99 (see *CMG Suppl.Or.* V.1, p. 75, 99–101, 193), *Hipp.Epid.II* 2.7 (*CMG Suppl.Or.* V.2, p. 309), *Hipp.Epid.III* XVIIa.502, 506, 515, *Hipp.Epid.VI* XVIIb.302, *Hipp.Aph.* XVIIb.562, *Hipp.Off. Med.* XVIIIb.654, *Ord.Lib.Prop.* XIX.57–8; pharmacology: *SMT* XII.15, *Comp.Med.Loc.* XII.385, 606, *Ant.* XIV.69–71. For further analysis of these interests, see Grmek and Gourevitch (1994), 1505–11.

[92] Galen, *AA* S230–1.

[93] Galen, *HNH* XV.68 (μηδ᾽ ἔγραψαν ... σύγγραμμα μηδέν) and 136, where he again confirms that Quintus "wrote neither any other book nor an anatomical one" (οὔτ᾽ ἄλλο τι βιβλίον οὔτ᾽ ἀνατομικὸν ἔγραψε), but adds that his students Satyrus and Lycus did.

[94] Galen, *Praen.* XIV.602 (βελτίων μὲν ὢν ἰατρὸς τῶν καθ᾽ἑαυτόν); *HNH* XV.68 (τῶν καθ᾽ ἡμᾶς ἐνδόξων ἰατρῶν Κόιντος); *Hipp.Epid.VI* XVIIb.151 locates him in Rome.

the patient's fever-stink, which is far nastier than winey breath.[95] His students were full of such reminiscences, and there were favorite stories among them; it is through them that Galen comes to convey not only Quintus' opinions on pharmacology and Hippocratic exegesis, but also his rude jokes.[96] All in all, Quintus appears to have been a larger-than-life figure, and his anatomical feats very probably enhanced his persona. The only specific instance that Galen relates is his memorable vivisection of the testicles of a goat. As I have explored already in Chapter 3, this was likely a public demonstration, which Quintus jazzed up by tying the goat upright on his hind legs to make the testicles appear as human as possible; one can imagine the ribald spin a man of his tastes might have put on the commentary.[97] His most spectacular moment in Rome, however, may have been his departure. In two different texts, Galen describes how a cabal of jealous rivals purportedly brought him up on charges of murdering his patients and had him ousted from Rome to live the remainder of his life in exile.[98] Where he went when he left Rome – like whence he came when he arrived, assuming he was not a native – is an open question; however, it is clear that the most noteworthy part of his career was in the capital city, and it is reasonable to suppose that many of his students learned from him there, making Rome an established powerhouse for anatomical education before Galen's arrival.[99]

---

[95] Galen, *Hipp.Epid.VI* XVIIb.151 (τινα τῶν πλουσίων τε καὶ πολὺ δυναμένων ἀνδρῶν). Palladius adopts this same anecdote in his sixth century commentary on *Epidemics VI* (II.113 Dietz); cf. Grmek and Gourevitch (1994), 1506.

[96] Because of his lack of writings, all of the medical and editorial opinions that Galen attributes to Quintus (see this chapter, n. 91) must have been orally transmitted. Galen passes on some jokes at *San.Tu.* VI.228 (cf. the analysis at Grmek and Gourevitch [1994], 1506–7) and adds, at *Ant.* XIV.69–71, that Satyrus, laughing, conveyed to him some of Quintus' pharmacological dictums and that he had heard one of them "not only from Satyrus, but also from others of Quintus' students" (οὐ παρὰ Σατύρου μόνον, ἀλλὰ καὶ ἄλλων μαθητῶν ἤκουσα τοῦ Κοίντου).

[97] See Chapter 3, "Performance for Public Display" at pp. 75–6.

[98] Galen, *Praen.* XIV.602; cf. *Opt.Med.Cogn.* 3.3 (*CMG Suppl.Or.* IV, p. 53). Schlange-Schöningen (2003), 77 suggests that Quintus rather took matters into his own hands and left before Rome became too hot to hold him.

[99] We know that Lycus traveled there in order to study with Quintus (see this chapter, "Quintus and His Students: Lycus" at p. 249) and that Quintus' student Antigenes was also established in Rome (see this chapter, n. 103); further, the fact that this same Antigenes also spent time with Marinus opens the interesting possibility that some of Marinus' teaching may have been located in Rome as well. Indeed, Schlange-Schöningen (2003), 74–5, 83 has suggested that Satyrus also came from Rome before taking up his teaching in Pergamon. On the possibility that Pergamon was Quintus' native city, see this chapter, n. 88; I incline towards the Arabic reading of that passage, but even if the Greek reading is true, it seems unlikely that he went to Pergamon after his departure from Rome without Galen having remarked as much.

Antigenes, Aiphicianos, and Satyrus

Galen was sufficiently impressed with Quintus' reputation for anatomy that he decided to reconstruct his unwritten teachings by systematically seeking out his students to learn from them.[100] He says that he "took great pains to meet" all of Quintus' students, travelling extensively for this purpose while pursuing his education and "shrinking neither from length of road nor of sea voyage."[101] Some of these students had substantial reputations in their own right, while others' significance did not go much further than their ability to give insight into Quintus' teachings. In this latter group we might put Satyrus, who was Galen's own teacher in Pergamon, Antigenes, and Aiphicianos. Aiphicianos is remarkable only for having inflected Quintus' teachings with Stoicism; Galen lists him among his teachers, perhaps in Corinth, but the man does not seem to have otherwise made much of an impression.[102] Antigenes appears to have been among Quintus' earlier pupils since he may also have studied directly with Marinus, whom Galen says he "associated with"; like his teacher, Antigenes also operated in Rome, where he reached the top of the medical scene, "treating all the very powerful people" in the city.[103] Far from seeking him out as a potential conduit to his master's thought, however, Galen's only interaction with him – as far as he tells us – was an unpleasant interchange at a patient's bedside; he rejoices in having bested him there and thereby

---

[100] Galen was not equally impressed with Quintus' work on Hippocrates (*Ord.Lib.Prop.* XIX.57–8).

[101] Galen, *AA* S232, II.470 (μήθ' ὁδοῦ μῆκος ὀκνήσας μήτε πλοῦν); cf. his travels in search of Numisianus, discussed in the following section.

[102] Galen, *Hipp.Off.Med.* XVIIIb.654, *Ord.Lib.Prop.* XIX.58, appearing both times in apposition to Satyrus; cf. *Hipp.Epid.III* XVIIa.575 (a difficult bit of text, edited, with input from the Arabic tradition, at *CMG* V.10.2.1, p. 59) and *Hipp.Epid.VI* (*CMG* V.10.2.2, p. 287). Both his Stoic predilections are not mentioned, but he is again in the company of Satyrus. Both Smith (1979), 70, and Mattern (2013), 41 have suggested that these Stoic leanings indicate that he may have been the Pneumatist teacher Galen mentions at *Hipp.Elem.* I.462–5. The spelling of his name is variable, but all of these instances likely refer to same person; see Moraux (1983) and Grmek and Gourevitch (1994), 1520–1. Galen says at *Hipp.Epid.III* XVIIa.575 (cf. *CMG* V.10.2.1, p. 59) that Aiphicianos, in addition to Satyrus, was his teacher (confirming the reconstruction of a passage in a Renaissance forgery of a Galenic commentary on the Hippocratic *Humors*, which may nevertheless draw on ancient information; see Moraux [1983], 86); this supports the likely transliteration of his name in a passage in a thirteenth-century Arabic text, which says that Galen traveled to Corinth to study with him (Grmek and Gourevitch [1994], 1514), though this interpretation is not without its own complications, as explored in this chapter, n. 116.

[103] Galen, *Praen.* XIV.613, where the association with Marinus is in contrast to his more clearly defined relationship as "one of the students of Quintus" (εἷς τῶν Κοίντου μαθητῶν, συγγεγονὼς δὲ καὶ Μαρίνῳ … ἅπαντάς τε τοὺς πολὺ δυναμένους ἰώμενος).

causing the downfall of his reputation.[104] This episode suggests, as his comments about Lycus will soon corroborate, that Galen's quest for Quintus' students was not as comprehensive as he paints it to be. His opinion that his teachers were "the very best of the students of Quintus and Numisianus" and that all of the others were too inferior to warrant mention has no doubt served to conceal the breadth and variety of the anatomical community springing from Marinus' influence.[105]

Satyrus, the last of this first group, was one of these exalted teachers. He is the most frequently mentioned of these three, no doubt because of Galen's connection to and affection for him as his student. Galen often introduces Satyrus as having been his teacher prior to his studies with Pelops, indicating that he considered his affiliation with Pelops, Numisianus' student, to be more important, more commonly known, or both.[106] Nevertheless, it is Satyrus who gets the credit for introducing Galen to anatomy and dissection, which would become the cornerstones of his future career. Satyrus taught him in Pergamon at the very beginning of his medical education, starting in around AD 145, and, even as a teacher, he remained a devoted disciple of Quintus.[107] Galen repeatedly remarks on his fidelity, saying that he "had a clearer recollection than anyone else of the theories of Quintus" and that he preserved them "with the greatest exactitude, without adding or removing anything."[108] His anatomical activities made a big impression on Galen. He recalls the epidemic, early in their studies together, of a necrotizing skin disease, which caused the muscles, tendons, and vasculature of some patients to be visible; Satyrus demonstrated the locations and functions of these internal parts to a group of his students, pressing home to a teenage Galen the unparalleled advantage that advanced practice in dissection conveys to a practitioner.[109] Nevertheless, looking back from the vantage point of a mature anatomist, Galen was not terribly impressed with the quality of his first teacher's work. He says briefly that Satyrus wrote a treatise on anatomy that was "neither final nor exhaustive"; while this text does not seem to have met with substantial renown nor to have had much

---

[104] Galen, *Praen.* XIV.613–14 and Chapter 3, "Performance to Discredit Rivals" at pp. 84–5.

[105] Galen, *AA* II.660 (οἱ κορυφαῖοι δ' ἦσαν οὗτοι τῶν Κοΐντου τε καὶ Νουμησιανοῦ μαθητῶν), S232; Grmek and Gourevitch (1994), 1513 come to the same general conclusion.

[106] Galen, *AA* II.217, *Hipp.Prorrh.* XVI.524, *Ord.Lib.Prop.* XIX.57.

[107] Galen, *AA* II.224.

[108] Galen, *AA* S231, *Ord.Lib.Prop.* XIX.58 (ἀκριβέστατα διασῴζειν τὰ Κοΐντου δόγματα μήτε προσθεὶς αὐτοῖς τι μήτ' ἀφελών).

[109] Galen, *AA* II.224–5 (cf. *Ven.Art.Diss.* II.803, though Satyrus is not mentioned directly there); see the discussions in Chapter 3, "Performance for Public Display" at p. 58 and Chapter 4, "Anatomical Subjects: Humans" at pp. 119–20.

lasting influence – he only mentions it one other time in passing – its very existence is indicative of the diversity of the anatomical literature circulating in this period.[110]

Numisianus, Heracleianus, Pelops, and Aelianus

Numisianus was, in Galen's opinion, by far Quintus' most successful pupil and one of those who had an independent reputation, generating many noteworthy students of his own.[111] Indeed, Galen couples him with Marinus as one of the premier names of the resurgence of interest in anatomy and describes him as "a man of profound learning, who had valuable ideas on the subject of anatomy."[112] Like Antigenes, he seems to have been old enough to have possibly benefited from Marinus' direct influence in addition to Quintus' more formal teaching; Galen tells us that he had "in Marinus' lifetime … already become preeminent in Alexandria."[113] Despite his evident high regard for him, Galen cites his opinions rarely and only in the context of Hippocratic exegesis, where they are often described as having been filtered through his student Pelops.[114] The reasons for this silence are apparently twofold. First, although Galen sought him out, in keeping with his quest to learn from all the students of Quintus, it is not at all clear that he met him before he died. Galen tells us that he went to Corinth in order to study with Numisianus and that he subsequently went to Alexandria where he learned that Numisianus was residing (according to the Greek tradition) or that a student of Quintus or Numisianus was residing (according to the Arabic).[115] While both versions have their

---

[110] Galen, *AA* S232; mentioned again at *HNH* XV.136, where it keeps the questionable company of Lycus' contribution. Satyrus, like all this group, also wrote many Hippocratic commentaries, but they proved even less popular than his anatomical work (*Hipp.Epid.VI* at *Epid.VI* 7.2 [V.338 Littré] [*CMG* V.10.2.2, pp. 412–13]); cf. Smith (1979), 70, 132 (though the translation he provides there does not faithfully correspond to Pfaff's German).

[111] The Arabic tradition has caused Garofalo (1986–2000), I.3 to downgrade Galen's description of him at *AA* II.217 as "the most notable student of Quintus" (ἐνδοξότατος ἦν τῶν Κοΐντου μαθητῶν) to merely "a notable student of Quintus" (ἔνδοξός τις), but not without some skepticism from Grmek and Gourevitch (1994), 1514, n. 86; regardless, Galen's other comments make clear that Numisianus had a reputation that surpassed that of any of Quintus' other students that he mentions. On the quantity of his students, which Galen compares to Marinus', see *HNH* XV.136.

[112] Galen, *HNH* XV.136; *AA* S231.

[113] Galen, *AA* S231; indeed, Smith (1979), 66 classes him as Marinus' student rather than Quintus' and Nutton (2013a), 219 implies this as well.

[114] Galen, *Hipp.Aph.* XVIIb.751, 837, *Hipp.Epid.II* 4.6 (*CMG Suppl.Or.* V.2, pp. 743–5, 749, 753), *Ord.Lib.Prop.* XIX.57.

[115] Galen, *AA* II.217–18; von Staden (2004), 206–9 walks through the evidence for and ramifications of the two versions carefully, taking into account the previous work of Nutton (1987) and Grmek and Gourevitch (1994), 1513–15.

difficulties, the information common to both – namely, that Galen had to follow another lead on Numisianus' whereabouts after arriving in Corinth, that he expended considerable time afterwards in attempting to get access to Numisianus' books, and that he never cites Numisianus directly, refers to him as a teacher, or references any of his anatomical teachings – leaves me with little doubt that Galen spent no meaningful time, if any at all, in Numisianus' company.[116]

The second, and apparently more aggravating, reason for Galen's comparative silence on his views is that Numisianus' writings were impossible to get hold of. Unlike his teacher Quintus, he did leave a large written legacy, but it would seem that it was considered to be esoteric: It did not circulate during his lifetime and was assiduously guarded by his students after his death. The two main intellectual gatekeepers were Numisianus' son, Heracleianus, and his star pupil, Pelops. Galen's relationship with Heracleianus was more calculated than sincere, and he vents at some length about his difficulties in trying to winkle the books out of him:

> [Numisianus] wrote many books, although during his lifetime these did not reach a wide public. Because of that, after his death, since his son Heracleianus wished to secure himself in the sole possession of all that his father left, none of these books were shown to anyone. Then, when Heracleianus also was on the point of death, they say that he destroyed them by fire, although he was otherwise one of those who, in the days of my residence in Alexandria, had given me the most hospitable reception.... I constantly rendered him the most zealous service, so much so that, contrary to my first impression, I almost admired him to adulation. But none of that availed to procure for me any of the writings of Numisianus, which had not yet been shown to many. For Heracleianus used to put off giving me those books, and he was continually hinting at reasons for this delay. He was not one of those who have no knowledge or any understanding of anatomy. Rather, he had views on anatomical science which he explained to me, just as did Satyrus, who had a clearer recollection than anyone else of the theories of Quintus.[117]

If Galen's account is not too embittered by the outcome, Heracleianus gloried in having inherited his father's position in Alexandria. Galen considers him to be an experienced anatomist in his own right, and it seems

---

[116] The trip to Corinth to seek out Numisianus is further complicated by a thirteenth-century Arabic biographical account of Galen by al-Mubassir, which asserts that Galen went to Corinth in order to study with Aiphicianos, not Numisianus, and agrees with the Arabic tradition of *AA* II.217–18 that he then went to Alexandria to seek out students of Quintus and Numisianus, not the latter himself; see Grmek and Gourevitch (1994), 1514 for a translation of the passage.

[117] Galen, *AA* S231.

probable that it was his reputation that drew him to study in Alexandria, where he "associated with him in no casual way."[118] It was likely with Heracleianus that he studied osteology on human bones, a set of teaching tools that were apparently only available in Alexandria.[119] The fact that Numisianus' texts did not circulate in his lifetime and that Heracleianus neither shared them, even among assiduous followers of his school, nor wrote any of his own, rather suggests that the anatomical reputation shared by father and son centered around performative dissections; this would further indicate that Numisianus' writings, so jealously guarded, may have included some in the genre of anatomical procedures. Anatomical facts suitable to a handbook, even when relayed orally, could be easily remembered by students regardless of their publication status, but the ways and means of impressive anatomical feats would have been harder to glean from observation. It would therefore have been more worthwhile to conceal procedural texts that described them, and doing so would have vouchsafed an unrivaled reputation to the possessors. Heracleianus' ultimate act of burning his inheritance on his deathbed, if true, would thus have protected the tricks of the trade and served to cement his own and his father's exceptionalism.[120]

Pelops' behavior confirms this general picture. While Heracleianus laid claim to Numisianus' legacy in Alexandria, Pelops seems to have taken his own copies of the texts to Smyrna with him, where he adopted the same protective approach to this privileged possession:

> Pelops also, who was the principal pupil of Numisianus, did not expound them, nor did he show any of them to anyone. For he preferred that certain theories, as yet unknown, should be attributed to himself. Pelops also wrote some very valuable books, but after his death all were destroyed by fire before anyone had copied them, since he used to keep them in his house and repeatedly postponed their publication.[121]

Again, Pelops was hesitant to reveal his secrets. Unlike Heracleianus, he apparently planned to enhance his legacy by unveiling his knowledge to the world later in life or after his death, but he was thwarted by the vagaries of fortune. This esoteric impulse evident in Numisianus' school

---

[118] That is, assuming it was Numisianus' student and not Numisianus himself he was seeking. *HNH* XV.136 (ᾧ συνεγενόμην ἐπὶ τῆς Ἀλεξανδρείας οὐκ ἐν παρέργῳ), where he also groups Heracleianus tightly with his father in anatomical reputation.

[119] Galen, *AA* II.220–21; see Chapter 4, "Anatomical Subjects: Humans" at p. 114.

[120] For the suggestion that Galen's comments about Aelianus, the author of a book on the anatomy of the muscles, is a mistranscribed reference to Heracleianus, see later on in this section.

[121] Galen, *AA* S232; on Pelops' location in Smyrna, see *Lib.Prop.* XIX.16, *AA* II.217.

adds an interesting wrinkle to the history of anatomical texts. Since the Hippocratic period, the medical profession, with its competitive marketplace and outcome-driven reputations, had harbored an inclination to guard professional secrets; the more theatrical medium of performative dissection would no doubt have especially rewarded this type of behavior.[122] While traditional anatomical handbooks and treatises combining anatomical and physiological topics would remain useful vehicles for laying claim to and broadcasting new discoveries and new theories, Marinus' novel format relayed the methods themselves, betraying the behind-the-scenes techniques that led to discoveries and noteworthy performances. They were thus a type of text that a practitioner less self-assured than the pioneering Marinus might particularly want to keep from his rivals – including potential ones like the young Galen, whose ambition must have been palpable.

Although he never succeeded in getting Numisianus' books from Pelops, Galen nevertheless imbibed a great deal from him and does seem to have been privy to some of his own writings. After losing his father, Galen travelled to Smyrna to study with Pelops, having already been impressed by his public engagements during a visit to Pergamon.[123] Galen received a broad medical education from him – he mentions his thoughts on humoral theory and on the treatment and analysis of various conditions, as well as his devoted Hippocratean outlook – but anatomical training was a dominating component.[124] A central element in Pelops' anatomical repertoire

---

[122] Both the Hippocratic *Oath* and *Law* allude to professional secrets that must be safeguarded by the practitioner.

[123] Galen says at *Lib.Prop.* XIX.16 that he went to Smyrna "for the sake of Pelops the doctor and Albinus the Platonist" (Πέλοπός τε τοῦ ἰατροῦ καὶ Ἀλβίνου τοῦ Πλατωνικοῦ χάριν); cf. *AA* II.217. While still in Pergamon, he recorded a two-day long debate between Pelops and Philip, an Empiricist physician, on whether or not medical theory could successfully be based on experience alone (*Lib.Prop.* XIX.16–17); the resulting text, *On Medical Experience*, survives in Latin translation; see Frede (1985). He also describes a debate between Pelops and Satyrus that likely occurred during the same period at *Nom.Med.* 99v–101r (Meyerhof and Schacht [1931]).

[124] Though no doubt Galen learned all sorts of other things from him that he does not mention, he names Pelops specifically in the context of humoral theory (*Atr.Bil.*V.112), theories on the mechanism and causation of epilepsy (*Loc.Aff.* VIII.194–8), serious head wounds (*Hipp.Aph.* XVIIIa.29), and the treatment of rabies (*Simp.Med.* XII.358–9, *Ant* XIV.172). He indicates that Pelops was also a dedicated Hippocratean, mentioning his interpretation of Hippocrates, which appears to have been extensive and to have remained influenced by the teachings of his master Numisianus (*Ord.Lib.Prop.* XIX.57, *Hipp.Art.* XVIIIa.541, *Hipp.Epid.II* 4.2, 6.7 [*CMG Suppl.Or.* V.2, pp. 707, 745–53], *Hipp.Epid.VI* 5.15 and at *Epid.VI* 7.2, 8.26 [V.338, 354 Littré] [*CMG* V.10.2.2, pp. 291, 412–13, 500]), and telling us that the text he distributed to all his students as a parting gift was called *Introduction to Hippocrates* (*AA* S232); for his work on Hippocratic texts, see Smith (1979), 69–70, and Manetti and Roselli (1994), 1591–3.

were his thoracic dissections. These appear to have been a signature set of procedures that all of his students observed and learned. Galen tells us that his own *On the Motion of the Lungs and Thorax*, now lost, contained "the doctrines of my teacher Pelops, with whom I was still passing my time in Smyrna when I wrote them."[125] Further, he wrote the text at the behest of a fellow student, who had completed his studies and felt the need of further support in order to feel confident in replicating his master's demonstrations and the accompanying patter back home.[126]

These thoracic procedures appear to have been the hallmark of an education under Pelops, but he in turn quite likely learned them from his own teacher Numisianus, who may himself have picked them up from Quintus: Galen mentions elsewhere that *On the Motion of the Lungs and Thorax* contains proof of muscular physiology that "[his] teachers – these being the preeminent students of Quintus and Numisianus – demonstrated and showed to [him]."[127] At the very least, this emphatically plural group must encompass both Pelops and Satyrus, but it likely included all the teachers from this school of anatomy that he had tracked down, making it probable that this was a signature dissection of Quintus or perhaps even Marinus himself.[128] While Pelops' dissections of the thorax appeared to have toed the party line, not all of his anatomical beliefs were so mainstream. Whether he was here branching out on his own or passing on some of Numisianus' unpublished theories that he deviously hoped to appropriate, he champions the unusual position that the veins and arteries originate from the brain rather than from the heart. Galen was not convinced; he

---

[125] *Lib.Prop.* XIX.17 (Πέλοπος ἦν τοῦ διδασκάλου δόγματα, παρ' ᾧ διατρίβων ἔτι κατὰ Σμύρναν ἔγραψα ταῦτα) (cf. *AA* II.217, 659–60); text according to Boudon-Millot (2007). He adds in *Lib. Prop.* that he later appended a few of his own more recent discoveries at the end of the final book. Marra (1966), 42–3 provides the text of a brief Latin passage that is attributed to this lost work.

[126] Galen characterizes his friend as "not himself capable of producing the display speeches" required for his demonstrations (μὴ δυναμένῳ δὲ αὐτῷ συντιθέναι λόγους ἐπιδεικτικούς) at *AA* II.217; he adds that, after his friend's death, an unscrupulous fellow acquired the text and "lectured from it as if it were his own" (ἀναγιγνώσκων ὡς ἴδια) at *Lib.Prop.* XIX.17; see the further discussion in Chapter 3, "Performance for Advertisement" at pp. 78–9. These passages suggest that this was neither a descriptive nor a prescriptive anatomical text – Galen's friend had learned perfectly well how to carry out the dissection – but that it contained a serviceable lecture on the physiology of the thorax, which the dissections could then have illustrated.

[127] *AA* II.660 (τῶν οὖν διδασκάλων τῶν ἡμετέρων, οἱ κορυφαῖοι δ' ἦσαν οὗτοι τῶν Κοΐντου τε καὶ Νουμησιανοῦ μαθητῶν ... ἀποδειξάντων τε καὶ δειξάντων ἡμῖν).

[128] Galen embraces this heritage, basing his debut dissections in Rome on this same theme, and thus, perhaps, marking himself as part of Marinus' and Quintus' intellectual legacy, though he is careful to indicate that he has modified and improved them to reflect his own innovations (*Loc.Aff.* VIII.53, *AA* II.663–6); see Chapter 3, "Performance for Public Display" at pp. 65–7.

says that even as a young man he thought this was nonsense, but his evident fondness for his teacher softens his reaction. His description of "our Pelops … very valiantly exerting himself" to prove this misguided claim is flavored more by bemused indulgence than the venomous outrage he would no doubt have unleashed on a less favored figure.[129] It seems likely that Pelops used dissections to try to prove this claim, but the only thing that Galen tells us for sure is that he wrote about them.

Though Galen indicates in the passage concerning Pelops' hoarding of Numisianus' work that all of Pelops' most substantial writings were posthumously lost to fire, a few of his treatises did continue to circulate after his death, and Galen had access to them. Some of these were Hippocratic commentaries, which Pelops apparently composed for every text in the corpus; however, he was characteristically cagey with these, and "only a very small part" circulated and survived.[130] The main texts available under his name were informal ones written for his students:

> The numerous books on anatomy by Pelops which are found in the hands of the public are only such writings as he used to hand over to his pupils, and to which he appended the work on the *Introduction to Hippocrates*; these he would present when his pupils wished to return to their homes, so that he might equip them with something of which, when they pleased, they might avail themselves in order to elucidate what they had gathered from him. But the *Anatomy* of Pelops had a far wider scope and greater usefulness than has this book which comprises these sections of his, though even his *Anatomy* is neither exhaustive nor final.[131]

Galen implies here that he had seen Pelops' more substantial anatomical text, but he never references it again, so it seems unlikely that he owned or had continued access to it; he received his own copy of the farewell text, and it is this that he twice cites, referring to it as the *Hippocratic Introductions*. In one of these references, we learn that the second book contained his physiological theories, including a discursive argument for his pet theory that the brain was the source of not just the nerves, but also the arteries and veins; the third book contained the anatomy, including a description of the veins that, as Galen triumphantly points out, inconsistently begins from the liver, not the brain.[132] The other reference confirms

[129] *PHP* V.543–4 (VI.5.22–3 De Lacy) (ὁ ἡμέτερος Πέλοψ … εὖ μάλα γενναίως ἀγωνισάμενος); cf. *PHP* V.527 (VI.3.26 De Lacy).
[130] *Hipp.Epid. VI* at *Epid. VI* 7.2 (V.338 Littré) (*CMG* V.10.2.2, p. 412) (nur ein ganz geringer Teil).
[131] *AA* S232.
[132] *PHP* V.544 (VI.5.23 De Lacy).

that the third book is the anatomical one: "Pelops in the third book of the *Hippocratic Introductions* together with all the other parts also dissects the muscles."[133] Galen singles out this treatment of the muscles as one of the three most popular in circulation in his time, better even than that of Marinus, which was too disjointed. He praises Pelops for sticking only to the anatomical facts, unlike Lycus, who added too much physiology. His unusual way of describing the book – that in it Pelops "dissected," rather than described, the parts of the body – potentially offers a glimpse into the authorial voice, which may have had a more procedural tone. Even if so, however, it was not sufficient to satisfy Galen's departing friend, who evidently felt that there was not nearly enough in it "to elucidate what he had gathered" from Pelops and desired that Galen write him a much more substantial memorandum of the thoracic dissections.

It is at this juncture that the mysterious Aelianus, whom Galen mentions only in *On the Dissection of the Muscles*, comes into the picture. He appears as the author of the third of these three most popular muscular anatomies, coming after Lycus, who followed Pelops: "Aelianus, in the book that he made as an epitome of the anatomical writings of his father, together with all the other parts also himself writes an anatomy of the muscles."[134] His position as the anatomical son of an anatomical father so famous that he required no introduction has led Nutton to suggest that the unknown Aelianus was none other than Heracleianus, mistranscribed, and that we have here evidence of an anatomical text that he wrote summarizing his father Numisianus' views – though this would contradict the dim picture of Heracleianus as intellectually secretive that Galen paints in the long passage from *Anatomical Procedures* previously quoted.[135] Garofalo rejects this theory, since the Arabic tradition does not support it; he instead suggests that Aelianus' father was Lycus, who is the nearest antecedent in the Greek.[136] Taking into account all of the evidence, however, both of these identifications seem implausible to me, and I would like to suggest a third – namely that Aelianus is Pelops' son. Two of the three times he is mentioned, after his initial introduction just quoted, he is closely paired with Pelops and in direct contrast to Lycus, making it far more probable

[133] *Musc.Diss.* XVIIIb.926 (ὁ μὲν οὖν Πέλοψ ἐν τῇ τρίτῃ τῶν Ἱπποκρατείων εἰσαγωγικῶν ἅμα τοῖς ἄλλοις ἅπασι μέρεσι καὶ τοὺς μῦς ἀνέτεμεν).
[134] *Musc.Diss.* XVIIIb.926–7 (Αἰλιανὸς δὲ κατὰ τὴν βίβλον ἣν ὥσπερ ἐπιτομὴν ἐποιήσατο τῶν τοῦ πατρὸς ἀνατομικῶν συγγραμμάτων, ἅμα τοῖς ἄλλοις ἅπασι μορίοις καὶ αὐτὸς ἔγραψε τὴν τῶν μυῶν ἀνατομήν); text according to Garofalo and Debru (2005).
[135] Nutton (1993), 18.
[136] Garofalo and Debru (2005), 118, nn. 4 and 7.

that he was epitomizing the former's views than the latter's.[137] Further, the description of Aelianus' text very closely mirrors that of Pelops' – "together with all the other parts … the muscles" – with the intensive pronoun (αὐτός) added, perhaps, to acknowledge the added contributions of the son. Finally, the fiery destruction of Pelops' writings after his death, as recounted by Galen, would be a strong motivation for his son to salvage what he could remember of the lost works in the form of an epitome, in an attempt to make his father's written legacy more reflective of the "wide scope and greater usefulness" to be found there. Certainly, Aelianus appears possessed of much more filial piety than Heracleianus ever had.

Lycus

The last of Quintus' students to discuss is Lycus, who was, in Galen's eyes, the black sheep of Marinus' legacy. Lycus hailed from Macedonia, where he apparently spent the beginning of his life in obscurity; at some point, he traveled to Rome to study under Quintus.[138] Before a year had passed, however, something – perhaps Quintus' hasty departure from Rome, which would suggest that Lycus arrived in the early 140s AD – brought their relationship to a close.[139] Lycus lived long enough after this to produce a good amount of written work and was still living, possibly in Rome, while Galen was travelling in pursuit of his medical education; however, Galen claims that he never thought to seek him out because "he was a man who, in his lifetime, had no great reputation with the Greeks."[140] Be that as it may, he was certainly dead by the time Galen returned to Rome in AD 169 and probably already at the time of his first arrival in AD 162 – at any rate, the two never met.[141] Lycus first comes

---

137 *Musc.Diss.* XVIIIb.927 (ἐμηκύνθη δὲ τὸ τοῦ Λύκου βιβλίον … Αἰλιανὸς μέντοι καὶ Πέλοψ…), 935 (καθάπερ Αἰλιανὸς καὶ Πέλοψ. ὁ Λύκος δ᾽…); texts according to Garofalo and Debru (2005). His third, solitary, appearance is at 986, where he is singled out as exemplary of a flaw common to anatomists.

138 *Hipp.Epid.VI* 5.14 (*CMG* V.10.2.2, p. 287). Wellmann (1900), 383–4 did not have access to this Arabic material when he made the suggestion – which it renders impossible – that Lycus was Pelops' son, basing himself on the entry "*Lupus Pelopis*" in a list of ancient medical authors appended to an eleventh-century manuscript of Celsus (cf. the already skeptical discussion in Kind [1927], 2408–9).

139 *Hipp.Epid.III* XVIIa.575 (*CMG* V.10.2.1, p. 155).

140 *AA* S232 (cf. II.470); Galen presents Lycus' trip to Rome and his death as consecutive events, suggesting, though hardly conclusively, that he stayed on in Rome after his studies for the remainder of his life (*Hipp.Epid.VI* 5.14 [*CMG* V.10.2.2, p. 287]) (er in Rom war und dann gestorben ist).

141 Galen says explicitly that they never met at *AA* II.470 and *Hipp.Epid.VI* 5.14 (*CMG* V.10.2.2, p. 287); the speculation in Scarborough (1971), 99, and Johnston and Horsley (2011), xviii that Lycus may have been Galen's teacher in Alexandria therefore seems quite impossible.

to his attention at some point after Galen's return to the capitol for the
second time, somewhere in the 170s AD, when Lycus' work was beginning to gain popularity after his death. The first of these texts that Galen
read was his anatomy of the muscles, which he repeatedly refers to in *On
the Dissection of the Muscles* and the first and fourth books of *Anatomical
Procedures*, all composed in roughly the second half of that decade. He
describes Lycus' book as having recently appeared on the scene and as
being very well regarded; though he groups it with the similar texts of
Pelops and Aelianus as all being "highly esteemed," he adds that Lycus
"was considered to have anatomized the muscles the most clearly and the
best of everyone."[142] Galen, needless to say, did not agree. He complains
that Lycus' text is too long, discursively off-topic, frequently incorrect,
and woefully incomplete.[143] He conceives of his own *On the Dissection of
the Muscles* – at the behest, he tells us, of his friends – in no small part
as a vehicle for directly supplanting Lycus' text, setting out to mention
everything he omitted and inexactly explained; sure enough, his discussions of the muscles both there and in the fourth book of *Anatomical
Procedures* are liberally sprinkled with direct criticisms of Lycus. Galen
refers to nothing else by him during this period, except to name him as
the proposer of what he considered to be a unique but outrageous theory
on urine production; he is aware that there are other books circulating,
but he says that he has not come across any but the anatomical ones and
has not read all of those.[144]

In the following decades, however, it would seem that Lycus' fans continued to promulgate his writings, which Galen perforce became familiar
with, and his posthumous fame grew apace. Popular among these were
his Hippocratic commentaries; Galen several times refers to the exegetical opinions of "those around Lycus," suggesting a devoted and productive following for these texts.[145] Galen, however, finds Lycus' handling
of Hippocrates so bad as to be unbearable: "Lycus is so ignorant about
the art of Hippocrates that—I swear to all the gods—after reading the
first interpretations from his books on the *Aphorisms*, I continued to read

---

[142] Recency of Lycus' book: *AA* II.227, 458, 470; good reputation: *Musc.Diss.* XVIIIb.926 (εὐδοκίμησεν),
928 (σαφέστατά τε καὶ κάλλιστα πάντων οὗτος ἀνατετμηκέναι μῦς πεπίστευται).
[143] *AA* II.227, *Musc.Diss.* XVIIIb.927.
[144] On the urine: *Nat.Fac.* II.70–1, *UP* III.366 (I.268H); Kind (1927), 2410 even suggests that this
theory about the urine may also have derived from the book on the muscles, being one of the
superfluous topics Galen complains about. On Lycus' books: *AA* II.470.
[145] *Hipp.Epid.III* XVIIa.515 (τοὺς περὶ τὸν Κόϊντον καὶ Λύκον), 534 (τοῖς περὶ Λύκον), *Hipp.Epid.VI*
XVIIa.957 (οἱ περὶ τὸν Λύκον).

no further."[146] This passage comes at the beginning of a small text Galen devotes exclusively to refuting Lycus' explanation of one of the aphorisms and to revealing his complete lack of understanding of Hippocrates on the relevant point.[147] Galen's criticisms of his work on Hippocrates abound even outside of this dedicated text: He finds his commentaries to be simultaneously derivative and debased.[148] There were indeed some substantive differences in their approach to exegesis – as we shall see, Lycus appeared to harbor some Empiricist tendencies that Galen distrusted – but it is hard to avoid the suspicion that his dislike was magnified by the contemporary popularity of Lycus' writings, which caused him to view Lycus as a direct rival, albeit a deceased one.[149]

Nowhere is this one-sided rivalry more apparent than in the realm of anatomy. Despite Galen's having dedicated space in *On the Dissection of the Muscles* and *Anatomical Procedures* to debunking his anatomical credibility, Lycus' works continued to flourish. Some fifteen years later, when Galen is writing the final books of *Anatomical Procedures*, he says that "Lycus' book on anatomy ... at the present time enjoys a wide circulation ... in this our own day I have seen [it] in the possession of many."[150] This book is likely not the same as the short (but, to Galen's taste, not short enough) book about the muscles, but rather an extensive text or set of texts similar to Marinus'. Indeed, Galen claims Lycus' anatomical works are little more than a spin-off of that important work: "it is clear that they are constructed out of the writings of Marinus, but they are full of errors, and are moreover less comprehensive even than the books Marinus himself."[151] Despite these aspersions, Galen finds himself in the frustrating situation where his own *On the Usefulness of the Parts* and the early books of his *Anatomical Procedures*, now both published and enjoying good popularity, are still having to compete

---

[146] *Adv.Lyc.* XVIIIa.198 (Λύκος δὲ εἰς τοσοῦτον ἄρα τῆς Ἱπποκράτους τέχνης ἀμαθής ἐστιν, ὥστ' ἐγὼ – θεοὺς ἅπαντας ἐπόμνυμι – τὰς πρώτας τῶν εἰς τοὺς ἀφορισμοὺς ὑπομνημάτων αὐτοῦ ἐξηγήσεις ἀναγνοὺς [ἀφορισμῶν] οὐκέθ' ὑπέμεινα ... γνῶναι...).

[147] *Against Lycus* (*Adv.Lyc.*); he remained either very proud of this text or very worked up about the topic, since he refers it repeatedly (*PHP* V.704–5 [VIII.7.13 De Lacy], *Hipp.Aph.* XVIIb.414–15, *Hipp.Epid.VI* XVIIb.179, 203–4, *Lib.Prop.* XIX.37).

[148] Galen describes Lycus' exegetical work as derivative of and yet worse than Marinus' and Quintus' at *Hipp.Epid.VI* 4.11, 5.14 (*CMG* V.10.2.2, p. 212, 287–8), *Hipp.Aph.* XVIIb.562, *Hipp.Epid.III* XVIIa.504, 507, and *Ord.Lib.Prop.* XIX.57–8. For Lycus' work on Hippocrates, all evidence for which comes through Galen's criticisms, see Kind (1927), 2412–14, and Manetti and Roselli (1994), 1582–8.

[149] For Lycus' Empiricism, see this chapter, "Anatomy in the Roman Intellectual Scene" at p. 268.

[150] *AA* S232; cf. *HNH* XV.136.

[151] *AA* S233; cf. *Hipp.Epid.VI* 5.14 (*CMG* V.10.2.2, p. 287–8) where he makes a very similar claim about Lycus' Hippocratic work, though Smith (1979), 67 thinks that he may simply have "for polemical effect ... transferred this judgement" from the anatomical sphere to the exegetical one.

with Lycus' older texts. Things come to a head after Galen is accused of
having included in those texts things that are simply impossible to see and
that he fabricated to improve his reputation. Outraged by this slander,
Galen's friends urge him to defend himself, and he proceeds to bring a pile
of books into a large performative arena and promise to prove, by bespoke
dissection, that his own take on every point of difference with a previous
author is demonstrably true. Some doctors pipe up from the crowd and tell
him not to bother with all the older authors, but to just compare himself
to Lycus, since he "wrote about everything that had been discovered up to
his day."[152] Galen no doubt relished the opportunity. He spent several days
vindicating himself at the expense of his defenseless opponent and then
summed everything up, at the request of these same conveniently solici-
tous friends, in a lost four-book treatise entitled *On the Ignorance of Lycus
in Anatomy*.[153] Apparently, though, he deemed even this insufficient, as he
subsequently added a further two books on his anatomical and physiological disagreements with Lycus, both also now lost.[154]

Reading between these aggressively polemical lines, we can infer that
Lycus' anatomical writing was broad and sophisticated. He evidently
inspired a great deal of respect among fellow physicians for decades after
his death; while Galen attempts to downplay his importance compared
to Marinus, it was Lycus' text that the anonymous audience members –
described as "important doctors" – considered to be state-of-the-art, not
the still-available text of his teacher's teacher.[155] Indeed, in addition to his
followers in exegetical circles, Lycus had a circle of anatomical admirers
dating back to the AD 170s; already in *On the Dissection of the Muscles*
Galen refers to the errors in anatomy of "those around Lycus."[156] Even
Galen, despite all his personal rivalry, considered Lycus' anatomical works
to be significant enough to merit a synopsis, like he made for Marinus',
and he deems them both equally worth mentioning among his anatomical
writing.[157] His list of the headings of this synopsis, recently restored by the
Vlatadon manuscript, allows us to attempt to reconstruct his writings.[158]

---

[152] *Lib.Prop.* XIX.21–2 (τὰ μέχρι τῶν καθ' ἑαυτὸν εὑρημένα πάντα ἔγραψεν); see the epigraph to
Chapter 6 for a significant portion of the relevant passage.

[153] *Lib.Prop.* XIX.22 and 4.40 (Boudon-Millot [2007]) (in a section not present in Kühn).

[154] *Lib.Prop.* 4.40 (Boudon-Millot [2007]).

[155] *Lib.Prop.* XIX.22 (τινες τῶν ἀξιολόγων ἰατρῶν).

[156] *Musc.Diss.* XVIIIb.938 (οἱ περὶ τὸν Λύκον); these two circles likely consisted of mostly the same
people.

[157] *Lib.Prop.* XIX.25.

[158] Galen's description of his summary of Lycus' work was missing in the single Greek manuscript on
which the modern knowledge of this text was based and was therefore lost until the rediscovery of

Galen's description of Lycus' work is much shorter than that of Marinus', even though it deals with nineteen books to the latter's twenty; part of this is no doubt because Galen's synopsis was half as long – only two books instead of four – but that very fact suggests that it is also in large measure an indication of the respective importance that he places on the two authors. In addition, Galen's wording in these two epitome-summaries is different. Although Lycus' books are arranged in a perfectly reasonable order and, in total, might be considered more or less comprehensive, it is not clear that we are dealing with a single work in nineteen books, comparable to Marinus' work in twenty. Galen represents each book as containing a discrete topic, in the following order: His first epitome volume contains the books on 1) the brain, 2) the nerves from the brain and its meninges, 3) the nerves from the spinal marrow, 4) the nerves from the eyes, 5) the "head of the throat,"[159] 6) the lungs in the dead animal, 7) the lungs in the living animal, 8) the heart, and 9) the diaphragm; the second volume of the epitome then contains 1) the liver, 2) the anatomy of the omentum and spleen, 3) the kidneys, 4) the bladder and genitals, 5) the uterus, 6) the pregnant womb in the dead animal, 7) the living embryo, 8) the dead embryo, 9) the testicles, and 10) the muscles. One is struck both by what is included and what is missing.

Most noticeably, there is no mention at all of the veins or the arteries, which usually occupy a prominent place in ancient anatomical texts – four of Marinus' twenty books are devoted to them, for example. It is quite likely that Lycus discussed them in the books on the heart and the liver, but their absence from the titles is nevertheless surprising. Again, the digestive tract is puzzlingly represented: There is no mention whatsoever of the stomach and the intestines, and yet the comparatively less significant omentum and spleen have an entire dedicated book. This is in keeping with the heightened level of detail that some of the books contain. The diaphragm and the "head of the throat" each get as much attention as the heart and the brain, while the reproductive organs dominate the oeuvre. The unusual weighting of all of these topics suggests that these are more likely to have been independent texts or groups of texts on questions of specific interest than to have been a considered and unified whole. Still more strikingly, Galen does not present these as numbered books, like Marinus' and like

---

the Vlatadon manuscript in 2005; see Boudon-Millot (2007), 33–4. It appears at *Lib.Prop.* 4.34–7 (Boudon-Millot [2007]).

[159] See Boudon-Millot (2007), 153, n. 1; she cites two other uses of this term in the text and concludes that Galen is referring to the area at the base of the tongue around the larynx and the tonsils.

the books of most other multivolume works that he refers to. He says that he wrote an epitome "of Marinus' anatomical books, being twenty in number," but that he wrote one of "all of Lycus'."[160] When he comes to enumerate them, he carefully introduces the book numbers included in each epitome of Marinus – "in the first epitome, the first six books ... are contained ... in the second of our treatises ... the seventh and eighth and ninth and tenth are contained ... etc." – whereas for Lycus he merely says, "the first book holds the epitome of nine of his books ... the second book of the epitome of Lycus' anatomical books contains an epitome of ten of the books ascribed to him."[161] Most tellingly, when he lists the books contained in the second part of the epitome, *he begins enumerating them again from one*, rather than treating them as a group consecutive to the first and picking up where he left off, in this case at ten, as he did when describing the work on Marinus.

While it is certainly possible that Lycus conceived of these nineteen books as parts of an overarching set, he never published them as such. Whether he had inherited the reticence for publication evident in Quintus and Numisianus and his followers or he was merely biding his time like Pelops, he did not see fit to assemble his anatomical wisdom into a polished and official whole. Rather, these texts appear to have remained in the hands of friends or students after his death and to have circulated independently of each other.[162] For example, the last book Galen includes, on the muscles, is likely identical to the one that he was so agitated about in the 170s. That text was clearly a distinctly operating unit. Galen describes it as "a single giant book" that "stretched to almost five thousand lines," boasting that his own was a third as long yet far more complete.[163] He explains that its length was due to the fact that "he describes everything rather tediously and mixes in logical inquiries to the anatomical data and, in addition to this, he spends a lot of time talking about illnesses, some of which are in no way relevant to the anatomy of the muscles."[164] This statement and his claim elsewhere that "they are all constructed out of the writings of Marinus" comprise the only direct description of Lycus' literary

---

[160] *Lib.Prop.* XIX.25.

[161] *Lib.Prop.* XIX.25, 27 (4.10, 17, 34, 36 Boudon-Millot [2007]).

[162] *AA* II.458.

[163] *Musc.Diss.* II.926 (ἓν μέγιστον βιβλίον); *AA* II.227 (μικροῦ δεῖν εἰς πεντακισχιλίους στίχους ἐκτετ αμένον).

[164] *Musc.Diss.* II.927 (ὅτι τε μακρότερον ἑρμηνεύει πάντα καὶ ὅτι λογικὰς ζητήσεις ἀνέμιξε τοῖς ἐξ ἀνατομῆς φαινομένοις· ἔτι τε πρὸς τούτοις ὅτι περὶ παθῶν ἐποιήσατο λόγους πολλούς, ὧν ἔνια κατ' οὐδὲν ᾠκείωται ταῖς τῶν μυῶν ἀνατομαῖς).

output, but, together with some tangential comments, they are sufficient to piece together a sketch of its character.

First, to use Galen's corpus as a frame of reference, it would seem that the book on the muscles was more akin to *On the Usefulness of the Parts* than to *On the Dissection of the Muscles* or *Anatomical Procedures*. Like Marinus, Lycus appears to have been happy to mix anatomy with more physiological topics, which is what I assume to have required the "logical inquiries" Galen objects to; indeed, it is difficult to imagine an entire book about the testicles that did not spend the bulk of its time on questions of physiology. In addition to this, he appears to have gone beyond the scope that Galen gave to his *On the Usefulness of the Parts* and to have fully integrated his anatomical work into his broader medical outlook, offering discussion of diseases as he deemed them relevant. Like Galen, he seems to have approached the organization of the body from a teleological outlook and, like Galen, to have been committed to addressing the theories of his predecessors, as suggested both by his work on Hippocrates and by the anonymous doctors' claim that his work touched on everything that had come before.[165] Galen also credits him with doing his own dissections, though he is determined to be unimpressed with his skill at it; he cautions against observing the results of dissection "carelessly, like Lycus" and twice indicates which muscles he thinks Lycus misobserved in order to come to the conclusions that he did.[166] Further, the pair of books on the subject of the lungs in the dead animal and the lungs in the living animal suggest that he, like Galen, used dissection as a training ground for more difficult acts of vivisection; the suite of books on embryos, living and dead, and their situations in the mother confirm that this was the case. These latter texts must have been quite detailed or must, like their counterpart on the muscles, have expanded to contain physiological and medical discussion as well as anatomical facts; Galen covers in a single book of *Anatomical Procedures* the generative topics that Lycus here spreads over five.[167] Interestingly, that book is also the only one in *Anatomical Procedures* outside of the fourth book, on the muscles, where Galen references Lycus' anatomical opinions, saying that his beliefs about the female reproductive tract are in contrast to the consensus of all other anatomists.[168] This confirms that reproductive topics were an area where Lycus' attention and reputation were particularly focused.

[165] For his rejection of a Nature without skill, *UP* III.366 (I.268H).
[166] *AA* II.451 (ἀμελῶς ... καθάπερ ὁ Λύκος); *Musc.Diss.* XVIIIb.949, 1007.
[167] The twelfth book of *AA* covers the uterus, the testicles, the pregnant womb in the dead animal, and both the dead and living embryo.
[168] *AA* S139–40.

While Lycus' anatomical writings must have been based on dissection, there is no hint of the degree to which they incorporated instructions.[169] Indeed, Galen's claim that his writing is entirely derivative from Marinus is more confusing than not. Which of Marinus' texts was he thinking of? There does not seem to be a candidate in the list of Lycus' texts to be equivalent to Marinus' *Procedures*, unless we are to think that all of Lycus' work was of that character, presaging Galen's multivolume version; on the whole, it seems very unlikely that Galen would not have mentioned this and attempted to aggressively assert the originality and superiority of his own version. On the other hand, the organizational structure of Lycus' work was certainly very different from that of Marinus' large anatomy, as was his focus on reproductive topics where Marinus clearly favored the brain and nervous system. Perhaps Galen was implying that the contents, not the arrangement, were the same; perhaps Marinus wrote a great deal on generation and reproductive that Galen failed to mention; or perhaps Galen was simply being meanspirited. No matter how we interpret it, a close look at everything he tells us about Marinus, Quintus, and all of their intellectual followers, including Lycus, makes it hard to avoid the conclusion that Galen was not as exceptional as he would paint himself. For at least two generations before him, others had been engaged in methodical dissection, in careful Hippocratic exegesis, and in producing extensive and varied literature of a character similar to the work that he would produce. It will fall to Chapters 8 and 9 to interrogate the degree to which his texts offered something new.

Pseudo-Galenic *Doctor: Introduction*

The idiosyncratically titled *Doctor: Introduction* circulated, perhaps from its very inception, under the name of Galen, but has long been recognized as a pseudonymous work. It is altogether possible that this text is the same one that features in the anecdote with which Galen opens *On My Own Books*, where he covertly witnesses an educated consumer at a bookstall refuting the Galenic authorship of a book for sale under the name *Galen's Doctor*.[170] Even if the two books are not identical, this surviving text probably dates to Galen's lifetime and is certainly not earlier than that.[171] As the subtitle

---

[169] Though it is worth noting that, like he did for Pelops (see this chapter, n. 133), Galen describes Lycus as "dissecting" the muscles in his text (*Musc.Diss.* XVIIIb.928).

[170] *Lib.Prop.* XIX.8.

[171] On the dating of the text and the possibility of its relationship to the Galen anecdote, see Petit (2009), xlii–li.

indicates, the text provides an introductory overview to the main topics of medicine, including a chapter on external anatomy, one on internal anatomy, and a third on osteology. These sections are of a piece with parallel passages in comparable texts, but there are identifiable authorial patterns and some unique moments. The author, certainly not himself an anatomist, therefore offers a window into the anatomical wisdom prevalent in medical circles outside of the dedicated anatomists we have just been considering.

Unlike Rufus, the closest extant parallel for these chapters, the author here has almost no interest in recording varied nomenclature and its sources. He only rarely gives more than one name for any given part. Rarer still are his direct attributions to authors: There are only three, two of which are not to medical authors at all, but, predictably, to Homer.[172] His only real linguistic concern manifests in a penchant for etymological explanations.[173] The most notable authorial characteristic for our purposes, though, is his lack of interest in anatomical description for its own sake. He rarely describes the form and aspect of organs, spending considerably more time explaining their physiology, a far more prominent concern in this treatise as whole. A reader relying on this text for anatomy would find himself at a loss if presented with a dissected animal. Indeed, not only does the author not mention dissection anywhere, he positively rules it out. With an attitude similar to the Hippocratic author of *Art*, he begins the chapter on internal anatomy by saying:

> Anatomy is not the showing of [the internal parts] to the eye, but the having knowledge of each of them, according to reason, and the understanding of the natural faculties, how they are accomplished through [the parts of the body], and the connections that the viscera and the other parts of the body have to each other through veins and arteries and nerves, through which the confluence and co-respiration of everything with everything is accomplished.[174]

---

[172] Homer: *Int.* XIV.703, 707; the third is a reference to Hippocrates' description of the eye (XIV.711–12), including a direct quotation, which, however, does not directly parallel anything in the modern corpus (see Petit [2009], 141–2). Hippocrates comes up again one other time in these chapters, together with Erasistratus and Plato, in a more physiological discussion of the nature and purpose of the brain (XIV.709–10); for the author's general Hippocrateanism, see Petit (2009), xxi–xxxvi.

[173] He gives etymology for the iris (*Int.* XIV.702), the bags under the eyes (703), the names of the fingers (704), the area and internal organs of the abdomen (705), the anus (706), the buttocks (707), and the tonsils (713).

[174] *Int.* XIV.709 (οὐ γὰρ τὸ τῇ ὄψει αὐτὰ δειχθῆναι ἀνατομή ἐστιν, ἀλλὰ τὸ μετὰ λόγου ἑκάστου αὐτῶν γνῶσιν λαβεῖν, τάς τε κατὰ φύσιν ἐνεργείας, ὅπως δι᾽ αὐτῶν ἀποτελοῦνται ἐκμαθεῖν καὶ τὰς κοινωνίας ἃς ἔχει πρὸς ἄλληλα τὰ σπλάγχνα καὶ τὰ ἄλλα μέρη τοῦ σώματος διὰ φλεβῶν

Not only does this definition preclude dissection as a valuable methodology and make the study of anatomy a purely literary, thought-based activity, it emphasizes the function and interactions of the organs almost to the exclusion of the descriptive element traditional to the topic.

This independent approach to anatomy is typical of the author. He also offers an idiosyncratic definition of the subject, namely that the term anatomy can only properly be applied to the study of the internal parts, not to the parallel description of the external parts.[175] Further, he presents his own history of anatomy; he frames Aristotle as the first to have conceived of it as an academic endeavor and is the single and precious witness to the contributions of the Erasistrateans Xenophon and Apollonius of Memphis.[176] He also supplies a few new anatomical terms, notably offering a new constellation of names for the cranial sutures, which overlaps only partially with those that Rufus attributed to the linguistically challenged Egyptians and includes one term that is unique.[177] Finally, his osteology has a different feel from the other two sections and from its ps.-Rufian and Galenic counterparts. Though arranged in the traditional *a capite ad calcem* format, it is organized more aggressively around numerical divisions, beginning with the two types (and three subtypes) of joints and then introducing each group of bones with their number. This format is characteristic of texts meant for memorization and suggests that the author here was drawing on a pedagogical source – unsurprising given the introductory agenda of the text.[178] In short, this author appears to have been tapping into an entirely different strand of anatomy than we have yet encountered, and either he or his sources placed less emphasis on dissection than Marinus and his school.

Anatomy in the Papyri

The medical papyri are able to further supplement our understanding of the breadth and diversity of anatomical writing; they offer glimpses, too, into the more practical, teaching-oriented texts – like those on which *Doctor:*

καὶ ἀρτηριῶν καὶ νεύρων δι'ὧν ἡ σύρροια καὶ ἡ σύμπνοια πάντων πρὸς ἅπαντα γίγνεται); text according to Petit (2009). For *Art.*, see Chapter 2, "Hippocratic Doctors" at pp. 14–15.

175 *Int.* XIV.709.
176 *Int.* XIV.699–700.
177 *Int.* XIV.720 and Petit (2009), 143 (n. 1 to p. 41); see also XIV.701 for his names of the parts of the ear and 703 for a nuance to the nomenclature of the acromion (with reference to the notes in Petit [2009], *ad loc*).
178 For the various sources employed by the author of this text, see Petit (2009), li–lxiv.

Introduction was likely drawing – which have otherwise left little trace. The corpus of medical papyri as a whole tends to focus on questions of more practical urgency for the working physician; there are, however, a cluster of anatomically related texts, indicating that this was a popular topic in its way. Surprisingly prominent among them is a focus on osteology. One text from the second or third century AD, whose careful layout and presentation suggests a library copy, offers a description of the bones of the foot, going into a level of detail comparable to the corresponding passages in the pseudo-Rufian *On Bones*, the pseudo-Galenic *Doctor: Introduction*, and Galen's *On Bones for Beginners*, but drawing on its own tradition.[179] This fragment offers a glimpse into a larger text that in all likelihood included a description of the entire skeleton, seemingly quite similar in character to the extant osteological parallels from the Roman period. The same larger context might also be argued for three of the other remaining fragments. One appears to be a fairly advanced discussion of the different types of joints, another discusses the bones of the pelvis, while a third differentiates bone marrow from spinal marrow, all using language that would be at home in Galen.[180] The complete erasure of these texts from the historical record, but for these small surviving scraps, is a reminder that the diversity that once characterized the field of anatomical handbooks has since been largely obscured.

Other osteological examples derive from less substantial treatments. A nicely presented text from the first century AD contains an extremely rapid enumeration of the bones in the body.[181] In the space of a mere twelve lines, it covers the spine, arms, hands, hips, legs, and feet; only a few of the bones are actually named, there being far greater emphasis on numbers, as for example in the description of the bones of the fingers, which reads simply, "of each finger, 3."[182] This emphasis on counting is similar to the section

---

[179] P.Lit.Lond. 176 (MP³ 2358); see Marganne (1987) for edition, translation, and commentary, including comparison to the relevant passages in the authors mentioned.

[180] P.Oxy. 74.4974 (MP³ 2345.21) (II/III cent. AD) (see Leith [2009*b*]), to which compare Galen, *Oss.* II.737–8; P.Köln 9.358 (MP³ 2357.15) (I cent. BC) (see Gronewald [2001]), to which compare Galen, *Oss.* II.755, 772 (Gronewald [2001], 19–21 rightly offers earlier comparanda since this text predates Galen by several centuries); P.Köln 7.291 (MP³ 2357.11) (I/II cent. AD) (see Gronewald and Maresch [1991]), to which compare Galen, *Mot.Musc.* IV.369–70 and *Temp.* I.600.

[181] PUG II.51 (MP³ 2345.2); see Andorlini (2006).

[182] These twelve lines are PUG II.51 l. 7–19, after which line 20 appears to open a new section; Andorlini (2006), 89–90 suggests that the new topic is the bones of the face, based on the word teeth in line 24, but I wonder if the teeth are brought in as a parallel for a type of jointure (ἁρμονίαν [l. 22, 26]) found in the bones of the lower extremities; cf. Galen, *Oss.* II.738 where the teeth are used as an example in this way (albeit for a different term), and P.Oxy. 74.4974, where I suspect something similar is going on. On the fingers: PUG II.51 l. 9 (ἑκά<σ>του δακ(τύλου) γ').

on bones in *Doctor: Introduction*, though the heightened brevity is more reminiscent of the even more compressed first chapter of the Hippocratic *On the Nature of Bones*.[183] All this suggests to me that the text here is not, in fact, from a dedicated osteology, but rather from the osteological section of a broader introductory text.[184] Another, still briefer, fragment from the third century AD provides what is basically a list of bones and parts of the arm and hand, with very little description or localizing information.[185] Its only structural similarity to the parallel passage in Rufus' *Names* is to introduce an alternative name for a bone with "some [call it]," as Rufus often does, though eliding the verb that he usually provides; otherwise, its complete lack of contextualization or description, combined with its rudimentary grammar and notably bad spelling, is more suggestive of a student's memorandum than an authored anatomical treatise.[186]

The study of bones dominates the surviving anatomical papyri, whether due to the vagaries of fortune or to a more intensive interest in this sub-topic, but other types of anatomy survive as well. One particularly nice example from the third or fourth century AD, whose script suggests a personal, rather than library, copy is couched in the question and answer format popular in medical pedagogy.[187] The passage that remains relates to the anatomy, as well as the physiology, of the lower digestive tract. The questions present the names of different elements – the caecum, the rectum, the sphincter – and query their etymology, location, qualitative characteristics, and function; the answers, variable in length, include an alternative name for one structure, as so often reported in the fully surviving texts, and possibly a reference to the work of Marinus, if Marganne's tempting conjecture is correct.[188] Another example of an anatomical catechism includes similar questions eliciting information about the location, alternative names, etymology, and, perhaps, function of the tonsils, as well

---

[183] Hippocrates, *Oss.* 1 (IX.168 Littré) (as noted by Andorlini [2006], 90); for this text, see Chapter 6, "The Hippocratic Corpus" at p. 173.

[184] I am, therefore, somewhat in disagreement with the conclusions in Andorlini (2006), 91.

[185] P.Bagnall 51 (P.Genav. inv. 512) (MP³ 2345.12); see Schubert (2012).

[186] P.Bagnall 51 col.ii.3 (οἱ δὲ); see Schubert (2012), 295–6 for the spelling and also his suggestion, similar to mine, that this might be a digest of Rufus or one of his sources.

[187] P.Lund. 1.7 (MP³ 2341); see Marganne (1987). For more on question and answer texts broadly, see Zalateo (1964), Kollesch (1973), 35–46, Andorlini (1999), Hanson (2003), Marganne (2004), 75–7, Leith (2009c). In addition to the papyrological evidence for anatomical texts in this genre, there is also a small anonymous anatomical text preserved in a tenth-century manuscript (Paris. suppl. gr. 446) that contains Galenic, pseudo-Galenic, and other medical texts; the tract covers the body from head-to-toe, followed by the bones, using a rudimentary question and answer format; see Kollesch (1973), 41–3, and, on the manuscript as whole, including its dating, Wilson (1987), 52–3.

[188] Marganne (1987), 198.

as the tail end of an answer that seems to relate to the pharynx.[189] A third includes a section on a uterine tunic, mentioning the investigations of a certain Demetrius of Apamea and another physician whose name is lost; however, this anatomical information is followed by a description of how the tunic in question bursts and oozes, which muddies the characterization of this text as purely anatomical, especially when combined with the fact that the preceding topic is clearly therapeutic in nature.[190]

We also find general anatomy in the papyri outside of catechisms, but it can be difficult there, too, to differentiate between anatomical aspects of broader medical discussions and dedicated anatomical texts. Pretty squarely on the latter end of the spectrum is a text dating to the second century AD, which offers the beginning of an introductory medical treatise written on the back of a copy of the *Iliad*.[191] This text opens by claiming that the "first and most necessary" thing for a student beginning the study of medicine is to learn the names of the internal and external parts of the body, and it therefore promises to provide them.[192] It is possible, though not completely clear, that the text, which is abruptly broken off, would then have gone on to other introductory topics; either way, the owner took the initial advice to heart, writing out some anatomical terms related to the head on the other side, in the wide gap that the original scribe left between the end of *Iliad* 23 and the end of the roll. Slightly more ambiguously, another text, this one dating to the second or first century BC, includes a column that handles the male and female genital tracts in some detail.[193] The language and level of information is quite similar to that found in Rufus, suggesting a full-scale anatomical text; however, the other columns, which are unfortunately far less well preserved, appear to discuss illnesses of these organs and their therapies, which would then point to a treatise on urogenital issues that included anatomical background information rather than to an anatomical handbook.[194] More ambiguous still is a text

---

[189] PSI 15.1510 (MP³ 2364.01); see Manfredi (1997).

[190] P.Gollenischeff (MP³ 2347) col. III.1–8, 23–IV.15; see Leith (2009a), 216 who also suggests that the gynecological section was a discrete unit appended to a completed therapeutic text. Compare the catechism in PSI III 252 (MP³ 2364), which includes an answer that mentions the vessels, perhaps of the lower limbs; it is clear from the rest of the contents, however, that this is not an anatomical manual, but a treatise on "the definition, aetiology, and treatment of a variety of individual conditions" (Leith and Maravela-Solbakk [2009], 201).

[191] PSI 12.1275 (MP³ 2345.1); see Manfredi (1951).

[192] PSI 12.1275, l. 3 (πρῶτ[ο]υ καὶ ἀναγκαιοτάτο[υ]).

[193] P.Iand. 5.82 (MP³ 2345); see Azzarello (2004).

[194] Azzarello (2004), 238–9 even suggests that Rufus may have used this text as one of his sources and speculates that it might be the work of an early Erasistratean, perhaps the Apollonius who *Doctor:*

that combines anatomical, psychological, and pathological comments on the branching veins of the pericardium, followed by a philosophical and philological introduction to the thymus.[195] Finally, trending now, I think, to the other end of the spectrum, another example mentions, in the space of a few lines, the brain, meninges, and vascular system and deploys the concept of man as a microcosm of the larger world; this same idea frames the introduction that was added to the *Parts of the Human Body* attributed to Rufus, but it was a popular trope in philosophical, medical, and, eventually, Christian circles.[196] The text in question certainly has a medical rather than philosophical flavor, but the close proximity of the brain and the vessels, together with what seems to be a mention of something "melting away," suggests a broader medical topic rather than an anatomical handbook.[197] All told, the papyri offer a picture of anatomy as a niche topic – one that was often incorporated, as relevant, into broader discussions and that merited a place, even if sometimes rudimentary, in introductory education. It was, nevertheless, a topic that also supported a circumscribed but robust subfield of specialized study; indeed, the papyrological evidence for these various anatomical texts over and above those we know of from the literary record serves to underscore just how robust it was.

Anatomy in the Roman Intellectual Scene

Having concentrated so far on individual authors and texts, I will now close the chapter by drawing a more holistic picture of the place of anatomical literature across the relevant intellectual landscapes in the period leading up to and including Galen's lifetime. Galen is acutely aware of the sectarian tendencies prevalent in both medical and philosophical circles; being himself a proudly independent thinker, he often scorns those who blindly adhere to their chosen sect – though, as with most polemical rhetoric in Galen, one suspects that he is exaggerating the degree of polarization.[198] Where anatomy is concerned, however, his outlook is somewhat

---

Introduction tells us was interested in exterior nomenclature; there seems to me insufficient evidence to make this latter claim, but it is certainly possible (see Chapter 2, n. 138). For interpretation of the seemingly nonanatomical columns, see Azzarello (2004), 239, 243–8.

[195] BKT X 23 (MP³ 2355.023); see Gronewald (2012).

[196] BKT IX 80 (MP³ 2355.01); see Hanson (1998) and (2001). Hanson (1998), 146–51 offers a detailed discussion of this trope, as well as her view that the author was a "philosophizing physician … rather than a medicalizing philosopher" (146); cf. the similar but briefer treatment in Hanson (2001), which provides a translation.

[197] BKT IX 80 l.7 (ἐκτηκομε-).

[198] For example, at *Lib.Prop.* XIX.13 and *Aff.Pecc.Dig.* V.42–3.

different. He conceives of "the anatomists" as a sort of supra-sect; they are a heterogeneous group with considerable internal disagreement, but nevertheless the main salient division is between those who dissect and those who do not.

As I have already explored in Chapter 3, Galen presents the anatomists as a fairly large group, and it is one with a deep history. His lost text *On Controversies in Anatomy* is dedicated to disentangling real versus semantic differences among the various opinions of previous anatomists; the scope seems to have been broad, and the necessity for such a text indicates the extent of the field.[199] In *Anatomical Procedures* he also frequently references the long-standing history of anatomists' thought, as well as the diversity of anatomists' established nomenclature, which offers a window into the variety of figures he includes under this term and the proliferation of texts they provided.[200] The title of anatomist, in this historical sense, thus seems to encompass most of the figures handled in Chapter 6, whether or not they would have self-identified as such. Modern anatomists were, for Galen, a distinct subgroup and are the ones most relevant here; he singles them out several times as "the newer anatomists" and discusses the modern anatomical scene at length.[201] He is also wary of the apparently numerous imposters to the title, scorning the practices of "all those affecting to be anatomists" and those who "deem themselves worthy to pursue anatomical research" without meeting Galen's own threshold for competency.[202]

In keeping with what we have already surmised about the performance-heavy nature of the anatomical work of Quintus and much of his school, Galen's explicit engagement with these modern anatomists centers largely on their active dissections; indeed, a healthy number of the group must

---

[199] On this text, see Chapter 8, "On Controversies in Anatomy" at pp. 292–3.

[200] A particularly rich section in this regard is the treatment of the eyes in the tenth book (*AA* S32–63), which makes frequent mention of varied nomenclature and the differing opinions of previous anatomists. His discussion of anatomists is by no means limited to this text; as highlighted throughout Chapter 8, he discusses them frequently and in similar ways across the anatomical texts, but also the nonanatomical texts, including the Hippocratic commentaries (see, e.g., *Hipp.Epid.II* 4.2 [*CMG Suppl.Or.* V.2, p. 695–9]).

[201] *AA* II.574 (ὑπὸ τῶν νεωτέρων ἀνατομικῶν), 590 (πρὸς τῶν νεωτερικῶν ἀνατομικῶν), S144–5 ("the current usage of anatomists"), 266 ("in our own time") (cf. S301), *Musc.Diss.* XVIIIb.934 (οἱ νεώτεροι), *Oss.* II.746 (ἅπασι τοῖς νεωτέροις ἀνατομικοῖς) (cf. II.735, where he mentions the anatomical nomenclature used by "the modern doctors" [ὑπὸ τῶν νεωτέρων ἰατρῶν]); he criticizes modern trends in anatomy particularly at *AA* II.287–91, 416–20.

[202] *AA* II.243 (παμπόλλων ἀνατομικῶν εἶναι προσποιουμένων), 291 (ὅσοι γε μεταχειρίζεσθαι τὴν ἀνατομικὴν θεωρίαν ἀξιοῦσιν).

have belonged to that intellectual heritage one way or another.[203] He does, however, also indicate contemporary literary output in the field, beyond just the particularly influential works by the named authors discussed earlier. He indicates a substantial library of osteological texts available to the novice desiring to learn about bones – "some entitle theirs *Osteologies*, others *Skeletons*, others simply *On Bones*" – corroborating the suspicion from the papyrological evidence that this was a particularly fertile area of publication.[204] He also alludes to a considerable number of authors working on the muscles; he mentions explicitly Marinus, Pelops, Lycus, and Aelianus as the authors of the best, or at least the most popular, versions, but he seems to refer to a wider field of substandard authors as well. He complains about authors, in whose number he pointedly includes Lycus, whose work indicates that they have not pursued serious or complete anatomical research on the muscles to support their writing; rather, the fact that they include some features but omit equally visible adjacent features leads him to the damning claim that "they seem to me ... to not engage with the dissection of these things thoroughly ... [but] to trust in reasoning without dissection and then to write in their treatises as if they had seen them."[205]

He repeats this complaint with regards to the nerves, accusing "a number of anatomists" of being too lazy to engage in this particularly difficult aspect of dissection and instead "adopting what others have said without having seen those nerves with their own eyes."[206] Others err through the more venial sin of having dissected too hurriedly, among whom are likely the "skilled anatomists" who nevertheless make erroneous claims about the nerves in their writings.[207] He refers, too, to the adjacent genre of books written by surgeons, which are also prone to errors when broaching anatomical topics.[208] Nor is it just Galen who is reading – and criticizing – modern anatomical literature. He reports that an otherwise unknown Theophrastus, who was clearly a contemporary, wrote an anatomical treatise disproving the claims of a third contemporary, and he expects his

---

[203] For this engagement, see Chapter 3, "Performance for Public Display" at pp. 70–6.

[204] *AA* II.220 (τινὲς μὲν ὀστολογίας ἐπιγράφουσιν, ἔνιοι δὲ σκελετούς, ἔνιοι δ᾽ ἁπλῶς περὶ ὀστῶν).

[205] *AA* II.459 (μοι δοκοῦσιν ... οὐδ᾽ ὅλως ἅψασθαι τῆς ἀνατομῆς αὐτῶν ... ἀποπιστεῦσαι τῷ λογισμῷ χωρὶς τῆς ἀνατομῆς, εἶτ᾽ ἐν τοῖς ὑπομνήμασι γράφειν ὡς ἑωρακότες). Other complaints about these subpar authors occur at *AA* II.469–70, 498–9.

[206] *AA* S228–9.

[207] *AA* S229, 291.

[208] *AA* S230, *Musc.Diss.* XVIIIb.996–7; cf. *Loc.Aff.* VIII.268, where he discusses the limits of anatomical knowledge among surgeons.

readers to be able to find it in current circulation.²⁰⁹ This was a dynamic literary landscape.

The anatomists' emphasis on dissection and the insight it provides into the body's normal functioning naturally earmarks them for a generally "Rationalist" or "Dogmatist" profile. The intense interest in commenting on Hippocrates that was characteristic of the foremost anatomists also suggests that many in this group could likely have been classified as "Hippocratean." However, the title of anatomist was not synonymous with any sectarian label, and interest in anatomy appears to have bled widely across borders in the medical community, even into areas where its presence is rather surprising.²¹⁰ Comparatively unsurprising is the anatomical activity on the part of the Roman Erasistrateans. Although for several centuries after Erasistratus his followers paid little attention to the topic – in keeping with the general disinterest of the later Hellenistic period – by the early second century AD a revival of their founder's anatomical studies had stirred among the sect. Galen tells us of a certain Martianus, a member of the previous generation who was still active on the medical scene in Rome as an old man when Galen first arrived: "He had a great reputation among the modern doctors as an extremely anatomical man, both at that time and also previously; two books of his anatomical work enjoyed great popularity."²¹¹

This popularity was not transient: Looking back from about two decades later, while writing *On My Own Books*, Galen says that "two of his books of anatomy, which at that time were greatly well-reputed, are still available and are currently in the possession of many."²¹² Martianus' sectarian allegiances are revealed by his claim that he considers Erasistratus, rather than Hippocrates, to be the leading ancient authority on anatomy – a claim that, no doubt as intended, whips Galen into a frenzy and results in his *Anatomy of Hippocrates* and *Anatomy of Erasistratus*.²¹³ Though perhaps

---

²⁰⁹ *AA* S166–7; see also the discussion in Chapter 3, "Performance for Public Display" at p. 71.

²¹⁰ At *Loc.Aff.* VIII.260–1 Galen criticizes the faulty anatomy deployed for partisan purposes.

²¹¹ *Praen.* XIV.615 (αὐτοῦ κατά τε τὸν χρόνον ἐκεῖνον ἔτι δὲ πρότερον ὡς ἀνατομικωτάτου δόξα μεγάλη παρὰ τοῖς ἰατροῖς νεανίσκοις ἦν. ἐσπουδάζετο δὲ δύο βιβλία τῶν ὑπ᾽ αὐτοῦ γεγραμμέν ων ἀνατομῶν); in addition to being admired for his anatomical skill, Martianus, much like Galen, was "considered to be not just a doctor but also a philosopher" (*Praen.* XIV.619) (οὐκ ἰατρὸς μόνον, ἀλλὰ καὶ φιλό<σοφο>ς εἶναι μαρτυρούμενος); following the text in Nutton (1979). On the correct spelling of Martianus' name, which appears as the equally plausible Martialius in *Lib.Prop.*, see Nutton (1979), 168–9, n. 84.2, and Boudon-Millot (2007), 185–6, n. 138.3. Smith (1979), 68 lists him as a student of Quintus, but there is no direct evidence for such an affiliation, which he probably assumed owing to Martianus' being mentioned in connection with Aelianus.

²¹² *Lib.Prop.* XIX.13.

²¹³ *Lib.Prop.* XIX.13–14, with quotation and discussion in Chapter 6, "Hippocractic Corpus" at pp. 176–7 and "Erasistratus" at pp. 202–3. Despite this provocative stance, he does appear to have

the most popular, Martianus was not the only Erasistratean writing about anatomy: Galen complains that "many have written anatomies of a sort, in which they announce that they will show arteries to be empty of blood … shamelessly lying in their anatomical writing."[214]

The Pneumatists are another group for whom anatomical interest would be a logical fit. Drawing inspiration from Stoicism, this line of medical thinking was premised on an understanding of the body that fore-grounded pneuma in its physiology and was cardiocentric, laying emphasis on sphygmology and the analysis of arterial motion.[215] A variety of topics are covered in the works attributed to doctors associated with this sect, including a number that deal with the pulse, some that handle embryology, and what Galen considers to be the best modern work on general medicine; anatomy would certainly be at home in this group, but there is no mention of it specifically.[216] The closest we come is with Aretaeus, who certainly shows himself conversant with internal anatomy, though he does not focus on it directly. His books on the causes and symptoms of chronic and acute diseases introduce each new condition with a discussion of the affected organs; often this is as simple as mentioning the main organ involved (lungs, heart, etc.) or offering a brief list if there is more than one, but he is sometimes more forthcoming, verging into descriptions suitable to a dedicated anatomical text. His account of the origin and branching paths of the vena cava, for example, is particularly detailed and includes an indication that dissection – whether by Aretaeus himself or by his source – was actively in the background: "for the name ['hollow vein'] is the same, since it is one and the same vein, having its origin from

---

generally been a proponent of the study of Hippocrates, using him to accost the upstart young Galen in another episode (*Praen.* XIV.619–20).

[214] *Art.Sang.* IV.735–6 (γεγράφασι μὲν γὰρ πολλοὶ τρόπους τινὰς ἀνατομῶν οἷς δείξειν ἐπαγγέλλονται κενὰς αἵματος εἶναι τὰς ἀρτηρίας … τούτων τοίνυν ἀναισχύντως ψευδομένων ἐν ταῖς ἀνατομαῖς).

[215] For an overview of the Pneumatists, see Kudlien (1968*b*), Gourevitch (1998), 115–17, and Nutton (2013*a*), 207–11, as well as the (now dated) collected fragments in Wellmann (1895); Harris (1973), 235–51 offers an in-depth account of their cardiocentrism and sphygmology. However, it is not always certain who should be classed as members of this sect, and Nutton (2013*a*), 211 offers the caveat that "one may have considerable doubts about its very existence as a sect in any strong sense of the word," adding that it might be "merely an ahistorical, classificatory term" (386, n. 30).

[216] Galen says of Athenaeus, whom he describes as the founder of the sect (*Caus.Cont.* 2.1 [*CMG Suppl.Or.* II, p. 55]) (cf. *Diff.Puls.* VIII.749), that "just about none of the modern doctors treated fully an entire account of the medical art" like he did (σχεδὸν οὐδεὶς τῶν νεωτέρων ἰατρῶν οὕτως ἅπαντα τὸν κατὰ τὴν ἰατρικὴν τέχνην ἐξειργάσατο λόγον ὡς ὁ Ἀθήναιος) (*Hipp.Elem.* I.457). He also mentions his work on pulse (*Diff.Puls.* VIII.646, 750–7) and on embryology (*Sem.* IV.612–14), among other topics; he similarly lists a variety of topics covered by Agathinus and Archigenes, including writing by both on the pulse (*Diff.Puls.* VIII.575–8, 591–4, 674, 748–54, with Archigenes appearing frequently elsewhere in the text as well).

the liver. For if one wished, one could thrust a probe both from the upper part of the hollow vein near the heart into the part near the spine and also from part by spine, through the liver, to the heart."[217] In addition to this evident anatomical familiarity on the part of Aretaeus, it is suggestive that Galen repeatedly marks Aiphicianos' work on Hippocrates as Stoically inflected.[218] That, combined with the fact that Aiphicianos was a student of Quintus and therefore likely a dissector, could indicate that he is an example of a Pneumatist anatomist – but this is admittedly flimsy straw with which to build bricks.

More surprising would be any connection between anatomy and the Empiricists. One of the core tenets of Empiricism was a rejection of theoretical understandings of the body and therefore also of systematic dissection as a means to understand the body and thus how to heal it. We have already seen Celsus' framing of this position as central to their differentiation from rival sects, and he is by no means the only source of evidence.[219] The pseudo-Galenic *Medical Definitions* says that there are "two types of dissection," the systematic type practiced by Dogmatists and then another, incidental kind, which "comes about by chance or through large wounds," but which "only the Empiricists use."[220] Galen offers valuable details on this particularly Empiricist brand of anatomy:

> [Knowledge of the anatomical arrangements of the arms and legs] is so necessary for doctors that not even those Empiricists who write entire books against dissection dare to condemn it, rather they agree that it is the most useful knowledge of all its kind. But they say that they have taught themselves the nature of these things sufficiently through wounds, whenever they happen.... Someone sitting high on his chair is able to say these things to his students, but he is not able to teach the actual facts of the art, being himself ignorant in the first place of all the parts of the animal organs mentioned here. For those of them who give a great impression of being skilled in this area know only such things as appear clearly through the skin.... Not only are "incidental dissection" and "wound observation"—these are their words—not capable of teaching exactly the nature of each of the parts,

---

[217] Aretaeus, *Caus.Sign.Acut.Morb.* II.8 (οὔνομα γὰρ τὸ αὐτό, οὕνεκεν μία καὶ ωὑτή ἐστὶν ἡ φλέψ, τὴν ἀρχὴν ἀπὸ τοῦ ἥπατος ἴσχουσα. εἰ γάρ τις ἐθέλοι, διελάσαι ἂν ἔλασμα καὶ ἀπὸ τῆς ἄνωθεν τῆς ἐπὶ τὴν καρδίην κοίλης φλεβὸς ἐς τὴν παρὰ τὴν ῥάχιν καὶ ἀπὸ τῆς ῥάχιος διὰ τοῦ ἥπατος ἐπὶ τὴν καρδίην). Compare the anatomical information appearing at *Caus.Sign.Acut.Morb.* I.10, II.2 and *Caus.Sign.Diut.Morb.* I.7, 9, 10, II.3, 9.

[218] See this chapter, n. 102.

[219] See Chapter 2, "The Later Hellenistic Period" at pp. 42–3.

[220] Ps.-Gal., *Def.Med.* XIX.358 (εἰσὶ τῆς ἀνατομῆς εἴδη δύο ... ἐκ συντυχίας ἢ ὑπὸ μεγάλης τρώσεως γινομένη. προσχρῶνται δὲ αὐτῇ μόνοι οἱ ἐμπειρικοί.).

it is not even so when they are given close attention unless with frequent practice on many specimens following the instructions which I am recounting in this work.[221]

In Galen's telling, then, there *are* some Empiricists who profess to being "skilled" experts of anatomy and even lecture on the subject, though deploying their own terminology and methods. These may even be the same figures who wrote the books dedicated to attacking the practice of dissection, perhaps framing them as an argument for their own style of anatomical inquiry instead.

Despite this firmly embedded tradition at the core of the sect, not all Empiricist doctors necessarily held the same view about the undesirability of systematic dissection. Notably, Galen repeatedly balks at Empiricist readings in Lycus' work on Hippocrates.[222] Surely Lycus – author of extensive anatomical writing and active dissector and vivisector – could not be less in harmony with the mainline Empiricist position on dissection. The received wisdom is therefore that Galen is exaggerating his Empiricist sympathies for rhetorical purposes; that reading like an Empiricist does not make one an Empiricist; in short, that everything else about Lycus makes it impossible that he is an Empiricist.[223] Yet one cannot escape the fact that Galen actually lists Lycus as an Empiricist in *Method of Healing*.[224] It is certainly possible that Lycus' Empiricist leanings were piecemeal and that he aligned with them in some areas, for example various exegetical readings, but not in others, like anatomy; indeed, this would be a version of the approach that Galen takes – he himself sometimes expresses Empiricist sympathies and has a grounding in Empiricist teachings, and, as always, we should never believe that Galen is quite as exceptional as he

---

[221] *AA* II.288–9 (ταῦτα γὰρ οὕτως εἰσὶν ἀναγκαῖα τοῖς ἰατροῖς, ὥστ᾽ οὐδ᾽ οἱ κατὰ τῆς ἀνατομῆς γράψαντες ὅλας βίβλους ἐμπειρικοὶ καταγνῶναι τῆς ἐπιστήμης αὐτῶν ἐτόλμησαν, ἀλλ᾽ ὁμολογοῦσιν, εἶναι χρησιμωτάτην ἁπάντων τῶν τοιούτων τὴν γνῶσιν· ἐκ δὲ τῶν ἑκάστοτε γιγνομένων τραυμάτων αὐτάρκως διδάσκεσθαί φασι τὴν φύσιν αὐτῶν. τούτους μέν γε θαυμάσειεν ἄν τις τῆς προπετείας ... ταῦτ᾽ οὖν ἐπὶ μὲν τοῦ θρόνου τις ὑψηλὸς καθήμενος δύναται λέγειν τοῖς μαθηταῖς, ἐπ᾽ αὐτῶν δὲ τῶν ἔργων τῆς τέχνης οὐ δύναται διδάξαι, πρῶτος αὐτὸς ἀγνοῶν ἅπαντα τῶν εἰρημένων ὀργάνων τοῦ ζῴου τὰ μόρια· μόνα γάρ, ὅσα προφανῶς ὑπὸ τῷ δέρματι φαίνεται, γινώσκουσιν οἱ πάνυ δοκοῦντες αὐτῶν εἶναι τρίβωνες ... οὐ μόνον ἡ κατὰ περίπτωσιν ἀνατομὴ καὶ τραυματικὴ θέα, ταῦτα γὰρ ἐκείνων τὰ ῥήματα, διδάσκειν ἀκριβῶς ἑκάστου τῶν μορίων τὴν φύσιν οὐχ οἷαί τέ εἰσιν, ἀλλ᾽ οὐδὲ κατ᾽ ἐπιτήδευσιν, ἄνευ τοῦ πολλάκις ἐπὶ πολλῶν γεγυμνάσθαι μετὰ παραγγελμάτων, ὧν ἐγὼ κατὰ τήνδε τὴν πραγματείαν διέρχομαι); cf. *Comp.Med.Gen.* XIII.604–9 for a similar tirade against the Empiricist anatomical methods.
[222] Empiricist readings at *Hipp.Epid.VI* 5.27 (*CMG* V.10.2.2, p. 308–9), *Hipp.Epid.III* XVIIa.515 (where Quintus is implicated too), *Hipp.Epid.III* XVIIa.726, *Hipp.Aph.* XVIIb.562.
[223] Kind (1927), 2416–17, and Manetti and Roselli (1994), 1588.
[224] *MM* X.143.

would make himself out to be.[225] All this suggests a fluidity to the sect that Galen's antagonistic rhetoric would deny and indicates that the embargo on intentional dissection among Empiricist doctors was perhaps not as unqualified as it might seem.

Finally, the Methodists are another sect where evidence for dissection might seem anomalous. Galen frames their simple – to his mind, simplistic – theory for understanding disease and treatment as leaving no room for anatomical inquiry. Indeed, he says that they "spit upon anatomy" and "keep away from [it] on the grounds that it is useless."[226] The evidence from Soranus (*fl.* AD 98–138), who is the only Methodist of antiquity whose writing survives in any substantive way, adds some additional nuance, though it is worth noting that both Galen and the author of *Doctor: Introduction* indicate that there was considerable internal dispute within the sect and give Soranus as an example of a somewhat unorthodox member.[227] Soranus is upfront about his attitude to dissection:

> Since we are about to shift to the discussion of female health, it will be necessary first to describe the female organs. Some of these are knowable directly, others through dissection. Even though this latter is useless, we nevertheless teach the things observed through it since it is a received part of general learnedness. For we will easily be believed when we say that anatomy is useless if we are first found to know about it and we will not leave ourselves open to the suspicion of having rejected out of ignorance something assumed to be serviceable.[228]

---

[225] Galen includes among his teachers "Aischrion the Empiricist," whom he describes as "an old man most experienced with drugs" at *Simp.Med.* XII.356–7 (Αἰσχρίων ὁ ἐμπειρικὸς ... φαρμάκων ἐμπειρικώτατος γέρων); he describes his sympathies for some Empiricist arguments at *Loc.Aff.* VIII.142–4.

[226] Galen, *MM* X.349 (τὴν ἀνατομὴν διαπτύουσι), 422 (ἀποστάντες ὡς ἀχρήστου τῆς ἀνατομῆς); cf. similar statements at *MM* X.319, 410–11, 928, *Sect.Int.* I.96.

[227] Caelius Aurelianus' Latin texts *On Acute Diseases* and *On Chronic Diseases*, which draw heavily from Soranus' lost work on these subjects, are another valuable window into Methodist thought, but date to probably the fifth century AD; see Drabkin (1950), xi. On the patchy survival of Soranus' texts, see Hanson and Green (1994), 969–81. On the diversity of views among the Methodists and Soranus' role in this, see Galen, *MM* X.53 and ps.-Galen, *Int.* XIV.684; Lloyd (1983), 182–200 also points out that Soranus himself confirms this characterization, periodically indicating that he is deviating from the opinions of previous Methodists (see especially p. 185, n. 256) (cf. Burguière, Gourevitch, and Malinas [2003], xl–xlvi).

[228] Soranus, *Gyn.* I.5 (ἐπειδὴ δὲ μεταβαίνειν ἐπὶ τὸν γυναικεῖον ὑγιεινὸν λόγον μέλλομεν, δεήσει πρῶτον τὴν φύσιν τῶν γυναικείων διηγήσασθαι τόπων. ἐξ ὧν τὰ μὲν αὐτόθεν καταλαμβάνεται, τὰ δὲ ἐξ ἀνατομῆς. ἥτις <εἰ> καὶ ἄχρηστός ἐστιν, ὅμως ἐπεὶ παραλαμβάνεται [ἐκ] χρηστομαθείας ἕνεκα, διδάξομεν καὶ τὰ ἐκ ταύτης ἐπιγνωσθέντα. ῥᾳδίως τε γὰρ πιστευθησόμεθα λέγοντες ἄχρηστον τὴν ἀνατομήν, εἰ πρότερον αὐτὴν εἰδότες εὑρεθείημεν, καὶ οὐ παρέξομεν ὑπόνοιαν τοῦ δι' ἄγνοιαν παραιτεῖσθαί τι τῶν ὑπειλημμένων εὐχρήστων).

On the one hand, this passage confirms the information from Galen that the study of anatomy was considered to be useless in Methodist doctrine; Soranus is clearly marking his allegiance to a matter of principle here. On the other, despite his sectarian posturing, he himself is actually quite open to engaging with the subject; while it is possible that this was an aspect in which his departure from the party line was idiosyncratic, his position generally suggests that Galen's imagery of spitting Methodists was overdrawn or overgeneralized or both.[229]

Soranus goes on to describe the anatomy of the female internal genitalia at some length. He includes attention to nomenclature, betraying an interest in etymology, and also mentions by name Herophilus, whose work he is perhaps relying on, and Diocles, whom he mentions only to disagree with.[230] In his disagreement with Diocles and once again a little later, he uses the evidence of dissection to disprove false theories, indicating a reliance on the soundness of anatomical science that belies his rhetorical, sectarian introduction to the topic.[231] Further, he bolsters the claims of anatomy with his own observations gleaned from medical practice, again evincing confidence in the reliability of anatomical data, but also indicating, unsurprisingly, that his own personal involvement is limited to chance observations and that his familiarity with anatomy has been acquired from books, not experience.[232] Outside of the gynecological texts, what traces

---

[229] Tecusan (2004), 31–2, 34–5 has argued that Galen's characterization of the sect as virulently anti-anatomy is more a strategic construct of his polemics than a reliable description of their beliefs. She points out that ps.-Soranus, *Quaest.Med.* 9 (Tecusan Fr. 295) is the only other ancient testimony (also negative) directly regarding Methodists and anatomy, but that it is "a very late source and probably influenced by [Galen's] *De Sectis*" (p. 32, n. 50). It is, however, the case that Celsus' description of Methodism as rejecting "conjecture about hidden things" (coniectura rerum latentium) (*DM* praef. 57) is strongly suggestive of a rejection of dissection, as is the evidence from Soranus here; it therefore seems plausible to me that Galen exaggerated the virulence, but not that he fabricated the position.

[230] Soranus, *Gyn.* I.6–18; he mentions Herophilus at I.10 and Diocles at I.14; Temkin (1956), xxxix and 11, n. 21 and Hanson and Green (1994), 982 suggest that his anatomy was to some degree reliant on Herophilus, though, in addition, the latter, as well as Burguière, Gourevitch, and Malinas (2003), xxiii and Nutton (2013a), 199, 219, suggest that he probably learned some anatomy during his time in Alexandria; while we can say with certainty that anatomy as being practiced there at around this time by Numisianus (see this chapter, "Quintus and His Students: Numisianus, Heracleianus, Pelops, and Aelianus" at pp. 243–4), there was other significant medical activity there as well and it does not follow as a given that any doctor who went there became adept in dissection – indeed, we know for a fact that the Methodists had a foothold of their own in the city, from Galen's discussion of his encounter with Julian there (*MM* X.53).

[231] Soranus, *Gyn.* I.14, 17.

[232] At *Gyn.* I.12 he says "we also have observed this with our own eyes on a certain woman suffering from intestinal hernia, in whose surgery the ovary prolapsed since the vessels that support and surround it were slackened" (καὶ ἡμεῖς δὲ τοῦτο ἐπὶ τῆς αὐτοψίας ἱστορήκαμεν ἐπί τινος ἐντεροκηλικῆς

we have of his other writing also show both conversance and comfort with anatomy; his text on the eyes appears to have included some anatomical discussion, and his etymology of the human body must surely have had some parallels with Rufus' *Names*.[233] More universally, his stance on dissection, quoted earlier, offers a broader look at the place of anatomy in the medical scene of his time. Soranus lived and worked in Rome in the early second century AD, having very likely also spent some educational time in Alexandria; he was, therefore, contemporary to and likely even moving in some of the same circles as Marinus, Numisianus, and a young Quintus.[234] His characterization of anatomy as an established element of medical knowledge and his belief that not even those who fundamentally disagreed with its utility could afford to ignore it is testament to the pervasive influence of the anatomists on the medical discourse in the Roman period.

This influence of the anatomists was not confined just to medicine. As we have seen, anatomy also features among the interests of some philosophical circles, specifically as it relates to the location and function of the soul within the body. Many philosophers would have engaged with anatomy on a mostly theoretical level; indeed, Galen observes that philosophers are particularly liable to being deceived on points of physiology that they might find relevant to their doctrine "since they are not at all knowledgeable about the things made apparent in the dissection of animals."[235] He congratulates himself on having convinced some Stoics that their position was false by leveraging the proofs of dissection and

---

γυναικός, ἐφ’ ἧς ἐν τῇ χειρουργίᾳ προέπιπτεν ὁ δίδυμος χαλασθέντων τῶν κατεχόντων αὐτὸν καὶ περιειληφότων ἀγγείων); cf. I.17 where he follows up evidence from dissection with further, observational evidence from medical practice.

[233] For the texts on the eyes and on etymology, see Hanson and Green (1994), 1039–40 and 1021–3 respectively. Tecusan (2004), 31 also argues that the descriptions of surgery in Soranus and Caelius are evidence that the Methodists did not ignore anatomy; while the operation Soranus describes of hernial surgery (see the previous note) is a good example of the basic familiarity with anatomy that surgery both entails and facilitates, I did not find her singling out of paracentesis (the draining of fluids by perforation and insertion of a catheter – not a procedure requiring advanced anatomical knowledge) to be particularly persuasive. One might also point to the chapters of the *Gynecology* on embryotomy (IV.9–13), which parallel the Hippocratic treatises discussed in Chapter 2, "Hippocratic Doctors" at pp. 21–2, but, though they undoubtedly indicate Soranus' familiarity with cutting apart bodies, they do not require or display any very specialized knowledge of anatomy.

[234] On Soranus' dates and location, see Hanson and Green (1994), 981–8.

[235] Galen, *Foet.Form.* IV.664 (ὡς ἂν οὐδὲν ἐπισταμένους τῶν ἐν ταῖς διαιρέσεσι τῶν ζώων φαινομένων); cf. 676–7, where he criticizes the Stoics for enquiring into the question of the source of perception and motion "without [using] the things made apparent from anatomy" (χωρὶς τῶν ἐξ ἀνατομῆς φαινομένων).

having them be "put to shame by anatomy."[236] Nevertheless, not all philosophers who disagreed with Galen's anatomy did so out of anatomical
ignorance.

Two of the dominant philosophical sects in the Roman period – the
Stoics and the Peripatetics – espoused a cardiocentric view of the body,
and this was no doubt a strong motivation for the small but determined group of cardiocentric anatomists operating in the Roman world.
Certainly, there were some medical sects with cardiocentric positions, like
the Pneumatists and the Praxagoreans, but there seems to have been a
decidedly philosophical influence at play as well. Galen complains about
philosophers' erroneous interpretations of the results of vivisectory experiments; he criticizes the audacity of a specific Peripatetic, who proposed
a detailed anatomical route for the heart's control of the nerves, despite
"having in no way engaged with dissection."[237] But even Galen cannot pretend that all of them were so hands off: He repeatedly mentions anatomists
performing public dissections that betray an idiosyncratically Peripatetic
interest in demonstrating that the heart has three chambers.[238] Indeed, he
feels the need to dedicate some of his own anatomical work to disproving
cardiocentric beliefs.[239]

Independent of these doctrinally driven dissections, philosophical
interests could also motivate general anatomical curiosity. The audiences
of Galen's own dissections prominently included philosophers, both
Peripatetic and Academic, and he dedicates several of his strictly anatomical texts to Boethus, a dilettante Peripatetic, and to Antisthenes, a
Platonist.[240] His *On the Usefulness of the Parts* also addresses a philosophical
audience and presupposes that they are attending – or even performing –
dissections; he later boasts that this text was very popular with "philosophers who follow Aristotle" and that some people find it "more profound

[236] *PHP* V.587 (VII.1.5 De Lacy) (ἡδέσθησαν ... ὑπὸ τῆς ἀνατομῆς).
[237] On the vivisections, *PHP* V.266–7 (II.6.17 De Lacy); on the Peripatetic, V.591–2 (VII.1.18 De Lacy) (οὐδ᾽ ὅλως ἀνατομῆς ἁψάμενος).
[238] *AA* II.619, S53.
[239] He describes a series of vivisections meant to convince wavering cardiocentrists at *PHP* V.185–7 (I.6.4–12 De Lacy) (see Chapter 3, "Performance for Public Display" at p. 69). Pelops' quixotic attempt to prove that the veins and arteries stem from the brain (see this chapter, "Quintus and His Students: Numisianus, Heracleianus, Pelops, and Aelianus" at p. 246) may also have been an overreaction to cardiocentrism's conspicuous presence in anatomical debates.
[240] Galen wrote the original version of *AA* at the behest of Boethus (*AA* II.216), to whom he also dedicated his *Hipp.Anat.* and *Er.Anat.*, among other more physiological texts (*Lib.Prop.* XIX.13); Antisthenes received *Ven.Art.Diss.*, *Nerv.Diss.*, and *Part.Hom.Diff.* (*Lib.Prop.* XIX.12 and *Part. Hom.Diff.* 1.1 [*CMG Suppl.Or.* III, p. 45]).

and valuable than what Aristotle wrote."[241] Indeed, Aristotle's zoocentric anatomy seems to have generated a particular species of dissection independent of medical motivations and not restricted to (or even particularly characteristic of) the official Peripatetic school.[242] Galen, who expresses some scorn for modern, party-line Peripatetics, intends to write a book devoted exclusively to the anatomy of animals, which he frames as completing Aristotle's project.[243] Apuleius, neither a Peripatetic nor a doctor, has a similar goal: As I explored in the introduction, he was inspired to dissect by Aristotle and made it his business to "write about the little bits of all the animals – about their situation, size, and purpose – and studiously investigate and add to the books of anatomy by Aristotle."[244] There was thus a distinct philosophical strand of dissection that developed alongside the medical revival.

In short, the Roman period nurtured the most vibrant, prominent, and widespread interest in dissection and anatomy to occur in all of Classical antiquity. Herophilus and Erasistratus have garnered more enduring fame, because of their unusual access to human subjects, and the vagaries of fortune have all but obliterated traces of the individuals involved in the Roman renaissance, but this was the background that produced Galen, the most influential of all anatomical authorities. He would assuredly not have become the same passionate anatomist had he not been embedded in this diverse ecosystem of anatomical activity, and his anatomical world would, conversely, be almost invisible to us today if it were not for his incessant interaction with it in his work. It is time now to turn to his own anatomical writings and see where they fit in the story.

---

[241] *Lib.Prop.* XIX.20 (τῶν φιλοσόφων τοῖς ἀπ' Ἀριστοτέλους); *Hipp.Epid.II* 4.2 (*CMG Suppl.Or.* V.2, p. 683); see Chapter 8, "Dissection Elsewhere in the Galenic Corpus" at pp. 305–11.

[242] Though not strictly anatomical, the Aristotelian *Problemata* (see Chapter 2, "The Later Hellenistic Period" at p. 45) encouraged a similar spirit of zoological and medical curiosity among those with a philosophical interest; see Meeusen (2018) for the ways it was read and used in the Roman period.

[243] *UP* III.328, IV.145 (I.241, II.286H), *AA* S193; see *Sem.* IV.516, 520 on contemporary Peripatetics.

[244] Apuleius, *Apol.* 40; see Chapter 1, pp. 1–2 for the full quote, with discussion.

CHAPTER 8

Galen's Minor Anatomical Works

First among these [works of anatomy] is the text *On Bones for Beginners*, after that come all the books for beginners, one of them concerning the anatomy of the veins and arteries, the other that of the nerves. And there is also a certain other, the anatomy of the muscles, which accurately and briefly teaches everything that is written about the muscles in *Anatomical Procedures*. If someone wished to immediately proceed to *Anatomical Procedures* after the anatomy of the bones, it is possible for him to skip the anatomies of the vessels and the nerves, just as, certainly, also that of the muscles. For all elements of anatomy are written about in the *Procedures*.... So, these are the necessary works on anatomical theory, but, in addition to these necessary ones, other useful ones are also listed here: the epitome of the twenty anatomical books of Marinus into four of my own, just as also all those of Lycus into two.... In these books the necessary and useful aspects of the anatomical art are contained; but others on this same art were also written in addition, among which are two books on *Controversies in Anatomy*, one *On the Dissection of the Dead* and two others *On the Dissection of the Living*; in this same category is also the text *On the Difference between the Homoeomerous Parts*. Concerning the *Anatomy of Hippocrates* and *of Erasistratus*, I have spoken earlier. *On the Ignorance of Lycus in Anatomy* in four books was added to these later as an addition; and later, after those, I wrote a certain two books about the disagreements between me and Lycus in our anatomical writings concerning the use and function of the parts of the body. So then, these are the books on the art of anatomy, teaching the parts of the body and what is the constitution of each one.

Galen, *On My Own Books*[1]

---

[1] *Lib.Prop.* XIX.23, 25 (4.1–2, 8–9, 38–40 Boudon-Millot [2007], whose text I follow) (πρῶτον μὲν ἐν τούτοις ἐστὶ τὸ περὶ τῶν ὀστῶν τοῖς εἰσαγομένοις γεγραμμένον, μετὰ τοῦτο δὲ ἔστιν ἄλλα τοῖς εἰσαγομένοις βιβλία, τὸ μὲν ἕτερον αὐτῶν φλεβῶν τε καὶ ἀρτηριῶν ἀνατομὴν περιέχον, τὸ δ' ἕτερον νεύρων· ἔστι δέ τι καὶ ἄλλο [μυῶν ἀνατομή] ἐν συντόμῳ διδάσκον ἅπαντα ἀκριβῶς, ὅσα κατὰ τὰς ἀνατομικὰς ἐγχειρήσεις γέγραπται περὶ μυῶν. εἰ δέ τις βούλοιτο μετὰ τὴν τῶν ὀστῶν ἀνατομὴν ἐπὶ τὰς ἀνατομικὰς ἐγχειρήσεις εὐθέως ἔρχεσθαι, δυνατόν ἐστιν αὐτῷ παρελθεῖν τὰς [περὶ] τῶν

274

Here, Galen provides his own introduction to his anatomical writings, which are the first genre that he broaches in *On My Own Books* and among the first books that he suggests his audience read in *On the Order of My Own Books*.[2] The largest and most important of these texts, *Anatomical Procedures* (henceforth *AA*), will be the subject of Chapter 9; this chapter will examine each of the minor works individually. In each case, I characterize the text and its relationship to the tradition of anatomical writing discussed in Chapters 6 and 7, keeping a particular focus on the role of dissection in each text. At the end of the chapter, I turn to Galen's deployment of dissection in the rest of his oeuvre and chart the chronological progression of the significance he accords it. Unlike Galen, who groups his anatomical writings based on importance into the three tiers of "necessary," "useful," and "additional," I have arranged my handling of these texts chronologically, insofar as the evidence allows, and I have added two titles that he does not include here.[3] The first is his *On the Dissection of the Uterus*, which, though unambiguously anatomical, he mentions among his juvenilia. The second is the original version of *Anatomical Procedures*, which is now lost and, at only two books, was quite different from – and substantially less detailed than – the surviving work in fifteen books; because he refers to both of these texts with the same title, I have dubbed the earlier, two-book version *AA*₁ to avoid ambiguity.

ἀγγείων τε καὶ νεύρων ἀνατομάς, ὥσπερ γε καὶ τὴν τῶν μυῶν· ἅπαντα γὰρ τὰ τῆς ἀνατομῆς ἐν ταῖς ἐγχειρήσεσι γέγραπται ... τὰ μὲν οὖν ἀναγκαῖα τῆς ἀνατομικῆς θεωρίας ταῦτ᾽ ἐστίν, ἐπὶ δὲ τοῖς ἀναγκαίοις ἄλλα χρήσιμα καὶ ταυτὶ γέγραπται· τῶν Μαρίνου βιβλίων ἀνατομικῶν εἴκοσιν ὄντων ἐν τέτταρσιν ἡμετέροις ἐπιτομή, καθάπερ καὶ τῶν Λύκου πάντων ἐν δυοῖν·... ἐν τούτοις μὲν ἡ ἀναγκαία τε καὶ χρήσιμος ἀνατομικῆς θεωρίας περιέχεται· γέγραπται δὲ καὶ ἄλλα τῆς αὐτῆς θεωρίας ἐκ περιουσίας ὧν ἐστι δύο μὲν περὶ τῆς ἀνατομικῆς διαφωνίας, ἓν δὲ περὶ τῆς τῶν τεθνεώτων ἀνατομῆς καὶ δύο ἄλλα περὶ τῆς ἀνατομῆς τῶν ζώντων· ἐκ τούτου δὲ τοῦ γένους ἐστιν καὶ τὸ περὶ τῆς τῶν ὁμοιομερῶν διαφορᾶς. περὶ δὲ τῆς Ἱπποκράτους καὶ Ἐρασιστράτου ἀνατομῆς ἔμπροσθεν εἴρηταί μοι. προσετέθη δὲ τούτοις ὕστερον ἐκ περιουσίας περὶ τῶν ἠγνοημένων Λύκῳ κατὰ τὰς ἀνατομὰς βιβλία τέτταρα· καί τινα μετὰ ταῦτα ὕστερον ἐγράφη δύο περὶ τῶν διαπεφωνημένων μοι πρὸς Λύκον ἐν τοῖς ἀνατομικοῖς συγγράμμασιν περί τε τῆς τῶν μορίων τοῦ σώματος ἐνεργείας τε καὶ χρείας· τῆς μὲν οὖν ἀνατομικῆς θεωρίας ταῦτ᾽ἐστὶν τὰ βιβλία διδάσκοντα τὰ μόρια τοῦ σώματος ταῦτα τίνος ἕκαστον ἐστιν κατασκευῆς).

2 *Ord.Lib.Prop.* XIX.54; see also *Ars Med.* I.408–9 and this chapter, "Dissection Elsewhere in the Galenic Corpus" at p. 304.

3 For chronologies of Galen's oeuvre, see Ilberg (1892) and Bardong (1942); Peterson (1977) argues cogently for the need for a thorough update of Galenic chronology. For the surviving works, unless otherwise indicated, I have generally followed the dates provided in the *Liste des Oeuvres Conservées de Galien* at the end of Boudon-Millot (2012), which she based largely on the three aforementioned articles. I have chosen not to include here the single book on "*Articulation of the First of the Cervical Vertebrae,*" which is listed among Galen's anatomical works in one of the two recensions of Hunayn

On the Dissection of the Uterus

The earliest book on anatomy that Galen wrote was his short *On the Dissection of the Uterus*, which he composed as a student in Pergamon prior to leaving for Smyrna to study with Pelops.[4] It offers a succinct description of the anatomy of the uterus, including a final section on the extra-embryonic membranes found during pregnancy. He groups it in *On My Own Books* with his juvenilia rather than his anatomical works, and it does indeed bear the hallmarks of an early effort: Galen shows himself to be much more reliant on his predecessors and much less willing to criticize them than in his later works.[5] He openly depends on earlier sources, saying, for example, "I say these things not having witnessed them myself, but learning from Praxagoras ... indeed, I know clearly from reports that these things are so," a statement that would be inconceivably unauthoritative in one of his later works.[6] While he is evidently still at the very beginning of his anatomical journey, the text nevertheless suggests that he has used his own experience with dissection to inform his writing. He explicitly mentions the act of dissection only once, but his descriptions throughout indicate some personal familiarity with the things he is discussing.[7]

---

ibn Ishaq's *Risala* (Lamoreaux [2016], 48, n. 34.2); while it is true that it is accompanied there by the genuinely Galenic *On the Difference between the Homoeomerous Parts*, which lends credibility to this disputed section, unlike that text, which Hunayn says he translated, the one in question does not receive any commentary at all from Hunayn, which strongly suggests it is an interpolation of some kind, especially since there is no other trace of a work on this topic and the title does not seem convincingly Galenic. Similarly, the *De anatomia* listed in Diels (1905), 115–16 is a sixteenth-century compilation of passages from *Int.* and *Ven.Art.Diss.*, not an original text; see Formentin (1977).

4 *Lib.Prop.* XIX.16; it thus dates to the period AD 145–9.

5 See, for example, *Ut.Diss.* II.905, where, after describing an erroneous belief held by Hippocrates, Diocles, and Praxagoras, he says, "therefore were they all wrong? But it is not right to think thus about such men" (ἆρ' οὖν πάντες ἠγνόηκασι; ἀλλ' οὐ θέμις ὑπὲρ ἀνδρῶν τηλικούτων οὕτω φρονεῖν). Ilberg (1892), 490–1 has suggested that the present version of the work is a second edition of sorts, having been reworked by Galen when he came back into possession of it after his return visit to Pergamon; however, as Nickel (1971), 61–3 shows, his reasoning is not persuasive; cf. Flemming (2000), 261, n. 19 on the sexism inherent in Ilberg's logic.

6 *Ut.Diss.* II.906 (λέγω δὲ ταῦτα οὐ μαντευσάμενος, ἀλλὰ παρὰ Πραξαγόρου μαθών ... σαφὲς ἤδη οἶμαι ἐκ τῶν εἰρημένων γεγονέναι).

7 He explicitly mentions dissection in his discussion of the coats of the uterus at *Ut.Diss.* II.896–7: "if you wish to separate this [layer], flaying it, there seem to you to be two uteri, which lie on one and the same cervix. For this, just like the [outer] membrane of the uterus, you are no longer able to separate in two" ([οἱ]ὸν εἰ θελήσαις ἀποδείρας χωρίσαι, δύο σοι φανοῦνται μῆτραι, ἐφ' ἑνὶ καὶ τῷ αὐτῷ αὐχένι κείμεναι. τοῦτον γάρ, ὥσπερ καὶ τῆς μήτρας τὸν χιτῶνα, εἰς δύο χωρίσαι οὐκέτι δυνήσῃ); following the text in Nickel (1971). His comments at, for example, II.892 also suggest hands-on familiarity: "you would not be able to separate these things without cutting them" (οὐκ ἂν αὐτὰ χωρίσαις ἄνευ τομῆς) (cf. II.893–4, 900, 907).

As far as contents and style, this short treatise – Galen refers to it as a "small booklet" – offers a run-through of anatomical data with no directions for or urgings toward dissection, making it a straightforward example of a Dioclean-style handbook in Galen's terminology.[8] To elicit some of its particular characteristics, a comparison with the relevant material in Soranus, which is on a similar scale, is helpful.[9] Galen shows considerably less interest in nomenclature and etymology than Soranus, but considerably more in comparative anatomy; while Soranus mentions the anatomy of animals only twice, briefly, Galen comes back to them repeatedly, indicating his embeddedness in the world of heuristic animal dissection.[10] In keeping, the extra length of Galen's work is largely owing to a greater level of anatomical detail and, in some cases, a more thorough understanding.[11] He also engages more explicitly and more frequently with earlier anatomical thought, though the two are drawing on a similar pool of authors; further, he feels less need to address popular beliefs that are at variance with observable anatomy, for example the idea of the womb as a wandering animal or the reputed presence of a transverse membrane in the vagina of virgins, both of which Soranus takes pains to refute.[12] Where Soranus has included anatomical sections in support of his larger, more general purpose, Galen clearly conceived of his text as part of the tradition of specialized anatomical discourse.

As for its intended use and audience, there are few hints in the text itself. Unlike Soranus, who includes some remarks on disease even in the purely anatomical chapters, Galen says nothing of a medical nature – indeed, he explicitly deems any such discussion outside the scope of the text.[13] He portrays even childbirth as a largely tangential concern.[14] In *On My*

---

[8] *Lib.Prop.* XIX.16 (μικρὸν βιβλίδιον).

[9] Soranus, *Gyn.* I.6–18, 57–8, which contains the topics covered here by Galen, is roughly two-thirds the length of this treatise.

[10] Soranus, *Gyn.* I.9, 58; Galen, *Ut.Diss.* II.890–1 (on the differences between the shape of and location of implantation in human uteri and those of various other species), 895–6 (on Herophilus' privileged knowledge of human versus animal anatomy), 905–6 (on cotyledons in nonhuman animals).

[11] Compare, for example, both authors on the attachment of the uterus to its surroundings (Soranus, *Gyn.* I.8; Galen, *Ut.Diss.* II.892–4) and on the extraembryonic membranes (Soranus, *Gyn.* I.57–8; Galen, *Ut.Diss.* II.902–8).

[12] Soranus' explicit engagement with previous sources is limited in these chapters to succinct references at *Gyn.* I.10, 14, 57; Galen cites and discusses earlier authors throughout, including direct and extensive quotations at *Ut.Diss.* II.888, 895, 903–6. Interestingly, they both cite Herophilus for the exact same statement, on the comparison of the cervix of multiparous women to the top of the trachea (*Gyn.* I.10 and *Ut.Diss.* II.897). For the refutation of the wandering womb and the vaginal membrane in virgins, see Soranus, *Gyn.* I.8 and 17 respectively.

[13] Soranus, *Gyn.* I.8, 12–13, 15, 17; Galen, *Ut.Diss.* II.898.

[14] Galen, *Ut.Diss.* II.898.

Own Books, he says that he gave the text "to a certain midwife," though it does not necessarily follow that he wrote it expressly for her.[15] This brief, unelaborated remark opens up all sorts of questions about the education, knowledge base, and activities of second-century midwives and about the potential involvement of women in the world of ancient anatomy. Given the strictly anatomical and descriptive focus of the text, it is not obvious to what practical use a midwife could have put it; however, Soranus does say that in order to be a suitable candidate for training as a midwife a woman should be "literate, in order to have the ability to learn the art through theory as well" and that the very best midwife is one who "has great experience with theory."[16] While it seems unlikely that dissection formed any part of the typical training in midwifery, it could be that the ability to speak knowledgeably about anatomy – or even the mere possession of an anatomical book of this sort – would have heightened a midwife's status among the doctors she worked with and the clients she served. At any rate, it is fascinating for the history of female medical practitioners that the young Galen at the beginning of his medical career considered this midwife to be a colleague of sorts, to the degree that either she felt emboldened to ask him for such a text, perhaps having heard him or his teacher use anatomical knowledge to his advantage at a bedside, or he, in his turn, was inspired to give it to her, whether as a follow-up to a professional conversation or as a token of respect and encouragement.

The First *Anatomical Procedures* (*AA₁*)

Among the earliest of what Galen classes as his anatomical works was the original version of *Anatomical Procedures* (*AA₁*), now lost. Galen tells us at the beginning of the extant version that he composed *AA₁* when he first came to Rome, at the start of Marcus Aurelius' reign; we can thus infer that he wrote it on the earlier end of his first stay in Rome, which lasted from AD 162 to 166.[17] He adds that Boethus, who had observed many of Galen's dissections during his stay in Rome and was getting ready to return to his native city, "requested these books as a reminder, fearing that he might forget the

---

[15] *Lib.Prop.* XIX.16 (μαίᾳ τινί).

[16] Soranus, *Gyn.* I.3 (γραμμάτων μὲν ἐντός [εἶναι], ἵνα καὶ διὰ θεωρίας τὴν τέχνην ἰσχύσῃ παραλαβεῖν), 4 (ἐν τοῖς θεωρήμασιν πολύπειρον). For an analysis of the idealizations at work in Soranus' description and for further evidence for the social and educational status of midwives, see Flemming (2000), 38–42, 231–2, and Laes (2010).

[17] *AA* II.215.

things he had seen."[18] Galen indicates, however, that he had multiple copies of the text in Rome, and he refers his readers to it in subsequent works from this period, meaning that he considered it to have been an official, edited text that was circulating, not a one-off composition for a friend.[19]

This original version was only two books long and must thus have been considerably less exhaustive than the subsequent fifteen-book version. In fact, assuming that each of the two books was roughly on a par with the average book length in Galen's surviving multibook volumes, the original text would have been similar to – perhaps even a bit shorter than – the combined length of *On the Dissection of the Muscles*, *On the Dissection of the Veins and Arteries*, and *On the Dissection of the Nerves*, suggesting that the level of detail to be found in *AA₁* was roughly comparable to that found there.[20] What distinguished *AA₁* from the other minor anatomical texts was its purpose. While *On the Dissection of the Veins and Arteries*, *On the Dissection of the Nerves*, and *On the Dissection of the Muscles*, as we shall see, centered on conveying the relevant anatomical facts as learned from dissection, the goal of *AA₁* was to describe the methods by which to dissect.

Galen seems to have modeled *AA₁* on, and perhaps named it in homage to, Marinus' pioneering *Anatomical Procedures*.[21] That text comprised "a single long book" and was therefore likely not too much shorter than, and plausibly even about the same length as, Galen's two-book

---

[18] *AA* II.216 (δεδιὼς δέ, μὴ λάθοιτό ποτε τῶν ὀφθέντων, ἐδεήθη τοιούτων ἀναμνήσεων). On Boethus, see Chapter 3, "Performance for Public Display" at pp. 60–2.

[19] *AA* II.216, where he mentions the "copies" (ἀντίγραφα) that he had in Rome. On the differences Galen sees between formal and informal work, see *Lib.Prop.* XIX.8–13 (cf. Chapter 4, "Other Requirements: Books" at pp. 133–4) and, most recently, the discussion in Cribiore (2019), 262–71.

[20] As I discuss later in this chapter, these three texts vary in length and offer differing levels of detail; by Galen's own account, *AA₁* likely offered more about the nervous and vascular systems and less about the musculature than is found in the parallel works for beginners. I achieved a rough proxy for average book length in Galen's surviving multibook volumes by taking the average of the average book length in each of the following works, using the word counts as reported in the *TLG* and adjusting book-counts to reflect the final, truncated book of *AA* as it survives in Greek, the similarly truncated first book of *PHP*, and the final, intentionally brief book of *UP*: *AA* (8.3), *Mot.Musc.* (2), *Nat.Fac.* (3), *PHP* (8.5), *UP* (16.3), *Temp.* (3), *Caus.Symp.* (3), *Loc.Aff.* (6), *MM* (14), *MMG* (2), *Alim.Fac.* (3), *San.Tu.* (6), *Di.Dec.* (3), *Cris.* (3), *Diff.Puls.* (4), *Dig.Puls.* (4), *Caus.Puls.* (4), *Praes.Puls.* (4), *Diff. Resp.* (3). The average book length comes to 10,352 words and the highest average across a single work is 11,956 words (*UP*). These numbers suggest that the two-book *AA₁* was likely on the order of between 20,704 and 23,912 words. The combined total of *Musc.Diss.* (14,747), *Ven.Art.Diss.* (7,540), and *Nerv.Diss.* (3,607) comes to a comparable 25,894 words. Note that I deliberately excluded the multivolume commentaries, namely *Hipp.Aph.* (7), *Hipp.Fract.* (3), *Hipp.Art.* (4), *Hipp.Prog.* (3), *Hipp.Epid.I* (3), *Hipp.Epid.III* (3), *Hipp.Epid.VI* (6), *Hipp.Prorrh.* (3), *HNH* (3), *Hipp.Off.Med.* (3), and pharmacological works, namely *SMT* (11), *Comp.Med.Loc.* (10), *Comp.Med.Gen.* (7), *Ant.* (2), because they have different basic formats and higher average book lengths: an average of 12,549 words for the commentaries and 13,556 words for the pharmacological texts.

[21] On Marinus' *Anatomical Procedures*, see Chapter 7, "Marinus" at pp. 235–6.

version.[22] Galen also tells us that AA_1 did not follow the same order as the extant version, but rather followed that used by Marinus.[23] Unfortunately, we can only guess at the order and contents of Marinus' book. If it was roughly keyed to his twenty-book anatomy, in the same way that Galen's *AA* follows the order of his *On the Usefulness of the Parts*, then we might expect it to begin with a discussion of the homoeomerous parts.[24] While it is not immediately obvious how much could be said in a general way about the dissection of these substances as opposed to specific organs, Galen does in fact indicate that this topic formed a part of AA_1. In his short work *On Uneven Distemper*, which was written in the same period as AA_1 and long before *AA*, he discusses the constituent parts of the body and describes how any given body part, for example a finger, is composed of

> bones and cartilage and ligaments and nerves and arteries and veins, membranes and flesh and tendons, nails and skin and fat. And it is possible to separate these no further into different things, but they are homoeomerous and primary, except the arteries and veins, for those are composed of fibers and membranes; there is discussion on this subject in *Anatomical Procedures*. And what is more, many spaces exist between these aforementioned homoeomerous and primary parts and there are many large ones in the midst of the organic and compound parts and sometimes even within a certain individual homoeomerous part, like in bone or skin; and there is discussion about all of this in *Anatomical Procedures*.[25]

---

[22] Galen, *AA* II.470 (ἓν … μέγα βιβλίον). At *Indol.* 28 (Boudon-Milot et al [2010]) Galen indicates that any book exceeding the equivalent of 4,000 hexameter lines is too long and should be broken into two more appropriately sized books. He complains about the length of Lycus' book on the anatomy of the muscles, which he calls "one extremely large book" at *Musc.Diss.* II.926 (ἓν μέγιστον βιβλίον) and says is "almost five thousand lines" at *AA* II.227 (μικροῦ δεῖν εἰς πεντακισχιλίους στίχους); in contrast he calls Marinus' book just "large" (μέγα) rather than "extremely large" (μέγιστον). We might therefore guess that Marinus' *AA* was something like 3,750 lines. At a rough estimation of an average 6.5 words per line, this would have made it somewhere in the ballpark of 24,375 words, making it comparable to the 20,704–23,912 range estimated earlier for the two book AA_1. By the same calculation, Lycus' book on the muscles would have been about 32,000 words, making Galen's estimation at *AA* II.227 that his own *Musc.Diss.* (14,747 words) was about a third as long verisimilar, if rather an unfair exaggeration – which is just about what we would expect of him.

[23] Galen, *AA* II.234.

[24] For the order of Marinus' twenty-book work on anatomy, see Chapter 7, "Marinus" at pp. 232–3.

[25] Galen, *Inaeq.Int.* VII.735 (ὀστᾶ καὶ χόνδροι καὶ σύνδεσμοι καὶ νεῦρα καὶ ἀρτηρίαι καὶ φλέβες, ὑμένες τε καὶ σάρκες καὶ τένοντες, ὄνυχές τε καὶ δέρμα καὶ πιμελή· ταῦτα δ' οὐκέτ' ἐγχωρεῖ τέμνειν εἰς ἕτερον εἶδος, ἀλλ' ἔστιν ὁμοιομερῆ τε καὶ πρῶτα, πλὴν ἀρτηριῶν τε καὶ φλεβῶν· αὗται γὰρ ἐξ ἰνῶν τε καὶ ὑμένων σύγκεινται, καθ' ὃ κἂν ταῖς ἀνατομικαῖς ἐγχειρήσεσιν ἐλέγετο. καὶ μὲν δὴ καὶ ὡς χῶραι πολλαὶ μεταξὺ τῶν εἰρημένων ὁμοιομερῶν τε καὶ πρώτων μορίων ὑπάρχουσι, καὶ τούτων ἔτι πλείους τε καὶ μείζους ἐν τῷ μέσῳ τῶν ὀργανικῶν τε καὶ συνθέτων, ἐνίοτε δὲ καὶ καθ' ἓν ὁτιοῦν ὁμοιομερὲς μόριον, ὡς ἐν ὀστῷ καὶ δέρματι· καὶ περὶ τούτων ἁπάντων ἐν ταῖς ἀνατομικαῖς ἐγχειρήσεσιν εἴρηται).

These references are further supported by similar statements in *On the Elements According to Hippocrates* – where he says that *Anatomical Procedures* explains how the compound organs are formed out of simple organs, which are themselves formed out of the homoeomerous parts – and by passages in *Method of Healing to Glaucon* and *On Unnatural Swellings* that refer the reader to it for the topic of naturally occurring spaces in bodily tissues.[26] It would seem, then, that AA_1 contained a general overview of the body's constituent materials, which would be consistent with a book that followed the order of Marinus' *AA*, assuming that was in turn patterned on his large anatomy. One could also imagine instructions for skinning, which were likely a part of AA_1, belonging to an opening section of this nature.[27]

As the passage from *On Uneven Distemper* shows, cross-references from other texts can offer valuable insight into the contents of this lost work. However, the situation is rendered enormously complicated by the fact that Galen sometimes edited his texts later in life and describes both versions of *Anatomical Procedures* by the same title without differentiation. Therefore, while it is safe to assume that all references to an *Anatomical Procedures* in texts that postdate the composition of the second version are to *AA*, we cannot be equally secure in assigning all references from texts that predate it to AA_1. *On Uneven Distemper* is a case where we can be fairly confident: It was composed in the same window as AA_1 (AD 162–6) and there is no indication that it was later reworked; further, the passages alluded to in the quote just given find no ready counterpart in the extant *AA*, reinforcing the likelihood that this – together with the parallels in the other texts – is a genuine insight into AA_1, which must indeed have been quite different from its later manifestation.[28] Later in that same text we also learn that AA_1 describes the great heat that is perceptible if you insert your fingers into the left ventricle of a still-living animal, indicating that it contained some description of vivisection as well as dissection.[29]

---

[26] Galen, *Hipp.Elem.* I.481, 493; *MMG* XI.112; *Tum.Pr.Nat.* VII.714.

[27] Galen, *Musc.Diss.* XVIIIb.928 indicates that an *Anatomical Procedures* contained such instructions, likely referring to AA_1, as I explore later in this section.

[28] The dating of *Hipp.Elem.* is less clear-cut, but it still securely predated *AA*; see De Lacy (1996), 43, though his note at the relevant passage (p. 197, n. 126.24) is rendered confused by his apparent conflation of the lost AA_1 and the lost books twelve to fifteen of *AA*, which were burnt previous to publication and had to be rewritten (*AA* S135); *Hipp.Elem.* is clearly referencing the former, not the latter. *MMG* is also prior to *AA* (Peterson [1977], 489, 492 dates it to the early 170s and no later than AD 174) and the similarities between the citation there and that in *Tum.Pr.Nat.* suggest that the latter is referring to the same passage.

[29] Galen, *Inaeq.Int.* VII.742.

Cross-references from the other texts that mention *Anatomical Procedures* but predate *AA* require more careful consideration. First, there are the two minor anatomical texts *On the Dissection of the Veins and Arteries* and *On the Dissection of the Nerves*; they were written in the same period as AA_1, but Galen also tells us that he later edited them when he returned to Rome for a second time.[30] On the whole, I am nevertheless inclined to believe that the references to *Anatomical Procedures* in these texts are to AA_1, for several reasons. First, Galen returned to Rome in AD 169 and did not begin work on *AA* until somewhere between AD 176 and 180; this leaves plenty of time for the revisions to predate *AA*, which seems the most likely scenario, both because he directly associates his repossession of the texts with his return to the city, suggesting revisions quite soon after AD 169, and because he would have been more likely to put the time into a reedition if he had not yet decided to revisit all of the material in the expanded *AA*.[31] Second, several of the citations refer, in the present or past tense, to discussions of material that is handled in the final books of *AA*, which were not published until after AD 192; this would imply that the edits on the minor books were pushed back more than twenty years after his return to the city, which seems highly unlikely.[32] Finally, some of the citations lack a clear counterpart in *AA*, which is not incontrovertible evidence by any means, but still weighs in favor of their pointing towards AA_1.[33] While we still cannot discount the possibility that some of these cross-references are later insertions – for example, the result of Galen engaging in yet another round of edits after *AA* was entirely complete – it seems more plausible than not that the cross-references in these two texts can offer genuine information on AA_1.

---

[30] Galen, *Lib.Prop.* XIX.11–12; for the revision of these two texts, see this chapter, "*On Bones*" at pp. 294–5.

[31] Indeed, he feels the need to explain at *Musc.Diss.* XVIIIb.927 why he is bothering to write a dedicated treatise on the subject of the muscles since he has already decided to embark on the writing of *AA*. On the dating of the first books of *AA*, see Garofalo (1986–2001), ix.

[32] *Ven.Art.Diss.* II.807, *Nerv.Diss.* II.837, 844–5, 849, 852–3. Ilberg (1892), 498, n. 3, and Garofalo (1994), 1798–9 believe Galen's use of the present tense in these passages is proof that they were added during the reworking of the texts and that this reworking was contemporary to the composition of the first books of *AA*. This reasoning seems to me flawed on three counts: 1) As I say here, several of these references are to parts of *AA* that were still far in the future in the timeframe under consideration; 2) the original versions of the texts were written more or less contemporarily with AA_1, which equally well explains the present tense, and there seems no reason to assume that Galen would have bothered to alter the tense in his rewrites, and 3) the one reference that is in the past tense (*Nerv.Diss.* II.844) is grammatically embedded in the paragraph where it appears, arguing against casual insertion later, and is one of the ones that refers to material from the final book of *AA*. By far the easiest solution here is to assume that AA_1 is meant.

[33] *Ven.Art.Diss.* II.819, *Nerv.Diss.* II.840, 853.

Operating on this assumption, we can add to our characterization of
*AA*₁. First of all, Galen says that *AA*₁ offers "a more exact description" of
the anatomy of the veins and arteries, whereas *On the Dissection of the
Veins and Arteries* is intended to be "useful as a synopsis for beginners."[34]
In keeping, he adds that *AA*₁ goes more fully into the confusing details of
the veins of the armpits, as well as the intricacies of how the vessels insert
into the various muscles and the various organs of the body, including a
detailed passage on the connection of the arteries of the brain to the sense
organs – all subjects that he deems unnecessarily complicated for the average doctor, beginner, or philosopher at whom *On the Dissection of the
Veins and Arteries* is targeted.[35] In the course of one of these asides, we learn
in addition that the description of the muscles in *AA*₁ precedes that of the
vessels, which is not surprising given that this is also true both of Marinus'
large anatomy and the surviving *AA*.[36]

Similarly, he describes *On the Dissection of the Nerves* as "an outline
and kind of synopsis of the things accurately described in [*AA*₁] ... useful
for beginners."[37] This text is shorter than *On the Dissection of the Veins
and Arteries* and includes comparatively more frequent references to *AA*₁.
We learn here that *AA*₁ offered more details on the fourth pair of cranial
nerves, on the nerves of the larynx, on the nerves that serve the intercostal,
thoracic, and other muscles, and on the nerves of the arms and legs.[38] On
this last topic, he specifies that *AA*₁ describes the ways in which the nerves
insert into the muscles; this parallels the description of the insertion of the
vessels into the muscles mentioned in *On the Dissection of the Veins and
Arteries* and rather suggests that, just as the first three books of *AA* do for
the arms and legs, *AA*₁ introduced a set of, or perhaps all of, the muscles
and then followed this immediately with information on the insertion
into them of relevant vessels and nerves. In addition to these straight anatomical facts, he says that *AA*₁ also included a more critical section on the
reasons for other anatomists' mistaken opinions on the spinal nerves.[39]

---

[34] *Ven.Art.Diss* II.788 (ἡ μὲν ἀκριβεστέρα διήγησις ἐν ταῖς ἀνατομικαῖς ἐγχειρήσεσιν λέγεται·
συνόψεως δὲ ἕνεκα χρησίμης τοῖς εἰσαγομένοις εἰρήσεται καὶ νῦν); following the text in Garofalo
and Debru (2008).

[35] *Ven.Art.Diss.* II.788, 804, 807, 819; on the limited expectations for his target audience, see *Ven.Art.
Diss.* II.804.

[36] *Ven.Art.Diss.* II.804.

[37] *Nerv.Diss.* II.855 (νυνὶ μὲν γὰρ ὅσον ὑποτύπωσίν τε καὶ οἷον σύνοψιν τούτων τῶν ἐν ἐκείνοις
ἀκριβῶς εἰρημένων ἐποιησάμεθα χρησίμην τοῖς εἰσαγομένοις ἐσομένην).

[38] *Nerv.Diss.* II.837, 841, 852–3, 855.

[39] *Nerv.Diss.* II.844. Similarly, at II.837 he says that his discussion of the fourth pair of cranial nerves
in *AA*₁ interrogates whether Marinus correctly understood them; comparing the statement here to

Finally, he indicates that AA_1 concerns itself with variations among different species, and says that in it he "show[s] that there are six classes" of animals suitable for dissection in a context like this; Garofalo has suggested that Galen himself came up with these six classes, which appear in a scattershot manner in AA, and it is conceivable that he articulated the concept for the first time in AA_1.[40]

As I will explore at the end of this chapter, Galen's decision to produce a second, larger edition of *Anatomical Procedures* solidified while he was in the midst of writing *On the Usefulness of the Parts*.[41] Some of the references in the later books of that text were definitely to AA from the outset, and even the earlier ones are rendered potentially suspect by the fact that he made substantive edits to *On the Usefulness of the Parts* after completing it: There are multiple references in it to other works that we know he composed after finishing it. It would be incautious, therefore, to try to read too much into any of these citations, but it is worth noting that, on the whole, they highlight similar themes to those already attributed to AA_1 by the other texts considered here: anatomical details, some instructions for how to proceed in specific dissections or vivisections, and discussion of why previous anatomists were incorrect in their beliefs.[42] The cross-references in *On the Doctrines of Hippocrates and Plato* are similarly problematic. Galen composed the first six books of this text in the same period as AA_1, but the final four date to the period from AD 169–76, and it appears that he went back and edited the original books while writing them.[43] Unlike the reediting of the minor anatomical works, this seems to have occurred in the later end of this window; three of the five references to *Anatomical Procedures* are directly linked to *On the Usefulness of the Parts*.[44] This suggests that any references to *Anatomical Procedures* in *On the Doctrines of*

Galen's discussion of this pair in the fourteenth book of AA suggests that he believed Marinus to be mistaken, but – notably – he does not mention Marinus there at all, further suggesting that this reference is to AA_1, not to AA.

[40] On the differences, see *Nerv.Diss.* II.845, 849; on the six classes, see II.840 (ἐξ ὑπάρχειν γένη δείκνυμι) and Chapter 4, n. 45.

[41] See this chapter, "Dissection Elsewhere in the Galenic Corpus" at pp. 310–11.

[42] Anatomical details at *UP* III.96, 502, IV.34, 238, 304, 308, 310, 333 (I.70, 366, II.205–6, 357, 405, 409–10, 428H); instructions at III.154, 439, 510, IV.117 (I.113, 320, 371, II.266H); discussions of previous anatomists at III.115, 231–2, IV.32, 253 (I.84, 169–70, II.205, 368H). This last category is particularly interesting, since many of these references do not have obvious counterparts in AA and several of them refer to disputes or mistakes in the enumeration of muscles, a topic that *Musc.Diss.* also likely assigns to AA_1 (see this chapter, n. 52).

[43] De Lacy (1978–84), 46–8.

[44] Reference to AA and *UP* at *PHP* V.196, 209 (in the future tense), 610 (I.7.39, 10.17, VII.3.34 De Lacy); to AA and *Mot.Musc.* at V.204 (I.9.2 De Lacy); to AA alone at V.604 (VII.3.14 De Lacy).

Plato and Hippocrates are too potentially entangled with the already conceived expansion of *AA* to offer reliable insight to *AA₁*.

The final text to consider is *On the Dissection of the Muscles*, which dates to the same period as *On the Usefulness of the Parts* and *On the Doctrines of Plato and Hippocrates*; indeed, Galen says in *AA* that he had just finished writing it "not long before" he began *AA*, and his citations in it of *On the Usefulness of the Parts* place it in the very brief window between the composition of that text and the start of *AA*.[45] However, the version of *On the Dissection of the Muscles* that survives dates to after the completion of the first books of *AA* – Galen says at the end of it that his friends were dissatisfied with the treatment of the muscles of the feet he had originally supplied and that he has therefore appended a passage lifted verbatim from the second book of *AA*.[46] The fact that this passage is tacked on at the very end as a deliberate appendix without any attempt at integrating it into the text suggest to me that Galen did not engage in any substantive rewriting in the body of the text when he made this addition. Nevertheless, this later fiddling, combined with the same timing issues at play for *On the Usefulness of the Parts* and *On the Doctrines of Hippocrates and Plato*, renders it a bit ambiguous whether references to *Anatomical Procedures* in this text refer to the planned rewrite or to the extant, but soon to be outdated, version.

We can be confident, however, that the very first reference to an *Anatomical Procedures* in *On the Dissection of the Muscles* must be to *AA₁* since it appears in contrast to the as yet unnamed *AA*. Galen says that he has already covered the action and use of the muscles in *On the Movement of the Muscles* and *On the Usefulness of the Parts* and that

> how one might best lay bare not just the muscles but also all the other parts of an animal is described in *Anatomical Procedures*. For which reasons I did not intend to write something specifically about the anatomy of the muscles. Rather, since I am collecting all the things I have discovered about anatomy into one text, I will also make clear in that undertaking the things omitted or not well said by earlier physicians about the muscles.[47]

---

[45] *AA* II.227 (γέγραπται δ'οὐ πρὸ πολλοῦ). See Garofalo and Debru (2005), 96–8 on the date of the text and its relationship to *UP*, which also cites it.

[46] *Musc.Diss.* XVIIIb.1024.

[47] *Musc.Diss.* XVIIIb.927–8 (ὡς ἄν τις κάλλιστα γυμνώσειεν οὐ τοὺς μῦς μόνον, ἀλλὰ καὶ τὰ ἄλλα πάντα τοῦ ζῴου μόρια, διὰ τῶν ἀνατομικῶν ἐγχειρήσεων λέγεται. ὅθεν οὐδὲ προῃρήμην ἰδίᾳ τι γράψαι περὶ μυῶν ἀνατομῆς· ἀλλ' ἐπειδὰν εἰς ἓν ἀθροίζω πάντα τὰ κατὰ τὰς ἀνατομὰς ὑφ' ἡμῶν εὑρημένα, τηνικαῦτα καὶ τὰ παραλελειμμένα τοῖς ἔμπροσθεν ἰατροῖς, ἢ μὴ καλῶς εἰρημένα περὶ μυῶν ἐγνώκειν δηλῶσαι); text according to Garofalo and Debru (2005).

He proceeds to say that this intention was overruled by his friends, anxious to have a dedicated text on the muscles as soon as possible. We can infer several things from this passage: First, the text that he says will collect all of his anatomical knowledge can be none other than *AA*, which, as we already know from *On the Usefulness of the Parts*, was at this point fully conceived of in his mind. Second, given that identification, there can also be little doubt that the already complete *Anatomical Procedures* he refers to by name at the beginning of the passage must be AA_1. Finally, this allows us to confirm that the purpose of AA_1 was to give instructions on *how* to dissect – "how one might lay bare" – and it also indicates that, unlike in the case of the texts on the vessels and the nerves, which refer to it as more precise, AA_1 was less comprehensive in its treatment of the muscles and especially in its engagement with the work of other anatomists than the dedicated discussion in *On the Dissection of the Muscles*.[48]

The identities of the rest of the references to *Anatomical Procedures* in the text must remain somewhat uncertain. However, I think it would be most logical to take a cue from this first case and assume that all of the others, barring the final one that introduces the appendix and was certainly added later, refer to AA_1. It would be odd if, having once referred to the original by name, he subsequently called the second by the same name without any attempt at differentiation.[49] There are six citations of the title bookended between the two already discussed. The first tells the reader that *Anatomical Procedures* contains instructions on how to drown and kill a monkey; there is certainly such a section in *AA*, but it is very reasonable to assume that there was an analogue in AA_1, given his description of it as teaching how to "lay bare" the parts of the body.[50] The next reminds the reader that *On the Dissection of the Muscles* relates only to monkey anatomy and that he talks "about the differences of all the animals from each other in *Anatomical Procedures*"; this accords better with the similar claim about

---

[48] The conclusion that the treatment of the muscles in AA_1 was less detailed than that in *On the Dissection of the Muscles* fits in well with the overall reconstruction of the lost text. *On the Dissection of the Muscles* is almost twice as long as *On the Dissection of the Veins and Arteries*, which is itself more than twice as long as *On the Dissection of the Nerves*. While the complexity of the subjects themselves will probably dictate a slight imbalance in their coverage toward the muscles, it is reasonable to assume that the topics were much more evenly distributed in AA_1, which was likely roughly equivalent in length to the sum of these three texts (see this chapter, n. 20); thus, the muscles must have appeared there in considerably less detail.

[49] This is, of course, assuming that all of these references date to the original composition and that he did not engage in more invasive edits when he appended the passage from *AA* at a later date.

[50] *Musc.Diss.* XVIIIb.928.

AA_I in *On the Dissection of the Nerves* than with anything in AA.[51] The remaining four all relate to explaining the ways in which other anatomists were incorrect or disagree, especially about the enumeration of the muscles in various parts of the body; again, this accords with the information about AA_I from the text on the nerves.[52]

In sum, by amalgamating the evidence from all of these cross-references, uncertain though any individual one may be, a picture of the contents and character of AA_I emerges. In addition to the three core subjects of muscles, vessels, and nerves, it almost certainly included an introductory section on the homoeomerous parts. It seems to have also contained thoughts about the comparative suitability of species for dissection – perhaps even his first articulation of the six classes of animals and their similarity to human anatomy – together with periodic comments on the anatomical variations among species. It engaged in some criticism of the opinions of previous anatomists, though not to the same degree to be found in *On the Dissection of the Muscles*. Finally, like its homonymous successor, it was framed differently from the descriptive minor works to which he compares it: It certainly offered anatomical facts, but they were framed within a manual for how to perform dissections, including some engagement with vivisection.

On the Dissection of the Dead and On the Dissection of the Living

These two texts, which are among those that Galen describes in *On My Own Books* as ancillary to the core anatomical texts, often appear as a pair, with the two-book *On the Dissection of the Living* acting as a sort of sequel to the one-book *On the Dissection of the Dead*.[53] He says in *Anatomical Procedures* that he composed them in the same period in which he composed AA_I, during his fruitful relationship with Boethus before the latter left Rome.[54] In addition, he refers to the contents of each independently

---

[51] *Musc.Diss.* XVIIIb.950 (περὶ δὲ τῆς τῶν ἄλλων ζῴων πρὸς τούτους διαφορᾶς ἐν ταῖς ἀνατομικαῖς ἐγχειρήσεσι).

[52] *Musc.Diss.* XVIIIb.937, 978, 1014, 1019. Garofalo (in Garofalo and Debru [2005], *ad loc.*) does not find parallels in *AA* for the last three of these and asserts that one of them (978) refers to AA_I, somewhat puzzlingly since he assumes that all the rest are from *AA* and does not give a specific reason why this one should be different.

[53] *Lib.Prop.* 4.38 (Boudon-Millot [2007]), *Ord.Lib.Prop.* XIX.55, *ArsMed.* I.408; they are presented as a pair in the latter two, while the first groups them in a trio with *Controversies in Anatomy* (as does Hunayn ibn Ishaq who says that he translated all three together at *Risala* 28–9; see Lamoreaux [2016], 44–6).

[54] *AA* II.216–17.

on at least one occasion.[55] Neither of them survives in Greek, but we are
fortunate to have two manuscripts containing an Arabic translation of
On the Dissection of the Dead.[56] From the information there, we can see
that this text served a markedly protreptic function, in contrast to the
other minor anatomical works, which are more akin to traditional handbooks. *On the Dissection of the Dead* opens by describing the goal of the
text, which is to lay out the basic principles of dissection, not the specific
details, which are covered elsewhere in the corpus. Galen characterizes the
practice of dissection as essential for doctors and differentiates the types of
knowledge that can be gleaned from the dissection of dead animals and
the dissection of living ones, foregrounding the dissection of the dead,
unsurprisingly in this context, as the more fundamental of the two. He
then goes on to enumerate the ways in which a knowledge of dissection
is helpful to practitioners in their medical therapies as well as in surgery.
Though providing some illustrative examples in each case, he again reiterates that his goal in this text is not to give the relevant detailed anatomical
information, but rather to lay out the basic principles and precepts, in
order, in Ormos' paraphrase, "to encourage his friends to the study and
practice of dissection."[57]

Much less is knowable about *On the Dissection of the Living*, but it is
tempting to infer a similar character for its contents since Galen treats
it as a companion text. Indeed, Hunayn ibn Ishaq, who translated both
works into Syriac in the ninth century AD, offers parallel summaries of
their contents: In the one, Galen "describes … what can be learned from
the dissection of dead animals, what kinds of things they are," while in
the other, "his purpose … is to show what can be learned from the dissection of live animals, what kind of things they are."[58] This summary
of *On the Dissection of the Dead* nicely encapsulates that text's overarching goal of giving principles and motivations for dissection, rather than
detailed findings and instructions – "what kind of things," not what things

---

[55] *Diss.Mort.* at *AA* II.396; *Diss.Viv.* at *Loc.Aff.* VIII.140, 271 and *Mot.Dub.* 11.1 (Nutton [2011]), where
in each case he refers to contents of the second book.
[56] See Ormos (1993); the same author is working on a forthcoming edition. My characterization of the
text is based on the brief summary of the contents provided at Ormos (1993), 171–2.
[57] Ormos (1993), 171 (seine Freunde zum Studium und zur Übung der Sektion anzuspornen). One
of the illustrative examples for surgery includes the potential danger to the adjacent nerves while
bloodletting in the elbow, which correlates exactly to the one reference to the content of this text
that we have in the surviving Greek texts of Galen (*AA* II.396), nicely confirming that the Arabic
text is indeed genuine; see Ormos (1993), 165, 172.
[58] Hunayn ibn Ishaq, *Risala* 28–9 (Lamoreaux [2016], 44–6).

exactly. The repetition of the same phrasing for the companion text on the living is suggestive of a similar motivation there. The two references that Galen makes to the contents of the text in *On Affected Parts* do not shed much light on the question; each offers a specific vivisectory example that is discussed there, one relating to the potential of multiple systems to be simultaneously affected by the same cause, the other to the muscles involved in respiration, the latter of which appears to be a favorite example since, he tells us, it also features in *On the Causes of Respiration* and *On the Voice*.[59] While neither of these is indicative of a protreptic character, the only internal Galenic reference to the contents of *On the Dissection of the Dead* similarly points to an example contained within it and, if we were reliant only on it, would offer little insight into the overarching structure and goals of the text.

Beyond these very brief remarks by Hunayn and the cross-references in Galen, there are two other potential sources of evidence for the contents of this treatise, both surviving in Latin translations. One is the medieval *On the Dissection of the Living* that sometimes circulated under the name of Galen and was included in the Giuntine editions of Galen's *Opera Latina*. While it is clearly not an ancient text – it likely dates to between AD 1210 and 1240 – it shows familiarity with a variety of Greek and Arabic sources including repeated references to Galen, and it is at least conceivable that some trace of the Galenic version might be discernible within it.[60] The opening sentence, at any rate, is similar in spirit to what we might expect from the original text:

> A knowledge of anatomy is necessary to physicians in order that they may understand how the human body is constructed to perform different movements and operations, and how the body is formed in many diverse parts and endowed with a soul from which proceed noble powers and numerous virtues, by which it is ruled and preserved and protected from corruption and sudden accident.[61]

The word Corner translates here as "anatomy" (*anatomicos*) could equally well mean "dissection," thus offering a protreptic rationale for the practice;

---

[59] *Loc.Aff.* VIII.140, 271.

[60] On the dating, see Corner (1927), 40. The text is also at times (equally erroneously) ascribed to Aristotle and to "Richard the Englishman"; see Corner (1927), 35, 41–3, Talbot and Hammond (1965), 271, n. 4, and Nutton (2011), 109, 352. For the text's citation and use of earlier authors, including Galen, Hippocrates, Aristotle, Ibn Sina (Avicenna), and al-Razi (Rhazes), see Corner (1927), 37–9 (discussion) and 87–110 (translation). Rocca (2003), 69, n. 107 reports, via G. Strohmaier, that Ivan Garofalo thinks it "may ... comprise genuine elements"; Gleason (2009), 103, n. 94 is more skeptical, pointing out that the Latin text "does not discuss dissection at all," as is Nutton (2011), 352, who feels that there is "no evidence that [the author] knew of the genuine text."

[61] Translation from Corner (1927), 87.

however, the contents of the remainder of the work, which provide an anatomically informed physiology of the body and arguments that are drawn from texts rather than observations, are not terribly encouraging for this interpretation.[62] On the whole, it seems quite unlikely that this text can yield any useful information about its homonymous Galenic forebear.

The second, more robust source for the contents of *On the Dissection of the Living* is the Latin *On Problematical Movements*, which Vivian Nutton has recently rehabilitated as a genuinely Galenic text.[63] There, after a chapter discussing involuntary movements such as coughing, sneezing, and the laughter attendant on tickling, he adds, "something which was said in the second book of *On Dissection in the Living* will be said again now."[64] The next sentence asserts that true expertise requires familiarity with a variety of examples; for the question now at hand – namely the cause of the movement of swallowed food through the esophagus – the first of these must be the dissection of the dead for ascertaining the pertinent anatomical underpinnings. After a brief description of these anatomical findings and then a longer discussion of various unnamed anatomists' theories for the relevant physiology, Galen adds that the best source for information on this question is to be found in the dissection of living animals, and he describes, in broad strokes, how one might perform a vivisection that would get to the heart of the matter. This same experiment appears in far greater detail, with specific step by step instructions, in *AA*; interestingly, immediately prior to the instructions there, Galen says that he intends to spend a longer time discussing the absurdities of other anatomists views on the subject in *On Problematical Movements*.[65] The fact that he chooses to reference forward to a new text, rather than backwards to *On the Dissection of the Living*, suggests both that the instructions in *AA* are far more comprehensive than those in the lost text and that the discussion of other anatomists' theories might be a new feature of *On Problematical Movements* not found in *On the Dissection of the Living*, meaning that the passage following the mention of

---

[62] Corner (1927), 36 provides the Latin text of the first line (medicorum anatomicos necesse est praecognoscere quod humanum corpus cum sit compositum…). My general characterization of the text is based on Corner's translation, which unfortunately omits selected paragraphs in the interest of space.

[63] Nutton (2011), 4–5.

[64] *Mot.Dub.* 11.1 (Nutton [2011]) (dictum quidem igitur est aliquid in secondo libro de anathomia que in animalibus, dicetur autem et nunc).

[65] *AA* S128–30.

the lost work might not be completely derivative from it.[66] On the other hand, the fact that he chooses in *On Problematical Movements* to refer back to *On the Dissection of the Living* rather than to *AA* suggests that the framing of vivisection there as an ultimate form of proof was more bite-sized and protreptic – and thus more germane to his needs in *On Problematical Movements* – than the practical details expressed at greater length in *AA*.[67] After this discussion of the vivisection of the throat, the chapter in *On Problematical Movements* moves on to speculate that other anatomists may have been misled by trusting too much in the potentially deceptive anatomy of monkeys and by not first thoroughly acquainting themselves with the organs in a wide variety of species and conditions of animals, closing with the general advice "the older and more emaciated the animal, the more easily you will be able to dissect all of its muscles carefully."[68]

It must remain unclear how much of the material in *On Problematical Movements* refers back to the contents of our lost text, but, on the whole, the material there aligns well with the basic description of the character of *On the Dissection of the Living* in Hunayn and with the links Galen draws between it and its companion text on the dead. This text, too, seems to have been concerned with the utility of dissection and especially vivisection for those who wish to accurately understand and effectively argue about the nature and functioning of the human body. It likely offered some examples of effective procedures, without getting too bogged down in the details, and also perhaps provided some fundamental guidelines – which kinds of animals to use and how many – to acquaint the reader with the basic parameters of the art. Thus, while the question must remain an open one, it seems not unreasonable to speculate that *On the Dissection of the Living* did indeed parallel its companion in style and purpose and that both offered arguments for the utility and benefits of practicing dissection

---

[66] Indeed, it is not universally agreed that this is an original Galenic reference to the original Galenic text, although the very tentative suggestion of Larrain (1994), 224, n. 95 that it is a reference to the medieval *On the Dissection of the Living* is surely not correct.

[67] On the comparative dating of *Mot.Dub.*, which is likely quite late, see Nutton (2011), 6–10.

[68] *Mot.Dub.* 11.22 (Nutton [2011]) (quanto autem animal fuerit magis antiquum et macrius, tanto melius poteris inscidere universos eius musculos diligenter). The next sentence offers a segue into other forms of proof, drawing, for example, on veterinary practice, and the chapter then goes on to cite *On Natural Faculties* as a source, suggesting that the passage dependent on the lost text might stop after 11.22. However, it should be noted that in two of the three traditions for the text there is another reference to vivisection at the very end of the chapter (which is the last in the treatise and which, according to Nutton, is "beset by errors, omissions, and expansions in all three textual traditions" [p. 370]), describing a similar experiment, but specifically on the neck of a cock, an animal Galen uses but rarely (Nutton [2011], 177, 370–1); this experiment also appears at *AA* S81–2 with the species unspecified.

for oneself. As a pair, the two texts would thus have formed a nice protreptic counterpart to the instructions provided in *AA*₁.

On Controversies in Anatomy

Another text that Galen several times mentions in conjunction with the above pair is his *On Controversies in Anatomy* in two books, also now lost.[69] He offers no indication of when he wrote it, but one might infer from this notional proximity that it also dates to his first stay in Rome; at any rate, he cites it in the sixth book of *On the Usefulness of the Parts* and in the first book of *AA*, suggesting that if it were not written in his first stay, it dates to early in the second. Galen himself explains the purpose of the text:

> Disagreement among doctors on points of anatomy did not originate first with me, but has existed among them since ancient times, for two reasons: both because some wrote falsely and because they used different manners of teaching, through which those who did not disagree with each other as to the actual understanding of the matter under observation gave the appearance of disagreement to those who had not read their books, let alone seen the things made apparent by dissection. More is said about all these sorts of things in the first book of *Controversies in Anatomy*.[70]

In the continuation of this passage, he describes some semantic disagreements in counting muscles. Elsewhere he adds that the first book contained discussion of the differences of opinion and expression in regard to the orifices of the heart and to the number of chambers that it contains.[71] He also indicates in *On Natural Faculties* that the text covers the disagreement among anatomists over how to enumerate the coats of various organs; this probably included the tunics of the eye, since he says in *AA* that *On Controversies in Anatomy* explains why it is that those who number

[69] *Ars Med.* I.408, *Ord.Lib.Prop.* XIX.55, *Lib.Prop.* 4.38 (Boudon-Millot [2007]). The Arabic version mentioned at Boudon (2002), 443, n. 4 must really refer to that of *Diss.Mort.*, which also appears in the note; see the correct discussion of the three texts in question at Boudon-Millot (2007), 154, n. 1.
[70] Galen, *AA* II.235–6 (οὐκ ἀπ' ἐμοῦ πρώτου κατὰ τὰς ἀνατομὰς ἤρξατο διαφωνεῖσθαι τοῖς ἰατροῖς, ἀλλ' ἐκ παλαιοῦ τοῦθ' ὑπῆρξεν αὐτοῖς διὰ διττὴν αἰτίαν, ὅτι τε ψευδῶς ἔγραψαν ἔνιοι, καὶ ὅτι διαφόροις ἐχρήσαντο τοῖς τρόποις τῆς διδασκαλίας, δι' οὓς οἱ μὴ διαφερόμενοι πρὸς ἀλλήλους, ὅσον ἐπ' αὐτῇ τῶν ἑωραμένων τῇ γνώσει, φαντασίαν διαφωνίας ἐκπέμπουσι τοῖς ἀναγινώσκουσι μὲν αὐτῶν τὰ βιβλία, μηδεπώποτε δὲ ἑωρακόσι μηδὲν τῶν ἐξ ἀνατομῆς φαινομένων. εἴρηται μὲν οὖν ἐπιπλέον ὑπὲρ τῶν τοιούτων ἁπάντων ἐν τῷ προτέρῳ τῆς ἀνατομικῆς διαφωνίας). Hunayn ibn Ishaq, *Risala* 27 (Lamoreaux [2016], 44) offers a very similar summary: "his purpose in it is to explain the differences of opinion among the earlier anatomists, such as are found in the books on anatomy: which were merely verbal and which were substantive, and what caused them."
[71] *AA* II.625 and *UP* III.462–3 (I.337–8H), which are very likely referring to the same part of the text.

these as two and those as four are equally correct in their understanding of the underlying anatomy, though expressing themselves differently.[72] This text, then, was more in defense of the art of anatomy than representative of it. Galen was anxious that the multiplicity of voices on the anatomical scene did not diminish its reputation as a reputable science with consistent results. The accusation that "some wrote falsely" may also indicate that he dedicated some space to denouncing inferior anatomists or those who attempt to broach anatomy otherwise than through dissection. This makes *On Controversies in Anatomy* a thematically fitting companion piece to the protreptic *On the Dissection of the Dead* and *On the Dissection of the Living*.

On the Difference between the Homoeomerous Parts

The last in this cluster of ancillary texts is *On the Difference between the Homoeomerous Parts*. While the modern reader would class this topic as a sort of proto-histology rather than gross anatomy, Galen considers it an anatomical subject, and this treatise is accordingly linked to his other anatomical texts in a variety of ways. First, and most explicitly, he lists it with *Controversies in Anatomy, On the Dissection of the Dead*, and *On the Dissection of the Living* in *On My Own Books* and describes it as "in the same category," that is, covering an additional rather than an essential anatomical topic.[73] Next, the text is addressed to the same person as *On the Dissection of the Veins and Arteries* and *On the Dissection of the Nerves*, a certain Platonist by the name of Antisthenes, who was an attendee at Galen's dissections.[74] Finally, the subject matter overlaps with that handled in AA_1, which appears to have concerned itself with the homoeomerous parts in a way that its later reworking did not. Because it fits so neatly into the nexus of texts that we have just been considering, I have chosen to discuss it here, even though its chronology is debatable.[75]

---

[72] *Nat.Fac.* II.182; *AA* S52.

[73] *Lib.Prop.* 4.38 (Boudon-Millot [2007]) (ἐκ τούτου δὲ τοῦ γένους); see the epigraph to this chapter for the full text.

[74] *Part.Hom.Diff.* 1.1 (*CMG Suppl.Or.* III, p. 45); see this chapter, "*On the Dissection of the Veins and Arteries* and *On the Dissection of the Nerves*" at pp. 297, 299.

[75] Strohmaier (1970), 32–4 sets its composition in the period AD 169–80 and is inclined to suspect that it belongs to the latter half of that window on the rather tenuous grounds that Galen misses several opportunities to cross-reference it in texts written in the early 170s. This dating is certainly possible, but I would argue that he was overhasty in rejecting a composition period during Galen's first stay in Rome, when the other texts to which I link it were likely or certainly written; indeed, this early period is the one to which Ilberg (1892), 497, 513 assigns it. Strohmaier points out that Galen only mentions two books that he gave to Antisthenes at *Lib.Prop.* XIX.12 – namely *Ven.Art.*

The short text, which survives in an Arabic translation, has an unsurprisingly different feel from Galen's other surviving minor anatomical works: The pervasive nature of the homoeomerous parts renders a piecemeal tour of the body impracticable. There are, however, very brief parallels for it in Rufus and the pseudo-Rufian *On the Anatomy of the Parts of the Human Body*, each of which includes a short treatment of these substances after going through the body as a whole; and there is, of course, a substantial precedent in Aristotle's *History of Animals*.[76] Galen's goal, though, is not simply to list and describe the homoeomerous parts, as these earlier authors did, but also to engage in the debate of what should and should not be classed as such. Dissection plays only a minor role in the text, though still an important one. He frames it as the only way through which knowledge of these parts can be gained and indicates that he is basing his facts on anatomical observations.[77] The other three texts to which Galen ties this one in *On My Own Books* offer arguments for the efficacy and validity of dissection as a science; in contrast, this one, though also subordinate to the core anatomical texts, provides a deeper dive into a fundamental, though somewhat ancillary, topic.

On Bones

With *On Bones* we return to what Galen considers to be his core works on anatomy. This text, together with *On the Dissection of the Veins and Arteries* and *On the Dissection of the Nerves*, dates securely to his first stay in Rome, though he revised all three early in his second stay:

> For I did not even possess copies of all of these [texts for beginners], which were dictated to young men starting their studies or also given to certain friends who valued them. Later, when I came to Rome for the second time, after they were returned to me for corrections, I retained possession of them and <gave them> the title <"for beginners."> ... Dictated to beginners were

---

Diss. and *Nerv.Diss.* – and concludes that he must therefore not yet have written this third one at the time in question; the context of that comment is quite specific, however, and Galen may well have intentionally mentioned only the two texts that he gave to Antisthenes that were subsequently returned to him, rather than all the texts he had written for Antisthenes. Indeed, in that same passage he fails to mention AA_1 among the list of works he wrote for Boethus, even though it is securely contemporaneous or even anterior to the books he does mention (*Lib.Prop.* XIX.13).

[76] Rufus, *Nom.Part.* 211–17, followed by a discussion of the humors and other bodily fluids at 218–27; ps.-Rufus, *Diss.Hum.* 65–75; Aristotle, *HA* 511b1–523a27. Interestingly, Galen only mentions Aristotle and his school once in this text and only to criticize their imprecision, at *Part.Hom.Diff.* 1.10 (*CMG Suppl.Or.* III, p. 47–9).

[77] *Part.Hom.Diff.* 2.1, 3.6, 4.1–3, 5.2 (*CMG Suppl.Or.* III, p. 51, 59–61, 67).

the text *On Bones* and the one *On the Pulse*; and during that [first] stay I also gave two introductory books to a Platonist friend, one containing the anatomy of the arteries and veins and one of the nerves, and an *Outline of the Empiricist Sect* to some other person. Although I possessed none of these works, I received them from those who had them when I came to Rome for the second time.[78]

Just before this passage, Galen emphasizes again that all of these texts originated as untitled, one-off productions that subsequently circulated "among many people," receiving a different name with each iteration.[79] It is ambiguous how far his "corrections" went beyond assigning them official, unified titles, but it is certainly the case that even in their finished state *On Bones*, *On the Dissection of the Veins and Arteries*, and *On the Dissection of the Nerves* have a sparer feel than their later and more intentionally composed counterpart, *On the Dissection of the Muscles*.

On Bones is Galen's contribution to what was already, as we have seen, a thriving subfield of anatomical literature.[80] He is well aware of this fact and engages frequently, though anonymously, with the multiplicity of other voices on the topic. The only figure he names in these comments is Hippocrates, whose terminological idiosyncrasies he addresses twice; otherwise, he is content to list variations in nomenclature with general terms like "some" and "others."[81] Despite this lack of specificity, he reflects the fact that the osteological subfield had a developed, though not completely uniform, system of terms and definitions. Galen's text opens with a detailed overview of the different types of joints found in the body; he was clearly not alone in including such a section, as, indeed, the briefer examples from *Doctor: Introduction* and the papyrological record already confirm.[82] He several times indicates that the specific names for the subdivisions of the different types of joints are "modern" terms and includes nuances that some, but not others, feel are necessary, indicating that he is drawing on an established tradition

[78] Galen, *Lib.Prop.* XIX.11–13 (ἐγὼ μὲν οὖν οὐδ' εἶχον ἁπάντων αὐτῶν ἀντίγραφα μειρακίοις ὑπαγορευθέντων ἀρχομένοις μανθάνειν ἢ καί τισι φίλοις ἀξιώσασι δοθέντων· ὕστερον δ' ὁπότε τὸ δεύτερον ἧκον ἐν Ῥώμῃ, κομισθέντων, ὡς εἴρηται, πρός με διορθώσεως ἕνεκεν, ἐκτησάμην τε καὶ τὴν ἐπιγραφὴν <τοῖς εἰσαγομένοις ἐποιησάμην.> ... τοῖς δ' εἰσαγομένοις ὑπηγορεύθη τὸ περὶ τῶν ὀστῶν καὶ τὸ περὶ τῶν σφυγμῶν, ἐδόθη δὲ καὶ φίλῳ Πλατωνικῷ κατὰ τὴν ἐπιδημίαν ταύτην εἰσαγωγικὰ δύο βιβλία, τὸ μὲν ἀρτηριῶν καὶ φλεβῶν, τὸ δὲ νεύρων ἔχον ἀνατομήν, καὶ τινὶ ἑτέρῳ τῆς ἐμπειρικῆς ἀγωγῆς ὑποτύπωσις· ὧν οὐδὲν ἔχων ἐγὼ παρὰ τῶν ἐχόντων ἔλαβον, ἡνίκα τὸ δεύτερον ἧκον εἰς Ῥώμην); following the text in Boudon-Millot (2007).

[79] *Lib.Prop.* XIX.10–11 (εἰς πολλούς).

[80] See Chapter 7, "Anatomy in the Papyri" at pp. 259–60; cf. Chapter 7, n. 204.

[81] *Oss.* II.734–5 (probably referring to Hipp. *Fract.*), 757 (referring to *Epid.II.*2.24 [V.96 Littré]); *Oss.* 741 (τινες), 755 (ἔνιοι δὲ), 757 (ἔνιοι), 765 (ἔνιοι ... τινὲς δὲ), 766 (τινες μὲν τῶν ἀνατομικῶν ... ἔνιοι δὲ ... οἱ μὲν ... οἱ δέ).

[82] Ps.-Galen, *Int.* XIV.720; P.Oxy. 74.4974 (MP³ 2345.21) (see Chapter 7, n. 180).

of discussions about joints.[83] Nor was this diversity of views limited to questions of nomenclature: His discussion of the number of bones involved in the upper jaw lists an impressive six different schools of thought.[84]

This last example brings up a feature of osteological texts that seems to be characteristic of the subgenre. All the surviving examples are organized, to greater or lesser degree, around numbers. The brief chapter actually dedicated to bones in the Hippocratic *On the Nature of Bones* is an extreme manifestation of this tendency, but it is also a clear organizing principle in the relevant chapter of *Doctor: Introduction* and, to a lesser degree, in ps.-Rufus *On Bones*.[85] Galen does not embrace this approach with the same intensity as some of his peers, but enumeration is still very prominent in this text, suggesting that his approach to osteology is firmly entrenched within the established tradition.

Indeed, despite Galen's subsequent positioning of it in *On My Own Books* as foundational reading for all those interested in anatomy, *On Bones* is generally the most blinkered of all the anatomical texts, addressing itself directly to physicians, specifically those who are just beginning their studies. He opens the work by saying "it is necessary for the doctor to understand the nature of each bone and how it stands in relation to the others if he is going to heal fractures and dislocations of them correctly," and he ends the work by saying that "these things seem to me sufficient for the beginner to understand about bones."[86] The contents are a quite straightforward description of the arrangement of the human skeleton, a part of the body that was comparatively easy and uncontroversial to examine.[87] As discussed in Chapter 4, skeletons were not subject to quite the same taboos as corpses, which meant that even human specimens could be decently handled in appropriate contexts.[88] Additionally, skeletons, both human

---

[83] Moderns: *Oss.* II.735, 738–9, 746; diversity: *Oss.* II.737. Compare also Rufus' discussion of the modern terms applied to the sutures of the skull at *Nom.Part.* 133–4 (see Chapter 7, "Rufus of Ephesus" at pp. 221-2 for translation and discussion).

[84] *Oss.* II.751.

[85] Hipp. *Oss.* 1 (IX.168 Littré), to which compare PUG II.51 (MP³ 2345.2) (see Chapter 7, "Anatomy in the Papyri" at p. 259); Ps.-Galen, *Int.* XIV; ps.-Rufus, *Oss.* 3, 8, 21, 23, 38–9.

[86] *Oss.* II.732 (τῶν ὀστῶν ἕκαστον οἷόν τί ἐστιν αὐτὸ καθ' ἑαυτὸ καὶ ὡς ἔχει τῆς πρὸς ἄλληλα συντάξεως, ἐπίστασθαί φημι χρῆναι τὸν ἰατρόν, εἴπερ γε ὀρθῶς μέλλοι τά τε κατάγματα αὐτῶν καὶ τὰ ἐξαρθρήματα ἰᾶσθαι) and II.777 (ταῦτα ἀρκεῖν μοι δοκεῖ τοῖς εἰσαγομένοις ὑπὲρ ὀστῶν ἐπίστασθαι); following the text in Garofalo and Debru (2005).

[87] Though the description is quite compatible with the human skeleton, there are a few indications that Galen was either basing himself on or incorporating elements from simian skeletons, as for example when he describes the lower jaw as two bones, which is true in some animals, but not in humans (II.754–5); see Garofalo and Debru (2005), 6.

[88] See Chapter 4, "Anatomical Subjects: Humans" at pp. 113–15.

and animal, can be kept for generations and can be passively studied, making them durable, versatile, and unexceptionable teaching tools; Galen tells us that human specimens were kept for study in Alexandria and that he himself kept an assortment of animal skeletons for the same purpose.[89] As a result, *On Bones* is perhaps the most easily approachable anatomical text from the point of view of subject matter. Despite this, although Galen's interests and experience make themselves known between the lines, he gives no indication that he expected or encouraged his readers to engage, or to have engaged, with anatomy in anything but a passive, scholarly way: There is not a single command or second person address, not even a suggestion that the reader look at a specimen in conjunction with the text, though this would certainly have been a feasible way of approaching it.[90] Thus, though dealing with the anatomical subject matter that is easiest to access, the text itself does not offer guidelines for any active practice; the reader's own context would have dictated how he put *On Bones* into use, whether as a guide to studying skeletal specimens, as a memorandum of bones he had observed previously with a teacher, or as a completely textual replacement for studying the bones themselves.

On the Dissection of the Veins and Arteries and *On the Dissection of the Nerves*

On the Dissection of the Veins and Arteries and *On the Dissection of the Nerves* are similar to each other in style and were likely written in close succession. *On the Dissection of the Veins and Arteries* opens with an address to Antisthenes, Galen's Platonist friend who also received *On the Difference between the Homoeomerous Parts*; he says that he wrote it as "a synopsis of the anatomy of the veins and arteries, dearest Antisthenes, for you who wished me to give it to you as a reminder of the things you saw demonstrated in the body of a monkey."[91] Antisthenes persists as the second person addressee, and Galen adds that the knowledge that

---

[89] Alexandrian skeletons at *AA* II.220; Galen's animal skeletons at *AA* S230.

[90] Galen's experience as a practiced dissector comes through in his references to excising bones at *Oss.* II.747, to the removal of membranes at 764, and to boiling bones for heuristic purposes at 754; he also gives some insight into the practicalities of teaching in this subject, indicating that he himself has consulted multiple skeletons (758–9, 762), but seeming to also suggest that some specimens have been used to the point of being worn down (750).

[91] *Ven.Art.Diss.* II.779 (σύνοψίν τινα φλεβῶν καὶ ἀρτηριῶν ἀνατομῆς Ἀντίσθενες φίλτατε, βουληθέντι σοι παρ' ἐμοῦ δοθῆναι μνήμης ἕνεκεν ὧν ἐθεάσω δεικνυμένων ἐν πιθήκου σώματι, διὰ τοῦδε τοῦ λόγου πεποίημαι); following the text in Garofalo and Debru (2008). On Antisthenes, see also *Lib. Prop.* XIX.12, where Galen refers to him as a "Platonist friend" (φίλῳ Πλατωνικῷ).

the text provides is useful not just for doctors but "much more for you philosophers, dearest Antisthenes."[92] Nevertheless, the text is aimed at all beginners, perhaps with a slant towards those in the medical profession, visible, for example, in the highlighting of veins that are encountered in phlebotomy.[93] Despite the text's self-professed origin from a private anatomy lesson, it noticeably lacks encouragement to the reader to dissect for himself; the few direct suggestions for how to get a firsthand view of blood vessels are either noninvasive or in the context of medical practice.[94] In fact, there is a pointed emphasis in this text on the passive observation of internal anatomy through the skin.[95] This is, of course, not surprising given the obvious visibility of the veins through the surface of the body – an ancient and approachable means of accessing the topic, though insufficient in and of itself, as Aristotle took pains to prove.[96]

 Indeed, the subject of angiology has as long a history as that of osteology, but it does not seem to have flourished as a dedicated subgenre to the same extent.[97] Unlike in *On Bones,* Galen has very little to say about predecessors in this text and only rarely engages with any other views. This is likely related to the minimal nomenclature associated with the various veins and arteries: Only a few very prominent vessels achieved their own names in antiquity – the aorta, the vena cava, the jugular veins, the portal veins, for example – and it is largely in reference to these and to other

---

92 *Ven.Art.Diss.* II.804 (πολὺ μᾶλλον ὑμῖν τοῖς φιλοσόφοις, Ἀντίσθενες ἄριστε).

93 Beginners as audience at *Ven.Art.Diss.* II.788 and 804; phlebotomy at II.793 and 815.

94 Galen only mentions dissection twice: at *Ven.Art.Diss.* II.794, where passive observation in humans is described as just as effective, and at 799, where the effect is more to describe what he has seen in his own work than to encourage or direct the readers in their own dissections. There is perhaps an indirect command to doctors to study monkeys before operating on the neck at II.803: "therefore any doctor who intends to perform surgery on the neck must understand the variety of veins there that I have described and he must have examined which arrangement the part to be operated on was formed most like" (ἰατρῶν μὲν οὖν ὅστις χειρουργεῖν μέλλει κατὰ τὸν τράχηλον ἀναγκαῖόν ἐστιν ἐπίστασθαί τε τὴν εἰρημένην ποικιλίαν τῶν κατ᾽ αὐτὸν φλεβῶν, ἐπισκέπτεσθαί τε κατὰ τίνα μάλιστα αὐτῶν ἰδέαν ὁ χειρουργούμενος διαπέπλασται). Though this could be interpreted as an injunction to surgeons to investigate the veins in the neck in a variety of monkeys, it seems more probable that the surgeon was meant to read Galen's account carefully or examine human necks under the noninvasive conditions that he describes just before this passage. Galen explains how doctors can see veins and arteries in the course of their work at II.793 (phlebotomy), 803 (surgery and putrefying conditions, like the Pergamene skin-disease epidemic), and 815 (phlebotomy).

95 *Ven.Art.Diss.* II.790 (skinny people), 794 (veins readily visible through the skin), 803 (veins in the neck of people singing or holding their breath while exerting themselves, like athletes), 814 (skinny people), and 823 (skinny people).

96 Aristotle criticizes his predecessors for basing their descriptions on emaciated people and slaughtered animals at *HA* 511b10–23 (see Chapter 6, "Aristotle" at p. 185).

97 The two are equally emphasized in the Hippocratic Corpus, for example; see Chapter 6, "The Hippocratic Corpus" at p. 175.

extraneous terms that Galen mentions earlier voices, though naming only the most famous of them.[98] On the whole, this text offers a comprehensive – though, as he takes pains to point out, not complete – survey of the veins, followed by a much shorter exposition of the arteries, taking into account both the differences between various species and the variations from individual to individual.[99]

On the Dissection of the Nerves does not mention a specific addressee, but Galen says in *On My Own Books* that it, too, was for Antisthenes.[100] While the text does occasionally use the second person singular to refer to the reader, the instances are far more generic than in *On the Dissection of the Veins and Arteries*.[101] Further, he makes it clear that he is intentionally aiming it not at Antisthenes specifically, but at anyone, including those who – in unspoken contrast to Antisthenes – have not seen him dissect.[102] In addition to being less personally tailored, this text is much shorter than its counterpart; he says explicitly at the end that he "wrote this as an outline and sort of synopsis of the things described in detail in [*AA*₁], so that it would be useful to beginners," and throughout the text he makes it clear that he is only providing a basic overview.[103] Indeed, the text positively peters out at the end, leaving the reader with the hasty assurance that the nerves of the legs are basically just like those of the arms and that all the details are to be found in *AA*₁.[104]

Though more petite in stature, *On the Dissection of the Nerves* is a far more pugnacious text than its companion: This is a younger and more actively evolving subfield of anatomy. Galen begins aggressively, saying

---

[98] More specifically, Galen names or refers to previous anatomists at *Ven.Art.Diss.* II.780 (Hippocrates and "the most famous of the anatomists" [οἱ δοκιμώτατοι τῶν ἀνατομικῶν] on the likening of the branching veins to branching roots; Aristotle versus "others" [οἱ δ᾽ἄλλοι] on the name for the aorta), 785 ("the ancients" [οἱ ἀρχαῖοι] on the portal veins), 801 (three different views on the jugular veins), 808 ("some of the ancients" [ἔνιοι τῶν παλαιῶν] on the term for veins so slight as to be just barely visible), 817 (Aristotle on the structure of the heart); the remaining references do not relate to vessels at all: II.780 (Herophilus on the name of duodenum), 797 (the anatomists on the thymus). Rufus' section on the vessels is similarly quite short, though it does include more nomenclature than Galen mentions (*Nom.Part.* 198–210).

[99] Between species: *Ven.Art.Diss.* II.787, 825; between individuals: 781, 799–803, 809, 820.

[100] *Lib.Prop.* XIX.12.

[101] The second person appears at *Nerv.Diss.* II.832, 834, 836, 840, and 847. With the qualified exception of the first two (see this chapter, n. 109), these are generic statements of a sort that Galen makes frequently throughout the corpus.

[102] *Nerv.Diss.* II.844.

[103] *Nerv.Diss.* II.855 (νυνὶ μὲν γὰρ ὅσον ὑποτύπωσίν τε καὶ οἷον σύνοψιν τούτων τῶν ἐν ἐκείνοις ἀκριβῶς εἰρημένων ἐποιησάμεθα χρησίμην τοῖς εἰσαγομένοις ἐσομένην); indications that details have been omitted occur at II.843, 844, 849.

[104] *Nerv.Diss.* II.855.

that, though all doctors agree that nerves are necessary to sensation and motion, some are ignorant of the fact that they originate from the brain and the spinal marrow, "even though the evidence from dissection holds that way."[105] What follows is peppered with references, again, almost completely anonymous, to other anatomists and their grievous flaws. Where *On Bones* and, much less frequently, *On the Dissection of the Veins and Arteries* bring in predecessors mostly on disputed questions of nomenclature, such moments in *On the Dissection of the Nerves* are easily outnumbered by criticisms of the factual errors and observational failures of other anatomists.[106] Marinus is the only one to be named directly, and even he does not come off with flying colors; Galen indicates that he follows his nomenclature only out of respect – because it is technically wrong – and hints that he can disprove Marinus' view on the fourth cranial nerve, though he leaves the denouement to be discovered in *Anatomical Procedures*.[107]

All of this aggressive rhetoric is implicitly predicated on the position that Galen is a more skilled dissector with a clearer understanding of the relevant anatomy. Yet dissection plays a fairly muted role in the text as a whole. He opens the text, as we already saw, with an appeal to the evidence of dissection as incontrovertible proof, but he rarely calls on it directly. Once he says that a set of nerves is arranged "in a different and astonishing way, which is not easy to describe and perhaps someone would not believe it if he were just hearing about it until he had seen the sight for himself."[108] He also twice indicates how something would appear "to you when you look" at it or when you look at it carefully.[109] But the only passage that explicitly references audience engagement with dissection puts the reader in a decidedly passive role and indicates that even such a position is more than he expects of most: "I am forced to mention my predecessors because it will appear unclear to those reading their books without having seen the things made apparent through dissection *with me* whether all of them are wrong or just me."[110] Even in the best-case scenario, he does not expect

---

[105] *Nerv.Diss.* II.831 (καίτοι τό γε κατὰ τὰς ἀνατομὰς φαινόμενον τοῦτον ἔχει τὸν τρόπον).

[106] Questions of nomenclature at *Nerv.Diss.* II.833, 837–8, 841; criticisms at II.835, 840–5, 848.

[107] *Nerv.Diss.* II.839, 837.

[108] *Nerv.Diss.* II.832–3 (θαυμαστὸν δέ τινα τρόπον ἕτερον, ὃν οὔτε εἰπεῖν ῥᾴδιον, οὔτε ἀκούσας τις ἴσως πιστεύσει, πρὶν αὐτόπτης γενέσθαι τοῦ θεάματος); following the text in Garofalo (2008), which puts this in the third person rather than the second, as in Kühn.

[109] *Nerv.Diss.* II.832 (σοι θεασαμένῳ), 834.

[110] *Nerv.Diss.* II.844 (διὰ τοῦτο δ' ἀναγκάζομαι τῶν ἐμαυτοῦ πρεσβυτέρων μνημονεύειν ὅτι τοῖς ἀναγινώσκουσιν αὐτῶν τὰ βιβλία χωρὶς τοῦ θεάσασθαι *παρ'ἐμοὶ* τὰ φαινόμενα κατὰ τὰς ἀνατομὰς ἄδηλον εἶναι δόξει, πότερον ἐκεῖνοι πάντες ἥμαρτον ἢ μόνος ἐγώ); following the text in Garofalo and Debru (2008), with my emphasis.

the readers of this text to have dissected, but only to have attended and observed one of his own dissections, as Antisthenes did.

On the Dissection of the Muscles

On the Dissection of the Muscles is the last and by far the longest of the core minor anatomical works. Galen finished writing it "not long before" *AA* in a period when he has already become dissatisfied with *AA*₁ and begun planning its revision and expansion.[111] Unlike the previous two works, he considers this to be an improvement on the treatment in *AA*₁ rather than a synopsis of it. He says that he had already dealt with the muscles – and explained his predecessors' errors about them – in *On the Motion of the Muscles, On the Usefulness of the Parts,* and *AA*₁ and is now planning an even more in-depth treatment of them in the new, expanded *AA*; he therefore had no intention of writing a dedicated book on the muscles, but was compelled to do it, as so often, by his adoring fans:

> But some of my companions, *wishing to practice for themselves,* asked to have some memoranda of the things they observed with me and impelled me to write this book.… They also demanded that I mention anything that Lycus left out or said inaccurately, since he is believed to have dissected the muscles most clearly and expertly of all.[112]

The italicized section here is a substantial step forward from the previous minor works in terms of engagement with dissection. It clarifies that the intended audience has not only observed a dissection with Galen, like Antisthenes in the work on the vessels, but, further, that they intend to embark on additional dissections independent of him. Similarly, Galen indicates in *AA* that "it is possible for anyone who wishes it to practice dissecting a monkey using [*On the Dissection of the Muscles*] too."[113]

Despite this framing, however, the text does not read at all like a manual. While it is considerably more detailed and descriptive than the two books for beginners on the vessels and the nerves, it does not offer procedural instructions and it completely lacks the directive tone that is so

---

[111] *AA* II.227 (γέγραπται δ'οὐ πρὸ πολλοῦ).

[112] *Musc. Diss.* XVIIIb.928 (τῶν δ'ἑταίρων ἔνιοι *γυμνάζεσθαι βουλόμενοι καθ᾽ ἑαυτοὺς* ὑπομνήσεις τινὰς ἔχειν ἠξίωσαν ὧν ἐθεάσαντο δεικνυμένων παρ᾽ ἐμοῦ, καὶ τοῦτο ἠνάγκασάν με γράψαι τὸ βιβλίον … ἐπιμνησθῆναι δέ με καὶ τῶν εἴ τι παρέλιπεν ἢ οὐκ ἀκριβῶς εἶπεν ὁ Λύκος ἠξίωσαν, ἐπειδὴ σαφέστατά τε καὶ κάλλιστα πάντων οὗτος ἀνατετμηκέναι μῦς πεπίστευται); my emphasis.

[113] *AA* II.228 (ὑπάρχει μὲν δὴ τῷ βουληθέντι κἀξ ἐκείνου τοῦ βιβλίου γυμνάζεσθαι, πίθηκον ἀνατέμνοντι).

characteristic of *AA*.[114] There are, in fact, very few direct references to the act of dissection, though it is manifestly in the background of the whole treatise. He starts off strong in the beginning, saying "whoever wishes to train himself on the anatomy of the muscles, having drowned a monkey, should first skin it," but then he gives up on the instructional tone, merely adding "as is described in *AA*₁," in lieu of offering further directions.[115] Evidently he thought that the guidance offered in *AA*₁ – or the example he had already given in person to his companions – was enough, as he makes no further attempts to facilitate his readers' anatomical activities. The closest he comes to engaging with the act of dissection in the rest of the text is to frequently, though succinctly, mention that one structure cannot be seen until another has been cut away; he also occasionally mentions dissection in order to point out various muscles that can be observed without it.[116] It is thus no surprise that he follows up his characterization in *AA* of *On the Dissection of the Muscles* as a suitable guide for someone dissecting a monkey by adding, "but one will certainly learn still better here [in *AA*] how it is best to proceed in the dissection of each part of the muscles."[117]

The second stated goal of the text, aside from facilitating his companions' study of the muscles, was, as we saw earlier, to "mention anything that Lycus left out or said inaccurately, since he is believed to have dissected the muscles most clearly and expertly of all." Galen does this with gusto. Indeed, although Lycus is his prime target, and he often highlights him either alone or as the sole named representative of a group of like-minded thinkers, he goes over and above the request of his companions and seems to feel compelled to point out the deficiencies of all previous anatomists on the muscles.[118] It is rare for there to be a stretch of more than a few pages without a reference to the faults of his predecessors and

---

[114] There are only a handful of uses of the second person singular (*Musc.Diss.* XVIIIb.949, 965–6, 977, 979, 1026), which is Galen's main method of conveying instructions in *AA*; all of them are more suggestive of an impersonal "you" than a direct address to the reader.

[115] *Musc.Diss.* XVIIIb.928 (ὅστις ἐθέλει γυμνάζεσθαι περὶ τὴν τῶν μυῶν ἀνατομὴν ἐν ὕδατι πνίξας πίθηκον ἐκδειράτω πρότερον αὐτὸν, ὡς ἐν ταῖς ἀνατομικαῖς ἐγχειρήσεσι λέγεται).

[116] *Musc.Diss.* XVIIIb.929, 937, 944–5, 965–6, 968, 984–5, 953, 955, 993, 1002–4, 1011; also XVIIIb.1018, though it is from the section appended from *AA* (see this chapter, "The First *Anatomical Procedures* (*AA*₁)" at p. 285). The example at XVIIIb.966, which is one of the few moments in the text couched in the second person, is the closest any of these come to feeling like an instruction. Muscles visible before (πρὸ) dissection at *Musc.Diss.* XVIIIb.929, 937, 943, 975.

[117] *AA* II.228 (μαθήσεται δὲ κἀντεῦθεν ἔτι δὴ καὶ μᾶλλον, ὅπως ἐγχειρεῖν προσήκει τῇ καθ' ἕκαστον μόριον ἀνατομῇ τῶν μυῶν).

[118] He singles Lycus out at *Musc.Diss.* XVIIIb.935, 939–40, 949, 1000; he names him as an exemplar of an erroneous school of thought at *Musc.Diss.* XVIIIb.933, 937–8, 943, 956, 1007.

his own superior knowledge.[119] Where the earlier texts, particularly *On the Dissection of the Uterus* and *On Bones*, read like contributions to a wider field, this text, more than any of the others, seems designed to render its rivals obsolete. It is completely clear here that Galen considers himself to be – and wants to be recognized as – the most authoritative anatomist of all time.

Texts on Others' Anatomical Works

In addition to all of these original compositions, Galen also wrote a suite of texts summarizing, compiling, or commenting on previous anatomical work. I have already discussed all of these in more detail in the sections relevant to each author in question, but I will contextualize them here briefly as well, since Galen considers them to be a part of his own anatomical oeuvre. Two of these texts – his summaries of Marinus' and Lycus' anatomies – he considers to be "useful," that is in the second tier of importance among his anatomical corpus, while the rest he includes as merely ancillary. The composition of these texts likely spanned a large swath of Galen's career. It seems probable that his summary of Marinus' anatomy is of quite an early date, perhaps even put together while he was still pursuing his education.[120] *On the Anatomy of Hippocrates* and *On the Anatomy of Erasistratus* both sprang from his contentious encounter with Martianus, which occurred very early in his first stay in Rome; these texts, then, were among the slew of minor anatomical works that Galen was composing between AD 162 and 166 and, like many of them, they were dedicated to Boethus.[121] The remaining three texts in this category all relate to Lycus. As we saw, Galen first began engaging with his work while writing *On the Dissection of the Muscles*, in the first decade of his second stay in Rome. Over the course of the 170s his familiarity with Lycus' corpus grew: He says in the fourth book of *AA* that he had only so far read some of his anatomical works, but fairly soon after writing that – likely at some point at the very end of the decade – he found himself in the position of publicly defending his own anatomical opinions against those of Lycus on every

[119] Other anatomists are anonymously faulted at *Musc.Diss.* XVIIIb.930–1, 933, 935, 937–8, 943, 947, 951, 953, 956, 969, 979, 986, 991, 993, 1000, 1007, 1023.

[120] See Chapter 7, n. 65.

[121] At *Praen.* XIV.614–15 Galen associates his interaction with Martianus with his cure of Eudemus, which took place in the winter of AD 162–3; see Boudon-Millot (2012), 346. At *Lib.Prop.* XIX.13 he mentions the dedication to Boethus, indicating that their composition was complete while the latter was still in Rome.

topic.[122] *On the Ignorance of Lycus in Anatomy* stemmed directly from this public event, and Galen tells us that it was subsequent to his summary of Lycus' works on anatomy but previous, by an unspecified amount of time, to his work on his disagreements with Lycus.[123]

Dissection Elsewhere in the Galenic Corpus

Even beyond this group of texts dedicated to the topic, anatomy permeates all of Galen's thinking and writing: It is central to his understanding of the body, how it functions, and, therefore, how it must be brought back to normal functioning when an illness or injury has afflicted it. Further, he sees the evidence from dissection as a concrete and unimpeachable starting point from which to argue for his theories. In short, he views the study of anatomy as foundational to the entire study of medicine. In *On the Order of My Own Books*, he tells his readers that after having read the books for beginners – *On the Sects for Beginners*, *On the Pulse for Beginners*, and *On Bones for Beginners* – they should proceed to read *AA*, since it is only "after having been trained in the appearance of [the parts of the body] through dissection" that one can move on to the study of their functions.[124] Similarly, in the briefer reading list he provides at the end of *Art of Medicine*, he says: "since the things made apparent through dissections are of no small service in the demonstration of these [other texts], it is fitting to be practiced in them first."[125] It is thus not surprising that *On My Own Books* begins its topic-based exposition of the corpus with the works on anatomy.[126] To trace the role of anatomy throughout the Galenic corpus would therefore be an extensive undertaking, made still more complicated by the sometimes fluid boundary between anatomy and physiology, which is another all-pervasive

---

[122] *Lib.Prop.* XIX.21–3; see Chapter 7, "Quintus and His Students: Lycus" at pp. 249–52.

[123] *Lib.Prop.* 4.40 (Boudon-Millot [2007]).

[124] *Ord.Lib.Prop.* XIX.54–5 (ὁ δ᾿ ἐν τῇ τούτων θέα κατὰ τὰς ἀνατομὰς γυμνασάμενος).

[125] *Ars Med.* I.408–9 (ἐπεὶ δὲ εἰς τὰς ἀποδείξεις αὐτῶν οὐ μικρὸν ὄφελός ἐστι τὰ διὰ τῶν ἀνατομῶν φαινόμενα, πρώταις ἐκείναις ἐγγυμνάσασθαι προσήκει); he then adds, "there are a good number of others in addition [to *AA*]: *On Controversies in Anatomy* in two books, *On the Dissection of the Dead* in one book, on which follows *On the Dissection of the Living* in two books; and in some others, which I wrote for beginners, [anatomy is approached] part by part: the one on the anatomy of the bones, the one on muscles, the one on nerves, and on arteries and veins, and some other such ones" (ἄλλαι δέ τινες ἐπ᾿ αὐταῖς πλείους ἐν δυοῖν μὲν περὶ ἀνατομικῆς διαφωνίας, ἐν ἑνὶ δὲ περὶ τῆς ἐπὶ τῶν τεθνεώτων ἀνατομῆς· οἷς ἐφεξῆς δύο περὶ τῆς ἐπὶ τῶν ζώντων. ἐν ἄλλοις δέ τισι κατὰ μέρος, ὅσα τοῖς εἰσαγομένοις ἐποιησάμεθα, τό τε περὶ τῆς ὀστῶν ἀνατομῆς, τό τε περὶ μυῶν, καὶ νεύρων, καὶ ἀρτηριῶν καὶ φλεβῶν, καί τινα τοιαῦτα ἕτερα); following the text in Boudon (2002).

[126] *Lib.Prop.* XIX.23–30.

topic in and of itself. Instead, I will offer here a survey of the role of dissection in Galen's corpus outside of the dedicated anatomical texts. That is, I will look not to the data the dissection provides, but to the moments when Galen describes or promotes the act of dissection itself.

The first and, I would argue, in many ways the most pivotal nonanatomical text to consider in relation to Galen's rhetoric about dissection is *On the Usefulness of the Parts*, his seventeen-book-long masterwork on teleology and the functional construction of the body. It is over the course of writing this treatise that Galen decides to embark on the massive expansion of *Anatomical Procedures* into an unprecedently detailed and instructive text. This resolution is reflected in and to a degree perhaps even prompted by his evolving expectations of the audience of *On the Usefulness of the Parts*, a work that is notably geared at a far wider field than just doctors. His eventual conviction that the intellectually driven and professionally diverse readers of that text would benefit greatly from – would, indeed, be remiss in abstaining from – personal experience with dissection forms the motivating context within which he undertook the ambitious rewrite of his anatomical work.

Galen intends *On the Usefulness of the Parts* to appeal to a far wider circle than just the medical community, specifically targeting philosophers and other medical laymen as likely readers.[127] Throughout, Galen assumes that he is addressing medical novices and, though he will include medical anecdotes to prove his points with some frequency, he offers all the requisite details in a manner easily understandable to laymen; in fact, in a strong indication that he is addressing a lay audience, he suggests that if his readers are interested, they should consult doctors for more details, either through their writings or in person.[128] He certainly in no way discourages

---

[127] Although he closes with statement that "the doctor will be helped most by this work in his healing" at *UP* IV.365 (II.451H) (μέγιστα δ᾽ ἰατρὸς ἐκ τῆς πραγματείας τῆσδε καὶ πρὸς τὰς ἰάσεις ὀνήσεται), earlier in the chapter he says that the book is useful "much more for the philosopher than for the doctor," and he ranks the work's usefulness in "diagnosing the affected parts in the depths of the body" as secondary to its ability to guide people "not as physicians but, what is better, as men needing to understand something about the power [responsible for] usefulness" at *UP* IV.360 (II.448H) (χρησίμη … πολὺ δὲ μᾶλλον ἰατροῦ φιλοσόφῳ) and IV.362–3 (II.449H) (ἓν μὲν δὴ τοῦτο μέγιστον κέρδος ἐκ τῆσδε τῆς πραγματείας οὐχ ὡς ἰατροῖς ἡμῖν ἐστιν, ἀλλ᾽ὅπερ τοῦδε βέλτιον, ὡς δεομένοις ἐπίστασθαί τι περὶ χρείας δυνάμεως … ἕτερον δὲ δεύτερον εἰς διάγνωσιν τῶν πεπονθότων μορίων ἐν τῷ βάθει τοῦ σώματος).

[128] Examples of medical analogies at *UP* III.228, 253–4, 286–7, 289, 330, 493–4, 533–5, 567, 618, 643, 664, 685, 760, 776, 785, 797–8, 805–6, 808, 849, 888, IV.4, 18, 187, 191–2, 221, 234 (I.167, 186, 210, 212, 242–3, 359, 387–9, 412, 448, 466, 481, II.2, 55, 67, 73–4, 82–3, 88, 90, 118, 145–6, 184, 194, 319, 322, 344, 354–5H); suggestions to consult doctors for more information at III.352 (I.258H) (writings) and III.533 (I.387–8H) (in person).

practitioners from reading, but his solicitousness of those with no medical background indicates that he does not have the former in mind as his primary audience while he writes.[129] Rather, he casts his readers as intelligent, motivated, and well-educated generalists.[130] He says that he is writing "for the sake of those few who are able to hear and judge correctly the things that are said," protesting, with an elegant Ovidian twist, that it is for the sake of this select audience that he has sent his poor book out to be abused like an orphan by any ignorant fool into whose hands it may fall.[131]

Indeed, more than just about any of his other texts, Galen seems to be particularly aiming *On the Usefulness of the Parts* at an elite audience with a cultural polish.[132] He makes frequent allusions to the fine arts, and it is in the context of one of these that he first references a recurrent theme of the text: his desire to turn his readers into proficient natural philosophers.[133] He says:

---

[129] This solicitousness is on display at, for example, *UP* III.18 (I.13H) where he explains a saying of Hippocrates that is "too obscure for most people" (ἀσαφεστέραν τοῖς πολλοῖς) (cf. IV.51 [II.218H]), III.46–7 (I.33–4H) where he distinguishes among ligaments, nerves, and tendons, III.91 (I.66H) where he defines the technical terms used for the parts of the arm "for the sake of clearness" (ἕνεκα σαφηνείας), III.410 (I.299H) where he explains the construction of thorax since it is necessary for that to be mastered before the rest of the discussion can be understood, III.703–4 (II.15H) where he explains the attachments of veins and arteries, and III.740–1 (II.42H) where he explains terms relevant to the nerves.

[130] See *UP* III.347, 350, 938, IV.58 (I.254, 256–7, II.181, 223H) for their logical ability; III.254, 301–2, 365 (I.187, 221, 267–8H) on their self-motivation; and III.275 (II.384H) on their erudite use of leisure time.

[131] *UP* IV.21–2 (II.196–7H) (οὕτως οὖν καὶ ἡμεῖς οὐκ ἀγνοοῦντες, ὡς ἐπηρεασθήσεται καὶ προπη|λακισθήσεται μυριάκις ὅδε ὁ λόγος, οἷα ταῖς ὀρφανὸς ἐμπεσὼν χερσὶ μεθυόντων, ὑπ᾿ἀφροσύνης τε καὶ ἀπαιδευσίας ἀνθρώπων, ὅμως ἐπιχειροῦμεν γράφειν τῶν ὀλίγων ἐκείνων ἕνεκα τῶν ἀκούειν ὀρθῶς καὶ κρίνειν δυναμένων τὰ λεγόμενα). Ovid uses similar language of a defenseless book entering into a hostile world to describe his *Tristia* in poems 1.1 and 3.1, a trope that seems to have developed in Latin literature of the imperial period (my thanks to Stephanie Frampton for discussing this with me). This may, therefore, be an allusion to Latin poetry, which, though completely in keeping with the tenor of the text, would be the only such example in Galen; see Nutton (2020), 40–1 for his lack of citation of Latin authors.

[132] The text is full of literary quotations and allusions: Pindar at *UP* III.169–75 (I.124–8H), Homer at *UP* III. 236, 268, 313, 535, 661, 787 (I.173, 196, 230, 389, 480, II.75H), Thucydides at III.218, 776 (I.159, II.67H), Xenophon at III.775, 777 (II.66, 68H), melic poets at IV.365–6 (II.451H), and Moses at III.905–7 (II.158–9H); on Galen's literary allusions generally, see Nutton (2009), 23–7 for prose and De Lacy (1966) for poetry. He also flaunts a little bilingualism, comparing the urethra to a "Roman sigma" and opining that the Roman name for the brain is more exact than the Greek at *UP* III.407 (I.298H) (τῷ Ῥωμαϊκῷ σίγμα). Despite Galen's long tenure in Rome, his proficiency with Latin has been subject to debate, but was probably at a higher level than he is often given credit for (see Nutton [2020], 41); nevertheless, he does not cite Latin authors and, indeed, rarely mentions Rome at all, making the references here more pointed. For Galen's broader relationship with Rome, see Swain (1996), 363–72 and Nutton (2020), 40–6.

[133] He compares nature to a skillful chorus organizer at *UP* III.871 (II.133H); to an actor with near-faultless delivery at IV.356 (II.444H); to an artist at IV. 248, 330, 352 (II.364, 425, 441–2H).

Examine the art of the creator of everything like you examine that of Phidias. Perhaps, indeed, the external decoration on the Zeus at Olympia strikes you—the glistening ivory and abundant gold, or the size of the whole statue—but if you saw such a figure made of mud, you would turn away disdainfully. But the man who is an artist and knows how to judge the art in a work does not do this, rather he praises Phidias to the same degree, even if he sees him fashioning cheap wood or unremarkable stone or wax or clay; for the beauty of the material strikes the amateur, but that of the art strikes the artist. Come then, you too become for me skilled in the ways of Nature, so that we may no longer call you amateur, but natural philosopher.[134]

This goal of turning his readers into perfect natural philosophers runs through *On the Usefulness of the Parts*.[135] He repeatedly holds up the natural philosopher as the ideal, describing the man "who alone is rightly called natural philosopher" as he "who is willing to leave none of the works of Nature unknown."[136] It is notable, however, that he is not addressing those who are already natural philosophers, but rather those who want to become them; he in fact distinguishes the methods that he employs in *On the Usefulness of the Parts* from those of "real natural philosophers."[137] Indeed, he goes so far as to frame the book as a kind of philosophical alternative to Greek religion. He refers to *On the Usefulness of the Parts* as a "sacred discourse" and "true hymn of praise of our Creator," which offers the path to "true piety"; in the final book, he waxes particularly enthusiastic, claiming that "all men who honor the gods ought to be initiated into this rite," which, he avers, is much superior to the mysteries of Eleusis and Samothrace.[138]

---

[134] *UP* III.238–9 (I.175H) (ὡς τὴν Φειδίου κρίνεις τέχνην, οὕτω καὶ τὴν τοῦ πάντων ἐξέταζε δημιουργοῦ. σὲ μὲν οὖν ἴσως ἐκπλήττει τοῦ κατὰ τὴν Ὀλυμπίαν Διὸς ὁ πέριξ κόσμος, ἐλέφας στιλπνὸς καὶ χρυσὸς πολύς, ἢ τὸ μέγεθος τοῦ παντὸς ἀγάλματος· εἰ δ'ἐκ πηλοῦ θεάσαιο τοιοῦτον, καταφρονήσας ἂν ἴσως παρέλθοις. ἀλλ'οὐχ ὅ γε τεχνίτης καὶ γνωρίζειν εἰδὼς ἐν ἔργοις τὴν τέχνην, ἀλλ'ἐπαινεῖ τὸν Φειδίαν ὡσαύτως, κἂν ξύλον εὐτελὲς κἂν λίθον τὸν τυχόντα κἂν κηρὸν κἂν πηλὸν ὁμοίως ἴδῃ κεκοσμημένον· ἐκπλήττει γὰρ ἰδιώτην μὲν τὸ τῆς ὕλης κάλλος, τεχνίτην δὲ τὸ τῆς τέχνης αὐτῆς. ἄγε δή μοι καὶ σὺ περὶ φύσιν γίγνου δεινός, ἵνα σε μηκέτ' ἰδιώτην, ἀλλὰ φυσικὸν ὀνομάζωμεν).

[135] He calls it to the forefront again at *UP* IV.56 (II.222H).

[136] *UP* III.921–2 (II.170H) (τὸν γε μηδὲν τῶν ἔργων τῆς φύσεως ἄγνωστον ἐθέλοντα καταλείπειν, ὅσπερ δὴ καὶ μόνος ἐστὶν ὁ δικαίως φυσικὸς ὀνομασθησόμενος). For similar examples, see III.899, IV.23, 165–6 (II.154, 197–8, 302–3H).

[137] *UP* III.465 (I.339H) (ὄντως εἰσὶ φυσικοί); he expects real natural philosophers to concern themselves with all the different causes of the parts of the body (final, efficient, material, instrumental, and formal), whereas "we" are content with just the final cause.

[138] *UP* III.237 (I.174H) (ἱερὸν λόγον ... ὕμνον ἀληθινὸν ... τὴν ὄντως εὐσέβειαν); IV.361 (II.448H) (κατ' αὐτὴν χρὴ τελεῖσθαι τὴν τελετὴν ἅπαντας ... ἀνθρώπους, ὅσοι τιμῶσι θεούς) (cf. IV.20–1 [II.196H]). Similarly, he describes Hippocrates as "hymning" nature at III.235 (I.172H) and says that one of his statements should be taken "as if from the voice of god" at III.22 (I.16H).

Yet, while these rhetorical moves affirm the intellectual importance of the book and the cultural superiority of its audience, Galen actually requires of his readers very little in the way of specific prerequisite knowledge. He does not assume any real physiological or medical background. Though he makes some flattering remarks about the probable mathematical superiority of some of his readers, when he gets into a geometric description of optics he does not in fact require any real mathematical knowledge.[139] He does not even assume that his readers have read or will read any of his other works, but whenever he needs to refer to something he has discussed in detail elsewhere, he allows them to take the contents proven there on faith.[140] In short, he treats his audience largely as passive listeners who are joining him for a tour of the physiological wonders of nature.

As the work goes on, however, Galen evinces an increasing impatience with the role he has apportioned his readers and a desire for more serious engagement on their part – a discontent that centers tightly on the subject of dissection. Where in the beginning he was happy to have his readers take his word for the marvelous intention to be seen in the composition of the parts of the body, as he moves further into the material he begins to insist, slowly at first, but with growing intensity, that one cannot truly understand teleology unless one has a deep and personal understanding of anatomy. In the second book, he is considerate of those of "my future readers" who "are not familiar with my other anatomical works," a stance that he maintains for the first two-thirds of the treatise.[141] But in the eleventh and twelfth books he engages in some revisionist history, saying that he does not need to repeat topics covered in "my anatomical commentaries" since "I have created the entire narrative of this discourse for those who already know the things made apparent through dissection," and "it is fitting for one to first be well-versed [in my anatomical works] – as I said at the beginning – if he hopes to accurately follow the things written here."[142] Then in the sixteenth and penultimate book, he reverts to a

---

[139] *UP* III.814 (II.94H); he asks his mathematical readers to be patient here and again at III.819 (II.97–8H).

[140] *UP* III.45, 230–1, 359, 413, 455, 463, 494, 522–3, 526, 590, 601–2, 625–6, 667–8, IV.10–11, 304, 310, 337–8 (I.32, 169, 263, 301, 332, 337–8, 360, 379, 382, 429, 437, 453, 484, II.188–9, 405, 410, 431H).

[141] *UP* III.97 (I.70–1H) (τῶν ἀναγνωσομένων ... ὅσοι ταῖς ἄλλαις ἡμῶν ἀνατομικαῖς πραγματείαις οὐχ ὡμίλησαν).

[142] *UP* III.936 (II.180H) (ἐν τοῖς ἀνατομικοῖς ὑπομνήμασι ... πρὸς εἰδότας ἤδη τὰ κατὰ τὰς ἀνατομὰς φαινόμενα ταύτην τοῦ λόγου τὴν διέξοδον ἅπασαν ἐποιησάμεθα) and IV.34 (II.206H) (ἐν οἷς πρώτοις, ὡς καὶ κατ᾽ ἀρχὰς εἴρηταί μοι, προγεγυμνάσθαι προσήκει τὸν ἀκριβῶς ἕπεσθαι τοῖς ἐνθάδε λεγομένοις ἐσπουδακότα).

nuanced version of the stance he took for the majority of the work, offering his anatomical writing as optional, though strongly recommended, background reading, saying "let this be sufficient" but "if the lover of truth goes to [my other texts] in order to examine the account of each muscle and nerve, I shall not object; indeed I urge him to do so."[143]

This ambivalence and increasing urgency about whether anatomy in written form is optional for the audience is even more pronounced in regard to observation of or participation in actual dissections. From the very beginning Galen is clear that all of the facts he is relaying result from his own studies of dissection, and therefore that the same things will also be visible to you, the reader, "if you wish to dissect," a phrase he uses repeatedly.[144] As he enters the latter half of the text, though, he becomes less accommodating. His suggestions that his readers try dissection for themselves become more frequent and more urgent – no longer "if you wish to dissect," but "when you dissect."[145] This more directive phrasing in the future tense rather than the optative or conditional does not appear at all until the sixth book, but from there it steadily overtakes the softer alternative. At the beginning of the seventh book, for example, he describes his account of the anatomy of the lungs as "reminding those who have dissected, and teaching *in advance* those who are wholly unfamiliar," a not-so-subtle suggestion that those who have never dissected should find in *On the Usefulness of the Parts* the inspiration to do so, signaling the emerging shift in his position.[146]

Yet even as Galen pushes more heavily for dissection on the part of his philosophical audience, he does not ever believe that *On the Usefulness of the Parts* is a suitable text to facilitate this dissection. Those who want

---

[143] *UP* IV.310 (II.410H) (ἀρκείτω … ἐφ᾿ ἃς οὐ μόνον οὐ κωλύω τὸν ἀληθείας ἐραστὴν ἰόντα καθ᾿ ἕκαστον μῦν καὶ νεῦρον ἐξετάζειν τὸν λόγον, ἀλλὰ καὶ παρακαλῶ).

[144] Phrases similar to "if you dissect" or "if you wish to" occur at *UP* III.229, 231, 235, 254, 379, 420, 430, 439, 510, 524, 769, 781–2, 863, 912, IV.117, 154, 195, 200, 204, 302, 309 (I.168, 169, 172, 187, 277, 307, 314, 320, 371, 380, II.62, 71, 128, 163, 266, 294, 325, 329, 332, 404, 410H).

[145] Galen assumes or commands future dissection at *UP* III.508, 657–8, 720, 939, IV.23, 158, 211, 239–40, 290–1, 315 (I.370, 477, II.27, 182, 197–8, 296, 337, 358, 396, 414H).

[146] *UP* III.517 (I.375H) (τοὺς μὲν ἀνατετμηκότας ἀναμιμνήσκοντας, τοὺς δ᾿ ὅλως ἀγνοοῦντας προδιδάσκοντας); my emphasis. A similar shift is visible in his discourse about monkeys: The monkey is a repeated figure of comic-relief in *UP*, described as "laughable" (γελοῖος) and a "caricature" (μίμημα γελοῖον) (III.80, 263–4, 847–8, IV.126, 251 [I.58–9, 194, II.117, 273, 366–7H]). In the final instance, however, located in the antepenultimate book where Galen's urgency on the subject of dissection has reached a high pitch, he explains that, despite the ridiculousness of the gluteal muscles in the monkey, the rest of the leg is very similar to man's and should be used to study muscular anatomy, pivoting the animal into the role of anatomical substitute that it plays – completely without humor – in the anatomical works.

to experience dissection need to look elsewhere, either to anatomists, like Galen, who offer public and private demonstrations of animal anatomy, or, preferably, to personally conducted research. Those who want to dissect an animal for themselves – which in Galen's view is the best way – must have recourse either to teachers or to handbooks to guide them through their dissections. Galen, of course, had just such a handbook in circulation: He refers his readers in *On the Usefulness of the Parts* frequently to AA_1, at first mostly as the location where he has recounted the details of anatomy that prove his various claims, which they can take on faith, and later also as a guide for those who want to investigate for themselves.[147]

However, Galen's conviction, which proved to be irrepressible, that dissection is the only way to truly appreciate nature and the perfection of its teleology, even for those who are approaching it from a purely philosophical point of view, leads him eventually to decide that AA_1 is insufficient as it stands. In the sixteenth book he proclaims that he has decided to rewrite and expand it. He says,

> it seems better to me now, having explained the goals of [the blood vessel's] construction to send you for the part-by-part description of them to the work *Anatomical Procedures*, in which many other things too that have been left out here will be completely gone through. For while I wrote it some time ago, in two books, I have now decided to make another, longer version containing a description of everything, part by part.[148]

As we shall see in Chapter 9, this expanded *Anatomical Procedures* addresses itself to an inclusive audience. Even more so than the minor texts dedicated to Boethus and Antisthenes, it does not presuppose a monochromatically medical agenda on the part of its readers. Rather, the driving goal of the entire text is to make dissection accessible: Galen clearly feels that all readers, no matter their purpose in life, would benefit from observing the marvelous inner workings of the body firsthand. In fact, he twice

---

[147] These references occur at *UP* III.96, 115, 154, 231, 232, 439, 502, 510, IV.32, 117, 238, 253, 304, 308, 310, 333 (I.70, 84, 113, 169, 170, 320, 366, 371, II.205, 266, 357, 368, 405, 409, 410, 428H). For the potential ambiguity surrounding which version of *AA* any individual reference in *UP* intends, see this chapter, "The First *Anatomical Procedures* (AA_1)" at p. 284.

[148] *UP* IV.328 (II.424H) (ἄμεινον οὖν μοι δοκεῖ τοὺς σκοποὺς τῆς κατασκευῆς εἰρηκότι τὴν κατὰ μέρος ἐξέτασιν αὐτῶν ἐπὶ τὴν τῶν ἀνατομικῶν ἐγχειρήσεων ἀναπέμψαι πραγματείαν, ἐν ᾗ καὶ ἄλλα πολλὰ τῶν παραλελειμμένων ἐνθάδε τελέως ἐξεργασθήσεται. πάλαι μὲν γὰρ ἐπεποιήκειν αὐτὰς ἐν δυσὶν ὑπομνήμασιν, ἔοικα δὲ νῦν ἑτέραν ποιήσασθαι μακροτέραν διέξοδον ἁπάντων τῶν κατὰ μέρος ἐχουσαν ἐξεργασίαν).

implies in *AA* that he considers it to be a sort of sequel or successor to *On the Usefulness of the Parts*, indicating that the audience of the latter was indeed a motivating factor in his framing of the rewrite.[149]

While the broader character of *On the Usefulness of the Parts* is unique, Galen's increasing urgency with regard to the practice of dissection that emerges over its course is also visible in some of the other texts from around the same period. Nonanatomical texts dating to his first stay in Rome and to the beginning of the second – the period dominated by his composition of the minor anatomical works – engage with anatomy merely as a practice in the background. It appears overwhelmingly as a notional cornerstone of medical thought or as a basis, to be accepted on faith, for other claims; only rarely do descriptions of dissection itself obtrude.[150] Even in the two texts from this period that he most closely ties to the minor anatomical works – namely, *On the Causes of Respiration* and *On the Voice* – he seems to have left dissection mostly as understood.[151] Both of these texts have suffered from nontraditional transmissions and survive only in very truncated form, but, in what remains, we can see a physiology informed by anatomical descriptions similar to those found in the minor anatomical works.[152] *On the Causes of Respiration*, as it survives, includes some basic anatomical descriptions, but no mention of dissection. The transmitted passages from *On the Voice* include more detailed discussion of anatomy, but only oblique references to the vivisectory experiments on voice production that Galen was so memorably

---

[149] He says at S18 "I have formed the opinion that I should construct the scheme of this work and the ordination of the subjects reviewed in it according to the principle and the scheme of the work *On the Uses of the Bodily Parts* – a work to which this one is a successor – conformably to the sequence of the matters reviewed in it"; similarly, at II.571 he says "but now [I will say] only what is useful in relation to the work *On the Usefulness of the Parts*" (νῦν γάρ, ὅσον ἐστί σοι χρήσιμον εἰς τὰ περὶ χρείας μορίων ὑπομνήματα μόνον). He maintains the same order of subjects in the two works, in order to facilitate cross-referencing; see Chapter 4, "Other Requirements: Books" at pp. 128–9.

[150] Examples of anatomy appearing mostly in the role of background assumption in texts prior to AD 175 occur in *Sect* (I.77, 96), *Dig.Puls.* (VIII.767, 811–12, 876, 895), *Symp.Diff.* (VII.63), *Trem. Palp.* (VII.604), *Mot.Musc.* (IV.374), *Art.Sang.* (IV.718, 732), *MMG* (XI.78), and *MM* (X.100, 319, 348–9, 409, 411, 422); it is given a bit more emphasis in *Temp.*, especially at I.579, 601, but see also the sarcastic reference at 632, where he points out that "of course I do not think that you should dissect a living person" (οὐ γὰρ δὴ ἀνατεμεῖν γε ζῶντας τοὺς ἀνθρώπους ἀξιῶ) to see whether a patient suffers from the anatomical abnormality he is describing, marking dissection as a strictly theoretical background in this instance.

[151] *AA* II.217, where he pairs them specifically with *Hipp.Anat., Er.Anat., Diss.Mort.*, and *Diss.Viv.*

[152] For a text and translation of the text surviving under the name *Caus.Resp.*, as well as a discussion of its probable status as a summary of the original Galenic text, see Furley and Wilkie (1984), 231–45. For a newly edited edition and translation of the *De voce* as it survives (seemingly in a Latin translation of an Arabic translation of extracts from the Greek), as well as an argument for the ultimately Galenic origins of its contents, see Nutton (2022).

performing during this early period.[153] On the whole, dissection's limited appearances in the texts from this period frame it just as an informative fait accompli.

In texts generally considered to center around the mid-170s, however – in the same period when he was working on *On the Usefulness of the Parts* and *On the Dissection of the Muscles* and when his plans for the new, longer version of *AA* were coalescing – dissection begins to surface more prominently in a variety of contexts. In *On Natural Faculties* Galen describes several dissections and vivisections that he has performed to prove his claims to opponents, offering detailed instructions on how to replicate them, as well as positive encouragement to his readers to do so.[154] In *On Semen*, too, he repeatedly appeals to the evidence of dissection to bolster his arguments, often explaining what his readers would see if they dissected for themselves; he clarifies at one point that these are not idle or rhetorical suggestions, adding "I wish that you, too, the one engaging with these writings … would put to the test the things I have said … going first to dissection and observing with accuracy."[155] Even *Marasmus*, which is a tiny text and a seemingly unlikely venue for this topic, contains a similar suggestion, saying "it is possible for you to observe this, if you wish, on other animals" and going on to recount what "you will discover" no matter which part of the animal "you wish to dissect, having first greatly emaciated it."[156]

On the Doctrines of Hippocrates and Plato, which Galen finished writing more or less contemporarily to *On the Usefulness of the Parts*, often uses dissection and vivisection as trump cards.[157] In his quarrel with Chrysippus and the Stoics and their cardiocentric view of the soul, his knowledge – and

---

[153] At *De voce* I.1–5, 24, 3.3–5, 4.8 (Nutton [2022]), he mentions the effects that result if various things are "cut" in a living creature. Interestingly, in the very first sentence, this activity is described in the first person singular in the active voice, "if I cut" (scissio); in all the rest, however, it is a passive construction (scindatur/scindantur/abscindatur). In keeping with dissection's background role in the period, the very final sentence of the treatise (4.9) asserts the role of Galen's own dissections as the source of the data in the rest of the treatise: "as is obvious from our dissection" (ut patet ex anatomia nostra).

[154] *Nat.Fac.* II.35–8, 155–6, 169, 175–6. On the dating of this text, Galen says at II.92 that, as he writes, he is "about to complete" *UP* (μελλούσης … περαίνεσθαι).

[155] *Sem.* IV.587 (βουλοίμην δ᾿ ἂν οὖν καὶ σὲ τὸν ὁμιλοῦντα τοῖσδε τοῖς γράμμασι … βασανίσαι τὰ λεγόμενα … πρῶτον μὲν ἐπὶ τὰς ἀνατομὰς ἐλθόντα, καὶ θεασάμενον ἀκριβῶς); compare to IV.521, 524, 566. This text postdates the first book of *UP* and *Nat.Fac.*, thus probably dating from AD 174–80, per De Lacy (1992), 47.

[156] *Marc.* VII.684 (θεάσασθαι δ᾿ ἔστι σοι τοῦτο βουληθέντι κἀπὶ τῶν ἄλλων ζῴων. ὅ τι γὰρ ἂν ἐθελήσαις ἐπιπλεῖστον λιμαγχονήσας ἀνατέμνειν … εὑρήσεις…); Theoharides (1971), 369 dates this text to "around 176 AD."

[157] The first six books of *PHP* date to AD 162–6; the remaining three date to AD 169–76 and it is likely that Galen edited the first six books in the same period, since they contain references to texts that postdate them; see De Lacy (1978–84), 46–8.

their ignorance – of the evidence from dissection and especially vivisection forms the core of his attack. He deploys dissection as proof throughout the course of the text, alluding to or describing his own performances and research. In the early books, he encourages his readers to achieve anatomical competence by attending his demonstrations, telling them, "it is possible for anyone who wishes it to learn this from me" and "let anyone who truly loves the truth come to us and learn clearly from the animals themselves."[158] However, he also offers some descriptions of and advice for how to perform dissections and what "you" will see and learn in the process, leaning increasingly on this type of framing as the text goes on.[159]

The Hippocratic commentaries from this period provide another interesting case study. The two most concerned with anatomy are, unsurprisingly, those for *On Fractures* and *On Joints*, but they have noticeably different expectations of their readers' exposure to dissection. Galen opens his commentary to *On Fractures* by assuming that "most of those reading this book are unschooled in anatomy."[160] This assumption seems consistent throughout, including when he cautions that the natural position of a joint is "not clear to a layperson, but only to anatomists" and when he says that he can speed through one area of anatomical description, at least, since it is apparent "even without dissection."[161] Even when he does suggest that his readers might benefit from further anatomical study, he directs them exclusively to texts.[162] In his subsequent commentary to *On Joints*, however, his expectations with regard to dissection have evolved.[163] First, he repeatedly insinuates that Hippocrates is an accomplished dissector, a persona that he does not highlight in relation to *On Fractures*; this is no doubt in reaction to the more anatomically focused content of *On Joints*, but it is also an interesting parallel to his second shift.[164] Where he opened the commentary to *On Fractures* with the assumption

---

158 *PHP* V.185 (I.6.4 De Lacy) (τοῦτ᾽ ἔνεστι τῷ βουλομένῳ μαθεῖν παρ᾽ ἡμῶν), 234 (II.4.32) (ὅστις οὖν ὄντως ἀληθείας ἐρᾷ, πρὸς ἡμᾶς ἡκέτω μαθησόμενος ἐναργῶς ἐπ᾽ αὐτῶν τῶν ζῴων).

159 *PHP* V.262–4, 562–3, 604–5, 607, 613, 623–5, 645 (II.6.3–8, VI.7.9–10, VII.3.14–18, 24, 4.8–10, 5.22–30, 8.7 De Lacy).

160 *Hipp.Fract.* XVIIIb.320 (τοὺς πλείστους τῶν ἀναγινωσκόντων τὸ βιβλίον ἀμαθεῖς ἀνατομῆς εἶναι).

161 *Hipp.Fract.* XVIIIb.346 (οὐκέτ᾽ ἰδιώτῃ δῆλον, ἀλλὰ μόνοις τοῖς ἀνατομικοῖς), 620 (καὶ πρὸ τῆς ἀνατομῆς).

162 *Hipp.Art.* XVIIIb.360–1, 434, 448–9.

163 On the dating of these texts, see Peterson (1977), 492–5, who places them in the period from AD 175–8; their comparative dating is clearly established by the opening sentence of *Hipp.Art.* (XVIIIa.300), which refers to *Hipp.Fract.* as a previous work.

164 On Galen's casting of Hippocrates as an accomplished anatomist, see Chapter 6, "The Hippocratic Corpus" at pp. 177–8.

that his readers would be ignorant of anatomy, he introduces that to *On Joints* with the suggestion that a reader hoping to get the most out of the Hippocratic text should "observe the arrangement of the joints on human bones or at least on simian ones" and that a similar degree of familiarity with muscles would not go amiss.[165] As the text goes on, he repeats this advice that the text can be fully appreciated only with a previous understanding of anatomy; as in the commentary to *On Fractures*, he admits that reading (his own) anatomical texts is a viable way of achieving this familiarity, but it is distinctly a second choice to personal observation.[166] He does not, however, press the point here as far as he does in *On the Usefulness of the Parts*; when he recommends or assumes audience experience with dissection, he expects them to have been merely spectators of his own or another's demonstration.[167]

In texts dating to later in his career – into the 180s and beyond, when the first five books of *AA* were complete and circulating, and he was engaged in composing the remaining ten – his expectations surrounding dissection, when they come up, continue this established tenor. His commentary to *Nature of Man* is unsparing in its mockery of the anatomically ignorant.[168] He insists that the basics of the interior of the body are not mysterious, but rather that their arrangement, once you have seen it through dissection, is as obvious as the fact that Crete is an island or that Rome has seven hills.[169] Nor is this recondite knowledge requiring deep commitment: It can be obtained "having observed dissections of animals for only a single day."[170] His text *On Problematical Movements* also assumes that everyone can and should have a familiarity with anatomy.[171] While he describes his own and others' dissections in the first half of the text, it is in the last and longest chapter that he clarifies the audience's role.[172] He says that it is of superlative utility for anyone interested in the topics in question to be able to describe the relevant anatomy "from dissection," and he goes on to describe what "you will see" if you dissect and manipulate an animal

---

[165] *Hipp.Art.* XVIIIa.304 (ἐπ' ἀνθρωπείων ὀστῶν θεάσαιτο τὰς κατὰ τὰς διαρθρώσεις συνθέσεις ἢ πάντως γε ἐπὶ πιθηκείων).

[166] *Hipp.Art.* XVIIIa.425–6, 529.

[167] This is most explicit at *Hipp.Art.* XVIIIa.597, but is also implied at 627, 632, 639.

[168] Bardong (1942), 639 dates *HNH* to around AD 189.

[169] *HNH* XV.133, 137.

[170] *HNH* XV.139 (ἡμέρᾳ μιᾷ τεθεαμένος ἀνατομὰς ζῴων).

[171] Nutton (2011), 8 considers this text to be very late, dating "into the 190s, or even the early third century."

[172] *Mot.Dub.* 1.7–17, 2.9–11 (Nutton [2011]).

in various ways, including some brief instructions and suggestions for the types and conditions of animals that "you should practice on."[173] *On the Affected Parts* is similarly rife with references to anatomy, and, while it does not contain instructions, it repeatedly assumes that its readers have observed or at least have access to observing dissections.[174] Even the pharmacological texts are not immune: *On the Composition of Drugs by Type* includes a brief but passionate digression on the urgency of the study of dissection.[175]

Galen's unbounded enthusiasm for dissection and his gradually confirmed conviction that it was a desideratum for all of his readers, whether of medical texts, commentaries, or philosophy, reaches its full maturity in the fifteen-book *Anatomical Procedures*. It was an unparalleled and ambitious undertaking, long in the making, and one that sought to transform anatomy into an independent and prominent study. Its lasting effects were not quite as Galen envisioned, but let that not deter us from first appreciating the motivations for and results of his labor.

---

[173] *Mot.Dub.* 11.2 (Nutton [2011]) (ex anathomia); 11.14–22 (exercitari oportet). The very end of the chapter also has a problematically preserved passage (11.39–41) that describes the vivisection of the neck of a cock in some detail, again using the second person and offering instructions; see Nutton (2011), 177, 370–1.

[174] References to the readers' familiarity with or personal observations from dissection occur at *Loc.Aff.* VIII.208–10, 228, 246, 259, 271, 273, 346; at VIII.168, he councils his readers not to turn to the gods for answers about the reasoning part of the soul, but rather to "learn from some anatomical man" (παρά τινι τῶν ἀνατομικῶν ἀνδρῶν παιδευθέντας). Bardong (1942), 640 dates *Loc.Aff.* to after AD 192. Though less emphatically, *Hipp.Prorrh.* XVI.602, *Hipp.Epid.VI* XVIIb.4, 202, 245–6, and *MM* X.730 also assume a certain personal familiarity with observing dissection.

[175] *Comp.Med.Gen.* XIII.603–8.

CHAPTER 9

Galen's Anatomical Procedures *and Its Innovations*

> It is likely that this work will not be kept in the hands of my compan-
> ions alone, but that it will circulate through the hands of many men.
>
> Galen, *Anatomical Procedures*[1]

The expanded version of *Anatomical Procedures* (*AA*) is unlike any other anatomical text to survive from antiquity. Not only is it exponentially longer
than any of its peers, its character is completely different. In contrast to the
descriptive texts that have so far dominated this discussion, the bulk of *AA*
consists of precise directions on how to dissect every part of a monkey, from
head to toe and from exterior to innermost depths – it is, in short, not a text
about anatomy, but rather one about dissection itself. While this seems to
have also been the general tone of Marinus' *Anatomical Procedures* and of
Galen's first attempt in the genre, the massive scale of *AA* – fifteen books to
those versions' one or two – makes it clear that the level of detail and com-
prehensiveness of these instructions dwarfs anything that came before. With
this text, Galen has embarked on a new undertaking with a new and, I will
argue, quite radical purpose: He is bypassing, perhaps even subverting, the
traditional model of anatomical education and making anatomy and dissection available to any and every interested reader. Here, for the first time, the
practice of dissection merges seamlessly with an anatomical text.

The best way to get a feel for the personal, hands-on tone that is characteristic of *AA* is to read some representative extended passages. In his
introduction to the temporal muscles, which control some movements of
the jaw, he instructs his reader:

> One must dissect each of these in the following way. Cut the fibers of the
> masseter muscles that extend from the upper jaw into the lower, but not

---

[1] *AA* II.504 (οὐκέτ' ἐν ταῖς τῶν ἑταίρων μόνων χερσὶ τὴν πραγματείαν ταύτην εἰκός ἐστι
φυλαχθήσεσθαι, πολλὰς δ' ἀμείψειν ἀνθρώπων χεῖρας).

all simultaneously, so that you can learn how they interweave with one another. Having first cut away those on the surface, then, inserting hooks, draw them up, and skin and dissect them up to the upper jaw, whence they originate, until you arrive at the underlying ones, which have a different orientation…. The movement of the lower jaw will be clearly visible to you if you stretch each of the heads [of this muscle] in turn. Pay attention now to me for how one ought to do this. For, mark you, the coming description is going to be applicable to all anatomical procedures in which we are investigating the movement of a part of a dead animal. Well then, it is necessary to strip all the flesh from those bones on which the observation is to be made each time, keeping only the muscles that move them; dissecting these, too, right up to their heads, cut them off of the bones from which they spring and, grabbing hold of them yourself, draw them up, pulling them towards the position in which they originally lay. In doing this properly, you will observe the movements of bones into which equipoised muscles are inserted.[2]

Much later in the text, he guides the reader through the study of the cranial nerves:

Now when the eye has been removed, and also the bone between the eye and the brain, that is, the bone in which the cavity which surrounds the eye is situated, first study carefully the whole of the path which the two nerves of the third pair follow until they reach the eyes. After that, see how this nerve splits up in the skull, and how the fourth pair soon after its origin combines with the third pair. The latter is far more massive and compounded of many roots. But the fourth pair is very small, and therefore as soon as it blends and unites with the third pair, it will be difficult for you to see how it cuts itself off from the other and separates. Now, in order that nothing may escape your scrutiny of these nerves which are interwoven, as soon as the third pair has united with the fourth, first expose with care and attention, in the manner which I have described for you, the whole course and path of the nerves. That you should do by removing the dura mater

---

[2] *AA* II.436–8 (ἑκάστην δὲ αὐτῶν ἀνατέμνειν ᾧδε χρή. τῶν μασητήρων μυῶν τέμνε τὰς καταπεφυκυίας ἶνας ἐκ τῆς ἄνω γένυος εἰς τὴν κάτω, μὴ πάσας ἅμα, χάριν τοῦ καταμαθεῖν, ὅπως ἀλλήλαις ἐπαλλάττονται. πρώτας οὖν ἀποτέμνων αὐτῶν τὰς ἐπιπολῆς, εἶτ᾽ ἄγκιστρα καταπείρων, ἀνάσπα, καὶ ἀνάδερε, καὶ ἀνάτεμνε μέχρι τῆς ἄνω γένυος, ὅθεν ἐκπεφύκασιν, ἄχρις ἂν ἐπὶ τὰς ὑποκειμένας ἀφίκῃ, διαφερούσας ἐχούσας τὴν θέσιν … καὶ μέντοι καὶ τείνοντί σοι τῶν κεφαλῶν ἑκατέραν ἐν μέρει σαφῶς ἡ τῆς κάτω γένυος ὀφθήσεται κίνησις. ὅπως δὲ χρὴ τοῦτο πράττειν, ἤδη μοι πρόσεχε τὸν νοῦν. ὁ γάρ τοι λόγος ὁ μέλλων ῥηθήσεσθαι κοινός ἁπάσης ἐστὶν ἀνατομικῆς ἐγχειρήσεως, ἐν ᾗ τεθνεῶτος τοῦ ζῴου κίνησιν ἐπισκοπούμεθα μορίου. χρὴ τοίνυν ἀφαιρεῖν ἁπάσας τὰς σάρκας ἐκείνων τῶν ὀστῶν, ὑπὲρ ὧν ἂν ἡ σκέψις ἑκάστοτε γίγνηται, μόνους φυλάττοντας τοὺς κινοῦντας αὐτὰ μῦς· ἀνατέμνοντας δὲ καὶ τούτους ἄχρι τῶν ὀρθίων κεφαλῶν ἀποτέμνειν μὲν ἐκείνας ἀπὸ τῶν ὀστῶν, ὧν ἐκπεφύκασιν, αὐτὸν δὲ μεταχειρισάμενον αὐτὰς ἐφέλκεσθαι, τείνοντα καθ᾽ ἣν ἐξ ἀρχῆς ἔκειντο θέσιν· ἐν γὰρ τῷ καλῶς τοῦτο πράττειν ὀφθήσονταί σοι τῶν ὀστῶν αἱ κινήσεις, οἷς ἰσόρροποι μύες ἐμπεφύκασιν); following the text in Garofalo (1986–2000).

from round the nerve, cutting it and freeing it with a sharp knife. Follow this by incising next that part of the layer spread out beneath the nerve. After this, raise it with a hook, and lay freely open the whole of this region, until you can see the bone that underlies it, and all that is to be found hereabouts. For this is the only way in which you will be able to see that one portion of the nerve between the two layers breaks off on the course which both nerves pursue, and that the dura mater is perforated, and beyond it also you will see the portion of the bone adjoining the dura mater there.[3]

Even more vivid and detailed are his instructions for vivisections:

Next begin another task, in the following manner. Insert a hook into the dura mater and draw it upwards. Then first cut through the piece of it that has been raised, so that it may not make contact with the part of the brain lying beneath it. Next insert two hooks, one on each side of the first hook, from the ends of the margins of the incision; also with these two hooks draw upon the dura mater found above, and cut through the whole raised portion of it, without touching any of the underlying parts of the brain. If you do this well, you can also introduce your fingers upwards beneath the part of the dura mater which you have incised, and you can split it until you have uncovered the whole of the brain lying beneath it.... When you have done that, then make an inspection and ascertain for yourself whether the animal is being deprived of respiration, voice, movement or sensation, or whether none of these defects is showing itself in it, either at the time when the incision was made upon it or else soon afterwards. The latter may quite well be the case, when it happens that the air is warm. But if the air is cold, then in a degree corresponding to the amount of the cold air streaming in upon the brain, each single one of these functions of the brain that we have mentioned weakens; the animal remains for a certain length of time unconscious, and then expires. Therefore it is best that you should take in hand the detachment of the dura mater from the skull in the summertime, or, if you perform it at another season, no matter which that season may be, you should heat the room in which you intend to dissect the animal and warm the air. Should the dissection be thus performed, then after you have laid open the brain, and divested it of the dura mater, you can first of all press down upon the brain on each one of its four ventricles and observe what derangements have afflicted the animal.[4]

This is not a description of the anatomy of the body. It is a guided tour.

One thing that becomes immediately evident to the persevering reader of this text is that it is almost impossible to follow without a visual reference. The utter disorientation resulting from attempting to read ten or fifteen

---

[3] *AA* S240–1.
[4] *AA* S21–2.

pages without an anatomical guide of some kind should convince any but the most well versed in anatomy of the futility of approaching it in this way. The modern reader's solution to this problem is, of course, illustrations.[5] While illustration was a live option for scientific work in antiquity – and even specifically for anatomical texts, as with Aristotle's *Anatomies* – there is no indication that Galen's text was ever illustrated.[6] Indeed, it seems quite clear that it was not meant to be.[7] His manifest assumption that his readers are actively following along on animal specimens precludes any need for illustration.[8] In fact, I suspect that Galen would have considered illustrations to be a jejune alternative and would have objected to them as doing his readers a disservice by standing between them and the personal familiarity with dissection that he considers essential.

Galen, in short, expects his readers to have an animal in front of them while they proceed through the text. This expectation is implicit on almost

---

[5] Modern-day readers can avail themselves of illustrated anatomy textbooks to provide a visual map with which to keep track of Galen's prose. For the most part, a book or atlas of human anatomy is adequate to maintain comprehension, but for more exact correlation books on the anatomy of the rhesus monkey are also available; for example Berringer, Browning, and Schroeder (1968) or Bast, Hartman, and Straus (1971). The English translation in Singer (1956) also has an appendix with pertinent plates of simian anatomy.

[6] On Aristotle's *Anatomies*, see Chapter 6, "Aristotle" at pp. 185–7. On scientific illustration generally, see Weitzmann (1952), 245–50, Stückelberger (1994), and Marganne (2004), 36–7. The surviving examples that we have of illustrated medical texts are mostly herbals, but it does seem that illustration was used more widely, including for teaching various medical procedures and anatomy (Marganne [2004], 42–7); cf. the illustrations in the epitome by Mustio (sixth century AD) of Soranus' *Gyn.*, which likely stem from models in Soranus (Hanson and Green [1994], 1023–4). The most famous anatomical illustrations with a possible connection to antiquity are the "five-figure series" depicting the venous, arterial, muscular, nervous, and skeletal systems respectively. There are over seventy examples of this series of illustrations, many attached to Persian and Arabic texts, but with Latin and Provençal examples as well; it is unclear how far back the antecedent for these images goes or where geographically they first arose, but conjecturing an antecedent from classical antiquity is not completely out of the question; see French (1984) and Savage-Smith (2007), 155–9.

[7] He periodically expresses his frustration with his inability to describe things as clearly as he would like "with words," implying that this was the only medium he was working in (*AA* II.606, 609, 616, 690, S89–90, 131); he also sometimes asks his readers to use their imaginations to augment his descriptions (S15, 101). The one potential exception to this lack of illustrations – and to modern sensibilities not an enormously helpful one – is the possible presence of line drawings to illustrate two geometrical descriptions, that of the triangular shape of the deltoid at II.274 and that of the triangular interface between the scapula and the coracoacromial ligament at S309, both of which he describes in terms of labeled points and line segments, as in a geometrical proof. However, it seems equally likely that these geometrical descriptions are there precisely in order to overcome the lack of illustrations for an area that might otherwise be difficult to visualize; thus, the reader may have been expected to produce his own diagram, not to find one provided in the text. Salas (2020), 25–7 also concludes that *AA* was not illustrated, though for different reasons.

[8] A few intrepid modern scholars, including Charles Singer and Christopher Cosans, have taken this assumption to heart and read the text while actually dissecting a monkey with good success; see Singer (1956), xxi, and Cosans (1998), 71.

every page, but he also declares it explicitly throughout. He begins the first book with a lengthy disparagement of those who attempt to learn the anatomy of the bones without studying an actual skeleton.[9] The instructional framing of the rest of the text makes it clear that his opinions are the same with regard to the more friable parts of the body as well. Indeed, text and specimen are intimately linked in his mind from the very moment of composition: He tells us that he writes his works on anatomy "with the animal placed in front of me, while I am looking at the things about which I am talking, especially when I am describing the method to be followed in their dissection."[10] Even taking simultaneous dissection as a given, as he does throughout, he nevertheless takes the time to periodically underscore its necessity. He frequently tells his readers that they will not understand a topic until they have done their own dissection, and he introduces many of his transitions from one operation to the next with a stated assumption that the reader has reached a given point in dissection; at one point he even spells out, "I order whoever is reading these words to judge these things, becoming personal observers of dissections."[11]

This directive and micromanaging tone, combined with the intimate and almost conversational feel that results from the consistent use of the second personal singular, has impacted the way in which scholars discuss the text. The original view was that *AA* derives, to one degree or another, from a transcription of a series of lectures that Galen delivered to students.[12] This is certainly a compositional method that we know him to have employed; however, I think we can be confident that it is not the

---

[9] *AA* II.220, 223–4.

[10] *AA* S136. Similarly, at II.498 he says that he will describe an area he mentions in passing more clearly when he dissects it, implying again that he is constructing and conceiving of the text with a sort of built-in illustration in the form of the animal he is concurrently dissecting.

[11] Understanding following on dissection at: *AA* II.592, 603, S89, 160 (cf. his direct requests to the readers to do things ["I want you to…"] at II.384, 662, and 684); assumptions about transitions at II.261, 328, 445, 447, S32, 91, 99, 144, 248, 261, 269, 285–6, 306; command at II.449 (ἃ παρακαλῶ κρίνειν τοὺς ἐντυγχάνοντας τοῖσδε τοῖς γράμμασιν, αὐτόπτας γιγνομένους τῶν ἀνατομῶν). See also at *Ord.Lib.Prop.* XIX.54–5 where he says that the reader may move on from *AA* to his other works only "once he is practiced in the observation of [the parts of the body] through anatomy" (ὁ δ'ἐν τῇ τούτων θέᾳ κατὰ τὰς ἀνατομὰς γυμνασάμενος ἑξῆς αὐτῶν τὰς ἐνεργείας μαθήσεται); cf. *Hipp.Epid.VI* XVIIa.1004, where he describes what "you saw" (ἐθεάσασθε) when learning about anatomy from *AA*.

[12] See Singer (1956), xiii and xx (cf. xxiv where he says that *AA* "has the unique distinction of preserving the very words of an ancient teacher"). Duckworth, Lyons, and Towers (1962), xi, though modifying this view to allow for a great deal of editing, do not reject it. Garofalo (1994), 1802, however, has significant reservations about this theory and argues for a substantial editing of any orality that underlies it, leaning in large part on the notable scarcity of hiatus in the text; cf. Garofalo (1986–2000), xvi.

method he used for this text.[13] Indeed, the assumption that it was obscures the brilliance and originality of his agenda. He is – deliberately and in full awareness – creating an intentionally crafted text that transcends oral teaching and strives to reach a broader audience.

The Composition of *Anatomical Procedures*

First, let us recall that *AA* is a rewrite. Galen already had an *Anatomical Procedures* in circulation (*AA₁*), and he refers to it frequently in the texts that predate and coincide with the composition of *AA*. As I explored in Chapter 8, the contents of *AA₁* were similar in scope and scale to those of the other minor anatomical works, most of which – namely, *On Bones, On the Dissection of the Veins and Arteries*, and *On the Dissection of the Nerves* – do indeed seem to have been dictations of oral teaching that he subsequently edited. Thus, it is not improbable that *AA₁* had a similar compositional style.[14] But he was not satisfied with these texts. His patent disillusionment with *AA₁*, and his desire to produce a bigger, more comprehensive version that included his most up-to-date discoveries, indicate that he is approaching *AA* in a different and more authorially calculated way.

Galen, however, somewhat obfuscates this fact. He introduces the text with a familiar motivational trope, namely that his friends asked him to write it:

> I wrote an *Anatomical Procedures* once already, when I arrived in Rome for the first time, when the Antonine who rules us even now was just beginning his reign; I have decided to write again this different version for two reasons. The first is this: because Flavius Boethus, a Roman consul, when he was leaving Rome for his native Ptolemais, entreated me to write the earlier *Procedures* for him—if any man ever keenly loved observing dissections, he did. I gave this Boethus other works too as he was leaving and, of course, the *Anatomical Procedures* in two books. For since, you see, he had observed an enormous number of things with me in a short amount of time he was worried that he would at length forget what he had seen, and he requested this sort of reminder. But since he has now died, and I do not have copies of the existing work to give to my companions, having lost those I had in

---

[13] Among the minor anatomical works, he specifically describes *Oss.* as having been transcribed in this manner (*Lib.Prop.* XIX.12). For other examples, see *Lib.Prop.* XIX.11, 14, 21–2, *Ord.Lib.Prop.* XIX.49–50, 56, *Ven.Sect.Er.* XI.194–5, *HVA* XV.748, *Praen.* XIV.630. Note that many of these instances are accompanied by a disclaimer that the resulting texts were not intended for widespread publication; see Chapter 4, "Other Requirements: Books" at pp. 133–4.

[14] Galen does seem to have edited it to a certain degree, however, since he kept copies of it for himself, a mark of what he considered to be a more finished text; see Chapter 8, n. 19.

Rome, for this reason, when my companions asked for it, it seemed better to me to write a new one. The second reason is because the work that I am now going to produce will be better by far than the earlier one, both because it will spread over more books in its narrative for the sake of clarity and because it will be more accurate than that one, since I have discovered many more anatomical theories in the intervening time.[15]

A parade of authorial modesty – combined with a very immodest desire to advertise in what high demand his work is held – has led Galen to claim that the primary reason for his return to this genre is the need to satisfy the requests of companions who are eager to see his previous effort but cannot find it. He paints the composition of *AA* as primarily a response to the loss of *AA₁*.

It takes only the slightest prodding to topple this façade. Remarks in his other texts from this period make it clear that the second reason in this passage was the genuine one, and that it was completely sufficient in and of itself: He was planning this bigger, better version already, even when he considered *AA₁* to be a readily accessible text. As we have already seen, in the sixteenth and penultimate book of *On the Usefulness of the Parts* he expresses dissatisfaction with *AA₁*, to which he has been referring his readers periodically throughout, and says "it now seems suitable that another, longer treatment should be made, containing a description of everything, part by part."[16] Similarly in *On the Dissection of the Muscles*, in which

---

[15] *AA* II.215–16 (ἀνατομικὰς ἐγχειρήσεις ἔγραψα μὲν καὶ πρόσθεν, ἡνίκα τὸ πρῶτον ἀνῆλθον εἰς Ῥώμην, ἐνάγχος ἄρχειν ἠργμένου τοῦ καὶ νῦν ἡμῖν ἄρχοντος Ἀντωνίνου, γράφειν δ᾽ αὖθις ἄλλας ἔοικα ταύτας διὰ διττὴν αἰτίαν. ἑτέραν μὲν τήνδε· ὅτι Φλάβιος Βοηθὸς ἀνὴρ ὕπατος Ῥωμαίων, ἐξιὼν ἐκ Ῥώμης εἰς τὴν ἑαυτοῦ πατρίδα Πτολεμαΐδα, παρεκάλεσέ με τὰς ἐγχειρήσεις ἐκείνας αὐτῷ γράφειν, δριμὺν ἔρωτα τῆς ἀνατομικῆς ἐρασθεὶς θεωρίας, εἴπερ τις καὶ ἄλλος τῶν πώποτε γεγενημένων ἀνθρώπων. τούτῳ τῷ Βοηθῷ καὶ ἄλλας μὲν ἔδωκα πραγματείας ἐξιόντι, καὶ μέντοι καὶ τὴν τῶν ἀνατομικῶν ἐγχειρήσεων ἐν δυοῖν ὑπομνήμασιν· ἐπεὶ γάρ τοι ἐτεθέατο πάνυ πολλὰ παρ᾽ ἡμῖν ἐν ὀλίγῳ χρόνῳ, δεδιὼς δέ, μὴ λάθοιτό ποτε τῶν ὀφθέντων, ἐδεήθη τοιούτων ἀναμνήσεων. ἐπεὶ δ᾽ ἐκεῖνος μὲν ἤδη τέθνηκεν, ἐγὼ δὲ οὐκ ἔχω τῶν γενομένων ὑπομνημάτων ἀντίγραφα διδόναι τοῖς ἑταίροις, [δι᾽ ἐγκαύσεως] ἀπολομένων ὧν εἶχον ἐν Ῥώμῃ, διὰ τοῦτο παρακαλεσάντων αὐτῶν, ἔδοξεν ἄμεινον εἶναι γράφειν ἕτερα. δευτέραν δ᾽ αἰτίαν, διὰ τὸ βελτίω μακρῷ τῆς τότε τὴν νῦν μοι γενησομένην ἀποδειχθήσεσθαι πραγματείαν, ἅμα μὲν εἰς διέξοδον ὑπομνημάτων πλειόνων ἐκταθεῖσαν ἕνεκα σαφηνείας, ἅμα δ᾽ ἀκριβεστέραν ἐκείνης ἐσομένην, ὡς ἂν πολλῶν ἐν τῷ μεταξὺ προσεξευρημένων μοι θεωρημάτων ἀνατομικῶν); following the text in Garofalo (1986–2000), which excludes δι᾽ἐγκαύσεως based on its absence in the Arabic tradition. See also II.218 where Galen describes *AA₁* as "falling far short of the one I am writing now, not only in clarity, but also in exactitude" (πολὺ τῶνδε τῶν νῦν μοι γραφησομένων ἀπολειπομένας, οὐ σαφηνείᾳ μόνον, ἀλλὰ καὶ ἀκριβείᾳ).

[16] *UP* IV.328 (II.424H) (ἔοικα δὲ νῦν ἑτέραν ποιήσασθαι μακροτέραν διέξοδον ἁπάντων τῶν κατὰ μέρος ἐχουσαν ἐξεργασίαν) (see Chapter 8, "Dissection Elsewhere in the Galenic Corpus" at p. 310 for further context). He subsequently refers to the work three more times, once (IV.333 [2.428H]) in the perfect tense, almost certainly referring to the existing version, since the other two (IV.332,

he frequently refers his readers to AA_1, he describes the new *Anatomical Procedures* as already a work in progress: "I am gathering all the things I have discovered about anatomy into one work."[17] These two passages, coming as they do in texts that both securely predate our *Anatomical Procedures* and that consistently refer their readers to the original *Anatomical Procedures* as an extant and accessible text, make it fairly unambiguous that Galen undertook the rewriting of this work as a considered project in response to the deficiencies he saw in the original version, rather than as a response to an external request prompted by its disappearance.[18]

This passage from *On the Dissection of the Muscles* also points to the method of *AA*'s composition: He describes himself as "gathering" all of his anatomical discoveries "into one work." Rather than suggesting the model of an oral teaching agenda being subsequently captured on paper, this comment implies a more strictly textual compositional approach.[19] Indeed, we know Galen to have had a collection of written material to supply the research for his composition of this new, authoritative work: He mentions on two separate occasions that he habitually makes written notes every time he dissects an animal. In the first instance, he is explicit that these notes constitute their own physical text discrete from any of his named works. He explains how he produced them as a piece of court evidence, saying:

> The observation of these things was useful for some well-known doctors who had been accused [of causing a paralysis] … for I, having made [the relevant points] clear to the accusers … freed the doctors from blame. And the doctors' accusers were convinced by me on these points not only by my

---

344 [II.427, 436H]), which are very nearby, describe future or promised discussion and thus look forward to this newly decided-upon rewrite.

[17] *Musc.Diss.* XVIIIb.927 (εἰς ἓν ἀθροίζω πάντα τὰ κατὰ τὰς ἀνατομὰς ὑφ' ἡμῶν εὑρημένα); see Chapter 8, "The First *Anatomical Procedures (AA₁)*" at pp. 285–6.

[18] The ad hoc nature of the circulation and copying of books was such that Galen may well have assumed while writing these texts that AA_1 was available to anyone who wanted to find it, only to later discover that no one could lay their hands on it. Indeed, he tells us at *Lib.Prop.* XIX.20 (see 3.9 [Boudon-Millot (2007)], which fills in a lacuna) that while he was completing *UP* and *PHP* he was actively searching for "some of the anatomical observations which I had given to Boethus" but could not find them (τινα τῶν ἀνατομικῶν θεωρημάτων, ἃ ἐδεδώκειν τῷ Βοηθῷ). This does not explain, however, what happened to the copies of AA_1 that he himself had, which he describes at *AA* II.216 as having been destroyed; see the comments, including some skepticism as to their actual destruction, at Garofalo (1986–2000), vol. I, p. vii and n. 5.

[19] To be sure, it is quite likely that some of the material that Galen drew on in composing *AA* was from the context of demonstrations for one or more people – and thus "lectures" – but some also likely arose from his own private study. Galen makes it clear that frequent solo dissections are useful and necessary to an anatomist; see *AA* II.289–90, 348, 515, 621, 674, S41, 45, 146, 157, 159–60, 199. Note that his private notes, too, were presumably all dictated: see S136 and this chapter, n. 10.

calling on knowledgeable colleagues as witnesses, but also by my exhibiting my documentation in *the anatomical notes that I make for every animal that I dissect* of the phenomenon in the vein which I just described.[20]

In the second instance, he is speaking more directly about his composition methods. He describes the disastrous fire at the Temple of Peace in AD 192, which consumed the warehouse in which he stored his books and medical supplies, and explains its consequences for his work program:

> There were also burnt many other books on anatomy which I had not revised sufficiently to allow me to publish them. For I used to write them and note them down *bit by bit in disconnected passages every time I was dissecting an animal,* not only animals belonging to the six classes of which the body and the construction are like the body and the construction of mankind, but also animals of the kind which crawl, those which move forwards by bringing the abdomen to their aid, water animals, and those which fly.[21]

While the notes directly in question here were not incorporated into *AA*, which had already been fully composed when the fire occurred, they nevertheless elucidate his note-taking habits and his layered approach to editing and publication.[22] Taken in conjunction with the description of "gathering into *one* work" all of his anatomical discoveries, these two passages strongly suggest that Galen composed *AA* by drawing on the notes he accumulated from various dissections over the course of his career.

The idea that Galen wove together notes from different source materials is also supported by places where the jointure is clumsy. There are moments where he is clearly adding to or subtracting from a preexisting account. At one point, for example, after a two-sentence explanation for an illusion that occurs during the dissection of the brain, he follows with a further paragraph, in which he repeats and expands on his original point, saying: "I know that it often happens that the abbreviated and condensed

---

[20] *AA* II.396–7 (καὶ τούτων ἡ θέα χρήσιμος ἐπί τινων ἰατρῶν γνωρίμων ἐγκαλουμένων γέγονεν … δηλώσας οὖν ἐγὼ τοῖς ἐγκαλοῦσιν … ἠλευθέρωσα τοῦ ψόγου τοὺς ἰατρούς. ἐπείσθησαν δέ μοι περὶ τούτων οἱ ἐγκαλοῦντες τοῖς ἰατροῖς, οὐ μόνον ἑταίρους τοὺς ἰδόντας ἐπικαλεσαμένῳ μάρτυρας, ἀλλὰ κἂν τοῖς ἀνατομικοῖς ὑπομνήμασιν, ἃ καθ᾽ ἕκαστον τῶν ἀνατεμνομένων ζῴων ἐποιούμην, ἐπιδείξαντι γεγραμμένον ὃ διῆλθον ἄρτι φαινόμενον ἐπὶ τῆς φλεβός); following the text in Garofalo (1986–2000), with my emphasis.

[21] *AA* S135; my emphasis. Galen gives more details on this fire and its consequences in his *Indol.*

[22] For the state of *AA* at the time of the fire, see this chapter, n. 28. It seems quite likely that the unpublished notes he refers to here were destined for his planned project dedicated to the comparative anatomy of animals; see *UP* III.328, IV.145 (I.241, II.286H) and *AA* S193. This layered approach to notetaking and composition is paralleled in other authors (see Dorandi [2000], 27–50); see also *Puer.Epil.* XI.359, where Galen reflects on his holistic approach to the composition of longer treatises.

statement detracts something from the confirmation of the intended meaning. And therefore it is necessary that I should still submit something in addition to that which I stated in regard to these two points."[23] This savors strongly of textual adaptation rather than the smooth flow of an oral dictation or bespoke composition. Also strikingly, his grammatical choices vis-à-vis himself and his readers are inconsistent and demonstrate a range of different understandings of his audience and his relationship to them. The vast majority of the descriptions of dissection are in the second person, but he occasionally suggests that he is dissecting as he dictates, or at least that he is present at the dissection.[24] Elsewhere, in contrast, he reserves for himself a completely verbal and passive role in the proceedings.[25] Again, though the majority of the procedures are couched in the second person, the imperative, or the impersonal, in one passage, he describes a vivisection entirely in the first person and the past tense, as if inserting a previously composed account rather than composing new instructions as he typically does.[26] In another, he launches into an extended series of indirect statements introduced by "I said."[27] He is explaining a series of veins that he has presumably already enumerated in another place, but it is quite unusual for him to quote himself in this way rather than recapping or providing a reference, and suggests a different form of composition.

In addition to drawing on these varied sources, Galen composed the text over a considerable span of time. He released *AA* to his readers serially in discrete sections rather than as a complete unit. In the final paragraph of the eleventh book he describes the losses that he sustained in the fire of AD 192; he says that at the time of the fire "I had already published eleven books of the present work … but as for the books which will follow these [i.e. Books XII–XV], and which were then burnt, I am returning to compose them for the second time."[28] Bardong, in his chronology of Galen's

---

[23] *AA* S20. For an example of subtraction, see S190.

[24] See *AA* II.331, 350, 468, 498, 526, 593–4, and S155.

[25] For what seems to be a purely verbal relationship to the dissections he is describing for his reader to do, see *AA* II.444, 550, 584, S101, and especially II.519, where he asks his reader to do an operation *for him*, using μοι in the dative of interest (τοῦτό μοι νῦν ἔμπαλιν πρᾶττε; my emphasis). At other times, he divorces himself entirely from the readers' procedure, granting their dissections independence from the ones he describes; he says that his reader can do procedures in different orders, in different ways, or in addition to the ones he covers, "if you wish": II.246 (ἐθέλοις), 262 (ἐθέλοις), 347 (βουληθῇς), 357 (τὸν βουλόμενον), 358 (ἐθέλῃς), 366 (ἐθελήσῃς), 440 (βούλοιο), 462 (βουληθείης), 490 (τρέποιο), S69–70.

[26] *AA* S267–9. The passage is from the section preserved only in Arabic; the translations provided by Duckworth, Lyons, and Towers (1962) and Garofalo (1991*b*) both construe it with a preterit.

[27] *AA* II.382–3 (ἔφην).

[28] *AA* S135.

oeuvre, splits the composition of *AA* into three sections with a time span of well over a decade, placing Books I–V under Marcus Aurelius, Books VI–XI under Commodus, and Books XII–XV under Septimius Severus.[29] Garofalo has further suggested, based on the content and introductions of the various chapters, that Galen released *AA* in eight separate sections, namely (1) Book I, (2) Book II, (3) Book III, (4) Books IV and V, (5) Book VI, (6) Books VII and VIII, (7) Books IX–XI and (8) Books XII–XV.[30]

While the natural variations in mindset and authorial purpose over this lengthy timeframe of composition – as well as the variety of scenarios from which he was drawing his notes – do result in some inconsistencies in content and style, the text as we have it nevertheless stands as a unified whole, in which Galen presents a strong and consistent editorial program.[31] Despite the piecemeal release of the book, he conceives of *AA* as a single text. He assumes that his readers will read it in its entirety and in the order that he writes it. At any given point in the text, Galen takes it for granted that his readers possess, both literally and internally, all of the previous books. He describes operations in terms of skills, methods, and physical structures that should be familiar to the readers from earlier in the work. He tells his readers to perform an operation "as you have learned" or "as I have described," sometimes giving a specific book, sometimes not.[32] He also mentions earlier locations where he has explained factual or descriptive material, often declining to repeat himself.[33] These internal references are not limited to neighboring books, but span the text from beginning to end; the fifteenth and final book contains references to skills learned as far back as the third and fifth.[34] Further, the cross references in the text are not all backwards-looking. Galen periodically mentions topics

[29] Bardong (1942), 631–2 (and see 633–40 for a complete timeline), where he updates Ilberg (1892), 513.
[30] Garofalo (1986–2000), viii.
[31] Galen's conception of the composition of his audience can shift subtly from section to section – he gives the needs of doctors greatest weight in the first five books, where he outlines the anatomy of the limbs and extremities, whereas in the later books he puts more emphasis on the goals of teachers and demonstrators – and his expectations about the capabilities of his readers can also vary dramatically from one area to another. For example, he delays his detailed instructions on the proper skinning of animals until the beginning of the third book (*AA* II.348), which lends credence to Garofalo's thesis that the first five books were released serially rather than as a unit; similarly, at S234–5 he gives a fairly elementary description of what ligaments, tendons, and nerves look like, though he has been using the words as given in preceding chapters.
[32] See *AA* II.328, 366 (ὡς ἔμαθες ἐν τῷ πρώτῳ γράμματι), 371, 389, 400, 518, 553, S32, 78 ("as I have described to you"), 88, 114, 140, 210, 236, 240, 261, 302.
[33] Declining to repeat at *AA* II.353, 360, 529, S209, 210, 236, 238, 281, 306, 317; he does offer brief summaries at II.626, S123, 134, 303.
[34] *AA* S302–3.

that he will cover at future points, indicating a strong vision of the finished product, even at the beginning of the extended compositional window.[35] Most strikingly, Galen maintains a consistent articulation of the overall purpose of the text. From the early books to the late books, he repeatedly inserts parenthetical remarks indicating that the goal of *AA* is to teach his readers to dissect, expose, and display to others all the parts of the body.[36] Unlike his minor anatomical texts, the purpose of *AA* goes far beyond just facilitating the memorization and recollection of anatomical facts; rather it teaches the method of obtaining the facts through dissection and equips the reader with the wherewithal to teach others in turn.

The Purpose of *Anatomical Procedures*

This decidedly instructional tenor is a major shift and, I would argue, an intentional move on Galen's part to disrupt the status quo. While books did have a role in medical education from an early date, it was typically a secondary one. Certainly, the literary and antiquarian interests of late Hellenistic and Roman intellectual circles had resulted in textual criticism, especially of Hippocrates, becoming a central element of elite medical discourse, but, even in circles where this was true, medicine remained a skill to be learned in person. Direct, oral instruction from a teacher was considered foundational for what was, essentially, an apprenticed art.[37] Indeed, teachers' names were the closest thing an ancient doctor had to the modern medical credential.[38] In general, early medical books acted as aids to memorization and served as supplements to oral teaching, to be used in tandem with lectures and guided practice; as such, they were necessary but insufficient for a complete medical education.[39] This conviction was firmly rooted, even outside medical circles; both Plato and Aristotle express the opinion that, while useful for the trained physician, medical literature is not in and of itself a path to medical knowledge: "men do not seem to become doctors from handbooks."[40]

[35] See *AA* II.314, 363, 444, 494, 499, S11, 95, 179.

[36] See *AA* II.243, 292, 659, 661, 664–65, 672, S32, 52–3, 70, 80, 95, 127, 131, 169.

[37] On medical education in antiquity, see Kudlien (1970), Clarke (1971), 109–12, André (1987), 41–58, Boudon-Millot (2008), 266–73, Wolff (2015), 90–93, and the collected articles in Horstmanshoff (2010); for the role of books specifically, see Cavallo (2002) and Marganne (2004), 15–27.

[38] See Boudon-Millot (2008), 273–4 and Massar (2010).

[39] See Dean-Jones (2003), who also argues that many of the texts in the Hippocratic Corpus that do not fit this paradigm, such as *VM*, *Morb.Sac.* and *Nat.Hom.*, were of polemical or protreptic rather than educational origin.

[40] Aristotle, *Nic.Eth.* 1181b1–12 (οὐ γὰρ φαίνονται οὐδ'ἰατρικοὶ ἐκ τῶν συγγραμμάτων γίνεσθαι); cf. Plato, *Phdr.* 268a–269a.

In the Hellenistic and Roman periods, as medical literature expanded, substantial books seem to have nevertheless remained largely in the hands of a minority of established doctors and to have been the tools of teachers rather than students.[41] Indeed, Galen laments the lack of bookishness among his colleagues in Rome, saying that "the majority of physicians who saw [me treating certain patients] did not know where to find written material on this or on other subjects."[42] Treatises aimed directly at students, motivated perhaps in part by the expense of book ownership, tended to be short and sweet.[43] Medical catechisms – series of questions with the answers appended – and lists of definitions dominate the examples of medical literature in the papyrological record and served to provide "summary information to apprentice physicians and succinct reminders to those in actual practice."[44] There were also introductory handbooks in circulation, like Galen's works for beginners, Pelops' *Introduction to Hippocrates*, the pseudo-Galenic *Doctor: Introduction*, and the various introductory texts that Galen says his contemporaries were in the habit of producing for their students; but these, too, were intended to act as supplementary reference works for students who were moving on from in-person training rather than complete introductions for the uninitiated.[45]

This general situation was all the more true of the specific subfield of anatomical books. As we have seen, Galen, with typical second-century nostalgia, believes that written guides to anatomy only began to be a necessity in the time of Hippocrates, when medical training ceased to be a life-long family endeavor.[46] This was the moment, reports Galen, when Diocles wrote his anatomical handbook, ushering in a new and popular

---

[41] For the expectation that medical books should be broached in the company of teachers, see *Hipp. Vict.* XV.175, *Hipp.Fract.* XVIIIb.321, 335, *San.Tu.* VI.114, *MM* X.8; cf. Andorlini (2003), 12–14.

[42] *Opt.Med.Cogn.* 3.17 (*CMG Suppl.Or.* IV, p. 61, trans. Iskandar); see also 5.1, 8.6, 9.22–4 (*CMG Suppl.Or.* IV, pp. 69, 97, 115–17), where he lambasts "many famous physicians in our time" (5.1) for their ignorance of and disdain for books. Indeed, the broader thrust of the text is that, unlike this sorry majority, the best doctors – those his readers are trying to identify – are the select few who embed themselves in the academic side of medicine.

[43] On the diverse needs of medical readers, see Cavallo (2002), 412–15.

[44] Hanson (2010), 192–7, quote from 197.

[45] Galen mentions at *Lib.Prop.* XIX.11 that his predecessors were accustomed to produce introductory texts for their students with names like "Outline" (ὑποτυπώσεις), "Sketch" (ὑπογραφάς), "Introduction" (εἰσαγωγάς), "Synopsis" (συνόψεις), and "Guide" (ὑφηγήσεις); see Boudon (1994) and Boudon-Millot (2004), 204–6 for the secondary relationship of these texts to oral teaching.

[46] II.280–1; see Chapter 6, "Diocles of Carystus" at p. 182. Celsus (*DM* proem.5), it is worth noting, believes the exact opposite, namely that "no distinguished men practiced medicine until literary studies began to be pursued with greater zeal" (nulli clari uiri medicinam exercuerunt, donec maiore studio litterarum disciplina agitari coepit).

support for the faulty memory of the post-Classical medical student. The link between the handbook and previous oral teaching remained a strong one; recall the framing of Rufus' *On the Names of the Parts of the Body*, which presents itself as a product or facsimile of an in-person lesson. Galen at first embraces this paradigm: All of his core minor anatomical works, and many of the ancillary ones, are explicitly bespoke creations, made for those who had previously attended his lectures and lessons and who wanted a way to remember them. Yet, as time passes, he seems to grow increasingly frustrated with it and ultimately comes to see *AA* as a means of subverting it.

Galen approached this task in a world in which distrust of the efficacy of the written word for training doctors was ingrained to the point of being proverbial. Already in the mid-second century BC, Polybius derides doctors who value book learning over practical training, saying that they are as incompetent as "pilots who steer by the book."[47] Several centuries later, Galen was still very aware of this proverb, using it repeatedly throughout the corpus, including in *AA*.[48] Though this frequent recurrence might seem to indicate that he generally valorized spoken over written education, the situation is more complicated, particularly in the anatomical context.[49] In the pilot similes and passages like them, Galen certainly concedes that learning out of books is not ideal, but he nevertheless believes that it is for some a necessity, and he seems to routinely have those readers in mind. In other words, he typically introduces the proverb only to address himself to the exceptions. In *On the Properties of Foodstuffs*, for example, he takes his firmest stance on the inadvisability of learning from books alone, yet concludes with encouragement for those who are doing just that, saying:

> And for this reason the common phrase seems to me to say it well, that the best teaching is that from the living voice, and that no one is able to become a helmsman, nor the practitioner of any other craft, out of a book. For these are memoranda of things already taught and already known, not a complete course of instruction for the novice. However, if any of the latter, whoever

---

[47] Polybius, XII.25d6 (εἰσὶ γὰρ ἀληθῶς ὅμοιοι τοῖς ἐκ βυβλίου κυβερνῶσιν). For detailed analysis of the proverb, see Roselli (2002) and Dunsch (2016). See also Alexander (1990), who explores a related proverb valorizing oral education – "the living voice" – which had widespread application beyond just medical circles.

[48] *AA* S12, *SMT* XI.796–7, *Lib.Prop.* XIX.33, *Alim.Fac.* VI.480, *Comp.Med.Gen.* XIII.605.

[49] Boudon-Millot (2004) unravels some of the tensions inherent in such a prolific author's holding a seemingly antitext position; cf. Alexander (1990), 228–31 and Asper (2005), 27–31.

is lacking a teacher, wish to carefully attend to things written clearly and in detail, as I am doing, they will benefit greatly, and all the more so if they do not shrink from reading them many times.[50]

Thus, even in areas such as pharmacology and dietetics where he recognizes that books alone are insufficient for learning a subject completely or optimally, he has trouble dismissing this method altogether, perhaps because of his deep-seated reservations about the quality of teachers.

Galen is generally skeptical of contemporary medical education. He deplores the factional tendencies of his peers, bemoaning that "the evil of partisan rivalry among the sects is so hard to get rid of, so exceedingly hard to scrub out, and more difficult to cure than any itch."[51] He ridicules the lazy reasoning behind many doctors' choice of allegiance and repeatedly characterizes those who follow their teachers blindly as slaves.[52] Instead, he views it as the moral obligation of the student to learn from all the sects, to take only so much from each as seems sound, and to distrust teachers until and unless they prove themselves worthy guides; he assures us that "even as an adolescent [he] looked down on many [of his] teachers."[53] His basic conviction is that success in any study is in the hands of the students themselves, through a combination of natural aptitude, broad-minded study, and tenacious work ethic.[54] It is no wonder, then, that he had difficulty dismissing the belief that a student might be better off poring over his own meticulous writing than listening to the lectures of one of his despised colleagues.[55]

---

[50] *Alim.Fac.* VI.480 (καὶ διὰ τοῦτό μοι δοκοῦσι καλῶς οἱ πολλοὶ λέγειν, ἀρίστην εἶναι διδασκαλίαν τὴν παρὰ τῆς ζώσης φωνῆς γιγνομένην, ἐκ βιβλίου δὲ μήτε κυβερνήτην τινὰ δύνασθαι γενέσθαι, μήτε ἄλλης τέχνης ἐργάτην· ὑπομνήματα γάρ ἐστι ταῦτα τῶν προμεμαθηκότων καὶ προεγνωκότων, οὐ διδασκαλία τελεία τῶν ἀγνοούντων. εἴ γε μὴν ἐθέλοιέν τινες καὶ τούτων, ὅσοι διδασκάλων ἀποροῦσιν, ἐντυγχάνειν ἐπιμελῶς τοῖς σαφῶς τε καὶ κατὰ διέξοδον, ὁποίαν ἡμεῖς ποιούμεθα, γεγραμμένοις, ὀνήσονται μεγάλως, καὶ μάλιστα ἐὰν πολλάκις ἀναγιγνώσκειν αὐτὰ μὴ ὀκνῶσιν); following the text in Wilkins (2013). Compare *SMT* XI.796–7, where he follows the proverb by considering the circumstances "if there is actually need of a book" (εἰ δὲ ἄρα καὶ δέοιτο τοῦ βιβλίου); for instances of this ambivalent treatment outside of the proverb passages, see *Comp.Med. Gen.* XIII.562–3 and the synopsis of *MM* cited at Garofalo (2006), 61.
[51] *Nat.Fac.* II.34 (οὕτως ἄρα δυσαπότριπτόν τι κακόν ἐστιν ἡ περὶ τὰς αἱρέσεις φιλοτιμία καὶ δυσέκνιπτον ἐν τοῖς μάλιστα καὶ ψώρας ἁπάσης δυσιατώτερον); cf. *Diff.Puls.* VIII.657.
[52] *Ord.Lib.Prop.* XIX.50; *Lib.Prop.* XIX.13, *Nat.Fac.* II.35.
[53] *Lib.Prop.* XIX.13, *Pecc.Dig.* V.42–3, *Loc.Aff.* VIII.143; *Pecc.Dig.* V.70 (πολλῶν διδασκάλων ἔτι μειράκιον ὢν ὑπερεφρόνησα) (cf. *AA* II.289 for his adult scorn of ignorant teachers).
[54] He repeatedly urges prospective doctors to cultivate a passion for study, as for example with his urgings to study night and day at *Nat.Fac.* II.179–80 and *CAM* I.244.
[55] The same general attitude comes across at *Ord.Lib.Prop.* XIX.54, where he says that a reader lacking in natural intelligence can trust Galen instead of trusting himself; cf. Mansfeld (1994), 119–26.

The need for personal dedication to study is particularly salient in the field of anatomy; Galen emphasizes that constant repetition is critical to achieving sufficient familiarity.[56] It is not surprising, then, that his two uses of the navigation simile in anatomical contexts are subtly different from its appearances elsewhere. His emphasis is on the repeated practical experience required of the student, not the means of their first introduction to the subject. In a brief digression on the benefits of anatomical study in *On the Composition of Drugs by Type*, he opines:

> Even more ridiculous than [the Empiricist doctrine of "chance anatomy"] is learning through anatomical handbooks, just like the so-called pilots from a book in the proverb. For how could it be that those having observed clearly the nerves and ligaments of the body demonstrated by a teacher are not able to accurately remember the places where they are situated unless they see the same things again a second time and a third and many times continually, if it were possible for someone, just by reading, to learn them at his leisure?[57]

His conclusion is not that books cannot teach anatomy, but rather that neither books nor live teachers can teach anatomy without hands-on practice and diligent repetition on the part of the student. In *AA*, tellingly, he does not even bother to mention teachers at all; rather he focuses only on whether or not his readers are practicing what they read: "whoever does not know [the solution to a seeming contradiction] is, as the proverbial expression goes, like a seaman who navigates out of a book. Thus he reads the books on anatomy, but he omits inspecting with his own eyes in the animal body the several things about which he is reading."[58] Where anatomy is concerned, it is irrelevant whether initial lessons are textual or oral: The body itself, not the teacher or the book, is the ultimate source of knowledge.

That an anatomical text should stand in distinction to other books appropriate for medical education is not surprising; despite Galen's protestations as to its fundamental necessity, deep training in anatomy was not a

---

[56] He often underscores the need for anatomists to practice, for example at *AA* II.289, 384–5, S16, 146, 159–60; indeed, he points out at II.621 that even the most experienced can continue to learn through continued repetition.

[57] *Comp.Med.Gen.* XIII.605 (ἔτι δὲ ληρωδεστέρα ταύτης ἡ διὰ τῶν ἀνατομικῶν συγγραμμάτων μάθησις ἐοικυῖα τοῖς κατὰ τὴν παροιμίαν λεγομένοις ἐκ βιβλίου κυβερνήταις. ὅπου γὰρ οἱ θεασάμενοι σαφῶς ὑπὸ διδασκάλου δεικνύμενα τὰ κατὰ τὸ σῶμα νεῦρα καὶ τοὺς τένοντας αὐτῶν, εἰ μὴ καὶ δεύτερον ἴδοιεν αὐτὰ καὶ τρίτον καὶ πολλάκις ἐφεξῆς, οὐ μνημονεύουσιν ἀκριβῶς τὸν τόπον ἐν ᾧ κεῖνται, σχολῇ δ' ἄν τις ἀναγνοὺς δυνηθείη μαθεῖν).

[58] *AA* S12.

given in the formation of doctors. His own rigorous anatomical education was not easily come by. Recall that, though he was lucky enough to begin his medical training in Pergamon under Quintus' own student Satyrus, his quest to continue his anatomical education with only the best anatomists was far-flung, time consuming, and often disappointing. He traveled widely around the Mediterranean in search of teachers – an option open, incidentally, only to the already wealthy would-be doctor – and was often disappointed in not finding the person he was seeking or in not gaining access to the details that he coveted.[59]

Indeed, it seems highly probable that the difficulties he experienced in acquiring his anatomical education must have been a large factor in Galen's decision to write *AA*. He is distressed by the trend to esotericism that he encounters in his attempts to collect the writings and knowledge of contemporary anatomists. He complains about Quintus, who relied solely on oral teaching to transmit his knowledge, saying that he thereby "concealed it from us and grudged it to us."[60] He is appalled by the inaccessibility and eventual destruction of Numisianus' written legacy, condemning the practices of Heracleianus, who hoarded those writings and, allegedly, burned them on his deathbed, and of Pelops, who was guilty of the same hoarding and who suffered the poetic justice of having all of his own works destroyed after having "repeatedly postponed their publication."[61] He is haunted by the idea that his own carefully cultivated knowledge and discoveries will meet the same fate as Numisianus', saying "already I see some of those who have been taught by me grudging to share their knowledge; and if they should die soon after me, these studies will die with them."[62] Creating a written course on anatomy ensured that his discoveries and doctrines could continue to be learned even after his own teaching days were over.[63] Approached from this perspective, it is hardly surprising that

---

[59] See Chapter 7, "Quintus and His Students" at pp. 240–6.

[60] *AA* S230; see Chapter 7, "Quintus and His Students: Quintus" at p. 238.

[61] *AA* S231–2; see Chapter 7, "Quintus and His Students: Numisianus, Heracleianus, Pelops, and Aelianus" at pp. 243–5.

[62] *AA* II.283 (τῶν δ' ὑπ' ἐμοῦ διδαχθέντων ἤδη τινὰς ὁρῶ φθονοῦντας ἑτέροις μεταδιδόναι, οἷς ἐὰν ἐξαίφνης ἀποθανεῖν συμβῇ μετ' ἐμέ, συναπολεῖται τὰ θεωρήματα); others of his students were apparently more reliable, since he describes some who teach anatomy to students of their own (*Comp.Med.Gen.* XIII.603) and others who would be able – always assuming they were willing – to reproduce one of his experiments after his death (*Sem.* IV.595).

[63] Even outside of anatomy, he several times expresses concern that his teachings are lost on his contemporaries and hope that his writing will fall into the hands of some exceptional and worthy future reader, as at *Dig.Puls.* VIII.826, *Nat.Fac.* II.179–80, and *MM* X.21; cf. Asper (2005) and Boudon-Millot (2008), 278–82.

Galen considers *AA* to be an outright substitute for oral teaching. In the second book, after describing the deficiencies of other available works on anatomy, he explains:

> since there is a danger, because of the small regard that men today have for the arts and, further, because men have ceased to practice from childhood, that these sorts of [anatomical] observations shall perish, I am justified in writing these memoranda, though, *if it were possible for men to preserve this [knowledge] by relaying it from person to person, it would be superfluous to write them.* Therefore, I share everything that I have learned from the beginning of my studies with those who need it, hoping, if possible, that all men learn these things.[64]

From the very beginning of its composition, Galen intended *AA* to be able to take the place of oral teaching, believing that in-person lecturing provided insufficient accuracy, permanency, and reach to be the sole conduit for the subject of anatomy.[65]

The Audience of *Anatomical Procedures*

A profoundly audience-oriented text, *AA* is custom-made for bypassing in-person instruction. As we saw, the initial framing of the text orients it toward a small group of companions who already have a personal relationship with Galen and have, presumably, attended his dissections – precisely the type of addressee typical of the minor anatomical texts and of a world predicated on in-person learning. Yet this group, addressed with the second person plural, surfaces only sporadically in the remainder of the text. When they do appear, they serve mostly as a means of showcasing Galen's fame and his expertise: The large majority of his uses of the second-person plural appear in circumstances where he is reminding the avowed addressees that they have already seen him perform the action that he is describing, usually on many occasions: "you have often seen me demonstrating

---

[64] *AA* II.282–3 (ἐπεὶ δὲ κίνδυνός ἐστι, διά τε τὴν ὀλιγωρίαν, ἣν ἔχουσιν οἱ νῦν ἄνθρωποι περὶ τὰς τέχνας, ἔτι τε διότι τῆς ἐκ παίδων ἀσκήσεως ἀπολείπονται, διαφθαρῆναι τὰ τοιαῦτα τῶν θεωρημάτων, εἰκότως ὑπομνήματα γράφομεν, ὡς, εἴ γε τῇ παρ᾽ ἀλλήλων διαδοχῇ τοῖς ἀνθρώποις ὑπῆρχε διασώζειν αὐτά, περιττὸν ἂν ἦν τὸ γράφειν. ἐγὼ μὲν οὖν ἁπάντων, ὧν ἐξ ἀρχῆς ἔγνων, ἐκοινώνησα τοῖς δεομένοις, βουλόμενος, εἰ οἷόν τε, πάντας ἀνθρώπους ἐκμαθεῖν αὐτά); my emphasis.

[65] See also *AA* II.449–50, 651 where he refers to the text as a "teacher" (διδάσκον) and II.417, where he explains that the order of the text is meant to prioritize what "the young" (τοὺς νέους) should learn first. Salas (2020) suggests a different but related motivation for this text, namely that it extends the credentialling mechanism of anatomical display beyond just the circles that are able to witness actual dissections, allowing Galen to broaden his reputation and authority.

the parts of [the arm]"; "you have, of course, seen me do this"; "you have seen me demonstrate all these things often both privately and publicly."[66] This strategy, in keeping with the already self-promotional stance of framing his writing as at the behest of this devoted group of followers, allows him to call upon this group as plural witnesses to his extensive experience and thus highlight it for the rest of his readers.[67]

Even as he addresses himself to these associates, however, Galen makes clear that his target audience is much larger and less familiar. He says "it is likely that this work will not be kept in the hands of friends only, but that the hands of many men will pass it along" and therefore that "it is necessary, for the sake of those men, to recall and state often things already known to friends," overriding the interests of his ostensible audience and aiming the level of discourse at strangers instead.[68] Again, three books later, acknowledging that the needs of strangers have first priority in his composition, he says:

> Since, as I have said before, it is not proposed for me to aim at you alone, for whom this work is a memorandum, but also at all others—whoever is zealous about anatomy—it is necessary to write this in such a way that, even for those who have not ever seen such things, they are as clear as possible.[69]

He is, thus, quite open about the fact that the plural "you," despite its positional importance, is not his intended audience. Indeed, he frequently mentions them only to highlight and prioritize those readers who, unlike them, have never seen him dissect and who might need further directions.[70] As the passages citing their repeated witnessing of his skills remind us, he has already reached these people. The real object of his concern are the readers who have not been able to access anatomical instruction in person; these are the "you" he is most targeting in the second person singular addresses that permeate the text.

---

[66] *AA* II.348 (κἀμὲ πολλάκις ἑωράκατε τὰ κατ' αὐτὴν δεικνύντα), 608 (ὁρᾶτε γὰρ δήπου καὶ ἐμὲ τοῦτο πράττοντα), 690 (πάντα τὰ τοιαῦτα δεικνύντα με ἐθεάσασθε πολλάκις ἰδίᾳ τε καὶ δημοσίᾳ); cf. II.478, 635, 677.

[67] Galen deploys this same strategy in other treatises as well; see Mattern (2008), 83–4.

[68] *AA* II.504–5 (οὐκέτ' ἐν ταῖς τῶν ἑταίρων μόνων χερσὶ τὴν πραγματείαν ταύτην εἰκός ἐστι φυλαχθήσεσθαι, πολλὰς δ' ἀμείψειν ἀνθρώπων χεῖρας ... χρὴ τοίνυν κἀκείνων ἕνεκα τὰ γιγνωσκόμενα τοῖς ἑταίροις ἀναμιμνήσκειν τε καὶ λέγειν πολλάκις).

[69] *AA* II.651 (ἐπεὶ δ' οὐχ ὑμῶν μόνον, οἷς ἀνάμνησίς ἐστιν ὁ λόγος ὅδε, πρόκειταί μοι στοχάσασθαι, καθότι καὶ πρόσθεν εἶπον, ἀλλὰ καὶ τῶν ἄλλων ἁπάντων, ὅσοι σπουδάζουσι περὶ τὰς ἀνατομάς, ἀναγκαῖόν ἐστιν οὕτως γράφειν αὐτόν, ὡς ἂν καὶ τοῖς μηδὲ πώποτε θεασαμένοις αὐτὰς ὅσον οἷόν τε μάλιστα γενέσθαι σαφεστάτας); following the text in Garofalo (1986–2000). He continues to be explicit about this wider audience, for example at S15 and 169.

[70] *AA* II.628, 690, S65, 128, 131.

Galen's consideration for these readers is paramount and he mentions them fairly frequently, though the fact that he feels the need to do so only underscores the conclusion that they would have been an atypical or unexpected part of the audience of a medical text of this nature. Over and over, across the span of the text, he encourages the teacherless reader to study the text, practice, and persevere: "I wrote this work for this reason: so that it might be able to teach hard-working men, even if they lack someone to demonstrate"; "whoever has not observed me, but comes to this [procedure] having learned about anatomy even from a book, will easily find [the structure in question]"; "I shall explain about these things in [the section on] the dissection of the nerves so clearly that any hard-working man, training himself by himself, will eventually be able to completely achieve the described dissection"; "if anyone has learnt that and studied it only from my words and my descriptions, he must exercise himself first on the body of a dead animal"; "as for those who have not seen how I performed it, I have reason to think that the reward of perseverance should benefit them also"; "as I have thought it right in this book to try to serve the advantage of those who have never been present or seen me when I was performing a dissection, I must describe this operation also in the clearest possible way"; "in my descriptions here also I shall propose as my intention and my aim to make my discourse clear and lucid to such a degree that it may be possible for one who studies them without ever having seen the dissection of an animal at all, after he has followed the account of the dissection of the veins and arteries as I have given it to him, to apply himself unaided to the study of them all."[71] Galen sets up the text to be an anatomical curriculum sufficient to itself.

While Galen's educational ideals shine through clearly, it is worth questioning the degree to which he adhered to them: Does he, in short, take care to write a book that could actually serve to teach any teacherless reader possessed of sufficient diligence and perseverance? To address this question, it is necessary to consider the audience that Galen addresses, both as he imagines them to be and as he assumes them to be – that is, the ways in which he describes and characterizes them, on the one hand, and the things that he actually expects of them, on the other.

---

[71] *AA* II.449–50 (ἐγὼ γὰρ διὰ τοῦτο τὴν πραγματείαν ἔγραψα ταύτην, ὥστ᾽ αὐτὴν διδάσκειν δύνασθαι τοὺς φιλοπόνους, ἐὰν ἀπορῶσι τῶν δειξόντων), 622 (καὶ ὅστις οὐκ εἶδεν ἡμᾶς, ἀλλὰ τῷ λόγῳ γε προδιδαχθεὶς ἐπὶ τὴν ἀνατομὴν ἦλθε … εὑρήσει ῥᾳδίως αὐτό), 694 (εἰρήσεται γὰρ ὑπὲρ αὐτῶν ἐν τῇ τῶν νεύρων ἀνατομῇ σαφῶς οὕτως, ὡς δύνασθαί τινα φιλόπονον, αὐτὸν ἐφ᾽ αὑτοῦ γυμνασάμενον, ἐργάσασθαι ποτε τὴν εἰρημένην ἄρτι τελέως ἀνατομήν), S65, 128, 131, 169.

Galen is consistent in his expectation that his readers will be drawn to the text by diverse motivations and from differing occupations. He says:

> Anatomical investigation has one use for a scientific man, who enjoys knowledge for its own sake, another for the man who does not practice it for its own sake, but rather to prove that nature does nothing in vain, still another for the man who provides data from anatomy for the understanding of a function, whether physical or psychical, and, beyond these, another for the man who is going to competently remove thorns or the points of weapons or cut anything out in a suitable way so as to correctly operate on ulcers or sores or abscesses.[72]

He here envisions a spectrum ranging from the serious intellectual and the philosopher to the research-oriented physician and the practitioner. Even outside of this programmatic passage, Galen gestures periodically to each of these four types of expected reader. Information and asides aimed at the practicing doctor are the most frequent, easiest to spot, and least surprising. In the first five books particularly, where he discusses the muscles of the body as well as the vessels and nerves of the limbs – topics of urgent relevance to the practitioner who must competently handle these sites of common injury – he singles out the doctors in his audience repeatedly and pointedly.[73] Indeed, the medical utility of anatomical knowledge is a cornerstone of his general approach to medicine, and it is no surprise that he reiterates this conviction frequently here, claiming that the uses to which doctors put anatomy are "the most essential ones."[74]

Distinct from these asides to the hard-working practitioner, Galen also targets the type of reader whom he described as approaching anatomy for the sake of providing "data for the understanding of a function, whether physical or psychical," that is, the research-oriented physician or the anatomist.[75] As befits their more intellectually driven motivations, he offers

---

[72] *AA* II.286 (ἄλλη μὲν γὰρ ἀνδρὶ φυσικῷ χρεία τῆς ἀνατομικῆς ἐστι θεωρίας, αὐτὴν δι᾽ ἑαυτὴν ἀγαπῶντι τὴν ἐπιστήμην· ἄλλη δὲ τῷ μὴ δι᾽ ἑαυτήν, ἀλλ᾽ ἵνα ἐπιδείξῃ μηδὲν εἰκῇ γεγονὸς ὑπὸ τῆς φύσεως· ἄλλη δὲ τῷ πρὸς ἐνεργείας τινὸς γνῶσιν, ἤτοι φυσικῆς, ἢ ψυχικῆς, ἐξ ἀνατομῆς ποριζομένῳ λήμματα· καὶ πρὸς τούτοις ἄλλη τῷ σκόλοπας ἢ βελῶν ἀκίδας ἐξαιρήσειν μέλλοντι καλῶς ἢ ἐκκόπτειν τι προσηκόντως, ὥστ᾽ οὖν ἢ κόλπους, ἢ σύριγγας, ἢ ἀποστήματα χειρουργήσειν ὀρθῶς).

[73] He includes particularly urgent appeals to doctors at or near the beginnings of three of these books (*AA* II.288–91, 340–6, 416–20), but similar comments occur throughout, as at II.284, 394–6, 634, and he will also occasionally direct his medical readers to supplement or relate their anatomical studies with their daily practice, as at II.229–30, 386–8, 391–2, 510, 551, S15–16, 55, 62–3, 75, 157–9, 297, 326.

[74] *AA* II.286 (ἀναγκαιότατα).

[75] He refers to the same group again at *AA* II.611 as "doctors who are clever about the natural world" (οἱ περὶ φύσιν δεινοὶ ... ἰατροί).

fewer direct instructions to this group and feels no need to harangue them into the study. Indeed, though he is happy to teach them the technical skills with which to collect their data, he makes it clear that the greater purpose of these readers is beyond his own agenda in *AA* and encourages them to "seek out at their leisure" the why and wherefore of anatomical and physiological questions.[76] Nevertheless, he has deep sympathy for this particular anatomical motivation and, even in sections where he is emphasizing the needs of the practitioner, he is careful not to omit points and suggestions that will only be of use to this more advanced group.[77] It also seems likely that the extensive instructions directed towards anyone reading *AA* in order to teach anatomy to his own students are aimed first and foremost at this type of reader.[78] As we saw in Chapter 7, the study of anatomy as a distinct discipline seems to have gone hand in hand with demonstration and instruction – to be an anatomist was also, almost inevitably, to be a teacher of anatomy.

In addition to these two types of medical readers, Galen is invested in promoting the profile of the lay audience to whom *AA* is equally addressed. These are the philosophers and the educated intellectuals – those who "enjoy knowledge for its own sake" – who also formed a core target audience for *On the Usefulness of the Parts*.[79] Indeed, I suggested in Chapter 8 that Galen's decision to expand *AA* into this compendious and reader-oriented second edition was motivated to some extent by his evolving conception of the needs of these very readers during his composition of that text. Philosophers, as we have seen, are not surprising candidates for anatomical study. Although its practice was neither mainstream nor always robustly represented in philosophical circles, philosophers were a core constituency in the history of dissection from its very beginnings. Galen reminds his readers of this long-established link, saying that in his idealized golden age of pre- and peri-Hippocratic dissection, "the ancients were zealous about anatomy to an appropriate degree, not just

---

[76] *AA* II.641 (ζητητέον ἐπὶ σχολῆς).

[77] See, for example, *AA* S155–6, where he encourages study beyond that strictly necessary for medical practice, "if you are one of those who take account of this [type of] detail," and subsequently sends such an "anatomist" to *UP* for even more details.

[78] The idea of equipping the reader to be a future teacher is pervasive throughout *AA*; see II.226, 242, 292, 351, 520, 564, 659, 661, 672, S81.

[79] See Chapter 8, "Dissection Elsewhere in the Galenic Corpus" at pp. 305–8 for Galen's vision of the audience of *UP*, and *Lib.Prop.* XIX.20 for his description of the actual audience it found during his lifetime, namely "practically every doctor who practices traditional medicine and those of the philosophers who follow Aristotle" (τοῖς ἰατροῖς σχεδὸν ἅπασιν, ὅσοι τὴν παλαιὰν ἰατρικὴν μετεχειρίζοντο, καὶ τῶν φιλοσόφων τοῖς ἀπ' Ἀριστοτέλους).

doctors, but philosophers also."[80] As indicated by his characterization of this group as those who want "to prove that nature does nothing in vain," he views the primary philosophical relevance of anatomy to be the study of teleology. Indeed, he believes that dissection will lead inevitably to the conclusion that "one art is the maker of all living creatures" even for those who at first disbelieve.[81] Although he certainly targets what we might call professional philosophers with these remarks, he also aims them to cast a wider net: He says that he is addressing *AA* to "all those who love knowledge," "whoever is zealous about anatomy," and "those who wish to instruct themselves about each one of the parts of the composite parts in the body," people he refers to more broadly as "intellectuals," "the educated," "amateurs of medicine," and "lovers of the medical art," who study it "in order to exercise their minds."[82] It is in this last class, of course, that Boethus belongs; maintaining his name in the introduction to the rewrite serves Galen to offer a sort of posthumous endorsement from a prominent reader of this class and a role model for other aspiring dilettante readers.

There was, to be sure, a certain amount of fluidity among these groups of readers – Galen would have self-identified with all four to greater or lesser degree – yet each represents a distinct agenda and set of skills that would be brought to the table by the readers within it. Whereas most philosophers would have had an extensive rhetorical and philosophical education and only a minimum of exposure to the medical arts, many doctors began medical training at quite a young age, sometimes bypassing much of the traditional educational system.[83] Galen's assertion, therefore, that "everyone is competent" to follow his directions is more complicated than it at first sight appears, and it is worth querying the assumptions that he makes throughout *AA* about his audience's preexisting knowledge of the

---

[80] *AA* II.280 (ἱκανῶς γὰρ ἐσπουδάκασιν οἱ παλαιοὶ τὴν ἀνατομήν, οὐκ ἰατροὶ μόνον, ἀλλὰ καὶ φιλόσοφοι); cf. *PHP* V.266 (II.6.17 De Lacy).

[81] *AA* II.541–2 (μίαν τέχνην ... τῶν ζώων ἀπάντων δημιουργὸν); cf II.544–5, 548–9. For a consideration of *AA* as a guide to "philosophy with a scalpel," see Cosans (1998), especially 63–70 and 75–80. Galen says that these philosophical questions are a driving purpose in his own study of anatomy (II.537–42) and, similarly to his tone in *UP*, he marvels throughout *AA* at the ingenuity of nature and even ascribes intentionality and logical thought to it (II.590).

[82] *AA* addressees at S15, II.651 (cf. II.573), and S168 respectively. Characterizations at II.351, 672 (φιλομαθαί); II.281 (πεπαιδευμένοι); *Praen.* XIV.619 and *San.Tu.* VI.449 (οἱ ἰδιῶται τῆς ἰατρικῆς τέχνης); *San.Tu.* VI.269 (φιλιάτρους ... ὡς γεγυμνάσθαι τὴν διάνοιαν); cf. *Comp.Med.Gen.* XIII.636, where φιλίατρος is paired with φιλοφάρμακος.

[83] For the variable educational level of doctors, see André (1987), 41–3 and Nutton (2013a), 254–78.

body and their basic education – that is, in short, whether or not he consistently follows through on his agenda.[84]

To begin with Galen's expectations of his audience's general educational background, the most obvious prerequisite for reading this text is the ability to read Greek fluently.[85] Greek was the standard language for medical study and for philosophy more generally, so it would not be hasty to assume that the vast majority of people with a medical or philosophical interest in anatomy would have spoken it. Regardless of their specific interests, Romans of a high social standing would also have attained a good degree of fluency in Greek over the course of their elite educations. Thus, it is difficult to imagine that many people with the time and interest to broach the subject would have been excluded from the text by Galen's language.[86] Literacy is a more vexed issue. In general terms, medicine, even in its humbler forms, was a comparatively book-dependent art; most doctors were likely literate to some degree.[87] Nevertheless, the medical audience that Galen had in mind was clearly restricted to those who had received a more academic medical training and therefore read with a level of fluency that would not have impeded their ability to derive benefit from his texts. Though he conceives of his readers as the type of people who read Herodotus for pleasure, he is certainly aware of the spectrum of abilities on this front.[88] His acerbic claim that most men who attend medical and philosophical lectures "cannot read well" is more complex than a condemnation of their basic literacy – such phrasing can equally refer to a lack of culture and educational refinement – rather it signals his observation of a gradation in competencies even among those seeking a more advanced medical education.[89] Unlike the impeccably cultured individual to whom

---

[84] *AA* II.512 (πᾶς ... ἱκανός ἐστι), a statement directly about the ability to skin specimens, but which is representative of his general attitude, as sketched earlier. Compare *Hipp.Fract.* XVIIIb.321, where he says explicitly that he is aiming his commentary "not at the best prepared nor the least ... [but at] those having an average level" (οὔτε τοῦ ἄριστα παρεσκευασμένου οὔτε τοῦ χείριστα στοχάζομαι ... τῶν μέσην ἕξιν ἐχόντων) and *Hipp.Epid.I* XVIIa.84–5, where he is aiming "neither only at those who are exceedingly unlearned nor only at those with sufficient preparation" (οὔτε μόνων τῶν ἐσχάτως ἀμαθῶν οὔτε μόνων τῶν ἱκανὴν ἐχόντων τὴν παρασκευήν).

[85] Alternatively, one could bypass literacy in Greek by means of a lector, though this would require a level of wealth that would in most cases already correlate to an elite education.

[86] Debru (1995), 73 does speculate, though, that Galen's larger public demonstrations would have attracted "tout comme les conférences des sophists, des personnes qui ne comprenaient pas toutes le grec."

[87] See Harris (1989), 82 and Hanson (2010), 189–90; cf. Lougovaya (2019), who argues that Galen's elite education was not anomalous in the broader medical community.

[88] For Herodotus, see *AA* II.393; cf. Dio Chrysostom, *Or.* XVIII.10, which also marks his works as pleasure reading.

[89] *Lib.Prop.* XIX.9 (οὐδ᾽ ἀναγνῶναι καλῶς δυνάμενοι); see Harris (1989), 5–6 on the interpretation of this phrase.

he compares them, these men have not received "a first-class education" with proper grammatical and rhetorical training.[90] Some of these maligned individuals would, no doubt, have been perfectly capable of reading and properly understanding *AA*, but we can probably exclude from its readership the less literarily proficient among them, a group very unlikely to have had the time or the resources to devote to the study anyway, even if they had the requisite literacy.

As far as other areas of general study are concerned, Galen does not mention any requirements for his readers, ideal or otherwise, which is fairly unexpected given his general insistence on the primacy of logic to all studies.[91] The only academic subject that he handles in *AA* in a way geared towards a reader with some previous study is geometry. Galen compares the trapezius muscle to a trapezoid, saying that the muscle is "a little short of a triangle, what the geometers call the trapezoid shape," instructing the reader that "you will understand what I mean more clearly if you cut through a right triangle with a straight line parallel to the base near the top of the triangle," clarifying further that in this figure one side is at right angles to the base and the new top while the other is oblique to those lines.[92] This description requires a decent understanding of triangles and lines, but it is predicated on the assumption that "trapezoid" is not a term that can be lightly bandied about.[93] He also expects his readers to be able to conceive of a simple geometrical figure via a Euclidean description of labeled points and line segments – nothing terribly advanced (or essential to his narrative), but nevertheless presupposing at least some basic familiarity with mathematical procedure on the part of the readers.[94]

Geometry would not typically have been taught to those receiving only an elementary education but was rather an aspect of secondary education.[95] It was believed to be useful in sharpening analytic skills and stimulating

---

[90] *Lib.Prop.* XIX.9 (τὴν πρώτην παιδείαν).

[91] At *Ord.Lib.Prop.* XIX.53 he recommends that his readers begin with his lost introduction to logic, *On Demonstration*; he does allow at XIX.53–4 that a man who was not "clever by nature and a friend of truth" (φύσει συνετοὶ καὶ ἀληθείας ἑταῖροι) could put his faith in Galen's logical ability and go directly to his other works, but says that he would only achieve correct information, not an exact knowledge.

[92] *AA* II.445–6 (ὀλίγου δεῖν τρίγωνος, οἷά περ οἱ γεωμέτραι καλοῦσι τὰ τραπέζια σχήματα. νοήσεις δ᾿ ὃ λέγω σαφέστερον, εἰ τρίγωνον ὀρθογώνιον διατέμνοις εὐθείᾳ γραμμῇ παραλλήλῳ τῇ βάσει <...>; following the text in Garofalo (1986–2000) and restoring the lacuna from Garofalo (1991*b*), which offers an Italian translation of the Arabic.

[93] Again, at *AA* II.458 Galen assumes that his readers know what he means by "equilateral triangle" (τρίγωνον ἰσόπλευρον).

[94] *AA* II.274, S309.

[95] See Marrou (1956), 176–9, 281–2, Clarke (1971), 45–52, Cribiore (2001), 41–2, and Sidoli (2015).

the mind and was thus considered part of the ideal liberal education. Quintilian, for example, despite banishing its place in the curriculum to "spare moments," claimed that "no orator can exist without geometry" and takes care to demonstrate his own familiarity with elementary problems, including a very simple exercise with areas and perimeters, which requires about the same level of skill as Galen's trapezoid construction.[96] Galen himself indicates that Euclid's *Elements* and *Data* were taught to the children of elite Romans, though he is scornful of their parents for not having progressed any further than that in mathematics.[97] Doctors, too – at least those supported by a wealthy family – might begin their studies with the basics of geometry, though it was not universally considered a necessary part of an academic medical education.[98] Thus a passing acquaintance with triangles that does not necessarily extend to comfortable familiarity with trapezoids seems a plausible level to expect of many of the types of reader that Galen targets.[99]

As for any assumed medical background, Galen lists *AA* in his autobibliographic texts as a first point of access for those interested in medicine, along with his works designated as "for beginners," indicating that he intended them to have a low bar for entry. In both *On My Own Books* and *On the Order of My Own Books*, he says that one may go directly from *On Bones* to

---

[96] Quintilian, *Inst.* I.12.13 (haec temporum velut subsiciva) and I.10.49 (nullo modo sine geometria esse possit orator). He demonstrates his familiarity with the subject in the section on the orator's need for geometry at I.10.34–49; cf. I.10.3, where he references constructing an equilateral triangle on a given line (Euclid, *Elem.* I.1).

[97] See Strohmaier (1993), 162 discussing the Arabic translation (as yet unpublished) of Galen's commentary on Hippocrates' *Airs, Waters, Places*. In fact, at *PHP* V.222–3 (II.3.14–15 De Lacy), Galen claims that many well-educated and intelligent people of his acquaintance even have trouble with arithmetic, and at *UP* III.814 (II.94H) he assumes that only a small minority even of the intellectually superior audience of *UP* "understand what a circle and a cone and an axis and all the rest of those sorts of things are, having been properly educated in mathematics and especially geometry" (νομίμως παιδευθέντες ἔν τε τοῖς ἄλλοις μαθήμασι καὶ γεωμετρίᾳ γιγνώσκουσι, τί ποτ' ἐστὶ κύκλος καὶ κῶνος καὶ ἄξων καὶ τῶν ἄλλων ἕκαστον τῶν ὁμοίων); cf. III.819 (II.98H).

[98] See Kudlien (1970), 22–3, and Clarke (1971), 111; Marasco (2010) describes the general education of doctors in late antiquity, offering examples where arithmetic and geometry were explicitly included (pp. 207, 214–15). Galen, heavily influenced by his architect father and the mathematically advanced education that he received from him (*Lib.Prop.* XIX.40), has a particularly high valuation of geometry; see, for example, *MM* X.5, 30–5, where he explains that the study of geometric proof and logical demonstration is necessary to the training of a competent doctor (cf. *Const.Art.Med.* I.244). His view is certainly not the universal one – indeed he criticizes the narrowmindedness of his peers on the subject at *Opt.Med.* I.53–4 – but it is by no means unique; the ps.-Hippocratic *Ep.* 22 contains an injunction to the son of the writer to study geometry as useful for medical thinking, and the introductory framing at Rufus, *Nom.Part.* 2–5 suggests that medical study keeps company with that of grammar and geometry.

[99] Compare Netz (2002), 210–16, who uses Polybius as an example of the sketchy nature of geometrical competency even among those who consider it valuable in theory.

AA.[100] Indeed, in the text itself the only two books Galen explicitly requires that his readers have read beforehand are *On Bones* and *On the Movement of the Muscles*, though, in practice, he only follows through on this expectation in regard to the former.[101] In fact, though he is not always consistent about the level to which he is pitching his discourse, Galen basically never assumes a degree of anatomical knowledge beyond that characteristic of a beginner familiar with the names of the vital organs and with the basic vocabulary of medical literature, unless the knowledge should have been learned earlier in *AA.*[102] He is fond of saying that "everyone knows" an anatomical fact, but, although this might hurt the self-esteem of an ignorant reader, the very act of announcing how elementary a fact is allows him to state that fact, to the advantage of the previously unaware.[103] Indeed, he takes considerable pains to make all of the entry points for dissection clear and easy to locate, as, for example, in his introduction to the dissection of the leg muscles in the second book, where he says: "you will find [the first muscles in question] easily, as I will show you, when you start your search from certain parts familiar to all men. For no one does not know the ham and the knee and the shin."[104] This is characteristic of his general commitment to ease of understanding in his descriptions and directions. He often refers to organs by their color, size, or shape in order to distinguish them from each other.[105] He takes care to orient the reader in terms of obvious

---

[100] *Lib.Prop.* XIX.23 and *Ord.Lib.Prop.* XIX.54.

[101] For *Oss.* see *AA* II.227, 267, 460, S64; for *Mot.Musc.* see II.458, 473, S234, 272. He does indeed expect some knowledge about the bones that *AA* itself does not provide, as at S4, where he expects the reader to know how to locate the so-called cribriform bone in the nose, but in the few places where he gestures toward his readers' existing knowledge of the movement of the muscles, he takes care to provide, in a tactful *praeteritio*, all of the information that the disobedient and unversed reader would need (II.464, 695).

[102] Galen will occasionally include mention of a structure or phenomenon in passing before he has described it in detail, but, as these are asides, this would not materially affect the reader's comprehension. For example, at *AA* II.358, before having taught the veins and arteries, he tells the reader to begin dissection of the arm at "the humeral vein" (τὴν ὠμιαίαν φλέβα), but he also describes the spot in terms of a muscle that he described in Book I and, therefore, one that the reader should already be familiar with, as he points out (ὡς ἔμαθες). Again, in Book VII (II.613), he mentions in passing the third and sixth pairs of cranial nerves, which he does not systematically explain and identify until Book IX (S9), but as the nerves were simply examples of a phenomenon this would not seriously affect the reader's ability to understand the point he was making.

[103] For example, *AA* II.572 (ἅπαντες ἤδη γιγνώσκουσιν) on the homogeneous nature of the intestines, S127 on the uses of the tongue, and S165 on the nomenclature of parts of the penis.

[104] *AA* II.293 (ἐξευρήσεις δὲ αὐτάς, ὡς ἐγὼ διδάξω, ῥᾳδίως, ἀπό τινων οἷον σκοπῶν ὁρμώμενος ἅπασιν ἀνθρώποις γνωρίμων. ἰγνύαν γὰρ καὶ γόνυ καὶ ἀντικνήμιον οὐδεὶς ἀγνοεῖ); following the text in Garofalo (1986–2000).

[105] For uses of descriptors rather than nomenclature, see *AA* II.300–1, 307, 312, 357, 363–4, 371, 401–2, 435, 480, 493, 496, 656, S17, 61, 94, 224.

or familiar landmarks in the body, saying things like "once you clearly see the angle of the triangle [formed by the deltoid muscle] on its outward facing side, raise up your glance."[106] He even attempts to give real-time feedback in the form of descriptions of what the reader should see if he has proceeded correctly and what he will see if he has not.[107]

Galen's evaluation of the technical skills of his readers is less consistent. He gives very detailed instructions on how to skin an animal properly – the necessary first step to many dissections – but not until the third book.[108] In the first two books, though he repeatedly instructs the reader to skin animals and dwells on the importance of doing the skinning oneself so as to be sure of its accuracy, he assumes that his readers can do it without detailed instruction.[109] Again, in an aside later on, he stops himself from assuming that all readers will be familiar with the tools his friends have seen him employ and promises to describe those needed for the exposure of the brain. Yet the fulfillment of this promise is to tell his readers to picture the "osteoclastic instrument which is commonly used and which everyone knows," and in his explanation of how to use it he says to hit it with the "hammer which one is generally accustomed to employ."[110] This is hardly an enlightening description to the unfamiliar reader. Similarly, though he generally gives very detailed instructions for dissection, he in various places assumes a great deal of previous experience – for example, that the reader is an old hand at removing vertebrae with a pair of chisels, describing the process only as to be done "as usual"; that the reader is "accustomed" to piercing skulls, even though he says this in the section where he is introducing the practice of exposing the brain for the first time; and that his readers will be able to "turn out and evacuate the uterus in which the fetus is contained, employing the current usage of anatomists" without any further instructions.[111]

A prime example of this inconsistency is at the beginning of the thirteenth book, which deals with veins and arteries. After a brief introduction in which he states that his aim is to make his discourse on the vessels clear enough so

---

[106] *AA* II.354 (ὅταν οὖν ἐναργῶς ἴδῃς τὴν κορυφὴν τοῦ τριγώνου κατὰ τὴν ἐκτὸς αὐτοῦ πλευράν, ἀνάβαινε τὴν θέαν). For more examples, see II.293, 325, 509, 513–14, 523, 550, 646–7, 719, 720–21, S13, 33, 95, 102–4, 152, 155, 172, 184, 250, 258, 278, 326.

[107] For descriptions of the correct outcome, see *AA* II.258, 437–8, 646–7, 665, S55, 60, 62, 117, 241, 242, 246, 275, 283, 285, 305, 327; for the results of errors, see II.251, 329, 485–6, 512–13, 515, 709, 714, 722–3, S93, 246, 315–16.

[108] *AA* II.348–52.

[109] He does mention that the sharp lancet is suitable to the task at *AA* II.244.

[110] *AA* S15–16.

[111] Chisels at *AA* II.686 (ὡς ἔθος); piercing the skull at S14; uterus at S144–5.

that "it may be possible for one who studies them without ever having seen the dissection of an animal at all" – that is, a complete novice – to learn them thoroughly with only the aid of this book, Galen goes on to say:

> *I do not think that anyone's lack of understanding of anatomy will extend so far that*, when he hears me say: "make an incision from the end of the sternum as far as the two pubic bones, an incision which passes straight over the body of the animal," he will not understand what I mean. Rather he will follow and keep to my instructions. *There is no one who does not know that* when he sets his hand to making an incision, in the first place the skin only will be incised, and that beneath the skin there extends a covering which intervenes between it and what is subjacent to it.[112]

The first italicized assumption that he makes seems to be a fair one: that everyone – and the readers of *AA* in particular, given his previous emphasis on the importance of reading *On Bones* – will be familiar with the location of the sternum and the pubic bones, and therefore that they will be capable of following this clear direction. The second assumption, however, is not so obviously correct. Perhaps Galen is assuming that no reader *who has made it this far* in *AA* would be unaware of this fact, something that is sure to be the case given the number of incisions such a reader would have made at this point. But the sentiment that the details of how to cut into animal flesh are elementary would also be typical of a man who casually assumes that his readers frequently use chisels to excise vertebrae. One gets the sense either that, caught up in his world of daily anatomical investigation, Galen has lost his consistent sense of what is normal and what needs explanation or that his conception and awareness of his audience fluctuates from book to book and chapter to chapter, making him decide in the third book to describe the skinning process in detail though he thought it unnecessary in the two that preceded.

An outline emerges of the basic qualifications that Galen assumes of the audience of this text. The reader must be a literate Greek speaker, ideally one who progressed far enough in his basic studies to have attained at least an elementary mathematical education. Though some previous experience with anatomy via lectures or medical procedures would no doubt be helpful, Galen takes pains to arrange his instructions so that it is not strictly necessary. A reader who had attained at least a moderate level of education and who had followed Galen's instructions to read *On Bones* carefully before approaching *AA* should have been able to follow the

---

[112] *AA* S169; my emphasis.

complete course on anatomy with no previous medical or scientific train-ing.[113] These assumptions about the audience, then, are largely consistent with his vision of the targeted readers: A practicing physician would find few intellectual barriers here, nor would an amateur enthusiast be materi-ally excluded by lack of previous medical experience. The main excluding factor would rather have been financial.

Galen in general assumes that the majority of his readers can acquire all the various items that he himself can afford and has access to, though he does take some steps to prevent this assumption from necessarily punish-ing those who cannot. He suggests that the readers' tools all be made of finest steel, but he does acknowledge the variety in the marketplace; he assumes that his readers will do the majority of their dissections on mon-keys, a comparatively expensive species, but he gives alternatives for those who cannot get them; he mentions a variety of books and authors in pass-ing, but he limits the essential reading to only two additional books, both of them short; he describes elaborate vivisections using trained assistants, but does not require that the reader employ more than the occasional extra pair of hands. Even factoring in the lower cost options, however, the expenses involved would likely have skewed the readership away from the average medical practitioner or student. The social status of doctors in antiquity was highly variable, but only a small fraction would have been as financially secure as Galen.[114] In a revealing reminiscence about his stu-dent days in Pergamon, where he studied under several well-respected and well-pedigreed doctors whose pupils would have been set up to become successful physicians, Galen says:

> Several of my fellow students said to me, "you enjoy both an excellent nature and a marvelous education because of your father's ambition, and you are still in a stage of life suitable to learning, and you have the wealth necessary to provide leisure time for study; we, on the other hand, have a different lot. For we were untaught in our early childhood and not sharp-witted like you, and we have no money to squander."[115]

---

[113] Compare to Mansfeld (1994), 169–71, where he discusses the basic qualities Galen expects of the readers of his commentaries on Hippocrates, namely that they "at least have had a proper liberal education and be intelligent" (p. 171).

[114] For Galen's wealth, see Schlange-Schöningen (2003), 31–9 and Mattern (2013), 28–9; for a survey of the social and financial situations of doctors in this period, see Pleket (1995) and Nutton (2013*a*), 254–78.

[115] *MM* X.560–1 (οὐκ ὀλίγοι τῶν … συμφοιτητῶν ἔφασάν μοι, σὺ μὲν καὶ φύσει διαφερούσῃ κέχρησαι καὶ παιδείᾳ θαυμαστῇ διὰ τὴν τοῦ πατρός σου φιλοτιμίαν, καὶ ἡλικίαν δυναμένην μανθάνειν ἔχεις ὅθεν τε δαπανᾶν χρὴ σχολάζοντα μαθήμασι κέκτησαι· τὸ δ'ἡμέτερον οὐχ ὧδ' ἔχει· καὶ γὰρ ἀπαίδευτοι τὴν πρώτην παιδείαν ἐσμὲν καὶ οὐκ ὀξεῖς τὴν διάνοιαν ὥσπερ σὺ καὶ ἀναλίσκειν οὐκ ἔχομεν).

These classmates were fortunate enough to be pursuing their education in a place where in-person anatomical instruction was a readily accessible option, but it is surely the case that their less geographically fortunate peers would have viewed investing in an extensive course of anatomical self-study to be a squandering of money and – relatedly – of time that might be spent in more lucrative pursuits.

In short, the expenditure involved in following the course set out in *AA* would have deterred the humblest segment of the medical profession, as well as those just beginning to study medicine without the support of a wealthy family. It would also probably have discouraged the majority of the doctors located in the midrange of financial success, like Galen's Pergamene friends. While they might benefit from the comparatively low-cost observation of in-person instruction, perhaps bolstered, if they were particularly keen, by written memoranda like Galen's own minor anatomical works, the time and expenditures involved in the in-depth study of anatomy that Galen proposes in *AA* would likely have outweighed the expected practical utility. Some extra ambitious doctors from this category might have performed a modified version of the course – for example, using less expensive animals throughout, or choosing to dissect only those parts of the body most relevant to their practice – but, by and large, *AA* would have been most appealing to doctors and aspiring doctors who already had a degree of financial security and to the various well-educated, nonmedical readers that Galen envisions.

These financial considerations notwithstanding, Galen delivers on his promises. He has indeed produced a text suited to teach anyone with the wherewithal to engage with it, regardless of their ability to find a competent teacher. In a direct repudiation to the frustrations of his own anatomical education, in which good texts were scarce and teachers, though numerous, were scattered and secretive, he has consolidated, curated, and perfected the anatomical knowledge of his day and published it for all to read. Galen uses *Anatomical Procedures* to initiate his readers into the process of dissection rather than merely presenting them with his own version of anatomy, and in doing so he seeks to upend the status quo of anatomical practice and anatomical literature.

Conclusions

This book has charted the development of the practice of dissection and the overlapping practice of anatomical writing. It began in the Classical period, when dissection as a scientific methodology was in its infancy in the Greco-Roman world. Certainly, the dissection of animals for heuristic purposes did occur, both in medical and philosophical circles, but it was a niche practice, neither universally valued nor, in all likelihood, impinging noticeably on public attention. Anatomical literature of the period was concomitantly unfocused: Anatomy received little dedicated attention and, when it did, dissection was only one way of approaching its contents and not necessarily even the dominant one. In the Hellenistic period, dissection began to thrive. Aristotle's ambitious zoological program extended its reach in one direction, while his medical peers, like Diocles and Praxagoras, expanded it in another; Herophilus and Erasistratus took this momentum to the extreme and for the first time applied systematic dissection to human bodies. While there is no way of knowing how public all of this activity was, it was certainly publicized. Dedicated anatomical texts became the norm and their contents came to be familiar to a broad reading public. However, dissection was by no means the only methodology at play in the field of anatomical literature. Philosophical resistance to its cephalocentric findings promoted alternative avenues to anatomical knowledge on the one side, while the new Empiricist trend in medical thinking cast doubt on dissection's authority from the other. A fallow period ensued, from the end of the third century BC to the first century AD, which saw neither sustained dissective research nor noteworthy anatomical writing.

Under the aegis of the Roman Empire, perhaps encouraged by the different contours of a new social context, the dissection of animals reemerged in a new and vibrant way. Now a respectably ancient practice, dissection came to the fore as the dominant avenue to anatomical knowledge: Even those who still contested its use and doubted its epistemic efficacy could not afford to ignore it. Indeed, their anatomist peers did not allow them to ignore it, maneuvering a brashly performative breed of dissection into the fields of patient recruitment, medical credentialling, and even streetside debates. Anatomical literature exploded in tandem. Though only a small fraction survives, there is sufficient evidence to catch glimpses of an extensive and diverse library of anatomical texts, ranging from succinct handbooks to lengthy and sophisticated tracts on dedicated topics by a wide range of authors. In this period, Marinus attempted for the first time to fuse practice and text, creating a new, procedural genre of anatomical writing. Galen takes things a step further. He was content in his early career to rival his peers in performative ingenuity and to contribute to anatomical literature by producing texts of updated substance but traditional style. Soon enough, however, no longer satisfied with reaching only the geographically and temporally limited public of Rome with his dissections, he retooled Marinus' recently developed genre of anatomical procedures into an ambitious legacy. Far from jealously guarding his own discoveries and dissective techniques in the way many of his predecessors had done, he published every detail in the zealous hope of spreading knowledge of this science, which he deemed to be of the utmost interest and utility to everyone, doctor or not. Dissection, at the pinnacle of its development and popularity in the ancient world, was thus, thanks to Galen, poised to become a fundamental aspect of medical research and education. But things did not turn out that way at all.

CHAPTER 10

Epilogue – A Waxing and Waning Art

Truly, all those who followed [Galen]—in whose number I include
Oribasius, Theophilus, the Arabic authors, and those of our own era
whom I have yet been able to read (and I say this relying on their
kind indulgence)—if they have handed down anything at all worth
reading, they borrowed it from Galen. And, by Jove, to a careful dissector, they do not seem to have less appetite for anything than for
the dissection of the human body ... Indeed, they add at the front of
their books that their own writings are completely patched together
from Galen's opinions and that everything that is theirs, is Galen's ...
And they all put such faith in him that no doctor has been found who
believes that even the tiniest error has been apprehended, much less is
able to be apprehended, in Galen's anatomical writings.

Vesalius, *On the Fabric of the Human Body*[1]

Vesalius (1514–64) is engaging in unabashedly polemical rhetoric here, but
his thesis is not without justification. A striking feature in the history of
anatomy is the dearth of evidence for investigative dissections in the period
between Galen's death and Vesalius' birth, some thirteen hundred years
later.[2] In short, Galen's efforts to make *Anatomical Procedures* an accessible,
stand-alone guide to dissection do not seem to have found a receptive audience. In many ways, we appear to be dealing, on a far larger scale, with a

---

[1] Vesalius, *Fabrica* 3r–3v (qui vero ipsum sunt secuti, in quorum classem Oribasium, Theophilum,
Arabes, & nostros quotquot legere hactenus mihi licuit, recenseo (illorum bona dixerim venia)
omnes, si modo quid lectu dignum tradiderunt, ex Galeno id sunt mutuati, & per Iovem studiose
secanti, nihil unquam minus aggressi videntur, quam humani corporis sectionem ... imo librorum frontibus adiiciunt, ipsorum scripta e Galeni placitis penitus consarcinata, suaque Galeni esse
omnia.... Atque ita huic omnes fidem dedere, ut nullus repertus sit medicus, qui in Galeni anat-
omicis voluminibus, ne levissimum quidem lapsum unquam deprehensum esse, multoque minus
deprehendi posse, censuerit).

[2] Certainly, dissection did take place in this period and is especially well attested from the twelfth century
onwards; however, these dissections resulted in minimal change to the contents of Galenic anatomy, in
contrast to the boom in anatomical and physiological development that Vesalius ushers in.

phenomenon similar to the puzzling hiatus in significant anatomical activity after the groundbreaking work of Herophilus and Erasistratus. There
were certainly factors at play in that earlier peak and fallow period that are
not relevant in this later one, and there are many more vagaries of time and
space implicated in the later one than in the earlier. But there are two com-
monalities that I find instructive. The first is the ineluctable influence of the
political and social landscape. Just as the Alexandrian anatomists enjoyed
a supportive relationship with the Ptolemies, who both provided a nurtur-
ing environment for their research and actively facilitated it, Galen and his
peers inhabited a world of political stability whose ruling elite placed an
emphasis on intellectual attainment and philosophical inquiry.[3] Yet even
in Galen's lifetime the sands were shifting under his feet. In his later writings, he comments on the stress of life under Commodus, and he certainly
experienced the chaos of AD 193 and likely lived through the turbulent reign
of Caracalla.[4] The people of Rome came to have more pressing things to
discuss on street corners than the thoracic nerves of the pig.

The second factor is, as Vesalius suggests, the tyranny of authority.
Although it has long been a puzzle that Galen, unlike Herophilus and
Erasistratus, did not have a school of followers to further his intellectual legacy, his texts still managed to dominate the field.[5] So persuasive
is Galen's self-promotion as the best anatomist of all time that it seems to
have eclipsed his encouragements to his readers to add to and refine his
vision of the body with dissections of their own. Just as the Herophileans
and Erasistrateans were largely content to rest on their teachers' laurels, it
would be easy for Galen's readers to assume – as Vesalius accuses them all
of doing – that his exemplary work had found all that there was to find,
rendering further research an unnecessary hassle. After all, it was Galen
himself who assured his less ambitious readers that, by putting their faith
in his superior intelligence and experience, they would be able to acquire
correct opinions from his writings without putting in any extra work on
their own.[6]

Yet the waning of anatomical interest and the dominance of Galenism
were certainly neither immediate nor complete. Vesalius is not an unbiased

---

[3] On the support of the Ptolemies and the possible political factors for its withdrawal, see von Staden
(1992a), 231–7, and the bibliography at Chapter 2, n. 118.
[4] On Commodus, see *Indol.* 54–7 (Boudon-Milot et al [2010]), and Nutton (2013b), 49–50. On the
date of Galen's death, see Boudon-Millot (2012), 241–4, Mattern (2013), 274, and Nutton (2020), 39.
[5] On the absence of a Galenic school, see Boudon-Millot (2008).
[6] Galen, *Ord.Lib.Prop.* XIX.53–4. In this case, he is specifically excusing these readers from the study
of logic.

guide. He is defending and promoting his own careful reading and enactment of Galen's instructions in *Anatomical Procedures*: having meticulously approached the text in the spirit that Galen envisioned but on the new medium of the human body, he had uncovered errors and oversights whose presence he has to justify to his militantly Galenic peers.[7] He is therefore painting the history of anatomical study with a distinctly biased brush and in the light of his own contemporary situation. The path that led from Galen's anatomical world to his is far longer and more winding than Vesalius implies, and the task of tracing its course is beyond the scope of this book. But to stop at the pinnacle of ancient dissective activity as if at a precipice does not seem a satisfying conclusion. I will therefore tread lightly (and I do not claim comprehensively) into the murky waters of anatomical study in Late Antiquity and see what became of Galen's legacy – and Marinus' and Quintus' and that of all his teachers and sources – in the centuries after his death.

Hardly anything of relevance survives from the third century, but in the fourth century we can catch glimpses of anatomical study. The most controversial glimpse is a fresco found among the extensive decorative program of a Christian catacomb under the Via Latina in Rome (Figure 10.1). The painting, which is in the company of dozens of scenes from the Old Testament, the New Testament, and pagan mythology, depicts a large group of men clothed in white and seated in front of and above a nude figure lying recumbent on the ground with a dark spot, perhaps a gaping wound, on his abdomen. The central seated figure, who is noticeably larger and the only one of the company to be bare-chested, appears to be in charge of the scene, while another figure, seated two places to his left, points at the chest of the naked body, to a place slightly above the dark spot, with a long, slender stick. The remainder of the seated men are in active conversation, gesturing to each other and to the body before them. The nude figure is markedly smaller than the seated ones; his eyes seem to be open, though he could well be dead. His arms rest at his sides, but his feet are arranged in a position evocative of crucifixion. Interpretations of this fresco have been numerous and diverse. Some see a resurrection scene, while others see a surgical one; some cast the largest figure as God, others as Aristotle.[8] One popular interpretation, transposed backwards from the

---

[7] On Vesalius' relationship to Galen, see Cunningham (1997), 88–142, and Salas (2020), 265–84.

[8] For the many different interpretations, beyond even these, see Proskauer (1958), Boyancé (1964), de Bruyne (1969–70), Fink (1976), Kötzsche-Breitenbruch (1976), 45, n. 265, Hillert (1990), 232–4, Scortecci (2000), and the diverse bibliographies in each.

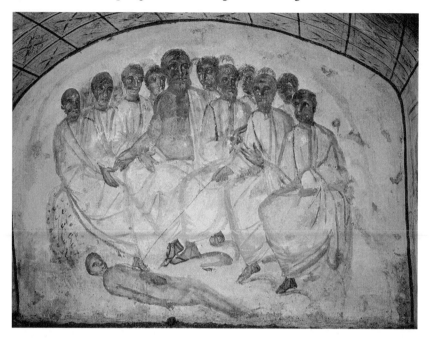

Figure 10.1   Fresco, Rome, hypogeum of Via Dino Compagni (Cubiculum Id), fourth
century AD. Image: © Album / Alamy Stock Photo.

educational practices of the fifteenth century, is that this a depiction of a
contemporary anatomy lesson: The central figure is the lecturing doctor,
while the man with the wand is the fourth-century equivalent of a medieval *ostensor*, pointing out the organs under discussion to the students.[9]
To me it seems much more probable, given the myth-historical settings
of the rest of the decorative program, that the scene depicts an idealized
lesson of the past, featuring some preeminent philosophical or medical
authority in the act of teaching.[10] It seems most plausible that the subject
of this lecture is a broad philosophical topic related to mortality or the
soul, but an ancient anatomical lesson is not impossible, especially given
that we have several examples of people from the first through fourth centuries AD who conceive of human dissection as a standard practice of "the

---

[9] This is the thesis of Proskauer (1958).
[10] This is also the general interpretation of Boyancé (1964) (who nominates Aristotle specifically), de
Bruyne (1969–70) (who prefers Socrates), and Gaiser (1980), 18–21 (who names Empedocles). It
is also certainly possible that the fresco has a religious meaning; Scortecci (2000) offers one of the
more persuasive solutions along these lines, arguing that it is a Creation scene.

ancients."[11] Though I do not think that we can learn anything about the practice of dissection in the fourth century here, it is certainly suggestive that the mind behind this fresco thought that this scene of anatomical contemplation – whether current or idealized, religious or secular – was a subject worthy of as much space as Christ's resurrection of Lazarus, Moses' parting of the red sea, or Hercules' rescue of Alcestis.

The textual evidence for dissection in this period is less fraught, but still not terribly enlightening. We learn from Eunapius (b. *c.* AD 345) that the fourth-century physician Ionicus of Sardis "was knowledgeable to the utmost about the parts of the body and fit to enquire into the nature of man."[12] This is certainly an indication that a knowledge of anatomy was considered laudable, if not necessarily proof of any personal acquaintance with dissection. Some of Ionicus' fourth-century peers evince similar interest, though, again, any evidence of actual anatomical investigations is lacking. Vindicianus (*fl. c.* AD 380) produced a small work on anatomy containing a brief description of all of the major parts of the body from head to toe, which became a popular anatomical text in the Middle Ages in the West.[13] In its preface, he says that "it was permitted for the older authorities, that is, for our antecedents practicing medicine in Alexandria … to dissect the dead in order to know how and from what they died, but it is not permitted for us to do this, because it is prohibited"; he offers no awareness of animal dissection as a possible alternative and says that he has collected all of his material from "Greek books."[14] Vindicianus'

---

[11] Rufus, *Nom.Part.* 10; Augustine, *De civ. Dei* 22.24; Vindicianus, *Gyn.* praef.; compare Galen's insistence that Hippocrates was a practiced dissector (see Chapter 6, "The Hippocratic Corpus" at pp. 177–9, especially n. 40 for the possibility that this conception included him using human subjects). I would also put in this company a passage from ps.-Eustathius (*Comm.Hex.* PG 18.788) that claims that "the best physicians" (οἱ ἄριστοι τῶν ἰατρῶν) dissect executed criminals; Bliquez and Kazhdan (1984) see it as evidence for fourth-century human dissection, but it maps onto the popular narrative about the ancients – assuredly the "best of the physicians" – so patly as to make that seem the likelier interpretation. The nude, like Rufus' slave, could also be a live model of external anatomy.

[12] Eunapius, *VS* 22.1.2 (τῶν τε τοῦ σώματος μορίων ἄκρως δαημονέστερος γενόμενος, καὶ τῆς ἀνθρωπίνης φύσεως ἐξεταστικός).

[13] This text, known misleadingly as the *Gynaecia*, survives through multiple manuscripts, belonging to two markedly divergent families; see Cilliers (2005) for the history of the text and an edition and translation, with commentary, of one exemplar. On the popularity of the text, see Langslow (2000), 64–5.

[14] There are several different versions of the preface, each containing different – but all to some degree imaginative – lists of "Alexandrians"; for different versions, see Vásquez Buján (1982), 32, von Staden (1989), 52, 60, 189, and Cilliers (2005), 166. The version of the preface that I translate here is from the edition in Cilliers (2005) (maioribus enim auctoribus, hoc est prioribus in Alexandria agentibus medicinam … licuit mortuos exenterare ut scirent unde vel quomodo morerentur. Sed hoc nobis facere iam non licet quia prohibitum est), except for the reference to "Greek books" (libris grecis), which occurs in a different manuscript (see Vásquez Buján [1982], 32).

contemporary to the East, the physician Posidonius of Byzantium (*fl.* late fourth century AD), engages with the anatomy of rational thought and reports a newly developed version of Galen's theory of the locations in the brain of the various functions of the rational soul, though this appears to be a theoretically rather than experimentally motivated change.[15] Nemesius of Emesa (*fl. c.* AD 400), too, offers sophisticated anatomical and physiological insights in his *Nature of Man*, drawing directly on Galen, whom he cites and quotes repeatedly in the text.[16]

Although *Anatomical Procedures* is not among the treatises that Nemesius references, it still held a position as an important anatomical text. Even in nonmedical circles its title resonated as that of an ultimate authority. A treatise attributed to Gregory of Nyssa, which laments the pervasive ignorance of the general public about their own internal structures, urges its audience to familiarize themselves with the many things that doctors have discovered about the human body "in their anatomical procedures," and chides them not to "despise the wonders inside [them]."[17] Though the author's pessimism implies that anatomy is not a booming field of study, his unusual phrasing is surely a direct allusion to Galen's *Anatomical Procedures*, whether or not he had actually read its contents.[18] On the medical side, its importance was secure. Oribasius (*c.* AD 320–*c.* 400), whose extensive compilations of passages from medical authors were widely popular in Late Antiquity, excerpts generously from *Anatomical Procedures* in the two chapters of his *Medical Collections* devoted to anatomy.[19] His organization and choice of selections, however, provide some of the most telling evidence for attitudes toward dissection in the fourth century. He has pieced together passages from across Galen into a traditional head-to-toe description of the body, running down the gamut of the internal organs in Book XXIV, from brain to genitals, and doing the same for the bones and

---

[15] Quoted in Aetius, VI.2 (125 Oliveri); see Rocca (2003), 245–7 for the development of this idea.

[16] For Nemesius' relationship to Galen, including a list of citations and allusions, see Sharples and van der Eijk (2008), 11–14, 20–1, 23–5.

[17] Gregory of Nyssa [*Sp.*], *Creat.Hom.Serm.Prim.* 4 (ἐν ταῖς ἀνατομικαῖς ἐγχειρήσεσιν ... μὴ καταφρόνει τοῦ ἐν σοὶ θαύματος).

[18] The pairing of the words ἀνατομικός and ἐγχείρησις is extremely rare outside Galen, making it likely that this is a direct allusion. Aside from this instance, its only other occurrences are in the passages of Stephanus of Athens and Theophilus Protospatharius discussed later in this chapter (pp. 357–8), both references to Galen's text, and in two twelfth-century medical authors: Michael Italicus, who deploys it abstractly, but within three lines of mentioning Galen's name (see this chapter, n. 43), and Joannes Bishop of Prisdrianon, who uses it to describe the human dissections of the ancients (including Galen) from which he believes all anatomical wisdom derives (*Ur.* 365).

[19] Oribasius, *Coll.Med.* XXIV–XXV.

musculature in Book XXV.[20] He is interested only in the anatomical facts and strips away instructions for dissection as inessential, removing all sense that anatomy is an art that should be practiced rather than memorized. Galenic anatomy has become static in Oribasius' hands: Galen is, for him, a calcified authority, and the convenience and popularity of Oribasius' work would only serve to keep him so.

Nevertheless, Galenic anatomy was not universally the standard in this period. Vindicianus, as we have seen, positions the "Alexandrians" as the ultimate authorities in the preface to his anatomical text – including in that group a generous variety of figures, from Hippocrates to Lycus and Pelops – and does not mention Galen at all.[21] Nemesius, though reliant on a distinctly Galenic understanding of the brain and nervous system, chooses, in his brief chapter devoted to an overview of the structure of the body, to refer readers seeking more information to Aristotle, not Galen.[22] Outside of medicine and philosophy, Ammianus Marcellinus (*c.* AD 330–95), the historian, hearkens all the way back to Democritus for his paradigmatic dissector, while Macrobius (*fl. c.* AD 400) includes in his Saturnalian dialogue a physician who has reportedly "studied [the layout of the body] even more than [the art of] medicine requires" and who claims to have "consulted the books of the anatomists," but has him offer up some highly dubious anatomy, stemming (on the most charitable interpretation) from a cardiocentric tradition.[23] Certainly, cardiocentric anatomy was still alive and well.[24] The Anonymous Brussels manuscript (*c.* fifth century AD) offers

---

[20] There is also a brief section on the nerves, arteries, and veins at the very end of Book XXV. Raeder indicates the Galenic sources for all of these passages in his edition for the *CMG* (VI.2.1), and Garofalo (1991*b*) italicizes all the sections excerpted by Oribasius in his translation of *AA*. Extracts from *AA* pervade these two books, but *UP* and the minor anatomical works are more dominant, further indicating that Oribasius is interested only in descriptive anatomy. Though the vast majority of text in these two books is Galenic, Oribasius does also include one selection from Rufus (XXV.1), one from Soranus (XXIV.31), and one from Lycus (XXIV.32).

[21] See this chapter, n. 14. Cilliers (2019), 126–7 argues that Galen, owing to his prolixity, was less popular with Vindicianus and the other Latin medical authors of North Africa than he was in the Greek-speaking East.

[22] Nemesius, *Nat.Hom.* 4.46.

[23] Ammianus Marcellinus, XXVIII.4.34, recalling the Hellenistic story about Democritus discussed in Chapter 2, "The 'Pre-Socratics'" at p. 13. Macrobius, *Sat.* VII.13.7–8 (doctrinam et ultra quam medicina postulat consecutus; libris anatomicorum … consultis) on the presence of a nerve stretching directly from the heart to the ring finger; cf. Gellius, *NA* X.10 for the same claim, attributed there to the Egyptians.

[24] Indeed, because of the influential ancient names who supported it, the heart would continue to rival the brain as the dominant organ of the body for centuries to come, including in the enormously popular work of Ibn Sina (Avicenna), who melded Galenic and Aristotelian models to create his own vision of the body. On the long legacy of Aristotelian anatomy, see Cunningham (1997), especially 167–87, and Fancy (2013), especially 69–95.

an account that acknowledges the role of the brain in perception and intelligence, but makes it firmly subordinate to an anthropomorphized heart, which provides the brain with the blood and heat necessary to do its work and which "is always vigilantly listening and understanding" with its little ears (auricles, the term for the cardiac atria).[25] Gregory of Nyssa (c. AD 330–95) is aware of these divergent traditions and weighs the relative merits of scientific and philosophical arguments on the question of the ruling organ before deciding on his own third way.[26] He paints the cephalocentrists as "devoting their time to anatomical study," but is equally happy to engage with the arguments of the cardiocentrists, who do not: Knowledge of the body and its workings is not, for Gregory, exclusively dependent on dissection.[27] Indeed, in the final chapter of his *Making of Man*, where he provides a summary of the constitution and function of the body, he says that he is basing himself on the written works of those who have studied such things, "some of whom learned how the things in us are situated through dissection, while others considered and described for what reason all the parts of the body came about."[28] Though the dissections practiced by Galen and his ilk are certainly important, the logical inferences employed by their anatomical rivals still have their place as well.

By the time we come to the fifth and sixth centuries, Galen squarely dominates medical education, but his emphasis on anatomy and dissection has not translated.[29] Arabic sources provide a retrospective view of the medical curriculum in Alexandria in this period: both Hunayn ibn Ishaq and Ibn Ridwan describe a set sequence of Galenic books that formed the foundation of medical lectures and exegesis there.[30] Anatomy is represented only by the minor anatomical works – *On Bones, On the*

---

[25] Anonymous of Brussels, 44 (semper vigilante, audiente et intelligente); cf. 17. On this text and its history in scholarship, see Debru (1996) and (1999), 453–6.

[26] For an analysis of Gregory's own solution and its relationship to his Greco-Roman sources, see Wessel (2009). On Gregory's engagement with anatomy more broadly, see Drobner (1996), 49–67.

[27] Gregory of Nyssa, *Op.Hom.* 12 (PG 44.156–64), with quoted text at PG 44.157 (τῶν ταῖς ἀνατομικαῖς θεωρίαις ἐσχολακότων).

[28] Gregory of Nyssa, *Op.Hom.* 30 (PG 44.240) (ὧν οἱ μὲν ὅπως ἔχει θέσεως τὰ καθέκαστον τῶν ἐν ἡμῖν, διὰ τῆς ἀνατομῆς ἐδιδάχθησαν· οἱ δὲ καὶ πρὸς ὅ τι γέγονε πάντα τὰ τοῦ σώματος μόρια κατενόησάν τε καὶ διηγήσαντο). Ultimately, he does describe a system in which the brain controls the nerves and thus sensation and voluntary action (*Op.Hom.* 30 [PG 44.244]), but his discussions of respiration and nutrition are based on a hybrid Aristotelian/Platonic model rather than a Galenic one (*Op.Hom.* 30 [PG 44.247–9]).

[29] Indeed, Fulgentius (late fifth or sixth century AD) refers to the doctors of Alexandria as "Galen's tribe" (*Galeni curia*) (*Myth.* I. praef).

[30] Hunayn ibn Ishaq, *Risala* 23 (Lamoreaux ([2016], 38–41) and Ibn Ridwan, *Useful Book on the Quality of Medical Education* (for the relevant passages see Iskandar [1976], 248–56; Garofalo (2019) offers a recent discussion of the Alexandrian school, with bibliography.

Dissection of the Muscles, On the Dissection of the Veins and Arteries, and *On the Dissection of the Nerves* – and *On the Usefulness of the Parts* does not appear either. In other words, the most potent of Galen's urgings towards dissection are absent. There continued to be some who studied the more advanced works. For example, Stephanus of Athens (late sixth–early seventh century AD), who lived and taught in Alexandria, references *Anatomical Procedures* and may even have written a commentary on it.[31] Indeed, he may have carried out his own dissections in addition to his exegetical work. He refutes the physiological opinion of an unknown predecessor on the reasons for whitened urine by appealing to dissection: "[Angeleuas' argument] requires certain discoveries that are not apparent *to us* in dissection. For no vessel connected from the glands to the bladder is apparent."[32] It is possible that Stephanus is simply getting his data here from Galen, but the more straightforward interpretation is that he has checked for himself.[33] Generally, though, there is minimal interest in engaging with anatomy and dissection, even in texts where one might expect it. Paul of Aegina (*fl.* seventh century AD), for one, despite a marked interest and skill in surgery, does not include any discussion of anatomy in his *Epitome of Medicine*.[34]

At this point my narrative must mimic the political schisms of late antiquity and split to the East and West. In the East, evidence for interest in

---

[31] Stephanus may be referencing such a commentary at *Comm.Hipp.Aph.* I.1 (*CMG* XI.1.3.1, p. 36), but no other trace survives. Agnellus of Ravenna (late sixth or seventh century AD) also offers a very Galenic discussion of the purposes of dissection and vivisection; his description of the circumstances in which dissection and vivisection can be performed, however, are medical or historical, and he shows no awareness of animal dissection as a methodology; see Westerink et al. (1981), 86–8. In addition to this continued engagement with Galenic anatomy, Garofalo (2019), 71–3 discusses some instances of anatomy derived from sources other than Galen that appear (for better or for worse) in Alexandrian scholarship of this period.

[32] Stephanus, *Comm.Gal.MMG* 20 (εὕρημά τι ζητεῖ παρ' ἡμῶν ἐν ταῖς ἀνατομαῖς μὴ φαινόμενον. οὐδὲ γὰρ φαίνεται κοινὰ τοῖς βουβῶσιν ἀγγεῖα πρὸς τὴν κύστιν); my emphasis; see Dickson (1998), 76–7 for text and comments.

[33] Stephanus also appeals to dissection at *Comm.Hipp.Aph.* IV.33 (*CMG* XI.1.3.2, p. 296), V.69–70, 72, VI.36, 52 (*CMG* XI.1.3.3, pp. 182–4, 188, 246, 266), but the phrasing in those instances, as well as the close parallels where the context is explicitly textual (*Comm.Hipp.Aph.* II.53 [εἴρηται], V.46 [τὰ εἰρημένα], 63 [a reference to *Ven.Art.Diss.*]), suggest that they are all references to Galen's anatomical texts rather than to Stephanus' own dissections. It is therefore possible that the reference in *Comm.Gal.MMG* is also textual, but the phrasing is sufficiently different to merit more serious consideration. Scarborough (2010), 249 believes that Stephanus' surgical instructions themselves imply familiarity with dissection.

[34] On Paul of Aegina and Byzantine surgical knowledge more generally, see Bliquez (1984) and Scarborough (2010). While the lack of an anatomical section does not preclude Paul himself from having had some experience with anatomy, it certainly indicates that he does not find it a practical necessity for his audience.

anatomy in the final centuries of the millennium is sparse but compelling. Meletius (*c.* ninth century AD) authors a religiously slanted *Constitution of Man* drawing on the work of earlier authors, both ancient and more recent; the text discusses anatomy and physiology, including etymologies for the names of the parts of the body, and was widely popular, inspiring abundant copies as well as an epitome soon after its appearance.[35] Theophilus Protospatharius, a Byzantine physician who likely dates to the late ninth or tenth century, seems to have been more hands-on than Meletius.[36] It is highly probable that he was dissecting animals; certainly, he was engaging closely with Galen's anatomical works. His text *On the Fabric of the Human Body* is closely modeled on – is, in fact, almost an epitome of – Galen's *Usefulness of the Parts*, and in it he also references multiple other Galenic texts, including *Anatomical Procedures* and the now lost *On the Dissection of the Dead*.[37] Despite his often word-for-word reliance on *Usefulness of the Parts*, his rhetoric surrounding dissection seems indebted but not derivative: He picks up from Galen the importance of practicing dissection, but he also seems to have acted on Galen's advice and to be advocating on his own authority that his readers do so too.[38] He indicates that some things should be learned from dissection itself and, in one passage, he even describes how to approach dissecting the brain.[39] There are two particularly striking moments. In the first, he says, "whoever wishes to fully understand, let him dissect or visit those who dissect"; the suggestion that a reader should attend a dissection performed by someone else is Galenic, certainly, but one that Theophilus presents as a feasible reality.[40] In the second, he urges his readers, "whoever wishes to be able to distinguish these sorts of ligaments, muscles, and tendons, let him dissect monkeys, if he has them; and if monkeys are not available, bears; and, if

---

[35] On Meletius, including his sources and the difficulties of his date, see Renehan (1984), Erismann (2017), especially p. 38, n. 1, and Bouras-Vallianatos (2019), 89–91, who also reports that there are some sixty extant witnesses to the text, indicating its wide dissemination. The epitome is the work of Leo the Physician (*c.* ninth century AD) and is also extant (*CMG* X.4); see Gielen (2018).

[36] On Theophilus' date, see Grimm-Stadelmann (2008), 36–42.

[37] Theophilus Protospatharius, *Corp.Hum.Fab.* I.9 for *AA* (and also *Mot.Musc.* and *PHP*) and V.4 for *Diss.Mort.* (in a passage transmitted in only one manuscript; see Grimm-Stadelmann [2008], 262). See Grimm-Stadelmann (2008), 43–7 for the text's relationship to *UP*; her edition and translation also italicize the direct verbal echoes.

[38] Indeed, Grimm-Stadelmann (2008) did not find parallels for any of the injunctions relating to dissection.

[39] Things to be learned from dissection at *Corp.Hum.Fab.* I.11–12, III.17; somewhat generic directions for dissection at IV.10.

[40] *Corp.Hum.Fab.* III.21 (ὅστις ἂν ἐθέλοι καταμαθεῖν, ἀνατεμνέτω ἢ φοιτάτω πρὸς ἀνατομικούς).

even these are absent, whatever animals he can find; at any event, let him dissect."[41] The insistence of the appeal and the emphasis on bears – an animal that Galen uses but rarely and that, unlike the monkey, is endemic to the region around Constantinople – suggest to me that Theophilus is speaking from experience.[42]

A few centuries later, this anatomical interest persists. Michael Italicus' eulogy of Michael Pantechnes (*fl.* AD 1118) mentions his skill in anatomy, though it is somewhat ambiguous there whether the research referred to was practical or textual.[43] Michael Choniates (AD 1138–*c.* 1222), however, offers engaging confirmation that Theophilus' anatomical interests were not unique, nor restricted only to medical circles. In one of his letters, he sends greetings to a doctor whose acquaintance he has made and whose exemplary learning has impressed him greatly. Michael hopes to welcome him for a visit soon, so that they can study some books in the doctor's possession, namely Galen's "*On the Method of Dissection*" and *On the Doctrines of Hippocrates and Plato* and Aristotle's *Parts of Animals*, and engage in dissections together to learn the wonders of God and philosophy through nature.[44] He promises that he will have "not just an abundance of leisure time, but also of animals to dissect – I do not mean *satyruses*, nor baboons,

---

[41] *Corp.Hum.Fab.* V.11 (ὅστις δὲ θέλει διαγνωστικὸς εἶναι τῶν τοιούτων συνδέσμων, μυῶν τε καὶ τενόντων, ἀνατεμνέτω, εἰ μὲν εὐπορεῖ, πιθήκους· εἰ δὲ μὴ πάρεισι πίθηκοι, ἄρκτους· εἰ δὲ ἀπορεῖ καὶ τούτων, ἐν τοῖς τυχοῦσι ζώοις· πάντως δὲ ἀνατεμνέτω); cf. V.4 where the version in one manuscript includes the line, "let whoever wishes to know these things exactly dissect many things and often" (ὅστις αὐτοὺς ἀκριβῶς θέλει γνῶναι, ἀνατεμνέτω πολλὰ καὶ πολλάκις).

[42] Galen does rank bears and other carnivores immediately after monkeys in his lists of the classes of animals that resemble humans (*AA* II.430, 535, 545, 548), but, in his practical instructions, he uses goats, pigs, and oxen as his primary alternatives to monkeys and never actually singles out a bear as the subject of a procedure; he mentions their features only a handful of times in the texts Theophilus is referencing (*AA* II.495; *UP* IV.161, 288 [II.298, 394H]).

[43] Michael Italicus, *Or.* 9, 114 (Gautier), where he says of Pantechnes, "oh, how great he was in anatomical procedures" (ὢ πόσος μὲν ἦν εἰς ἀνατομικὰς ἐγχειρήσεις); in the subsequent sentences, however, he describes Pantechnes as rivaling Galen specifically in his studies of the soul, not anatomy, and emphasizes his extensive scholarship and devotion to uncovering little-known texts of the ancients. It would therefore be tenable to argue that Pantechnes had only an academic familiarity with *Anatomical Procedures*, but I am content to credit him with actual anatomical experience. Stathakopoulos (2019), 149 however, is skeptical of the depth of Italicus' Galenic allusions and questions his or even Pantechnes' familiarity with *AA*. Browning (1985), 520 suggests that this passage is evidence for human dissection, but his only reason for assuming human rather than animal subjects is the implicit reference to *AA*, which "recommends the use of human cadavers" – a wildly misleading characterization that does not offer sufficient grounds for this claim.

[44] Michael Choniates, *Epist.* 102.12 (Περὶ μεθόδων ἀνατομικῶν). The fact that he has got the name of *AA* wrong is very interesting, but the title he provides, as well as the specific animals he names (see the following note), suggest that he is indeed familiar with the character and contents of the text we know.

nor monkeys, nor even bears"; he explains how difficult all of these animals are to procure where he lives – "even the last [i.e. bears]" – but proposes to have pigs ready and waiting to be dissected should his new friend come to visit.[45] The reference to the *satyrus* – a term that Galen uses in a highly unusual way to refer to a specific type of monkey – confirms that Michael is indeed acquainted with the contents of *Anatomical Procedures*, while the insistence on bears recalls Theophilus' instructions and suggests that they may have been local dissectors' animal of choice. The Byzantine world thus provides the best evidence so far for *Anatomical Procedures* guiding precisely the type of dissections that Galen hoped it would foster, nearly a millennium after he wrote it.

In addition to this evidence for work on animals, we must consider whether human dissection had become a more viable option in Byzantium in this period. Bliquez and Kazhdan have collected three references, made in passing by nonmedical writers of the eighth to twelfth centuries, which lead them to conclude that human dissection was a consistent and approved practice in the East.[46] The earliest reference, though somewhat sensational, is straightforward. Theophanes the Confessor (*c.* AD 759/60–817/18) records in his *Chronicles* that in the year AD 763/4 a taskforce of the emperor arrested a Christian apostate, cut off his arms and legs, and then, with the cooperation of some doctors, "dissected him alive from his genitals to his chest in order to understand the construction of man" before burning him.[47] Less lurid but also less convincing is the reference in Symeon the Theologian (AD 949?–1022). In discussing the dispassionate observation of shameful human emotions and the search for their origins and cures, he compares the process to that practiced by doctors: "exactly as we hear that doctors also proceed and as we have heard about the ancients. For they dissected the dead in order to understand the arrangement of the body, so that they might learn from these [the dead]

---

[45] Michael Choniates, *Epist.* 102.13 (οὐ σχολῆς μόνον ἡμῖν ἀφθονία, ἀλλὰ καὶ ζῴων τῶν ἀνατμηθησομένων, οὐ Σατύρων, λέγω, οὐ κυνοκεφάλων, οὐ πιθήκων, ἀλλ᾽οὐδὲ ἄρκτων. καὶ αὐταί...). The use of the term *satyrus* in reference to a monkey is very unusual and has clearly stumped someone in the chain of transmission of this text, leading to its persistent capitalization; Galen uses it at *AA* II.430, but it also appears at Aelian, *NA* 16.21, where it is described as an exotic Indian animal (cf. Pausanius, I.23.6).

[46] Bliquez and Kazhdan (1984). I do not find the fourth passage that they include, a reference to human dissection in the fourth-century ps.-Eustathius, *Comm.Hex.* PG 18.788, to be convincing, as I discussed in this chapter at n. 11.

[47] Theophanes Confessor, *Chron.* 436 (τοῦτον ἀνέτεμον ζῶντα ἀπὸ ἥβης ἕως τοῦ θώρακος πρὸς τὸ κατανοῆσαι τὴν τοῦ ἀνθρώπου κατασκευήν).

what is inside of living humans."[48] The phrasing of this passage makes it problematic as evidence for eleventh-century human dissection rather than just for dissection on the part of the ancients.[49] The final instance has more potential. George Tornikios (*c.* AD 1110–1156/7), in his eulogy for the emperor's daughter, describes her perspicacity as similar to that of "wise doctors, who, with certain wonderous and well-suited instruments of their art, dissect and analyze the bodies of humans in an analysis more horrifying than the syllogism, and lay bare each part from its neighbor in order to show its position and shape and structure."[50] While we are again dealing with the trope of the superior, dissecting doctor, which is often deployed nostalgically, George's use of the present tense and his more detailed descriptions, including the remark about the tools, suggest that he is describing something current, albeit "horrifying." The evidence from Theophilus and Michael Choniates indicates that animals remained standard subjects of dissection, but I think it would be hasty to completely rule out the idea that the doctors of Constantinople in these centuries could occasionally receive permission to dissect human bodies, as in the punitive example from Theophanes. It is, after all, within a few generations of George Tornikios that human dissection enters the mainstream in the West, this time to remain there.[51]

---

[48] Symeon Neotheologus, *Or.Eth.* 6.1.269–74 (καθὰ καὶ ἰατροὺς ποιοῦντας ἀκούομεν καὶ περὶ τῶν παλαιῶν ἀκηκόαμεν. ἀνέτεμον γὰρ τοὺς νεκρούς, ἵνα τὴν θέσιν κατανοήσωσι τοῦ σώματος, ὅπως ἐξ ἐκείνων γινώσκοντες ὦσι τῶν ζώντων ἀνθρώπων τὰ ἔνδοθεν).

[49] I see two reasons for skepticism. First, there is a deliberate grammatical break between the contemporary doctors and the ancient ones, and the aorist verb that follows ("they dissected") most reasonably refers only to the latter: We thus have modern doctors on the one hand, who dispassionately assess causation and treatment, and ancient doctors on the other, about whose activities Symeon has heard another interesting thing, namely that they practiced dissection. Second, he does not clarify the species of the "dead" being dissected, except to contrast them with "living *humans*"; thus, even if one wanted to conflate the two groups of doctors and argue that this is proof for contemporary dissection, one would still be short of proving contemporary *human* dissection, especially since the need to specify that the living beneficiaries are human – coupled with the evidence given earlier for animal dissection as a known practice in this period – rather suggests that the dead subjects were not. It would surely be more noteworthy that humans were being dissected than that human welfare was the goal.

[50] George Tornices, *Or.* 14, p. 225 (Darrouzès) (κατὰ τοὺς σοφοὺς τῶν ἰατρῶν οἵ, θαυμασίοις τισὶ καὶ εὐφυέσιν ὀργάνοις τῆς τέχνης τὰ τῶν ἀνθρώπων ἀνατέμνοντες ἢ ἀναλύοντες σώματα ἀνάλυσιν τῆς τῶν συλλογισμῶν φρικωδεστέραν, ἕκαστον μέλος ἀπογυμνοῦσι τοῦ γείτονος, ἵνα καὶ θέσιν αὐτοῦ καὶ σχῆμα καὶ σύστασιν παραστήσαιεν).

[51] Mondino de' Liuzzi (Mundinus) introduced the dissection of human bodies to the medical school curriculum in Bologna at some point during the first decades of the fourteenth century; see Cunningham (1997), 42–54, and French (1999), 35–54. Dissections unrelated to medical education, namely for legal postmortem analysis and religious embalming, are attested already in the late thirteenth century; see French (1999), 34 and Park (2010), 39–76.

From the eighth to the eleventh centuries, however, the West shows no interest.[52] I am not aware of any indications of anatomical study there, let alone of dissection, until the turn of the twelfth century, when the physicians in Salernum, freshly energized by the possession of newly translated Arabic texts, begin dissecting pigs.[53] Indeed, it is the pivotal work of Hunayn ibn Ishaq (d. AD 873) and his peers and successors that moves the history of anatomy and dissection forward. Hunayn, a Nestorian Christian from al-Hirah, was at the heart of the translation movement in Baghdad in the mid-ninth century, during which an enormous number of Greek scientific and philosophical texts were collected and translated into Arabic under the patronage of eager caliphs and courtiers.[54] He has access to many of Galen's ancillary works on anatomy that do not survive to the present day. In fact, the only ones that were lost by his time were some of the texts excerpting or reacting to other anatomists, namely Galen's summary of Marinus and all of his work related to Lycus: another indication that Galen's authority excluded interest in other voices.[55] A complete copy of *Anatomical Procedures* was also in circulation – a boon to modern scholarship, which relies on the Arabic tradition for the final six and a half books, now lost in Greek – and its translation into Syriac and then Arabic made Galen's knowledge of anatomy available to whole new audiences.[56] Though these audiences were voraciously and productively

---

[52] Vivian Nutton suggested to me that this stark split between the situation in the East and that in the West is indicative that even in antiquity anatomy was, essentially, a Greek concern – in other words, that, while Romans in multicultural centers (like Rome) or with multicultural educations (like Apuleius) engaged with dissection and anatomical debates, Roman doctors with less of an affiliation to Greek influences may well have operated with different educational and professional norms. I think that this must surely be to some extent true, especially given the patterns in Late Antiquity, both as discussed here and in n. 21 to this chapter. However, as I argue throughout and particularly in Chapter 5, I do think that it is nevertheless the case that the thriving of anatomical activities, both written and performative, in the first two centuries AD was not solely a Greek, but rather a distinctly Greco-Roman phenomenon. Though its entrenchment in the Greek language does seem to have impeded its lasting impact on the Latin-speaking world, the Roman context within which Galen and his immediate forerunners were working was an important factor in the development of anatomical study.

[53] Corner (1927), 19–30 discusses three small Salernian anatomical texts, which he dates to the first half of the twelfth century, each of which is written to accompany the dissection of a pig; he also provides a translation of one and an edition and translation of another (48–66).

[54] On the translation movement, see Gutas (1998); on Hunayn specifically, see Lamoreaux (2016), xii–xviii.

[55] Hunayn describes his inability to find these texts at *Risala* 25–6, 32–3 (Lamoreaux [2016], 42–5, 48–9).

[56] Hunayn reports at *Risala* 24 (Lamoreaux [2016], 42–3) that he corrected a Syriac translation by Job of Edessa that was already in circulation; the Arabic translation that survives appears to have been translated from this corrected Syriac version by Hunayn's nephew Hubaish, in consultation with his uncle; Garofalo (1986–2000), xxiv.

interested in Galen's anatomical and medical wisdom, their relationship to dissection and their role in the further dissemination of anatomical knowledge belongs to the next chapter of this history. It is at this point, therefore, that I must turn over the thread of the story to other, more competent hands.[57]

---

[57] The bibliography here is vast, but an interested reader might start with Nutton (1988) and (2020), 145–50, Savage-Smith (1995), Sawday (1995), Cunningham (1997) and (2010), Carlino (1999), French (1999), Park (2010), Quigley (2012), and Guerrini (2015).

Works Cited

Abou-Aly, A. M. A. (1992): *The Medical Writings of Rufus of Ephesus*. Dissertation; University College, University of London.

Adorno, F. (ed.) (1989): *Corpus dei Papiri Filosofici Greci e Latini*. Vol. I (Florence: Olschki).

Alexander, L. (1990): 'The living voice', in Clines, Fowl, and Porter (eds.) (1990): 221–47.

Algra, K., Barnes, J., Mansfeld, J., and Schofield, M. (eds.) (1999): *The Cambridge History of Hellenistic Philosophy* (Cambridge: Cambridge University Press).

Allen, M. (ed.) (2019): *The Role of Zooarchaeology in the Study of the Western Roman Empire* (Portsmouth, RI: Journal of Roman Archaeology).

Anderson, G. (1989): 'The *pepaideumenos* in action: Sophists and their outlook in the early empire', *Aufstieg und Niedergang der Römischen Welt* 2.33.1: 79–208.

Anderson, J. K. (1985): *Hunting in the Ancient World* (Berkeley: University of California Press).

Andorlini, I. (ed.) (1997): *'Specimina' per il corpus dei papiri greci di medicina. Atti dell'incontro di studio (Firenze, 28–29 marzo 1996)* (Florence: Instituto Papirologico G. Vitelli).

(1999): 'Testi medici per la scuola: Raccolte di definizioni e questionari nei papiri', in Garzya and Jouanna (eds.) (1999): 7–15.

(ed.) (2001): *Greek Medical Papyri I* (Florence: Istituto Papirologico G. Vitelli).

(2003): 'L'esegesi del libro tecnico: Papiri di medicina con scoli e commenti', in *Papiri Filosofici: Miscellanea di Studi* 4 (Florence: Olschki): 9–29.

(ed.) (2004): *Testi Medici su Papiro* (Florence: Istituto Papirologico G. Vitelli).

(2006): 'Frammento di una trattazione *De ossibus*: Rilettura di PUG II 51 (I d. C)', in Boudon-Millot, Jouanna, Garzya, and Roselli (eds.) (2006): 83–92.

(ed.) (2009): *Greek Medical Papyri II* (Florence: Istituto Papirologico G. Vitelli).

(2016): 'Crossing the borders between Egyptian and Greek medical practice', in Harris (ed.) (2016): 161–72.

André, J. (1987): *Être Médecin à Rome* (Paris: Belles Lettres).

(1991): *Le Vocabulaire Latin de l'Anatomie* (Paris: Belles Lettres).

Annoni, J.-M. and Barras, V. (1993): 'La découpe du corps humain et ses justifications dans l'antiquité', *Canadian Bulletin of Medical History* 10.2: 185–227.

Armour-Chelu, M. (1997): 'Appendix 8: Faunal remains', in Barker et al. (eds.) (1997): 350–64.

Asper, M. (2005): 'Un personaggio in cerca di lettore. Galens *Großer Puls* und die "Erfindung" des Lesers', in Fögen (ed.) (2005): 235–52.

Ast, R., Cuvigny, H., Hickey, T. M., and Lougovaya, J. (eds.) (2012): *Papyrological Texts in Honor of Roger S. Bagnall* (Durham, NC: American Society of Papyrologists).

Azzarello, G. (2004): 'PIand V 82: Trattato sull'apparato genitale e renale (?)', in Andorlini (ed.) (2004): 237–50.

Bailey, J. F., Henneberg, M., Colson, I. B., Ciarallo, A., Hedges, R. E. M., and Sykes, B. (1999): 'Monkey business in Pompeii: Unique find of a juvenile Barbary macaque skeleton in Pompeii identified using osteology and ancient DNA techniques', *Molecular Biology and Evolution* 16.10: 1410–14.

Baillet, J. (1926): *Inscriptions Grecques et Latines des Tombeaux des Rois ou Syringes à Thèbes* (Cairo: Imprimerie de l'Institut Français d'Archéologie Orientale).

Baldwin, B. (1984): 'Beyond the house call: Doctors in early Byzantine history and politics', *Dumbarton Oaks Papers* 38: 15–19.

Balme, D. M. (1987): 'The place of biology in Aristotle's philosophy', in Gotthelf and Lennox (eds.) (1987): 9–20.

(1991): *Aristotle. History of Animals. Books 7–10* (Cambridge, MA: Harvard University Press).

Bardinet, T. (1995): *Les Papyrus Médicaux de l'Égypte Pharaonique* (Paris: Fayard).

(2018): *Médecins et Magiciens à la Cour du Pharaon: Une Étude du Papyrus Medical Louvre E 32847* (Paris: Éditions Khéops).

Bardong, K. (1942): 'Beiträge zur Hippokrates- und Galenforschung', *Nachrichten von der Akademie der Wissenschaften in Göttingen: Philologisch-Historische Klasse* 7: 577–640.

Barker, P., White, R., Pretty, K., Bird, H., and Corbishley, M. (eds.) (1997): *The Baths Basilica Wroxeter: Excavations 1966–90* (London: English Heritage).

Barry, W. D. (2008): 'Exposure, mutilation, and riot: Violence at the *Scalae Gemoniae* in early imperial Rome', *Greece & Rome* 55.2: 222–46.

Barton, T. S. (1994): *Power and Knowledge: Astrology, Physiognomics, and Medicine under the Roman Empire* (Ann Arbor, MI: University of Michigan Press).

Bartsch, S. (2001): *Ideology in Cold Blood* (Cambridge, MA: Harvard University Press).

Bast, T. H., Hartman, C. G., and W. L. Straus (eds.) (1971): *The Anatomy of the Rhesus Monkey: Macaca Mulatta* (New York: Hafner Publishing Co.).

Bates, D. (ed.) (1995): *Knowledge and the Scholarly Medical Traditions* (Cambridge: Cambridge University Press).

Baykan, D. (2012): *Allianoi Tip Aletleri. Studia ad Orientem Antiquum 2* (Istanbul: Institutum Turcicum Scientiae Antiquitatis, Türk Eskiçağ Bilimleri Enstitüsü).

Beard, M. (2002): 'Did the Romans have elbows?', in Moreau (ed.) (2002): 47–59.

Beard, M. and North, J. A. (eds.) (1990): *Pagan Priests: Religion and Power in the Ancient World* (London: Duckworth).

Beard, M., North, J. A., and Price, S. R. F. (eds.) (1998): *Religions of Rome* (Cambridge University Press).

Belayche, N. (2007): 'Religion et consumation de la viande dans le monde romain: Des réalités voilées', *Food & History* 5.1: 29–43.

Bell, S. W. and Holland, L. L. (eds.) (2018): *At the Crossroads of Greco-Roman History, Culture, and Religion. Papers in Memory of Carin M. C. Green* (Oxford: Archaeopress).

Berrey, M. (2014): 'Chrysippus of Cnidus: Medical doxography and Hellenistic monarchies', *Greek, Roman, and Byzantine Studies* 54.3: 420–43.

(2017): *Hellenistic Science at Court* (Berlin: De Gruyter).

Berringer, O. M., Browning, F. M., and Schroeder, C. R. (1968): *An Atlas and Dissection Manual of Rhesus Monkey Anatomy* (Tallahassee, FL: Anatomy Laboratory Aids).

Bertier, J. (1972): *Mnésithée et Dieuchès* (Leiden: E. J. Brill).

Bethe, E. (1900): *Pollucis Onomasticon* (Leipzig: Teubner).

Bidez, J. and Leboucq, G. (1944): 'Une anatomie antique du cœur humain: Philistion de Locres et le "Timée" de Platon', *Revue des Études Grecques* 57: 7–40.

Blanck, H. (1992): *Das Buch in der Antike* (Munich: Beck).

Blank, D. L. and Dyck, A. R. (1984): 'Aristophanes of Byzantium and problem-solving in the Museum: Notes on a recent reassessment', *Zeitschrift für Papyrologie und Epigraphik* 56: 17–24.

Bliquez, L. J. (1984): 'Two lists of Greek surgical instruments and the state of surgery in Byzantine times', *Dumbarton Oaks Papers* 38: 187–204.

(2014): *The Tools of Asclepius: Surgical Instruments in Greek and Roman Times* (Leiden; Boston: Brill).

Bliquez, L. J. and Jackson, R. (1994): *Roman Surgical Instruments and Other Minor Objects in the National Archaeological Museum of Naples* (Mainz: Verlag Philipp von Zabern).

Bliquez, L. J. and Kazhdan, A. (1984): 'Four testimonia to human dissection in Byzantine Times', *Bulletin of the History of Medicine* 58.4: 554–7.

Bloomer, W. M. (2015): *A Companion to Ancient Education* (Malden, MA: Wiley and Sons).

Blümner, H. (1918): *Fahrendes Volk im Altertum* (Munich: G. Franzschen Verlags).

Bodnár, I. and Fortenbaugh, W. W. (eds.) (2002): *Eudemus of Rhodes. Rutgers University Studies in Classical Humanities. Vol. XI* (New Brunswick, NJ; London: Transaction Publishers).

Bomgardner, D. L. (2000): *The Story of the Roman Amphitheatre* (London: Routledge).

Boudon, V. (1994): 'Les œuvres de Galien pour les débutants ("De sectis", "De pulsibus ad tirones", "De ossibus ad tirones", "Ad Glauconem de methodo medendi" et "Ars medica"): Médecine et pédagogie au IIᵉ s. ap. J.-C.', *Aufstieg und Niedergang der Römischen Welt* 2.37.2: 1421–67.

(ed. and trans.) (2002): *Galien. Exhortation à l'Étude de la Médecine; Art Médical* (Paris: Belles Lettres).

Boudon-Millot, V. (2004): 'L'oral et l'écrit chez Galien', in Jouanna and Leclant (eds.) (2004): 199–218.

(ed. and trans.) (2007): *Galien. Sur l'Ordre de ses Propres Livres; Sur ses Propres Livres; Que l'Excellent Médecin est Aussi Philosophe* (Paris: Belles Lettres).

(2008): 'Un étudiant sans école, un maître sans disciples: L'exemple paradoxal de Galien de Pergame', in Hugonnard-Roche (ed.) (2008): 265–82.

(2012): *Galien de Pergame. Un Médecin Grec à Rome* (Paris: Belles Lettres).

(2018): 'Galen's Hippocrates', in Pormann (ed.) (2018): 292–314.

Boudon-Millot, V., Jouanna, J., Garzya, A., and Roselli, A. (eds.) (2006): *Ecdotica e Ricezione dei Testi Medici Greci. Atti del V Convengo Internazionale (Napoli 1–2 Ottobre 2004)* (Naples: M. D'Auria).

Boudon-Millot, V., Jouanna, J., and Pietrobelli, A. (eds.) (2010): *Galien. Ne pas se Chagriner* (Paris: Belles Lettres).

Boulogne, J. and Drizenko, A. (eds.) (2006): *L'Enseignement de la Médecine selon Galien* (Lille: Presses de l'Université Charles de Gaulle Lille 3).

Bouras-Vallianatos, P. (2019): 'Galen in Byzantine medical literature', in Bouras-Vallianatos and Zipser (eds.) (2019): 86–110.

Bouras-Vallianatos, P. and Xenophontos, S. (eds.) (2018): *Greek Medical Literature and its Readers. From Hippocrates to Islam and Byzantium* (New York; London: Routledge).

Bouras-Vallianatos, P. and Zipser, B. (eds.) (2019): *Brill's Companion to the Reception of Galen* (Leiden: Brill).

Bowersock, G. W. (1969): *Greek Sophists in the Roman Empire* (Oxford: Oxford University Press).

Boyancé, P. (1964): 'Aristote sur une peinture de la Via Latina', *Mélanges Eugène Tisserant* 4.1: 107–24.

Brancacci, A. and Morel, P.-M. (eds.) (2006): *Democritus: Science, the Arts, and the Care of the Soul. Proceedings of the International Colloquium on Democritus, Paris, 18–20 September 2003* (Leiden; Boston: Brill).

Brandeburg, H., Heid, S., and Markschies, C. (eds.) (2007): *Salute e Guarigione nella Tarda Antichità* (Vatican City: Pontificio Istituto di Archeologia Cristiana).

Brockmann, C., Brunschön, W., and Overwien, O. (eds.) (2009): *Antike Medizin im Schnittpunkt von Geistes- und Naturwissenschaften. Internationale Fachtagung aus Anlass des 100-jährigen Bestehens des Akademienvorhabens Corpus Medicorum Graecorum/Latinorum* (Berlin; New York: De Gruyter).

Browning, R. (1985): 'A further testimony to human dissection in the Byzantine world', *Bulletin of the History of Medicine* 59.4: 518–20.

Brunt, P. (1994): 'The bubble of the second sophistic', *Bulletin of the Institute of Classical Studies* 39: 25–52.

van den Bruwaene, M. (1978): *Cicéron. De Natura Deorum. Livre II* (Brussels: Latomus).

de Bruyne, L. (1969–70): 'Aristote ou Socrate? À propos d'une peinture de la Via Latina', *Rendiconti della Pontificia Accademia Romana di Archeologia* 42: 173–93.

Bubb, C. (2022): 'A new interpretation of the medical competitions at Ephesos (I. *Ephesos* 1161–69)', *Zeitschrift für Papyrologie und Epigraphik* 221: 152–6.

(forthcoming *a*): 'Ancient conceptions of the human uterus: Italic votives and animal wombs.' *Journal of the History of Medicine and Allied Sciences*.

(forthcoming *b*): 'The movement of fluids in Hippocratic *Places in Man* and the Egyptian vessel system', in Schiødt, Jacob, and Ryholt (eds.) (forthcoming).

Bubb, C. and Peachin, M. (eds.) (forthcoming): *Medicine and the Law in the Roman Empire* (Oxford: Oxford University Press).

Buecheler, F. (1963): *Petronii Saturae* (Berlin: Wiedmannsche Verlagsbuchhandlung).

Burguière, P., Gourevitch, D., and Malinas, Y. (eds. and trans.) (2003): *Soranos d'Éphèse. Maladies des Femmes* (Paris: Belles Lettres).

Burnard, E. D. and James, L. S. (1961): 'Radiographic heart size in apparently healthy newborn infants: Clinical and biochemical correlations', *Pediatrics* 27.5: 726–39.

Burrell, B. (2009): 'Reading, hearing, and looking at Ephesos', in Johnson and Parker (eds.) (2009): 69–95.

Byl, S. (1990): 'Le vocabulaire hippocratique dans les comédies d'Aristophane et particulièrement dans les deux dernières', *Revue de Philologie, de Littérature et d'Histoire Anciennes* 64: 151–62.

(2006): 'Autour du vocabulaire médical d'Aristophane: Le mot sans son contexte', *L'Antiquité Classique* 75: 195–204.

(2011): *La Médecine à l'Époque Hellénistique et Romaine: Galien: La Survie d'Hippocrate et des Autres Médecins de l'Antiquité* (Paris: Harmattan).

Calder, L. (2011): *Cruelty and Sentimentality: Greek Attitudes to Animals 600–300 BC* (Oxford: BAR Publishing).

Calder, W. M. (ed.) (1992): *Werner Jaeger Reconsidered. Proceedings of the Second Oldfather Conference, University of Illinois, April 26–28, 1990* (Atlanta, GA: Scholars Press).

Cambiano, G. (1999): 'Philosophy, science, and medicine', in Algra, Barnes, Mansfeld, and Schofield (eds.) (1999): 585–613.

Campbell, G. L. (2014): *The Oxford Handbook of Animals in Classical Thought and Life* (Oxford: Oxford University Press).

Capelle (1927): 'Lykon', *Paulys Realencyclopädie der classischen Altertumswissenschaft* XIII.2: col. 2303–9.

Capponi, F. (1995): *L'Anatomia e la Fisiologia di Plinio* (Genoa: Università di Genova).

Carbon, J.-M. (2017): 'Meaty perks: Epichoric and topological trends', in Hitch and Rutherford (eds.) (2017): 151–77.

Carbone, A. L. (2011): *Aristote Illustré. Représentations du Corps et Schématisation dans la Biologie Aristotélicienne* (Paris: Classiques Garnier).

Carlino, A. (1999): *Books of the Body: Anatomical Ritual and Renaissance Learning* (Chicago: University of Chicago Press).

Cavallo, G. (ed.) (1987): *Le Strade del Testo* (Bari: Adriatica).

(2002): 'Galeno e la levatrice: Qualche riflessione su libri e sapere medico nel mondo antico', *Medicina nei Secoli* 14.2: 407–16.

Champlin, E. (1987): 'The testament of the piglet', *Phoenix* 41.2: 174–83.

Chan, L., Rao, B. K., Jiang, Y., Endicott, B., Wapner, R. J., and Reece, E. A. (1995): 'Fetal gallbladder growth and development during gestation', *Journal of Ultrasound in Medicine* 14: 421–5.

Chantraine, P. (1975): 'Remarques sur la langue et le vocabulaire du corpus hippocratique', in *La Collection Hippocratique et son Rôle dans l'Histoire de la Médicine: Colloque de Strasbourg, 23–23 Octobre 1972* (Leiden: Brill): 35–40.

Cilliers, L. (2005): 'Vindicianus's "Gynaecia": Text and translation of the Codex Monacensis (Clm 4622)', *The Journal of Medieval Latin* 15: 153–236.

(2019): *Roman North Africa: Environment, Society and Medical Contribution* (Amsterdam: Amsterdam University Press).

Cioffi, R. L. (2013): *Imaginary Lands: Ethnicity, Exoticism, and Narrative in the Ancient Novel.* Dissertation; Harvard University.

Clarke, M. L. (1971): *Higher Education in the Ancient World* (London: Routledge).

Clauss, J. J. and Cuypers, M. (eds.) (2010): *A Companion to Hellenistic Literature* (Chichester: Wiley Blackwell).

Clines, D. J. A., Fowl, S. E., and Porter, S. E. (eds.) (1990): *The Bible in Three Dimensions* (Sheffield, England: JSOT Press).

Cohn-Haft, L. (1956): *The Public Physicians of Ancient Greece* (Northampton, MA: Department of History of Smith College).

Cole, F. J. (1944): *A History of Comparative Anatomy from Aristotle to the Eighteenth Century* (London: Macmillan).

Coleman, K. M. (1990): 'Fatal charades: Roman executions staged as mythological enactments', *Journal of Roman Studies* 80: 44–73.

(2006): *M. Valerii Martialis Liber Spectaculorum* (Oxford: Oxford University Press).

Collins, D. (2008): 'Mapping the entrails: The practice of Greek hepatoscopy', *American Journal of Philology* 129.3: 319–45.

Colson, F. H. (1939): *Philo. On the Special Laws, Book 4. On the Virtues. On Rewards and Punishments* (Cambridge, MA: Harvard University Press).

Connell, S. M. (ed.) (2021): *The Cambridge Companion to Aristotle's Biology* (Cambridge: Cambridge University Press).

Contadini, A. (ed.) (2007): *Arab Painting: Text and Image in Illustrated Arabic Manuscripts* (Leiden; Boston: Brill).

Cook, J. G. (2014): *Crucifixion in the Mediterranean World* (Tübingen: Mohr Sierbeck).

Corbier, M. (1989): 'The ambiguous status of meat in ancient Rome', *Food and Foodways* 3.3: 223–64.

Corner, G. W. (1927): *Anatomical Texts of the Earlier Middle Ages: A Study in the Transmission of Culture* (Washington, DC: Carnegie Institute of Washington).

Cosans, C. E. (1998): 'The experimental foundations of Galen's teleology', *Studies in History and Philosophy of Science* 29.1: 63–80.

Craik, E. M. (1998): *Hippocrates. Places in Man* (Oxford: Clarendon Press).

(2001): 'Medical references in Euripides', *Bulletin of the Institute of Classical Studies* 45: 81–95.

(2006): *Two Hippocratic Treatises, On Sight and On Anatomy* (Leiden; Boston: Brill).

(2015): *The 'Hippocratic' Corpus: Content and Context* (New York; London: Routledge).

Cribiore, R. (2001): *Gymnastics of the Mind: Greek Education in Hellenistic and Roman Egypt* (Princeton, NJ: Princeton University Press).

(2019): 'The dissemination of texts in the high empire', *American Journal of Philology* 140.2: 255–90.

Cross, J. (2018): *Hippocratic Oratory: The Poetics of Early Greek Medical Prose* (New York; London: Routledge).

Cunningham, A. (1997): *The Anatomical Renaissance: The Resurrection of the Anatomical Projects of the Ancients* (Aldershot, UK: Scholar Press).

(2010): *The Anatomist Anatomis'd: An Experimental Discipline in Enlightenment Europe* (Farnham, UK: Ashgate).

Curtis, T. (2016): 'Author, argument and exegesis: A rhetorical analysis of Galen's *In Hippocratis de natura hominis commentaris tria*', in Dean-Jones and Rosen (eds.) (2016): 399–420.

Daremberg, C. and Ruelle, C. E. (eds., trans.) (1879): *Œuvres de Rufus D'Éphèse* (Paris: L'Imprimerie Nationale).

Dasen, V. and Ducaté-Paarmann, S. (2006): 'Hysteria and metaphors of the uterus', in Schroer (ed.) (2006): 239–61.

Dean-Jones, L. (2003): 'Literacy and the charlatan in ancient Greek medicine', in Yunis (ed.) (2003): 97–121.

(2012): 'Clinical gynecology and Aristotle's biology: The composition of HA X', *Apeiron* 45.2: 180–99.

(2017): 'Aristotle's heart and the heartless man', in Wee (ed.) (2017): 122–41.

(2018): 'Galen and the culture of dissection', in Bell and Holland (eds.) (2018): 229–48.

Dean-Jones, L. and Rosen, R. M. (eds.) (2016): *Ancient Concepts of the Hippocratic: Papers Presented at the XIIIth International Hippocrates Colloquium, Austin, Texas, August 2008* (Leiden, Boston: Brill).

Debru, A. (1994): 'L'expérimentation chez Galien', *Aufstieg und Niedergang der Römischen Welt* 2.37.2: 1718–56.

(1995): 'Les démonstrations médicales à Rome au temps de Galien', in van der Eijk, Horstmanshoff, and Schrijvers (eds.) (1995): 69–81.

(1996): 'L'*Anonyme de Bruxelles*: Un témoin latin de l'hippocratisme tardif', in Wittern and Pellegrin (eds.) (1996): 311–27.

(1999): 'Doctrine et tactique doxographique dans l'*Anonyme de Bruxelles*: Une comparaison avec l'*Anonyme de Londres*', in van der Eijk (ed.) (1999*a*): 453–71.

De Carolis, S. (ed.) (2009): *Ars Medica. I Ferri del Mestiere. La Domus 'del Chirurgo' di Rimini e la Chirurgia nell' Antica Roma* (Rimini: Guaraldi).

Decouflé, P. (1964): *La Notion d'Ex-voto Anatomique chez les Étrusco-Romains. Analyse et Synthèse* (Brussels: Latomus).

De Grossi Mazzorin, J. and Minniti, C (2019): 'The exploitation and mobility of exotic animals: Zooarchaeological evidence from Rome', in Allen (ed.) (2019): 85–100.

De Haro Sanchez, M. (ed.) (2015): *Écrire la Magie dans l'Antiquité* (Liège: Presses Universitaires de Liège).

Deichgräber, K. (1930): 'Marinos 4', *Paulys Realencyclopädie der classischen Altertumswissenschaft* XIV.2: col. 1796.

(1965): *Die griechische Empirikerschule: Sammlung der Fragmente und Darstellung der Lehre* (Berlin: Weidmann).

De Lacy, P. (1966): 'Galen and the Greek poets', *Greek, Roman and Byzantine Studies* 7: 259–66.

(1978–84): *Galen. On the Doctrines of Hippocrates and Plato.* CMG V.4.1.2 (Berlin: Akademie Verlag).

(1992): *Galen. On Semen.* CMG V.3.1 (Berlin: Akademie Verlag).

(1996): *Galen. On the Elements According to Hippocrates.* CMG V.1.2 (Berlin: Akademie Verlag).

De Ligt, L. and Northwood, S. (eds.) (2008): *People, Land, and Politics: Demographic Developments and the Transformation of Roman Italy 300 BC–AD 14* (Leiden; Boston: Brill).

De Puma, R. D. and Small, J. P. (eds.) (1994): *Murlo and the Etruscans: Art and Society in Ancient Etruria* (Madison, WI: University of Wisconsin Press).

De Ruyt, C. (2007): 'Les produits vendus au *macellum*', *Food & History* 5.1: 135–50.

Desclos, M.-L. and Fortenbaugh, W. W. (eds.) (2011): *Strato of Lampsacus. Text, Translation, and Discussion* (New Brunswick, NJ: Transaction Publishers).

Devereux, D. and Pellegrin, P. (eds.) (1990): *Biologie, Logique et Métaphysique chez Aristote. Actes du Séminaire C.N.R.S.-N.S.F. Oléron 28 juin-3 juillet 1987* (Paris: Éditions du CNRS).

Di Benedetto, V. (1986): *Il Medico e la Malattia. La Scienza di Ippocrate* (Turin: Einaudi).

Dickson, K. M. (1998): *Stephanus the Philosopher and Physician: Commentary on Galen's Therapeutics to Glaucon* (Leiden; Boston: Brill).

Dieleman, J. and Moyer, I. S. (2010): 'Egyptian literature', in Clauss and Cuypers (eds.) (2010): 429–47.

Diels, H. (1905): 'Die Handschriften der antiken Ärzte', *Abhandlungen der Königlich Preussischen Akademie der Wissenschaften. Philosophisch-historische Classe* 3: 1–158.

Diels, H. and Kranz, W. (eds.) (1951–2): *Die Fragmente der Vorsokratiker* (Berlin: Weidmann).

Dionisotti, A. C., Grafton, A., and J. Kraye (eds.) (1988): *The Uses of Greek and Latin: Historical Essays* (London: The Warburg Institute).

Dix, T. K. (1994): '"Public libraries" in ancient Rome: Ideology and reality', *Libraries & Culture* 29.3: 282–96.

Dodds, E. R. (1965): *Pagan and Christian in an Age of Anxiety: Some Aspects of Religious Experience from Marcus Aurelius to Constantine* (Cambridge: Cambridge University Press).

Dombrowski, D. L. (1984): *The Philosophy of Vegetarianism* (Amherst, MA: University of Massachusetts Press).

(2014): 'Philosophical vegetarianism and animal entitlements' in Campbell (ed.) (2014): 535–55.

Dorandi, T. (2000): *Le Stylet et la Tablette: Dans le Secret des Auteurs Antiques* (Paris: Belles Lettres).

Drabkin, I. E. (ed. and trans.) (1950): *Caelius Aurelianus. On Acute Diseases and On Chronic Diseases* (Chicago: University of Chicago Press).

Draycott, J. and Graham, E.-J. (eds.) (2017*a*): *Bodies of Evidence. Ancient Anatomical Votives Past, Present and Future* (London; New York: Routledge).

(2017*b*): 'Introduction: Debating the anatomical votive', in Draycott and Graham (eds.) (2017*a*): 1–19.

Drobner, H. R. (1996): *Archaeologia Patristica: Die Schriften der Kirchenväter als Quellen der Archäologie und Kulturgeschichte: Gregor von Nyssa, Homiliae in Ecclesiasten* (Vatican City: Pontificio Istituto di Archeologia Cristiana).

Duckworth, W. L. H., Lyons, M. C., and Towers, B. (1962): *Galen on Anatomical Procedures. The Later Books* (Cambridge: Cambridge University Press).

Duminil, M.-P. (1983): *Le Sang, les Vaisseaux, le Cœur dans la Collection Hippocratique; Anatomie et Physiologie* (Paris: Belles Lettres).

(2003): *Hippocrate. Tome VIII. Plaies, Nature des Os, Cœur, Anatomie* (Paris: Belles Lettres) (second ed.).

Dunbabin, K. M. (1986): '*Sic erimus cuncti* … The skeleton in Graeco-Roman art', *Jahrbuch des Deutschen Archäologischen Instituts* 101: 185–255.

Duncan-Jones, R. (1982): *The Economy of the Roman Empire: Quantitative Studies* (Cambridge: Cambridge University Press) (second ed.).

Dunsch, B. (2016): 'ἐκ βιβλίου κυβερνᾶν? Ein Topos in antiker Medizin, Philosophie und Historiographie und die Existenz verschrifteter κυβερνητικαὶ τέχναι', *Antike Naturwissenschaft und ihre Rezeption* 26: 67–96.

Düring, I. (1950): 'Notes on the history of the transmission of Aristotle's writings', *Göteborgs Universitets Årsskrift* 56: 37–70.

Edelstein, L. (1932): 'Die Geschichte der Sektion in der Antike', *Quellen und Studien zur Geschichte der Naturwissenschaften und der Medizin* 3: 50–106.

(1935): 'The development of Greek anatomy', *Bulletin of the History of Medicine* 3.4: 235–48.

Edelstein, L. and Kidd, I. G. (1972): *Posidonius. Volume I: The Fragments* (Cambridge: Cambridge University Press).

Edwards, I. E. S. (1960): *Oracular Amuletic Decrees of the Late New Kingdom* (London: Trustees of the British Museum).

Egidi, R. (2010): 'L'Area di Piazza Venezia. Nuovi Dati Topografici', in Egidi, Filippi, Martone (eds.) (2010): 93–124.

Egidi, R., Filippi, F., and Martone, S. (2010): *Archaeologia e Infrastrutture. Il Tracciato Fondamentale della Linea C della Metropolitana di Roma: Prime Ingadini Archeologiche* (Florence: L. Olschki).

Eichholz, D. E. (1951): 'Galen and his environment', *Greece & Rome* 20.59: 60–71.

van der Eijk, P. J. (ed.) (1999*a*): *Ancient Histories of Medicine: Essays in Medical Doxography and Historiography in Classical Antiquity* (Leiden: Brill).

(1999*b*): 'The Anonymus Parisinus and the doctrines of "The Ancients",' in van der Eijk (ed.) (1999*a*): 295–332.

(2000–1): *Diocles of Carystus. A Collection of the Fragments with Translation and Commentary* (Leiden; Boston: Brill).

(2009): '"Aristotle! What a thing for you to say!" Galen's engagement with Aristotle and Aristotelians', in Gill, Whitmarsh and Wilkins (eds.) (2009): 261–81.

(2016): 'On "Hippocratic" and "non-Hippocratic" medical writings', in Dean-Jones and Rosen (eds.) (2016): 17–47.

van der Eijk, P. J., Horstmanshoff, H. F. J., and Schrijvers, P. H. (eds.) (1995): *Ancient Medicine in its Socio-Cultural Context: Papers Read at the Congress Held at Leiden University, 13–15 April 1992* (Amsterdam: Rodopi).

Ekroth, G. (2014): 'Animal sacrifice in antiquity', in Campbell (ed.) (2014): 324–54.

Ellis, S. J. R. and Devore, G. (2010): 'The fifth season of excavations at VIII.7.1–15 and the Porta Stabia at Pompeii: Preliminary report', *Fasti Online Documents and Research* 202: 1–21.

Engelmann, H. (1990): 'Ephesische Inschriften', *Zeitschrift für Papyrologie und Epigraphik* 84: 89–94.

(1993): 'Celsusbibliothek und Auditorium in Ephesos (IK 17.3009)', *Jahreshefte des Österreichischen Archäologischen Institutes in Wien* 62: 105–11.

Epplett, C. (2001): 'The capture of animals by the Roman military', *Greece & Rome* 48.2: 210–22.

(2003): 'The preparation of animals for Roman spectacula: Vivaria and their administration', *Ludica: Annali di Storia e Civiltà del Gioco* 9: 76–92.

Erbse, H. (1969): *Scholia Graeca In Homerum Iliadem (Scholia Vetera)* (Berlin: De Gruyter).

Erismann, C. (2017): 'Meletius Monachus on individuality: A ninth-century Byzantine medical reading of Porphyry's logic', *Byzantinische Zeitschrift* 110.1: 37–60.

Ernout, A. and Pepin, R. (2003): *Pline l'Ancien. Histoire Naturelle. Livre XI* (Paris: Belles Lettres) (second ed.).

Erskine, A. (ed.) (2003): *A Companion to the Hellenistic World* (Oxford: Oxford University Press).

Fagan, G. G. (2011): *The Lure of Arena: Social Psychology and the Crowd at the Roman Games* (Cambridge: Cambridge University Press).

Fagan, G. G., Fibiger, L., Hudson, M., and Trundle, M. (eds.) (2020): *The Cambridge World History of Violence. Volume 1: The Prehistoric and Ancient Worlds* (Cambridge: Cambridge University Press).

Fancy, N. A. G. (2013): *Science and Religion in Mamluk Egypt: Ibn al-Nafis, Pulmonary Transit and Bodily Resurrection* (London; New York: Routledge).

Faraone, C. A. (1993): 'The wheel, the whip and other implements of torture: Erotic magic in Pindar *Pythian* 4.213-19', *The Classical Journal* 89.1: 1–19.

Fink, J. (1976): 'Die römische Katakombe an der Via Latina', *Antike Welt* 7.1: 2–14.

Fischer, K. D. (1988): 'Ancient veterinary medicine: A survey of Greek and Latin sources and some recent scholarship', *Medizinhistorisches Journal* 23.3/4: 191–209.

(1997): 'Was ist das δελτάριον in POxy lix 4001', in Andorlini (ed.) (1997): 109–113.

Fischer, K.-D., Nickel, D., and Potter, P. (eds.) (1998): *Text and Tradition. Studies in Ancient Medicine and its Transmission. Presented to Jutta Kollesch* (Leiden: Brill).

Flemming, R. (2000): *Medicine and the Making of Roman Women: Gender, Nature, and Authority from Celsus to Galen* (Oxford: Oxford University Press).

(2003): 'Empires of knowledge: Medicine and health in the Hellenistic world', in Erskine (ed.) (2003): 449–63.

(2008): 'Commentary', in Hankinson (ed.) (2008*a*): 323–54.

(2016): 'Anatomical votives: Popular medicine in republican Italy?', in Harris (ed.) (2016): 105–25.

(2017): 'Wombs for the gods', in Draycott and Graham (eds.) (2017*a*): 112–30.

Fögen, T. (ed.) (2005): *Antike Fachtexte – Ancient Technical Texts* (Berlin: De Gruyter).

Formentin, M. (1977): 'Galenus, De anatomia internarum et externarum partium', *Annali della Facoltà di Lettere e Filosofia. Università di Padova* 2: 83–92.

Forsén, B. (1996): *Griechische Gliederweihungen. Eine Untersuchung zu ihrer Typologie und ihrer religions- und sozialgeschichtlichen Bedeutung* (Helsinki: Suomen Ateenan-instituutin säätiö).

Forshaw, R. (2016): 'Trauma care, surgery and remedies in ancient Egypt: A reassessment', in Price et al. (eds.) (2016): 124–41.

Fortenbaugh, W. W. and White, S. A. (eds.) (2006): *Aristo of Ceos. Text, Translation, Discussion*. Rutgers University Studies in Classical Humanities. Vol. XIII (New Brunswick, NJ: Transaction Publishers).

Fortenbaugh, W. W., Huby, P. M., Sharples, R. W., and Gutas, D. (eds.) (1992): *Theophrastus of Eresus. Sources for his Life, Writings, Thought, and Influence* (Leiden; New York: Brill).

Foucault, M. (1976): *Histoire de la Sexualité* (Paris: Gallimard).

Fraser, P. M. (1969): 'The career of Erasistratus of Ceos', *Rendiconti del Istituto Lombardo, Classe di lettere e scienze morali e storiche* 103: 518–37.

(1972): *Ptolemaic Alexandria* (Oxford: Oxford University Press).

Frayn, J. (1993): *Markets and Fairs in Roman Italy* (Oxford: Oxford University Press).

(1995): 'The Roman meat trade', in Wilkins, Harvey, and Dobson (eds.) (1995): 107–14.

Frede, M. (1985): *Galen. Three Treatises on the Nature of Science: On the Sects for Beginners, An Outline of Empiricism, On Medical Experience* (Indianapolis, IN: Hackett).

(1987): *Essays in Ancient Philosophy* (Oxford: Clarendon Press).

French, R. K. (1978): 'The thorax in history', *Thorax* 33: 10–18, 153–66, 295–306, 439–56, 555–64, 714–27.

(1984): 'An origin for the bone text of the "Five Figure Series",' *Sudhoffs Archiv* 68.2: 143–56.

(1994): *Ancient Natural History. Histories of Nature* (London; Routledge).

(1999): *Dissection and Vivisection in the European Renaissance* (Aldershot: Ashgate).

Fuld, E. (1922): 'Prähomerische Sektionen?', *Münchener Medizinische Wochenschrift* 50: 1731.

Furley, D. J. and Wilkie, J. S. (1984): *Galen on Respiration and the Arteries* (Princeton, NJ: Princeton University Press).

Gagarin, M. (1996): 'The torture of slaves in Athenian law', *Classical Philology* 91.1: 1–18.

Gaillard-Seux, P. (2009): 'Un pseudo-Démocrite énigmatique: Bolos de Mendès', in Le Blay (ed.) (2009): 223–43.

(2015): 'Sur la distinction entre médecine et magie dans les textes médicaux antiques (Iᵉʳ-VIᵉ siècles)', in De Haro Sanchez (ed.) (2015): 201–23.

Gaiser, K. (1980): *Das Philosophenmosaik in Neapel. Eine Darstellung der platonischen Akademie* (Heidelberg: Carl Winter Universitätsverlag).

Garcia Barraco, M. E. (2020): *Larvae Conviviales. Gli Scheletri da Banchetto nell'Antica Roma* (Rome: Arbor Sapientiae).

Garnsey, P. (1999): *Food and Society in Classical Antiquity* (Cambridge: Cambridge University Press).

Garofalo, I. (1986–2000): *Galenus: Anatomicarum Administrationum Libri qui Supersunt Novem. Earundem Interpretation Arabica Hunaino Isaaci Filio Ascripta* (Naples: Brill).

(1988): *Erasistrati Fragmenta* (Pisa: Giardini Editori e Stampatori).

(1991a): 'L'anatomia umana in Galeno', *Nuova civiltà delle machine* 9: 101–111.

(1991b) (trans.): *Galeno: Procedimenti Anatomici* (Milan: Biblioteca Universale Rizzoli).

(1991c): 'The six classes of animals in Galen', in López Férez (ed.) (1991): 73–87.

(1994): 'Note filologiche sull'anatomia di Galeno', *Aufstieg und Niedergang der Römischen Welt* 2.37.2: 1790–1833.

(2006): 'L'enseignement de l'anatomie chez Galien', in Boulogne and Drizenko (eds.) (2006): 59–65.

(2019): 'Galen's legacy in Alexandrian texts written in Greek, Latin, and Arabic', in Bouras-Vallianatos and Zipser (eds.) (2019): 62–85.

Garofalo, I. (ed. and trans.) and Debru, A. (trans.) (2005): *Galien. Les Os pour les Débutants. L'Anatomie des Muscles* (Paris: Belles Lettres).

(2008): *Galien. L'Anatomie des Nerfs. L'Anatomie des Veines et des Artères* (Paris: Belles Lettres).

Garofalo, I. (ed.) and Fuchs, B. (trans.) (1997): *Anonymi Medici. De Morbis Acutis et Chroniis* (Leiden: Brill).

Garzya, A. and Jouanna, J. (eds.) (1999): *I Testi Medici Greci. Tradizione e Ecdotica, Atti del III Convegno Internazionale (Napoli, 15–18 Ottobre 1997)* (Naples: d'Auria).

(eds.) (2003): *Trasmissione e Ecdotica dei Testi Medici Greci: Atti del IV Convengo Internazionale (Parigi 17–19 Maggio 2001)* (Naples: d'Auria).

Gautherie, A. (2017): *Rhétorique et Thérapeutique dans le De Medicina de Celse* (Turnhout: Brepols).

Ghalioungui, P. (1973): *The House of Life (Per Ankh): Magic and Medical Science in Ancient Egypt* (Amsterdam: BM Israel).

(1983): *The Physicians of Pharaonic Egypt* (Cairo: Al-Ahram Center for Scientific Translations).

Gielen, E. (2018): 'Physician versus physician: Comparing the audience of *On the Constitution of Man* by Meletios and *Epitome on the Nature of Men* by Leo the Physician', in Bouras-Vallianatos and Xenophontos (eds.) (2018): 153–179.

Gigon, O. (1987): *Aristotelis Opera. Volumen Tertium, Librorum Depereditorum Fragmenta* (Berlin: De Gruyter).

Gilhus, I. S. (2006): *Animals, Gods and Humans: Changing Attitudes to Animals in Greek, Roman and Early Christian Ideas* (London: Routledge).

Gill, C., Whitmarsh, T., and Wilkins, J. (eds.) (2009): *Galen and the World of Knowledge* (Cambridge: Cambridge University Press).

Giroire, C. and Roger, D. (2007): *Roman Art from the Louvre* (New York: American Federation of Arts in association with Hudson Hills Press).

Gleason, M. (1999): 'Truth-contests and talking corpses', in Porter (ed.) (1999): 287–313.

(2009): 'Shock and awe: The performance dimension of Galen's anatomy demonstrations', in Gill, Whitmarsh, and Wilkins (eds.) (2009): 85–114.

Goebel, V. and Peters, J. (2014): 'Veterinary medicine', in Campbell (ed.) (2014): 589–606.

Gold, B. K. (ed.) (1982): *Literary and Artistic Patronage in Ancient Rome* (Austin: University of Texas Press).

Goldhill, S. and Osborne, R. (eds.) (2006): *Rethinking Revolutions through Ancient Greece* (Cambridge: Cambridge University Press).

Gotthelf, A. (ed.) (1985): *Aristotle on Nature and Living Things: Philosophical and Historical Studies. Presented to David M. Balme on his Seventieth Birthday* (Pittsburgh, PA: Mathesis Publications, Inc.).

Gotthelf, A. and Lennox, J. G. (eds.) (1987) (eds.): *Philosophical Issues in Aristotle's Biology* (Cambridge: Cambridge University Press).

Gourevitch, D. (1998): 'The paths of knowledge: Medicine in the Roman world', in Grmek (ed.) (1998): 104–38.

Gourevitch, M. and Gourevitch, D. (1965): 'Anatomie et religion chez les Étrusques', *La Presse Medicale* 73.51.27: 2961–2.

Grant, M. (2000): *Galen on Food and Diet* (London: Routledge).

Grapow, H. (1954): *Anatomie und Physiologie. Grundriss der Medizin der Alten Ägypter I* (Berlin: Akademie Verlag).

Grilli, A. (1988): 'Iatrosophistes', *Rendiconti. Instituto Lombardo, Accademia di Scienze e Lettere* 122: 125–8.

Grimm-Stadelmann, I. (2008): *Theophilos Der Aufbau des Menschen. Kritische Edition des Textes mit Einleitung, Übersetzung und Kommentar.* Dissertation; Ludwig-Maximilians-Universität.

Grmek, M. (ed.) (1980): *Hippocratica. Actes du Colloque Hippocratique de Paris (4–9 Septembre 1978)* (Paris: Éditions du CNRS).

(1996): *Il Calderone de Medea: La Sperimentazione sul Vivente nell'Antichità* (Rome: Laterza).

(ed.) (1998): *Western Medical Thought from Antiquity to the Middle Ages* (Cambridge, MA; Harvard University Press).

Grmek, M. and Gourevitch, D. (1994): 'Aux sources de la doctrine médicale de Galien: L'enseignement de Marinus, Quintus et Numisianus', *Aufstieg und Niedergang der Römischen Welt* 2.37.2: 1491–1528.

Gronewald, M. (2001): '358. Medizinisch', *Kölner Papyri* 9: 18–21.

(2012): '23. Anatomische Schrift über Herzbeutel (περικάρδιος ὑμήν) und Thymusdrüse (θύμος)', in Reiter (ed.) (2012): 200–6.

Gronewald, M. and Maresch, K. (1991): '291. Medizinisch: über Knochenmark', *Kölner Papyri* 7: 27.

de Grummond, N. T. (2013): 'Haruspicy and augury: Sources and procedures', in Turfa and Tambe (eds.) (2013): 539–56.

Guarducci, M. (1989–90): 'Il cippo sepolcrale di un "bubularius de sacra via"', *Bullettino della Commissione Archeologica Comunale di Roma* 93.2: 325–8.

Guerrini, A. (2015): *The Courtiers' Anatomists: Animals and Humans in Louis XIV's Paris* (Chicago: University of Chicago Press).

Gundert, B. (1992): 'Parts and their roles in Hippocratic medicine', *Isis* 83.3: 453–65.

Gutas, D. (1998): *Greek Thought and Arabic Culture* (London: Routledge).

Habermann, W., Scholz, P., and Wiegandt, D. (eds.) (2015): *Das Kaiserzeitliche Gymnasion* (Berlin: De Gruyter).

Halfmann, H. (1979): *Die Senatoren aus dem östlichen Teil des Imperium Romanum bis zum Ende des 2. Jahrhunderts n. Chr.* (Göttingen: Vandenhoeck & Ruprecht).

Hankinson, R. J. (1995): 'The growth of medical empiricism', in Bates (ed.) (1995): 41–59.

(ed.) (2008a): *Cambridge Companion to Galen* (Cambridge: Cambridge University Press).

(2008b): 'The man and his work', in Hankinson (ed.) (2008a): 1–33.

Hanson, A. E. (1995): 'Uterine amulets and Greek uterine medicine', *Medicine nei Secoli. Arte e Scienza* 7: 281–99.

(1998): 'In the shadow of Galen: Two Berlin papyri of medical content (*BKT* IX 80 and 81)', in Fischer, Nickel, and Potter (eds.) (1998): 145–59.

(2001): 'Anonymous treatise on the brain (BKT IX 80)', in Andorlini (ed.) (2001): 95–100.

(2003): 'Text and context in papyrus catechisms on afflictions of the head', in Garzya and Jouanna (eds.) (2003): 199–217.

(2010): 'Doctors' literacy and papyri of medical content', *Studies in Ancient Medicine* 35: 187–204.

Hanson, A. E. and Green, M. H. (1994): 'Soranus of Ephesus: *Methodicorum princeps*', *Aufstieg und Niedergang der Römischen Welt* 2.37.2: 968–1075.

Harden, A. (2014): 'Animals in Classical art', in Campbell (ed.) (2014): 24–60.

Harris, C. R. S. (1973): *The Heart and Vascular System in Ancient Greek Medicine* (Oxford: Clarendon Press).

Harris, W. V. (1989): *Ancient Literacy* (Cambridge, MA: Harvard University Press).

(1994): 'Child-Exposure in the Roman Empire', *Journal of Roman Studies* 84: 1–22.

(ed.) (2016): *Popular Medicine in Graeco-Roman Antiquity: Explorations* (Leiden; Boston: Brill).

Harris, W. V. and Ruffini, G. (eds.) (2004): *Ancient Alexandria between Egypt and Greece* (Leiden; Boston: Brill).

Hartnett, J. (2017): *The Roman Street: Urban Life and Society in Pompeii, Herculaneum, and Rome* (Cambridge: Cambridge University Press).

Hatzimichali, M. (2021): 'The early reception of Aristotle's biology', in Connell (ed.) (2021): 228–45.

Haumesser, L. (2017): 'The open man: Anatomical votive busts between the history of medicine and archaeology', in Draycott and Graham (eds.) (2017*a*): 165–92.

Haupt, M. (1869): 'Analecta', *Hermes* 3.2: 205–29.

Hellmann, O. (2004): '"Multimedia" im Lykeion? Zu Funktionen der Anatomai in der aristotelischen Biologie', *Antike Naturwissenschaft und ihre Rezeption* 14: 65–86.

(2006): 'Peripatetic biology and the *Epitome* of Aristophanes of Byzantium', in Fortenbaugh and White (eds.) (2006): 329–59.

Helmreich, G. (ed.) (1907–9): *Galeni De Usu Partium Libri XVII* (Leipzig: Teubner).

Henrichs, A. (2000): 'Drama and *dromena*: Bloodshed, violence, and sacrificial metaphor in Euripides', *Harvard Studies in Classical Philology* 100: 173–88.

Hillert, A. (1990): *Antike Ärztedarstellungen* (Frankfurt am Main: P. Lang).

Hirt Raj, M. (2006): *Médecins et Malades de l'Égypte Romaine. Étude Socio-légale de la Profession Médicale et de ses Praticiens du Ier au IVe Siècle ap. J.-C.* (Leiden; Boston: Brill).

Hitch, S. and Rutherford, I. (eds.) (2017): *Animal Sacrifice in the Ancient Greek World* (Cambridge: Cambridge University Press).

Hodgson, G. W. I. (1990): *Catterick 433: Animal Bone Report.* Ancient Monuments Laboratory Report 2404 (London: Historic Buildings and Monuments Commission for England).

Hogan, L. P. (1992): *Healing in the Second Temple Period* (Fribourg: Academic Press; Göttingen: Vandenhoeck & Ruprecht).

Hollander, D. B. (2018): *Farmers and Agriculture in the Roman Economy* (London; New York: Routledge).

Holleran, C. (2011): 'The street life of ancient Rome', in Laurence and Newsome (eds.) (2011): 245–61.

—— (2012): *Retail Trade in the Late Republic and the Principate* (Oxford: Oxford University Press).

Holmes, B. (2010): *The Symptom and the Subject: The Emergence of the Physical Body in Ancient Greece* (Princeton, NJ: Princeton University Press).

—— (2018): 'Body', in Pormann (ed.) (2018): 63–88.

Hope, V. M. (2000): 'Contempt and respect: The treatment of the corpse in ancient Rome', in Hope and Marshall (eds.) (2000): 104–27.

Hope, V. M. and Marshall, E. (eds.) (2000): *Death and Disease in the Ancient City* (London; New York: Routledge).

Horstmanshoff, H. F. J. (1990): 'The ancient physician: Craftsman or scientist?', *Journal of the History of Medicine* 45: 176–97.

—— (ed.) (2010): *Hippocrates and Medical Education* (Leiden; Boston: Brill).

Houston, G. W. (2009): 'Papyrological evidence for book collections and libraries in the Roman empire', in Johnson and Parker (eds.) (2009): 233–67.

Hughes, J. (2017): *Votive Body Parts in Greek and Roman Religion* (Cambridge: Cambridge University Press).

Hughes, J. D. (2007): 'Hunting in the ancient Mediterranean world', in Kalof (ed.) (2007): 47–70.

Hugonnard-Roche, H. (ed.) (2008): *L'Enseignement Supérieur dans les Mondes Antiques et Médiévaux. Aspects Institutionnels, Juridiques et Pédagogiques (Actes du Colloque International de Paris, 6–8 Octobre 2005)* (Paris: J. Vrin).

Hunink, V. (1997): *Apuleius of Madauros. Pro Se De Magia* (Amsterdam: Gieben).

Ikeguchi, M. (2017): 'Beef in Roman Italy', *Journal of Roman Archaeology* 30: 7–37.

Ilberg, J. (1892): 'Über die Schriftstellerei des Klaudios Galenos', *Rheinisches Museum für Philologie* 47: 489–514.

—— (1930): *Rufus von Ephesos. Ein griechischer Arzt in trajanischer Zeit* (Leipzig: S. Hirzel).

Immerwahr, H. R. (1992): 'New wine in ancient wineskins: The evidence from Attic vases', *Hesperia* 61.1: 121–32.

Irby-Massie, G. L. (ed.) (2016): *A Companion to Science, Technology, and Medicine in Ancient Greece and Rome* (Chichester: Wiley Blackwell).

Irigoin, J. (1980): 'La formation du vocabulaire de l'anatomie en grec: Du mycénien aux principaux traités de la Collection hippocratique', in Grmek (ed.) (1980): 247–57.

Irmer, D. (1980): 'Die Bezeichnungen der Knochen in *Fract.* und *Art.*', in Grmek (ed.) (1980): 265–84.

Iskandar, A. Z. (1976): 'An attempted reconstruction of the late Alexandrian medical curriculum', *Medical History* 20.3: 235–58.

(ed. and trans.)(1988): *Galeni De optimo medico cognoscendo. CMG* Suppl. Or. IV (Berlin: Akademie Verlag).

Israelowich, I. (2015): *Patients and Healers in the High Roman Empire* (Baltimore, MD: Johns Hopkins University Press).

Jackson, R. (1994): 'The surgical instruments, appliances, and equipment in Celsus' *De Medicina*', in Sabbah and Mudry (eds.) (1994): 167–209.

(2003): 'The domus "del chirurgo" at Rimini: An interim account of the medical assemblage', *Journal of Roman Archaeology* 16: 312–22

(2009): 'Lo strumentario chirurgico della domus rimanese/The surgical instrumentation of the Rimini Domus', in De Carolis (ed.) (2009): 73–91.

Jaeger, W. (1940): 'Diocles of Carystus: A new pupil of Aristotle', *Philosophical Review* 49.4: 393–414.

Jannot, J.-R. (1998): *Devins, Dieux et Démons: Regards sur la Religion de l'Etrurie Antique* (Paris: Picard).

Jennison, G. (1937): *Animals for Show and Pleasure in Ancient Rome* (Manchester: Manchester University Press).

Johnson, W. (2010): *Readers and Reading Culture in the High Roman Empire* (Oxford: Oxford University Press).

Johnson, W. and Parker, H. (2009) (eds.): *Ancient Literacies: The Culture of Reading in Greece and Rome* (Oxford: Oxford University Press).

Johnston, I. and Horsley, J. H. R. (eds. and trans.)(2011): *Galen. Method of Medicine* (Cambridge, MA; Harvard University Press).

Johnston, S. I. (2008): *Ancient Greek Divination* (Malden, MA; Oxford: Wiley-Blackwell).

Jones, C. P. (1986): *Culture and Society in Lucian* (Cambridge, MA: Harvard University Press).

Jouanna, J. (2004): 'Médecine égyptienne et médecine grecque', in Jouanna and Leclant (eds.) (2004): 1–21.

(2012): *Greek Medicine from Hippocrates to Galen. Selected Papers* (Leiden: Brill).

(2013): 'Médecine et philosophie: La réception de la science aristotélicienne chez Galien', in Lehmann (ed.) (2013): 159–82.

(2017): *Hippocrate. Édition Mise à Jour.* (Paris: Belles Lettres).

Jouanna, J. and Leclant, J. (eds.) (2004): *La Médecine Grecque Antique, Cahiers de la Villa 'Kérylos' n. 15* (Paris: Belles Lettres).

Jouanna-Bouchet, J. (2016): *Scribonius Largus. Compositions Médicales* (Paris: Belles Lettres).

Kádár, Z. (1978): *Survivals of Greek Zoological Illuminations in Byzantine Manuscripts* (Budapest: Akadémiai Kiadó).

Kalbfleisch, K. (1896): *Galeni Institutio Logica* (Leipzig: Teubner).

Kalof, L. (ed.) (2007): *A Cultural History of Animals in Antiquity* (Oxford: Berg).

Keil, J. (1905): 'Ärzteinschriften aus Ephesos', *Jahreshefte des Oesterreichischen Archäologischen Instituts in Wein* 8: 128–38.

Kenney, E. J. (1982): 'Books and readers in the Roman world', in Kenney and Clausen (eds.) (1982): 3–32.

Kenney, E. J. and Clausen, W. V. (eds.) (1982): *The Cambridge History of Classical Literature. II: Latin Literature* (Cambridge: Cambridge University Press).

Kevorkian, J. (1959): *The Story of Dissection* (New York: Philosophical Library).

Kind, F. E. (1927): 'Lykos 52', *Paulys Realencyclopädie der classischen Altertumswissenschaft* XIII.2: col. 2408–17.

King, H. (2006): 'The origins of medicine in the second century AD', in Goldhill and Osborne (eds.) (2006): 246–62.

Kirova, N. (2002): 'Specialized medical instruments from Bulgaria in the context of finds from other Roman provinces (I–IV c. AD)', *Archaeologia Bulgarica* 6.1: 73–94.

Kollesch, J. (1973): *Untersuchungen zu den pseudogalenischen Definitiones Medicae* (Berlin: Akademie Verlag).

(1981): 'Galen und die Zweite Sophistik', in Nutton (ed.) (1981): 1–11.

(1992): 'Zur Mundlichkeit hippokratischer Schriften', in Lopez Ferez (ed.) (1992): 335–42.

(1997): 'Die anatomischen Untersuchungen des Aristoteles und ihr Stellenwert als Forschungsmethode in der aristotelischen Biologie', in Kullmann and Fölinger (eds.) (1997): 367–73.

Kollesch, J. and Nickel, D. (eds.) (1993): *Galen und das hellenistische Erbe. Sudhoffs Archiv Beiheft* 32 (Stuttgart: F. Steiner).

Körner, O. (1922): 'Wie entstanden die anatomischen Kenntnisse in Ilias und Odyssee?', *Münchener Medizinische Wochenschrift* 42: 1484–7.

(1929): *Die ärztlichen Kenntnisse in Ilias und Odyssee* (Munich: Bergmann).

Kosak, J. C. (2004): *Heroic Measures: Hippocratic Medicine in the Making of Euripidean Tragedy* (Leiden; Boston: Brill).

Kötzsche-Breitenbruch, L. (1976): *Die neue Katakombe an der Via Latina in Rom: Untersuchungen zur Ikonographie der alttestamentlichen Wandmalereien* (Münster Westfalen: Aschendorffsche Verlagsbuchhandlung).

Kowalski, G. (1960): *Rufi Ephesii De corporis humani partium appellationibus*. Dissertation; University of Göttingen.

Krön, G. (2008): 'The much maligned peasant', in De Ligt and Northwood (eds.) (2008): 71–119.

Kudlien, F. (1968a): 'Anatomie', *Paulys Realencyclopädie der classischen Altertumswissenschaft. Supplementband* XI: col. 38–48.

(1968b): 'Pneumatische Ärzte' *Paulys Realencyclopädie der classischen Altertumswissenschaft. Supplementband* XI: col. 1097–1108.

(1969): 'Antike Anatomie und menschlicher Leichnam', *Hermes* 97.1: 78–94.

(1970): 'Medical education in classical antiquity', in O'Malley (ed.) (1970): 3–37.

Kühn, C. G. (ed.) (1821–33): *Claudii Galeni Opera Omnia* (Leipzig: C. Cnobloch) (re-issued 2011, Cambridge University Press).

Kullmann, W. (1990): 'Bipartite science in Aristotle's biology', in Devereux and Pellegrin (eds.) (1990): 335–43.

(1998): 'Zoologische Sammelwerke in der Antike', in Kullmann, Althoff, and Asper (eds.) (1998): 121–139.

Kullmann, W., Althoff, J. and Asper, M. (eds.) (1998): *Gattungen wissenschaftlicher Literatur in der Antike* (Tübingen: Narr).

Kullmann, W. and Föllinger, S. (eds.) (1997): *Aristotelische Biologie: Intentionen, Methoden, Ergebnisse* (Stuttgart: Steiner Verlag).

Künzl, E. (1983): *Medizinische Instrumente aus Sepulkralfunden der römischen Kaiserzeit* (Cologne: Rheinland Verlag).

(1998): 'Instrumentenfunde und Ärzthäuser in Pompeji: Die medizinische Versorgung einer römischen Stadt des 1. Jahrhunderts n.Chr.', *Sartoniana* 11: 71–152.

Kuriyama, S. (1999): *The Expressiveness of the Body and the Divergence of Greek and Chinese Medicine* (New York: Zone Books).

Kyle, D. G. (1995): 'Animal spectacles in ancient Rome: Meat and meaning', *Nikephoros* 7: 181–205.

(1998): *Spectacles of Death in Ancient Rome* (London: Routledge).

Laes, C. (2010): 'The educated midwife in the Roman Empire. An example of differential equations', in Horstmanshoff (ed.) (2010): 261–86.

Lambros, S. P. (1885): *Excerptorum Constantini de natura animalium libri duo. Aristophanis historiae animalium epitome subiunctis Aeliani, Timothei aliorumque eclogis*. Supplementum Aristotelicum 1. (Berlin: Reimer).

Lamoreaux, J. C. (2016): *Hunayn ibn Ishaq on his Galen Translations: A Parallel English-Arabic Text* (Provo, UT: Brigham Young University Press).

Lang, P. (2013): *Medicine and Society in Ptolemaic Egypt* (Leiden; Boston: Brill).

Langslow, D. R. (2000): *Medical Latin in the Roman Empire* (Oxford: Oxford University Press).

Langslow, D. R. and Maire, B. (eds.) (2010): *Body, Disease and Treatment in a Changing World: Latin Texts and Contexts in Ancient and Medieval Medicine* (Lausanne: Éd. BHMS).

La Regina, A. (ed.) (2001): *Sangue e Arena* (Milan: Electa).

Larrain, C. J. (1994): 'Galen, De motibus dubiis, die lateinische Übersetzung des Niccolò da Reggio', *Traditio* 49: 171–233.

Laurence, R. and Newsome, D. J. (eds.) (2011) (eds.): *Rome, Ostia, Pompeii: Movement and Space* (Oxford: Oxford University Press).

Le Bas, P. and Waddington, W. H. (1870): *Voyage Archéologique en Grèce et en Asie Mineure, Fait par Ordre du Gouvernement Français pendant les Années 1843 et 1844 III. Inscriptions Grecques et Latines* (Paris: Chez Firmin Didot).

Le Blay, F. (ed.) (2009): *Transmettre les Savoirs dans les Mondes Hellénistique et Romain* (Rennes: Presses Universitaires de Rennes).

Le Breton, D. (1993): *Le Chair à Vif. Usages Médicaux et Mondains du Corps Humain* (Paris: Éditions A. M. Métailié).

Leca, A.-P. (1971): *La Médecine Égyptienne au Temps des Pharaons* (Paris: Dacosta).

Lefebvre, G. (1952): *Tableau des Parties du Corps Mentionnées par les Égyptiens* (Cairo: Imprimerie de l'Institut Français d'Archéologie Orientale).

Lehmann, Y. (ed.) (2013): *Aristoteles Romanus: La Réception de la Science Aristotélicienne dans l'Empire Gréco-romain* (Turnhout: Brepols).

Lehoux, D. (2017): 'Observation Claims and Epistemic Confidence in Aristotle's Biology', *Isis* 108.2: 241–58.

Leith, D. (2009*a*): 'A note on the Greek medical fragment PGolenischeff', in Andorlini (ed.) (2009): 211–18.

(2009*b*): '4974. Osteological fragment', *The Oxyrhynchus Papyri* 74: 70–3.

(2009*c*): 'Question-types in medical catechisms on papyrus', in Taub and Doody (eds.) (2009): 107–24.

Leith, D. and Maravela-Solbakk, A. (2009): 'Notes on PSI III.252', in Andorlini (ed.) (2009): 201–9.

Lennox, J. G. (1994): 'The disappearance of Aristotle's biology: A Hellenistic mystery', *Apeiron* 27.4: 7–24.

(2001*a*): *Aristotle's Philosophy of Biology* (Cambridge: Cambridge University Press).

(2001*b*): 'Divide and explain: The *Posterior Analytics* in practice', in Lennox (2001*a*): 7–38.

(2001*c*): 'Putting philosophy of science to the test: The case of Aristotle's biology', in Lennox (2001*a*): 98–109.

Leunissen, M. (2021): 'Empiricism and hearsay in Aristotle's zoological collection of facts', in Connell (ed.) (2021): 64–82.

Lewis, N. (1965): 'Exemption of physicians from liturgy', *Bulletin of the American Society of Papyrologists* 2.3: 87–92.

Lewis, O. (2017): *Praxagoras of Cos On Arteries, Pulse, and Pneuma. Fragments and Interpretation* (Leiden: Brill).

Lewis, S. and Llewellyn-Jones. L. (2018): *The Culture of Animals in Antiquity: A Sourcebook with Commentaries* (New York: Routledge).

Lind, L. R. (1978): 'Popular knowledge of anatomy and medicine in Greece before Hippocrates', *Archivio Italiano di Anatomia e di Embriologia* 83: 33–52.

Lindberg, N. (2019): 'The emperor and his animals: The acquisition of exotic beasts for imperial *venationes*', *Greece & Rome* 66.2: 251–63.

Lloyd, G. E. R. (1975*a*): 'Alcmaeon and the early history of dissection', *Sudhoffs Archiv* 59.2: 113–47.

(1975*b*): 'A note on Erasistratus of Ceos', *Journal of Hellenic Studies* 95: 172–5.

(ed.) (1978): *Hippocratic Writings* (Harmondsworth; New York: Penguin Books).

(1979): *Magic, Reason and Experience* (Cambridge: Cambridge University Press).

(1983): *Science, Folklore and Ideology* (Cambridge: Cambridge University Press).

(1987): *Revolutions of Wisdom* (Berkeley: University of California Press).

(1988): 'Scholarship, authority, and argument in Galen's *Quod Animi Mores*', in Manuli and Vegetti (eds.) (1988): 11–42.

(1991): *Methods and Problems in Greek Science* (Cambridge: Cambridge University Press).

(2006): 'Diogenes of Apollonia: Master of ducts', in Sassi (ed.) (2006): 237–57.

Lones, T. E. (1912): *Aristotle's Researches in Natural Science* (London: West, Newman & Co.).

Longrigg, J. (1981): 'Superlative achievement and comparative neglect: Alexandrian medical science and modern historical research', *History of Science* 19.3: 155–200.

(1993): *Greek Rational Medicine: Philosophy and Medicine from Alcmaeon to the Alexandrians* (London; New York: Routledge).

Lonie, I. M. (1964): 'Erasistratus, the Erasistrateans and Aristotle', *Bulletin of the History of Medicine* 38: 426–43.

(1973): 'The paradoxical text *On the Heart*', *Medical History* 17.1: 1–15 and 17.2: 136–53.

(1978): 'Embryology and anatomy', in Lloyd (ed.) (1978): 315–53.

López Férez, J. A. (ed.) (1991): *Galeno, Obra, Pensamiento e Influencia: Coloquio Internacional Celebrado en Madrid, 22-25 de Marzo de 1998* (Madrid: Universidad Nacional de Educación a Distancia).

(ed.) (1992): *Tratados Hipocráticos (Estudios Acerca de su Contenido, Forma e Influencia)* (Madrid: Universidad Nacional de Educación a Distancia).

Lougovaya, J. (2019): '*Medici docti* in verse inscriptions' in Reggiani 2019: 139–59.

Louis, P. (2002): *Aristote. Histoire des Animaux. Livres I-IV* (Paris: Belles Lettres) (second ed.).

Lusnia, S. (2020): 'Representations of war and violence in ancient Rome', in Fagan, Fibiger, Hudson, and Trundle (eds.) (2020): 654–83.

Lüthy, C. (2000): 'The fourfold Democritus on the stage of Early Modern science', *Isis* 91.3: 443–79.

MacKinnon, M. R. (2004): *Production and Consumption of Animals in Roman Italy: Integrating the Zooarchaeological and Textual Evidence* (Portsmouth, RI: Journal of Roman Archaeology).

(2006): 'Supplying exotic animals for the Roman amphitheatre games: New reconstructions combining archaeological, ancient textual, historical and ethnographic data', *Mouseion (Canada)* 6.2: 137–61.

(2014): 'Hunting', in Campbell (ed.) (2014): 203–15.

Majno, G. (1975): *The Healing Hand: Man and Wound in the Ancient World* (Cambridge, MA: Harvard University Press).

Malomo, A. O., Idowu, O. E., and Osuagwu, F. C. (2006): 'Lessons from history: Human anatomy, from the origin to the Renaissance', *International Journal of Morphology* 24.1: 99–104.

Manetti, D. (1999): '<Aristotle> and the role of doxography in the Anonymus Londiniensis (PBrLibr inv. 137)', in van der Eijk (ed.) (1999a): 95–141.

(2011): *Anonymus Londiniensis. De medicina* (Berlin: De Gruyter).

Manetti, D. and Roselli, A. (1994): 'Galeno commentatore di Ippocrate', *Aufstieg und Niedergang der Römischen Welt* 2.37.2: 1529–1635.

Manfredi, M. (1951): '1275. Hom. Ψ 877-897', *Papiri Greci e Latini. Vol. 12. Pubblicazioni della Società Italiana per la Ricerca dei Papiri Greci e Latini in Egitto* (PSI): 112–13.

(1997): 'PSI XV.1510: Questionario sui παρίσθμια', in Andorlini (ed.) (1997): 75–9.

Mansfeld, J. (1994): *Prolegomena: Questions to be Settled Before the Study of an Author or a Text* (Leiden: Brill).

Manuli. P. and Vegetti, M. (eds.) (1988): *Le Opere Psicologiche di Galeno* (Naples: Bibliopolis).

Marasco, G. (2010): 'The curriculum of studies in the Roman Empire and the cultural role of physicians', in Horstmanshoff (ed.) (2010): 205–19.

Marganne, M.-H. (1987): 'Une description des os du tarse: P. Lit. Lond. 167', *Bulletin of the American Society of Papyrologists* 24.1–2: 23–4.

———(1998): *La Chirurgie dans l'Égypte Gréco-Romaine d'après les Papyrus Littéraires Grecs* (Leiden: Brill).

———(2004): *Le Livre Médical dans le Monde Gréco-romain* (Liège: CEDOPAL).

Marra, P. (1966): 'Galeno 'Del movimento del torace e del polmone.' Traduzione e commento', *Medicina nei Secoli* 3–4 (suppl.): 38–43.

Marrou, H. I. (1956): *A History of Education in Antiquity*. Trans. G. Lamb (New York: Sheed and Ward).

Marshall, A. J. (1976): 'Library resources and creative writing at Rome', *Phoenix* 30.3: 252–64.

Massar, N. (2001): 'Un savoir-faire à l'honneur: "Médecins" et "discours civique" en Grèce hellénistique', *Revue Belge de Philologie et d'Histoire* 79.1: 175–201.

———(2010): 'Choose your master well. Medical training, testimonies and claims to authority', in Horstmanshoff (ed.) (2010): 169–86.

Mattern, S. (2008): *Galen and the Rhetoric of Healing* (Baltimore, MD: Johns Hopkins University Press).

———(2013): *The Prince of Medicine: Galen in the Roman Empire* (Oxford: Oxford University Press).

———(2017): 'Galen', in Richter and Johnson (eds.) (2017): 371–88.

May, M. T. (1968): *Galen. On the Usefulness of the Parts of the Body* (Ithaca, NY: Cornell University Press).

May, R. (1991): 'Les jeux d'osselets', in *Jouer dans l'Antiquité* (Marseille: Musées de Marseille, Réunion des Musées Nationaux): 100–5.

Mayhew, R. (2011): *Aristotle. Problems. Books 1–19* (Cambridge, MA: Harvard University Press).

———(2020): 'Athenaeus' Deipnosophistae 7 and Aristotle's Lost Zoïka or On Fish', in Mesquita, Noriega-Olmos, and Shields (eds.) (2020): 109–39.

Mazzini, I. (1999): *A. Cornelio Celso. La Chirurgia* (Macerata: Università degli Studi di Macerata, Facoltà di Lettere e Filosofia).

McCabe, A. (2007): *A Byzantine Encyclopedia of Horse Medicine: The Sources, Compilation, and Transmission of the Hippiatrica* (Oxford: Oxford University Press).

McClellan, A. M. (2019): *Abused Bodies in Roman Epic* (Cambridge: Cambridge University Press).

McDermott, W. C. (1938): *The Ape in Antiquity* (Baltimore, MD: Johns Hopkins University Press).

Meeusen, M. (2018): 'Aristotelian *Natural Problems* and imperial culture: Selective readings', Σχολή 12.1: 28–47.

Meijer, F. (2010): *Chariot Racing in the Roman Empire*. Trans. L. Waters (Baltimore, MD: Johns Hopkins University Press).

Meneghini, R. and Rea, R. (eds.) (2014): *La Biblioteca Infinita. I Luoghi del Sapere nel Mondo Antico* (Milan: Electa).

Menetrier, M. P. (1924): 'A propos du traité du pouls attribué à Rufus d'Ephèse et de la sphygmologie des anciens', *Bulletin de la Société française d'histoire de la médecine* 18: 97–8.

(1930): 'Comment Aristote et les anciens médecins hippocratiques ont-ils pu prendre connaissance de l'anatomie humaine?', *Bulletin de la Société française d'histoire de la médecine* 24: 254–62.

Mesquita, A., Noriega-Olmos, S., and Shields, C. (2020): *Revisiting Aristotle's Fragments: New Essays on the Fragments of Aristotle's Lost Works* (Berlin; Boston: De Gruyter).

Meyerhof, M. (1929): 'Autobiographische Bruchstücke Galens aus arabischen Quellen', *Sudhoffs Archiv* 22.1: 72–86.

Meyerhof, M. and Schacht, J. (1931): 'Galen über die Medizinischen Namen. Arabisch und Deutsch herausgegeben', *Abhandlungen der preussischen Akademie der Wissenschaften* 3: 1–43.

Michler, M. (1968): *Die Alexandrinischen Chirurgen. Eine Sammlung und Auswertung ihrer Fragmente* (Wiesbaden: Franz Steiner Verlag).

Miles, G. C. (ed.) (1952): *Archaeologica Orientalia in Memoriam Ernst Herzfeld* (Locust Valley, NY: J. J. Augustin).

Miller, H. W. (1945): 'Aristophanes and medical language', *Transactions of the American Philological Association* 76: 74–84.

Moraux, P. (1973–2001): *Der Aristotelismus bei den Griechen* (Berlin; New York: De Gruyter).

(1983): 'Ein unbekannter Lehrer Galens', *Zeitschrift für Papyrologie und Epigraphik* 53: 85–8.

(1985): 'Galen and Aristotle's *De partibus animalium*', in Gotthelf (ed.) (1985): 327–44.

Moreau, P. (ed.) (2002): *Corps Romains* (Grenoble: Éditions Jérôme Millon).

Moss, C. (2021): 'Infant exposure and the rhetoric of cannibalism, incest, and martyrdom in the early church', *Journal of Early Christian Studies* 29.3: 341–69.

Most, G. W. (1981): 'Callimachus and Herophilus', *Hermes* 109.2: 188–96.

(ed.) (1999): *Commentaries/Kommentare* (Göttingen: Vandenhoeck und Ruprecht).

Mudry, P. (ed.) (1999): *Traité des Maladies Aigües et des Maladies Chroniques de Caelius Aurelianus* (Nantes: Université de Nantes).

Nelson, E. (2016): 'Tracking the Hippocratic woozle: Pseudepigrapha and the formation of the corpus', in Dean-Jones and Rosen (eds.) (2016): 117–140.

Netz, R. (2002): 'Greek mathematicians: A group picture', in Tuplin and Rihll (eds.) (2002): 196–216.

Newmyer, S. T. (2011): *Animals in Greek and Roman Thought: A Sourcebook* (Abingdon; New York: Routledge).

Nicholls, M. (2011): 'Galen and libraries in the *Peri Alupias*', *Journal of Roman Studies* 101: 123–42.

Nickel, D. (1971): *Galeni De Uteri Dissectione*. CMG V.2.1 (Berlin: Akademie Verlag).

(2009): 'Pseudepigraphisches zur Anatomie bei Rufus von Ephesos', in Brockmann, Brunschön, and Overwien (eds.) (2009): 63–74.

North, J. (1990): 'Diviners and divination at Rome', in Beard and North (eds.) (1990): 51–71.

Nunn, J. F. (1996): *Ancient Egyptian Medicine* (London: British Museum Press).

Nutton, V. (1977): '*Archiatri* and the medical profession in antiquity', *Papers of the British School at Rome* 45: 191–226.

(ed. and trans.) (1979): *Galen: On Prognosis*. CMG V.8.1 (Berlin: Akademie Verlag).

(ed.) (1981): *Galen: Problems and Prospects* (London: Wellcome Institute for the History of Medicine).

(1987): 'Numisianus and Galen', *Sudhoffs Archiv* 71.2: 235–9.

(1988): '"*Prisci dissectionum professores*": Greek texts and Renaissance anatomists', in Dionisotti, Grafton, and Kraye (eds.) (1988): 111–26.

(1993): 'Galen and Egypt', in Kollesch and Nickel (eds.) (1993): 11–32.

(1995): 'The medical meeting place', in van der Eijk, Horstmanshoff, and Schrijvers (eds.) (1995): 3–26.

(ed.) (2002): *The Unknown Galen* (London: Institute of Classical Studies).

(2006): 'Rufus [5]', in *Brill's New Pauly* (Brill). Available at: https://referenceworks .brillonline.com/browse/brill-s-new-pauly (last accessed 27 March 2020).

(2008): 'Rufus of Ephesus in the medical context of his time', in Pormann (ed.) (2008): 139–58.

(2009): 'Galen's library', in Gill, Whitmarsh, and Wilkins (eds.) (2009): 19–34.

(2011): *Galen: On Problematical Movements. With an edition of the Arabic Version by Gerrit Bos* (Cambridge: Cambridge University Press).

(2013*a*): *Ancient Medicine* (London; New York: Routledge) (second ed.).

(2013*b*): 'Avoiding distress', in Singer (ed.) (2013): 45–106.

(2014): 'Allianoi: A missing link in the history of hospitals?', *Medical History* 58.1: 122–5.

(2019): 'Punishing the incompetent physician: Some neglected cases', in Reggiani (ed.) (2019): 133–8.

(2020): *Galen: A Thinking Doctor in Imperial Rome* (Abingdon; New York: Routledge).

(2022): 'Galen and the Latin *De voce*: A new edition and English translation', in Raiola and Roselli (eds.) (2022): 141–64.

Ogden, D. (2014): 'Animal magic', in Campbell (ed.) (2014): 294–309.

Ogle, W. (1882): *Aristotle On The Parts of Animals* (London: Kegan Paul, Trench & Co.).

O'Malley, C. D. (ed.) (1970): *The History of Medical Education* (Berkeley: University of California Press).

Oppermann, H. (1925): 'Herophilus bei Kallimachos', *Hermes* 60.1: 14–32.

Ormos, I. (1993): 'Bemerkungen zur editorischen Bearbeitung der Galenschrift "Über die Sektion toter Lebewesen"', in Kollesch and Nickel (eds.) (1993): 164–72.

Osen, E. (2022): 'Marinus of Alexandria: Galen's anatomical forefather, or: How do you solve a problem like Marinus?', *Studies in the History and Philosophy of Science* 92: 224–38.

Pahl, W. M. and Parsche, F. (1991): 'Rätselhafte Befunde an anthropologischem Untersuchungsmaterial aus Ägypten: Addenda zu Herodots 'Historie', Lib. II, 86–88 und zum ägyptischen Sparagmos?', *Anthropologischer Anzeiger* 49.1/2: 39–48.

Palombi, D. (2007): 'Medici e medicina a Roma tra Carine, Velia e Sacra Via', in Brandeburg, Heid, and Markschies (eds.) (2007): 53–78.

(2014): 'Medici al *templum Pacis*?', in Meneghini and Rea (eds.) (2014): 336–42.

Park, K. (2010): *Secrets of Women: Gender, Generation, and the Origins of Human Dissection* (New York: Zone Books).

Parker, R. (1983): *Miasma: Pollution and Purification in Early Greek Religion* (Oxford: Clarendon Press).

Patriquin, H., Lefaivre, J.-F., Lafortune, M., Russo, P., and Boisvert, J. (1990): 'Fetal lobation. An anatomo-ultrasonographic correlation', *Journal of Ultrasound in Medicine* 9.4: 191–7.

Peck, A. L. (1965): *Aristotle. History of Animals. Books 1–3* (Cambridge, MA: Harvard University Press).

(1970): *Aristotle. History of Animals. Books 4–6* (Cambridge, MA: Harvard University Press).

Peck, A. L. and Forster, E. S. (1937): *Aristotle. Parts of Animals, Movement of Animals, Progression of Animals* (Cambridge, MA: Harvard University Press).

Perilli, L. (2006): 'Democritus, zoology, and the physicians', in Brancacci and Morel (eds.) (2006): 143–79.

Persaud, T. V. N. (1984): *Early History of Human Anatomy* (Springfield, IL: Charles C. Thomas).

Persaud, T. V. N., Loukas, M., and Tubbs, R. S. (eds.) (2014): *A History of Human Anatomy. Second Edition* (Springfield, IL: Charles C. Thomas).

Peterson, D. W. (1977): 'Observations on the chronology of the Galenic corpus', *Bulletin of the History of Medicine* 51.3: 484–95.

Petit, C. (2009): *Galien. Le médecin. Introduction* (Paris: Belles Lettres).

(2018): *Galien de Pergame ou la Rhétorique de la Providence: Médecine, Littérature et Pouvoir à Rome* (Leiden: Brill).

Phillips, J. J. (1985): 'Bookprices and Roman literacy', *Classical World* 79.1: 36–8.

Picaud, S. (2004): 'Les représentations des jeux de la balle et des osselets dans les terres cuites, céramiques et reliefs', *Pallas* 65: 49–55.

van der Plas, M. (2020): 'Corpse mutilation in the *Iliad*', *Classical Quarterly* 70.2: 459–72.

Pleket, H. W. (1995): 'The social status of physicians in the Graeco-Roman world', in van der Eijk, Horstmanshoff, and Schrijvers (eds.) (1995): 27–34.

Popescu, E. (1956): 'Consideratii asupra Educatiei Tineretului la Histria in Legatura cu Trei Inscriptii Inedite', *Studii Si Cercetari de Istorie Veche* 7.3–4: 343–65.

Pormann, P. E. (2005): 'The physician and the other: Images of the charlatan in medieval Islam', *Bulletin of the History of Medicine* 79.2: 189–227.

(ed.) (2008): *On Melancholy: Rufus of Ephesus* (Tübingen: Mohr Siebeck).

(ed.) (2018): *The Cambridge Companion to Hippocrates* (Cambridge: Cambridge University Press).

Porter, J. I. (ed.) (1999): *Constructions of the Classical Body* (Ann Arbor: University of Michigan Press).

Potter, P. (1976): 'Herophilus of Chalcedon: An assessment of his place in the history of anatomy', *Bulletin of the History of Medicine* 50.1: 45–60.

(1993): 'Apollonius and Galen on "Joints,"' in Kollesch and Nickel (eds.) (1993): 117–23.

(ed. and trans.) (2010): *Hippocrates. Coan Prenotions. Anatomical and Minor Clinical Writings* (Cambridge, MA: Harvard University Press).

Powell, O. (2003): *Galen: On the Properties of Foodstuffs* (Cambridge: Cambridge University Press).

Price, C., Forshaw, R. Chamberlain, A., Nicholson, P., Morkot, R., and Tyldesley, J. (eds.) (2016): *Mummies, Magic and Medicine in Ancient Egypt: Multidisciplinary Essays for Rosalie David* (Manchester: Manchester University Press).

Priuli, S. (1991): 'ILLRP no.45a', in *Epigrafia: Actes du Colloque international d'Épigraphie Latine en Mémoire de Attilio Degrassi pour le Centenaire de sa Naissance* (Rome: Université de Roma-La Sapienza/Ecole française de Rome): 288–99.

Proskauer, C. (1958): 'The significance to medical history of the newly discovered fourth century Roman fresco', *Bulletin of the New York Academy of Medicine* 34.10: 672–86.

Quack, J. F. (2003): 'Methoden und Möglichkeiten der Erforschung der Medizin im Alten Ägypten', *Medizin Historisches Journal* 38.1: 3–15.

Quigley, C. (2012): *Dissection on Display. Cadavers, Anatomists and Public Spectacle* (Jefferson, NC: McFarland & Co.).

Raiola, T. and Roselli, A. (eds.) (2022): *Nell' Officina del Filologo. Studi sui Testi e i loro Lettori. Per Ivan Garofalo* (Pisa; Rome: Fabrizio Serra).

Rea, R. (2001*a*): 'Il Colosseo, teatro per gli spettacoli di caccia. Le fonti e reperti', in La Regina (ed.) (2002): 223–43.

(2001*b*): 'Gli animali per la venatio: Cattura, trasporto, custodia', in La Regina (ed.) (2002): 245–75.

(2014): 'Gli *auditoria* pubblici nel mondo romano', in Meneghini and Rea (eds.) (2014): 133–54.

Recke, M. (2013): 'Science as art: Etruscan anatomical votives', in Turfa and Tambe (eds.) (2013): 1068–85.

Regenbogen, O. (1956): 'Bemerkungen zur Historia animalium des Aristoteles', *Studi Italiani di Filologia Classica* 27–8: 444–9.

Reggiani, N. (ed.) (2019): *Greek Medical Papyri: Text, Context, Hypertext* (Berlin: De Gruyter).

Reiter, F. (2012): *Literarische Texte der Berliner Papyrussammlung. Berliner Klassikertexte 10* (Berlin: De Gruyter).

Renehan, R. (1984): 'Meletius' chapter on the eyes: An unidentified source', *Dumbarton Oaks Papers* 38: 159–68.

Richter, D. S. and Johnson, W. A. (ed.) (2017): *The Oxford Handbook to the Second Sophistic* (Oxford: Oxford University Press).

Riddle, J. M. (1985): *Dioscorides on Pharmacy and Medicine* (Austin: University of Texas Press).

Ritner, R. K. (2000): 'Innovations and adaptions in ancient Egyptian medicine', *Journal of Near Eastern Studies* 59.2: 107–17.

——— (2006): 'Cardiovascular system in ancient Egyptian thought', *Journal of Near Eastern Studies* 65.2: 99–109.

Robert, L. (1970): *Études Anatoliennes: Recherches sur les Inscriptions Grecques de l'Asie Mineure* (Amsterdam: A. M. Hakkert).

Robert, J. and Robert, L. (1958): 'Bulletin épigraphique', *Revue des Études Grecques* 71.334–8: 169–363.

Rocca, J. (2002): 'The brain beyond Kühn: Reflections on *Anatomical Procedures*, Book IX', in Nutton (ed.) (2002): 87–100.

——— (2003): *Galen on the Brain: Anatomical Knowledge and Physiological Speculation in the Second Century AD* (Leiden; Boston: Brill).

——— (2016): 'Anatomy and physiology', in Irby-Massie (ed.) (2016): 345–59.

Roselli, A. (1979): 'Un frammento dell' epitome περὶ ζῴων di Aristofane di Bisanzio. P. Lit. Lond. 164', *Zeitschrift für Papyrologie und Epigraphik* 33: 13–16.

——— (1989): 'Aristophanis Byzantii Aristotelis Historiae Animalium Epitome, 2.169–77', in Adorno 1989: 338–45.

——— (2002): 'ΕΚΒΙΒΛΙΟΥ ΚΥΒΕΡΝΗΤΗΣ: I limiti dell'apprendimento dai libri nella formazione tecnica e filosofica (Galeno, Polibio, Filodemo)', *Vichiana* 4.1: 37–50.

Ross, D. (1995): *Aristotle* (New York: Routledge).

Ross, W. D. and Nutton, V. (2016): 'Marinus', in *The Oxford Classical Dictionary. Fourth Edition* (Oxford: Oxford University Press).

Russell, D. A. (1983): *Greek Declamation* (Cambridge: Cambridge University Press).

Sabbah, G. and Mudry, P. (eds.) (1994): *La Médicine de Celse, Aspects Historiques, Scientifiques et Littéraires* (Saint-Étienne: Publications de l'Université de Saint-Étienne).

Sabbatini Tumolesi, P. (1988): *Epigrafia Anfiteatrale dell'Occidente Romano, Vol. I: Roma* (Rome: Quasar).

Sahin, S. (1999): *Die Inschriften von Perge. Inschriften griechischer Städte aus Kleinasien 54* (Bonn: Dr. Rudolf Habelt GMBH).

Salas, L. A. (2020): *Cutting Words: Polemical Dimensions of Galen's Anatomical Experiments* (Leiden; Boston: Brill).

Samama, E. (2003): *Les Médecins dans le Monde Grec. Sources Épigraphiques sur la Naissance d'un Corps Médical* (Geneva: Droz).

Sanchez, G. M., Meltzer, E. S. and Smith, E. (eds.) (2012): *The Edwin Smith Papyrus: Updated Translation of the Trauma Treatise and Modern Medical Commentaries* (Atlanta, GA: Lockwood Press).

Sarton, G. (1927): *Introduction to the History of Science. Volume I. From Homer to Omar Khayyam* (Baltimore, MD: The Williams & Wilkins Company).

Sassi, M. M. (ed.) (2006): *La Costruzione del Discorso Filosofico nell'Età dei Presocratici* (Pisa: Normale).

Saunders, K. B. (1999): 'The wounds in *Iliad* 13–16', *Classical Quarterly* 49.2: 345–63.

Savage-Smith, E. (1995): 'Attitudes toward dissection in medieval Islam', *Journal of the History of Medicine and Allied Sciences* 50.1: 67–110.

(2007): 'Anatomical illustrations in Arabic manuscripts', Contadini 2007: 147–59.

Sawday, J. (1995): *The Body Emblazoned: Dissection and the Human Body in Renaissance Culture* (London: Routledge).

Scarborough, J. (1971): 'Galen and the gladiators', *Episteme*, 5.2: 98–111.

(1985): 'Galen's dissection of the elephant', *Koroth* 8.11–12: 123–34.

(2010): 'Teaching surgery in late Byzantine Alexandria', in Horstmanshoff (ed.) (2010): 235–60.

Scheid, J. (2007): 'Le statut de la viande à Rome', *Food & History* 5.1: 19–28.

Schiefsky, M. (2005): *Hippocrates On Ancient Medicine: Translated with Introduction and Commentary* (Leiden; Boston: Brill).

Schiødt, S. (2021): *Medical Science in Ancient Egypt: A Translation and Interpretation of Papyrus Louvre-Carlsberg (pLouvre E 32847 + pCarlsberg 917)* (Copenhagen: Det Humanistiske Fakultet, Københavns Universitet).

Schiødt, S., Jacob, A., and Ryholt, K. (eds.) (forthcoming): *Scientific Traditions in the Ancient Mediterranean and Near East: Joint Proceedings of the 1st and 2nd Scientific Papyri from Ancient Egypt International Conferences, May 2018, Copenhagen, and September 2019, New York* (New York: ISAW Monographs).

Schlange-Schöningen, H. (2003): *Die römische Gesellschaft bei Galen* (Berlin: De Gruyter).

Schmitz, T. (1997): *Bildung und Macht: Zur sozialen und politischen Funktion der zweiten Sophistik in der griechischen Welt der Kaiserzeit* (Munich: C. H. Beck).

Schroer, S. (ed.) (2006): *Images and Gender: Contributions to the Hermeneutics of Reading Ancient Art* (Fribourg: Academic Press; Göttingen: Vandenhoeck & Ruprecht).

Schröder, H. O. (1934): *Galeni In Platonis Timaeum Commentarii Fragmenta*. CMG Suppl. I (Leipzig: Teubner).

Schubert, P. (2012): 'P.Gen.inv. 512: List of the parts of the forearm and hand', in Ast, Cuvigny, Hickey, and Lougovaya (eds.) (2012): 295–8.

Schulze, C. (1999): *Aulus Cornelius Celsus—Arzt oder Laie?: Autor, Konzept und Adressaten der De medicina libri octo* (Trier: Wissenschaftlicher Verlag).

Scortecci, D. (2000): 'La creazione dell'uomo psichico da parte dei Sette Arconti e degli Angeli', *Vetera Christianorum* 37.1: 93–111.

Sharples, R. W. (1995): *Theophrastus of Eresus. Sources for his Life, Writings, Thought, and Influence. Commentary Volume 5: Sources on Biology (Human Physiology, Living Creatures, Botany: Texts 328–435)* (Leiden: Brill).

(2006): 'Natural philosophy in the Peripatos after Strato', in Fortenbaugh and White (eds.) (2006): 307–27.

(2011): 'Strato of Lampsacus: The sources, texts, and translations', in Desclos and Fortenbaugh (eds.) (2011): 5–229.

Sharples, R. W. and van der Eijk, P. J. (eds. and trans.) (2008): *Nemesius: On the Nature of Man* (Liverpool: Liverpool University Press).

Shaw, J. R. (1972): 'Models for cardiac structure and function in Aristotle', *Journal of the History of Biology* 5.2: 355–88.

Shelton, J.-A. (2014): 'Spectacles of animal abuse', in Campbell (ed.) (2014): 461–77.

Sideras, A. (1994): 'Rufus von Ephesos und Sein Werk in Rahmen der antiken Medizin', *Aufstieg und Niedergang der Römischen Welt* 2.37.2: 1077–1253.

Sidoli, N. (2015): 'Mathematics education', in Bloomer (ed.) (2015): 387–400.

Sigerist, H. E. (1967): *A History of Medicine* (Oxford: Oxford University Press).

Simon, M. (ed. and trans.) (1906): *Sieben Bücher Anatomie des Galen: Anatomikōn egcheirēseōn, bibliōn Th-IE: zum ersten Male veröffentlicht nach den Handschriften einer arabischen Übersetzung des 9. Jahrh. n. Chr.* (Leipzig: J. C. Hinrichs'sche Buchhandlung) (re-issued 1996, Frankfurt am Main).

Singer, C. (1925): *The Evolution of Anatomy: A Short History of Anatomical and Physiological Discovery to Harvey* (New York: Knopf).

(trans.)(1956): *Galen On Anatomical Procedures* (Oxford: Oxford University Press).

(1957): *A Short History of Anatomy from the Greeks to Harvey* (New York: Dover).

Singer, P. N. (ed.) (2013): *Galen: Psychological Writings* (Cambridge: Cambridge University Press).

Singer, P. N. and van der Eijk, P. J. (2018): *Galen: Works on Human Nature. Volume I: Mixtures (De Temperamentis)* (Cambridge: Cambridge University Press).

Skeat, T. C. (1995): 'Was papyrus regarded as "cheap" or "expensive" in the ancient world?" *Aegyptus* 75: 75–93.

Slater, W. J. (1982): 'Aristophanes of Byzantium and Problem-Solving in the Museum', *Classical Quarterly* 32.2: 336–49.

Smith, S. (2014): *Man and Animal in Severan Rome* (Cambridge: Cambridge University Press).

Smith, W. D. (1979): *The Hippocratic Tradition* (Ithaca, NY: Cornell University Press).

(1990): *Hippocrates. Pseudepigraphic Writings: Letters, Embassy, Speech from the Altar, Decree* (Leiden: Brill).

Solmsen, F. (1961): 'Greek philosophy and the discovery of the nerves', *Museum Helveticum* 18.3+4: 150–97.

Sorabji, R. (1993): *Animal Minds and Human Morals: The Origins of the Western Debate* (Ithaca, NY: Cornell University Press).

    (ed.) (1997): *Aristotle and After* (London: Institute of Classical Studies, School of Advanced Study, University of London).

Sprengel, K. (1829–30): *Pedanii Dioscorides Anzarbei. Medicorum Graecorum Opera Quae Extant.* Vols. XXV and XXVI.2 (Leipzig: Car. Cnoblochius).

von Staden, H. (ed.) (1989): *Herophilus, the Art of Medicine in Early Alexandria* (Cambridge: Cambridge University Press).

    (1992*a*): 'Discovering the body: Human dissection and its cultural contexts in ancient Greece', *Yale Journal of Biology and Medicine* 65.3: 223–41.

    (1992*b*): 'Jaeger's "Skandalon der historischen Vernunft": Diocles, Aristotle, and Theophrastus', in Calder (ed.) (1992): 227–65.

    (1994): 'Media quodammodo diversas inter sententias: Celsus, the "rationalists", and Erasistratus', in Sabbah and Mudry (eds.) (1994): 77–101.

    (1995): 'Anatomy as rhetoric: Galen on dissection and persuasion', *Journal of the History of Medicine*, 50.1: 47–66.

    (1997): 'Galen and the second sophistic', in Sorabji (ed.) (1997): 33–54.

    (1998): 'Gatung und Gedächtnis: Galen über Wahrheit und Lehrdichtung', in Kullmann, Althoff, and Asper (eds.) (1998): 65–94.

    (1999*a*): 'Caelius Aurelianus and the Hellenistic epoch: Erasistratus, the Empiricists, and Herophilus', in Mudry (ed.) (1999): 85–119.

    (1999*b*): 'Celsus as historian?', in van der Eijk (ed.) (1999*a*): 251–94.

    (2004): 'Galen's Alexandria', in Harris and Ruffini (eds.) (2004): 179–216.

    (2010): 'How Greek was the Latin body? The parts and the whole in Celsus' Medicina', in Langslow and Maire (eds.) (2010): 3–23.

Stanton, G. R. (1973): 'Sophists and philosophers: Problems of classification', *American Journal of Philology* 94.4: 350–64.

Starr, R. J. (1987): 'The circulation of literary texts in the Roman world', *Classical Quarterly* 37.1: 213–23.

    (1991): 'Reading aloud: *Lectores* and Roman reading', *Classical Journal* 86.4: 337–43.

Stathakopoulos, D. (2019): 'Galen in non-medical Byzantine texts, 600-1453', in Bouras-Vallianatos and Zipser (eds.) (2019): 140–59.

Steckerl, F. (1958): *The Fragments of Praxagoras of Cos and his School* (Leiden: Brill).

Stewart, A. F. (1990): *Greek Sculpture: An Exploration* (New Haven, CT: Yale University Press).

van Straten, F. T. (1981): 'Gifts for the gods', in Versnel (ed.) (1981): 65–151.

Strohmaier, G. (1970): *Galen. Über die Verschiedenheit der Homoiomeren Körperteile. CMG* Suppl. Or. III (Berlin: Akademie Verlag).

    (1993): 'Hellenistische Wissenschaft im neugefundenen Galenkommentar zur hippokratischen Schrift "Über die Umwelt"', in Kollesch and Nickel (eds.) (1993): 157–64.

Stückelberger, A. (1993): 'Aristoteles illustratus: Anschauungshilfsmittel in der Schule des Peripatos', *Museum Hellveticum* 50.3: 131–43.

(1994): *Bild und Wort. Das illustriert Fachbuch in der antiken Naturwissenschaft, Medizin, und Technik* (Mainz: P. von Zabern).

(1998): 'Vom anatomischen Atlas des Aristoteles zum geographischen Atlas des Ptolemaios: Beobachtungen zu wissenschaftlichen Bilddokumentationen', in Kullmann, Althoff, and Asper (eds.) (1998): 287–307.

Swain, S. (1996): *Hellenism and Empire* (Oxford: Clarendon Press).

Swain, S. and Boys-Stones, G. R. (2007): *Seeing the Face, Seeing the Soul: Polemon's Physiognomy from Classical Antiquity to Medieval Islam* (Oxford: Oxford University Press).

Syrkou, A. (2021): *Horrorscope: The Gallery of Tortures in Late Antiquity* (Pisa; Rome: Fabrizio Serra).

Tabanelli, M. (1962): *Gli Ex-voto Poliviscerali Etruschi e Romani. Storia, Ritrovamenti, Interpretazione* (Florence: L. S. Olschiki).

Talbot, C. H. and Hammond, E. A. (1965): *The Medical Practitioners in Medieval England: A Biographical Register* (London: Wellcome Historical Medical Library).

Tamm, B. (1963): *Auditorium and Palatium. A Study on Assembly-rooms in Roman Palaces during the 1st Century B.C. and the 1st Century A.D.* (Stockholm: Almquist & Wiksell).

Taub, L. and Doody, A. (eds.) (2009): *Authorial Voices in Greco-Roman Technical Writing* (Trier: Wissenschaftlicher Verlag).

Tecusan, M. (2004): *The Fragments of the Methodists, Volume One: Text and Translation* (Leiden: Brill).

Temkin, O. (ed. and trans.) (1956): *Soranus' Gynecology* (Baltimore, MD: Johns Hopkins University Press).

Theoharides, T. C. (1971): 'Galen on marasmus', *Journal of the History of Medicine and Allied Sciences* 26.4: 369–90.

Thompson, D. W. (1910): *Historia Animalium. The Works of Aristotle Translated into English Under the Editorship of J. A. Smith and W. D. Ross, Volume IV* (Oxford: Clarendon Press).

Thomssen, H. (1994): 'Die Medizin des Rufus von Ephesos', *Aufstieg und Niedergang der Römischen Welt* 2.37.2: 1254–92.

Tieleman, T. L. (1996): *Galen and Chrysippus on the Soul: Argument and Refutation in the 'De placitis' Books II–III* (Leiden: Brill).

Toynbee, J. M. C. (1973): *Animals in Roman Life and Art* (Ithaca, NY: Cornell University Press).

Trapp, M. (forthcoming): 'How Does Philosophy Compare?', in Bubb and Peachin (eds.) (forthcoming).

Trümper, M. (2015): 'Modernization and change of function of Hellenistic gymnasia in the Imperial period: Case-studies Pergamon, Miletus, and Priene', in Habermann, Scholz, and Wiegandt (eds.) (2015): 167–221.

Tucci, P. L. (2017): *The Temple of Peace in Rome* (Cambridge: Cambridge University Press).

Tuplin, C. J. and Rihll, T. E. (eds.) (2002): *Science and Mathematics in Ancient Greek Culture* (Oxford: Oxford University Press).

Turfa, J. M. (1994): 'Anatomical votives and Italian medical traditions', in De Puma and Small (eds.) (1994): 224–40.

Turfa, J. M. and Tambe, A. (eds.) (2013): *The Etruscan World* (Abingdon; New York: Routledge).

Ullmann, M. (1994): 'Die arabische Überlieferung der Schriften des Rufus von Ephesos', *Aufstieg und Niedergang der Römischen Welt* 2.37.2: 1293–1349.

Vallance, J. T. (1999): 'Galen, Proclus, and the non-submissive commentary', in Most (ed.) (1999): 223–44.

Vásquez Buján, M. E. (1982): 'Vindiciano y el tratado *De natura generis humani*', *Dynamis* 2: 25–56.

Vegetti, M. (1979): *Il Coltello e lo Stilo* (Milan: Il Saggiatore).

Versnel, H. S. (ed.) (1981): *Faith, Hope, and Worship: Aspects of Religious Mentality in the Ancient World* (Leiden: Brill).

Walker, J. H. (1996): *Studies in Ancient Egyptian Anatomical Terminology* (Warminster: Aris and Phillips).

Walzer, R. (1944): *Galen. On Medical Experience* (Oxford: Oxford University Press). Reprinted in Frede (1985).

Watson, L. C. (2019): *Magic in Ancient Greece and Rome* (London: Bloomsbury Academic).

Watson, P. (2019): 'Animals in magic', in Watson, L. C. (2019): 127–65.

Webster, C. (forthcoming): *Tools and the Organism: Technologies and the Body in Greek and Roman Medicine* (Chicago: University of Chicago Press).

Wee, J. Z. (ed.) (2017): *The Comparable Body: Analogy and Metaphor in Ancient Mesopotamian, Egyptian, and Greco-Roman Medicine* (Leiden; Boston: Brill).

Wehrli, F. (1944–59): *Die Schule des Aristoteles. Texte und Kommentare* (Basel: B. Schwabe).

Weitzmann, K. (1952): 'The Greek sources of Islamic scientific illustrations', in Miles (ed.) (1952): 244–66.

Wellmann, M. (1895): *Die pneumatische Schule bis auf Archigenes* (Berlin: Weidmannsche Buchhandlung).

(1900): 'Zur Geschichte der Medicin im Alterthum', *Hermes* 35.2: 349–84.

(1901): *Die Fragmente der sikelischen Ärzte Akron, Philistion und des Diokles von Karystos* (Berlin: Weidmann).

(1907): 'Erasistratos (2)', *Paulys Realencyclopädie der classischen Altertumswissenschaft* VI.1: col. 333–50.

(1931): *Hippokratesglossare* (Berlin: Springer).

Wessel, S. (2009): 'The reception of Greek science in Gregory of Nyssa's *De hominis opificio*', *Vigiliae Christianae* 63.1: 24–46.

West, M. L. (1971): 'The cosmology of "Hippocrates", *De hebdomadibus*', *Classical Quarterly* 21.2: 365–88.

Westendorf, W. (1999): *Handbuch der altägyptischen Medizin* (Leiden; Boston: Brill).

Westerink, L. G. et al. (eds. and trans.) (1981): *Agnellus of Ravenna: Lectures on Galen's de sectis* (Buffalo: Department of Classics, State University of New York at Buffalo).

White, P. (2009): 'Bookshops in the literary culture of Rome', in Johnson and Parker (eds.) (2009): 268–87.

White, S. A. (2002): 'Eudemus the naturalist', in Bodnár and Fortenbaugh (eds.) (2002): 207–41.

Whitmarsh, T. (2005): *The Second Sophistic* (Oxford: Oxford University Press).

Wilhelm, A. (1974): *Akademieschriften zur Griechischen Inschriftenkunde* (Leipzig: Zentralantiquariat der Deutschen Demokratischen Republik).

Wilkins, J. (ed. and trans.) (2013): *Galien. Sur les Facultés des Aliments* (Paris: Belles Lettres).

Wilkins, J., Harvey, D., and Dobson, M. (1995) (eds.): *Food in Antiquity* (Exeter: University of Exeter Press).

Williams, M. H. (2002): 'Alexander, bubularus de marcello: Humble sausage-seller or Europe's first identifiable purveyor of kosher beef?', *Latomus* 61.1: 122–33.

Wilson, N G. (1987): 'Aspects of the transmission of Galen', in Cavallo (ed.) (1987): 47–64.

Winter, T. N. (1969): 'The publication of Apuleius' *Apology*', *Transactions and Proceedings of the American Philological Association* 100: 607–12.

Wiseman, T. P. (1982): 'Pete nobiles amicos: Poets and patrons in Late Republican Rome', in Gold (ed.) (1982): 28–49.

Wistrand, M. (1992): *Entertainment and Violence in Ancient Rome: The Attitudes of Roman Writers* (Gothenburg: Acta Universitatis Gothoburgensis).

Wittern, R. and Pellegrain, P. (eds.) (1996): *Hippokratische Medizin und antike Philosophie* (Hildesheim: Olms-Weidmann).

Wolff, C. (2015): *L'Éducation dans le Monde Romain du Début de la République à la Mort de Commode* (Paris: Picard).

Wolters, P. (1908): 'ἀρχιατρὸς τὸ δ', *Jahreshefte des Oesterreichischen Archäologischen Instituts in Wein* 9: 295–7.

Wootton, D. (2006): *Bad Medicine. Doctors Doing Harm since Hippocrates* (Oxford: Oxford University Press).

Yunis, H. (ed.) (2003): *Written Texts and the Rise of Literate Culture in Ancient Greece* (Cambridge: Cambridge University Press).

Zalateo, G. (1957): 'Un nuovo significato della parola δοκιμασία', *Aegyptus* 37.1: 32–40.

(1964): 'Papiri di argomento medico in forma di domanda e risposta', *Aegyptus* 44. 1/2: 52–57.

Zimonyi, A. (2014): 'The context of medical competitions in Ephesus', *Acta Antiqua Academiae Scientiarum Hungaricae* 54.4: 355–70.